NUTRITION ACROSS THE LIFE SPAN

MARY KAY MITCHELL, PhD, RD

Associate Professor
Department of Human Nutrition
The Ohio State University
Columbus, OH

W.B. SAUNDERS COMPANY

A Division of Harcourt Brace & Company

Philadelphia • London • Toronto • Montreal • Sydney • Tokyo

W. B. SAUNDERS COMPANY

A Division of Harcourt Brace & Company

The Curtis Center
Independence Square West
Philadelphia, Pennsylvania 19106

Library of Congress Cataloging-in-Publication Data

Mitchell, Mary Kay.
    Nutrition Across the Life Span / Mary Kay Mitchell.
        p. cm.
    ISBN 0–7216–3784–1
    1. Nutrition.   2. Children—Nutrition.   3. Aged–Nutrition.
I. Title.
    [DNLM: 1.　Nutrition.   QU 145 M6812n 1997]
QP141.M53   1997
612.3—dc21
DNLM/DLC   96–37236

Cover photo © 1994 Paul Barton/The Stock Market

NUTRITION ACROSS THE LIFE SPAN   ISBN 0–7216–3784–1

Printed in the United States of America

Last digit is the print number: 9   8   7   6   5   4   3   2   1

To Irv, for endless patience, support, and humor

PREFACE

The study of nutrition is interesting and rewarding. **Nutrition Across the Life Span** is directed to students and health care professionals who require more in-depth knowledge of nutritional needs for their work with individuals from embryo to old age. Physiologic and biochemical principles and results of current research are used to build a foundation for exploration of nutrition across the stages of growth and development, maturation, and aging. These serve as the basis for consideration of the social, economic, physiologic, and life style factors that influence nutrition status, food choices, and specific life stage concerns. Particular attention is paid to using the principles of nutrition in planning and implementing recommendations for dietary change.

ORGANIZATION

The overall organization of the book is presented in the Table of Contents. Part I, Foundations, provides a basic introduction to nutrition principles and applications across the life span. Chapter 1 reviews energy and nutrient needs and includes important tools such as dietary standards, food guidelines, dietary goals, nutrition labeling, and legislation for dietary supplements. Chapter 2 introduces the nutrition assessment skills used in later chapters that address the stages of growth, reproduction, and maturation. The concept of "intervention" or the use of nutrition counseling to change dietary habits and health behaviors is explored in Chapter 3.

Part II, Growth and Development, contains four chapters that cover the life span from birth through adolescence. A chapter of the nutrition needs and care of low-birth-weight and preterm infants has been included in this section.

Part III, Reproduction, addresses the nutrition needs and unique concerns of pregnancy, postpartum mothers, lactation, and breast-feeding. The chapter on high-risk pregnancy focuses on the nutrition-related factors that increase the risk of a poor pregnancy outcome.

The two chapters in Part IV, The Adult Years, cover the period from maturation to old age. This part emphasizes meeting nutrition needs and establishing dietary intakes that promote optimum health.

The chapters in Part V, Special Concerns Across the Life Span, address nutrition issues associated with eating disturbances, physical activity, and developmental delays and disabilities. These chapters address specific issues that influence nutrition status and food-related behaviors across more than one stage of the life span.

FEATURES

Each chapter begins with an *outline* of topics and ends with a list of *Concepts to Remember*. Within the chapters, each major section is preceded by a list of *review questions*. The outline and the questions give students an idea of the material to be covered in the chapter, and together with the *Concepts to Remember* they provide a useful review tool.

Chapters in Parts II through V are introduced with *vignettes* that illustrate the importance of nutrition and provide a better perspective for the reader. In each chapter, *key terms*, essential to understanding the content, appear in boldface type in the text and are defined in boxes on the spread where the term is first used. Extensive use of tables and illustrations facilitates assimilation of concepts and principles. In Chapters 4 through 15, boxed *Research Updates* provide state-of-the-art information on emerging issues in nutrition as they relate to various stages of the life span.

Following each chapter, an *Application* provides guidelines for using and applying nutrition principles of a particular life span group. For example, in Chapter 8, *Pregnancy*, the Application demonstrates the techniques of nutrition assessment and intervention used during pregnancy.

INSTRUCTOR'S MANUAL AND AUXILIARY AIDS

The *Instructor's Manual* accompanying this text was prepared by Kay Witt, PhD. In addition to containing learning objectives and lecture outlines, the manual includes student handouts of key terms and concepts. The many suggestions for learning activities include case studies for each stage of the life span to assist with problem-based learning. Examination questions and transparency masters are provided to enhance teaching and learning.

Mary Kay Mitchell

ACKNOWLEDGMENTS

I wish to acknowledge the efforts of those individuals who helped with the preparation of **Nutrition Across the Life Span.** They include Susie Wood, Amy Pearse, Jean Mitchell, and Sharon Hartley. Their suggestions have been especially helpful, and I am grateful to each for her contributions. Manuscript prepraration would have been impossible without the time, skill, and patience of Anne Schweininer, Mindy Smith, and Karla Reicher.

I also would like to thank the many persons at W.B. Saunders Company who worked so tirelessly in the various phases of planning and producing this book. I am particu-larly grateful to Daniel T. Ruth, formerly of Saunders, for his support, encouragement, and helpful ideas—especially the "what ifs" that defined the development of this text. Special gratitude goes to Maura Connor, Nursing Editor, and her staff, who provided input, assistance, and encouragement whenever it was needed. A special thanks goes to Peggy Gordon and her staff for generous assistance throughout the production process.

I am particularly indebted to the professors who served as critical reviewers. The insight, perspective, encouragement, and valuable ideas of the reviewers are most appreciated.

CONTRIBUTORS

Diane L. Habash, PhD, RD
Sports Nutrition Consultant
Lecturer, Otterbein College
Westerville, OH

Betty Kozlowski, PhD
Associate Professor Emeritus
Human Nutrition and Food Management
The Ohio State University
Columbus, OH

Martha Orabella, MS, RD
Nutrition Consultant
Detroit, MI

Melody Thompson, MS, RD
Neonatal Nutritionist
Children's Hospital
Columbus, OH

Kathryn Witt, PhD, RD
Assistant Professor, Nutrition and Dietetics
Department of Natural Sciences
Messiah College
Gratham, PA

REVIEWERS

Carmen Boyd, MS, LPC, RD, NBCC
Southwest Missouri State University
Department of Biomedical Science
Springfield, MO

Tracey L. Carlyle, MS, RD
Loyola University
Department of Food and Nutrition
Chicago, IL

Harriet H. Cloud, MS, RD
Professor Emeritus
University of Alabama
Department of Nutritional Sciences
College of Health Related Professions
Birmingham, AL

Rachel M. Fournet, PhD, MS, LDN, RD
Professor
University of Southwestern Louisiana
College of Applied Life Sciences
Lafayette, LA

Patricia M. Garrett, MS, RD, LDN
University of Tennessee
Department of Human Ecology
Chattanooga, TN

Mary Jacob, PhD, MS, RD
Professor
California State University
Department of Home Economics
Long Beach, CA

Michele W. Keane, PhD, RD
Assistant Professor
Department of Dietetics and Nutrition
College of Health
Florida International University
Miami, FL

Karen Kubena, PhD, RD, LD
Associate Professor
Texas A&M University
Department of Animal Science–Human Nutrition
    Section
College Station, TX

Suzanne Martin, PhD, RD
College of the Ozarks
Home Economics Department
Point Lookout, MO

Marcia Nahikian-Nelms, PhD, RD, Med
Director, Didactic Program in Dietetics
Southeast Missouri State University
Department of Human Environmental Studies
Cape Girardeau, MO

Annette L. Pedersen, MS, RD, LD, CDE
Notre Dame College
South Euclid, OH

Carol A. Perlmutter, MS, RD
Kansas State University
Manhattan, KS

Janet Faye Pope, PhD, RD
Assistant Professor
Louisiana Tech University
College of Human Ecology
Ruston, LA

Marsha H. Read, PhD, RD
University of Nevada
Department of Nutrition
Reno, NV

Marilyn Y. Sampley, PhD, RD, LD
Professor
Morehead State University
Department of Human Sciences
Morehead, KY

Patricia Sanders, MS, MBA, RD, LD
Texas A&M University
Department of Human Services
Kingsville, TX

Jacqueline E. Reddick Scherger, PhD, RD
Consultant in Private Practice
Huttonsville, WV

Ann C. Shetler, MA, RD
Goshen College
Department of Foods and Nutrition
Goshen, IN

Linda R. Shoaf, PhD, RD
Dietician in Private Practice
Rutherford, TN

Kaye Stanek, PhD, RD, CN
Associate Professor
University of Nebraska
Department of Nutritional Science and Dietetics
Lincoln, NE

Alice C. Williams, PhD, RD
Andrews University
Department of Nutrition
Berrien Springs, MI
and
Berrien County Health Department
Benton Harbor, MI

Kathleen Yadrick, PhD, RD, LD
University of Southern Mississippi
School of Home Economics
Hattiesburg, MS

CONTENTS

PART III Reproduction

CHAPTER 8

Pregnancy 191

CHAPTER 9

High-Risk Pregnancy 223

CHAPTER 10

Lactation and Breast-Feeding 250

PART IV The Adult Years

CHAPTER 11

Adulthood   277

CHAPTER 12

Aging and Older Adults   309

PART V Special Concerns Across the Life Span

CHAPTER 13

Eating Disturbances: Dietary Restraint, Purging, and Excessive Consumption   345

PART I

FOUNDATIONS

CHAPTER 1

INTRODUCTION TO NUTRITION AND THE LIFE SPAN

Nutrition is important at every stage of the life span. In recent years international news reports and fundraising organizations have vividly portrayed the devastation of undernutrition and disease in Third World nations. Severe undernutrition, particularly apparent in infants and young children, contributes to high mortality rates. For youngsters who survive malnutrition, decreases in growth and physical and mental development are common. Although the observable effects are less dramatic in adults, undernutrition compromises health and endurance and increases susceptibility to infection. Marginal food intake places millions of people throughout the world at nutritional risk. These populations are often pushed over the edge to starvation by natural disasters of famine, flood, and drought and human conflicts created by economic and political strife.

In North America overt signs of undernutrition are encountered infrequently, and classic "deficiency diseases" such as scurvy or pellagra are almost unknown. Here the effects of undernutrition are subtle, but they still affect health and performance of adults and impair the growth and development of infants and children. Particularly vulnerable segments of the population are young children, adolescents, pregnant women, and older adults.

In 1900, the life expectancy of a newborn infant in the United States was approximately 47 years. Mortality rates have declined dramatically, increasing the average life expectancy to approximately 75 years (Gibbons, 1990). This change primarily reflects decreases in infant mortality and in deaths due to infectious diseases. Other contributing factors include immunizations, improved health care and sanitation, and increases in the availability and quality of the food supply.

Today there is substantial evidence that the food essential for sustenance and well-being may, depending on the choices people make, contribute to the development and progression of some chronic diseases. Diet-related obesity, coronary heart disease, hypertension, and cancer, often referred to as the diseases of affluence, are leading causes of mortality and morbidity. Therefore, further increases in life expectancy and improvement of the health status of Americans will depend not only on providing adequate quantities of nutritious food but also on making food choices that reduce the risk of chronic diseases.

Americans have become increasingly aware of the importance of nutrition in all aspects of their lives. This is due in part to nutrition education and greater media coverage of nutrition research and issues. Foods, diets, and related products form a multimillion-dollar industry that pitches an almost overwhelming array of goods and services to consumers. Marketing and advertising range from the reliable to questionable to outright fraudulent. Advertising runs the gamut, from human milk substitutes and progressive foods for infants, to foods and snacks aimed at children who watch Saturday morning cartoons, to fast foods for teenagers, to "healthy" foods and supplements, to quick weight-loss diets for young and middle adults, and programs and products to relieve constipation or diarrhea for older adults. Thousands of products are promoted. It is apparent that understanding nutrition needs and the factors that influence food and health behavior is an important basis for providing reliable nutrition information and guidelines for food consumption at all stages of life.

It is assumed that the student using this text has a background in nutrition. This chapter offers a review of some basic concepts and tools used in nutrition, including nutrition needs, dietary standards and guidelines for food choices, nutrition labeling, national health objectives, and nutrition monitoring. This is followed by a brief introduction to the life span, the stages of which will be discussed in detail in future chapters.

NUTRITION NEEDS

■ What determines energy needs?

■ Outline the major roles of macronutrients and micronutrients in the body.

■ What are the essential nutrients?

Nutrition is a complex science that involves more than 40 nutrients. Nutrients are those substances that are essential to growth and health. From a practical standpoint these nutrients fall into six categories: carbohydrate, lipid, protein, water, vitamins, and minerals. Nutrients perform one or more of the following functions: they provide energy; form structural components of the body; and/or regulate body functions. Some nutrients, such as protein, fulfill all three functions, whereas others, such as vitamins, which function only as regulators, fulfill only one.

Food Energy

The fuel or energy obtained from food is measured in kilocalories or **joules**. The term "calorie" is often substituted for kilocalorie in popular literature. In fact, the Nutrition Facts Panel required for nutrition labeling lists the energy content of foods in "calories" (see page 14). The three components of energy expenditure are basal metabolism or basal energy need, the thermic effect of food, and physical activity. For adults the basal energy need is estimated to be between 1300 and 1800 kilocalories per day (National Research Council, 1989), which, depending on activity levels, represents one-half to three-fourths of total energy expended. A small portion (6% to 10%) of the daily energy is expended as the thermic effect of food. The remainder, physical activity, can be highly variable. Individual levels of expenditure depend on the individual's body weight as well as the intensity and duration of the activity.

Macronutrients

The major function of dietary carbohydrate and lipid is to provide energy (Table 1–1). Dietary protein also yields energy, but its primary role is to provide amino acids for synthesis of body proteins. Although alcohol provides energy, it represents predominantly "empty calories" providing few other nutrients, and, in excess, alcohol can have detrimental effects on nutrition status and health.

PROTEIN   Protein performs many important functions in the body. A major role is building and maintaining structural body tissues such as muscle, bone matrix, and connective tissue. Other body proteins include serum proteins such as albumin, some hormones and enzymes, as well as those proteins complexed with nucleic acids (DNA), carbohydrates (glycoproteins or mucoproteins), chromophores (rhodopsin for vision in dim light), lipids (lipoproteins), and metals (hemoglobin). Through this variety of structures, forms, and locations, proteins are essential to a multitude of functions in the body.

In the typical American diet, protein provides from 12% to 17% of the energy. In diets that provide sufficient energy to maintain body weight, this level meets and exceeds recommended levels of intake.

Carbohydrate

Carbohydrate is of prime importance in the diets of people throughout the world. It provides quick energy as well as the largest proportion of energy in the total diet. It is available in an abundance of foods and is the least expensive source of energy. Carbohydrate is obtained primarily from plant foods and is usually divided into simple (sugars) and complex (starches). Dietary fiber is a complex mixture of many indigestible substances, of which most, but not all, are carbohydrates. Epidemiologic research on dietary fiber suggests that it may be important in the prevention of constipation, diverticulosis, and colon cancer

TABLE 1–1 The Macronutrients

Nutrient	Major Functions	Food Sources
CARBOHYDRATE		
Disaccharides	Provide energy (4 kcal/g)	Sugars, fruits, honey, syrup, milk
Polysaccharides	Provide energy (4 kcal/g)	Grains, fruits, vegetables
Fiber		
Insoluble cellulose, most hemicelluloses, ligins (noncarbohydrate)	Modulates gastrointestinal function	Whole grains, bran, some vegetables, fruits, dried beans
Soluble	May reduce serum cholesterol, blood glucose	Oat and rice bran, some fruits and vegetables, dried beans
LIPID		
Triglycerides	Provide energy (9 kcal/g)	Vegetable oil, shortening, margarine, butter fat, lard, meats, fish, poultry, eggs, olives
Essential fatty acids	Membrane formation	Vegetable oils (except coconut)
PROTEIN		
Amino acids	Synthesis of body proteins; structural, serum and contractile immune proteins; hormones, enzymes; fluid, acid-base balance; provide energy (4 kcal/g)	Dried beans and peas, legumes, meat, fish, poultry, eggs, milk, cheeses, yogurt

(Willett et al, 1990), and may also be a factor in lowering blood lipid and glucose levels.

Lipid

Lipid is an important source of energy to the body and provides fatty acids for the synthesis of many body compounds. Most dietary lipid is in the form of triglycerides. The characteristics of individual dietary fats are determined by which fatty acids are present. Fatty acids have been classified, based on structure, as saturated (no double bonds between the carbon chains), monounsaturated (one double bond), and polyunsaturated (two or more double bonds). Polyunsaturated fatty acids are further classified by the location of the double bonds in the carbon chain. Fatty acids essential for humans are derived from linoleic acid (18 carbons, 2 double bonds) and linolenic acid (18 carbons, 3 double bonds). Linoleic acid is referred to as an omega-6 fatty acid and linolenic acid as an omega-3 fatty acid, indicating that the double bond occurs at the sixth and third carbons from the methyl (-CH$_3$) end of the fatty acid, respectively. Recently, attention has been focused on the potential health benefits of omega-3 fatty acids, which are found in fish and fish oils (Berdanier, 1994).

Over the last several decades the role of the kind and amount of dietary fat in the development and/or progression of chronic diseases has been studied extensively. This research is summarized in Chapter 11.

CHOLESTEROL Cholesterol is a fat-like substance that is found in foods of animal origin and also is synthesized in the human body. It is an important component of cell membranes and is found in many tissues, such as the brain and nervous system. Cholesterol and its derivatives are also precursors of vitamin D and various hormones and bile acids.

LIPOPROTEINS Because cholesterol is not soluble in water, it moves through the bloodstream as a component of lipoprotein molecules. Most of the cholesterol is transported by three types of lipoproteins: high-density lipoprotein (HDL), low-density lipoprotein (LDL), and very-low-density lipoprotein (VLDL). Cholesterol found in each of these lipoproteins is referred to, respectively, as HDL cholesterol, LDL cholesterol, and VLDL cholesterol. The sum of cholesterol in the lipoproteins is the total serum cholesterol. Numerous studies have established that both high total serum cholesterol and high LDL cholesterol levels are related to increased risk of coronary

 K E Y   T E R M S

joule: the international unit of energy defined as work done by the force of 1 newton acting over distance of 1 meter

artery disease and that high HDL-cholesterol levels are inversely related to risk (Schaefer, 1993).

Water

Although it is often overlooked, water is the most immediate of the nutrient needs and is essential for almost every body function. For most individuals thirst mechanisms automatically ensure adequate fluid intake, but under circumstances of rapid water loss from the body or impairment of the thirst sensation fluid levels can become depleted, which may lead to dehydration.

Minerals

The minerals that are essential in human nutrition are as diverse as their functions in the body. They are constituents of body compounds such as bone, hemoglobin, and enzymes. Minerals also function as free ions in hundreds of body reactions. Table 1–2 lists major functions and food sources of the minerals that are significant in human nutrition.

Vitamins

Vitamins occur in food and the body in exceedingly small quantities, have diverse chemical structures, and are essential as regulators of body metabolism. Those vitamins significant in human nutrition are listed in Table 1–3. A vitamin may participate in one, several, or even hundreds of reactions in the body. The absence of any vitamin can lead to lowered tissue levels and, eventually, negative effects on health and, in extreme circumstances, death.

Nutrition is an evolving science. As research continues to expand our understanding of food and its relationship to health, recommendations for dietary intake are constantly changing. There is evidence that some substances that do not meet current criteria for a nutrient may be required in certain circumstances or for very specialized functions. Some dietary components currently under investigation that may, in the future, be considered essential in human nutrition include phytochemicals, carotenoids, carnitine, and glutamine.

DIETARY STANDARDS

■ What are dietary standards?

■ How are the Recommended Dietary Allowances formulated?

■ What are their current and future uses?

How many calories do I need to eat to maintain my weight?

How much protein does a football player need while training?

An analysis of my diet shows that I eat 10 grams of fiber a day. Is that good?

How much formula should I feed my baby each day to make sure he gets all he needs to grow?

These questions about nutrient needs are representative of the myriad questions asked of dietitians each day. In most instances, responses to such questions are formulated using levels of energy and nutrients established in dietary standards. For more than 50 years the Recommended Dietary Allowances (RDAs) have been the American "gold standard" for recommending food intake to meet nutrient needs and against which dietary intakes are evaluated. Recommended Dietary Allowances, established by the Food and Nutrition Board, National Research Council, Institute of Medicine, National Academy of Sciences, are levels of nutrient intake assumed to be sufficient to meet the needs of most healthy individuals.

The original edition of the RDA, published in 1943, included only eight nutrients. As the discipline of nutrition has expanded and evolved, the RDA have been revised approximately every 5 years. Over time, specific nutrient recommendations have been modified and the number of nutrients included has increased. In the current (1989) edition, RDAs have been established for energy, protein, and most vitamins and minerals. Recommended energy Intake levels for the various age and gender groups (Table 1–4) are based on median heights and weights for the United States population from the Second National Health and Nutrition Examination Survey (NHANES II). The recommended energy levels represent average requirements for resting energy expenditure and an allowance for light to moderate activity. They must be adjusted for individual body size and activity level.

The RDAs established for protein, vitamins, and minerals are listed by age and gender in the summary table that appears inside the front cover of this text. These levels, determined from average requirements, are adjusted to meet the needs of most healthy individuals and to provide the most efficient utilization of the specific nutrient from dietary sources. Two additional tables, Estimated Sodium, Chloride, and Potassium Minimum Requirements of Healthy Persons and Estimated Safe and Adequate Daily Dietary Intakes, which present a range of intake levels for vitamins and minerals considered essential but for which data are insufficient for determination of a recommended allowance are found in Appendices 1A and 1B.

Although specific amounts of individual nutrients are listed in the RDA tables, it is assumed that these nutrients will be consumed as part of a normal diet composed of a variety of foods that provide adequate energy.

The Canadian Dietary Standards, known as the Recommended Nutrient Intakes (RNI), are listed in Appendix 2.

TABLE I–2 Minerals in Human Nutrition

Mineral	Major Functions	Significant Food Sources
Calcium	Constituent of bones and teeth; muscle contraction, blood coagulation; transmission of nerve impulses; cell membrane permeability; enzyme activation	Milk, cheese, milk-based foods; tofu and soy milk; sardines, canned salmon and other fish with bones; legumes; dark green vegetables
Chloride	Major anion in extracellular fluid; fluid, acid-base balance; component of hydrochloric acid in the stomach	Table salt; fish; eggs; meats; milk; large amounts in processed foods
Chromium	Co-factor for insulin in glucose uptake by cells; glucose tolerance factor	Whole grains; legumes; brewer's yeast; animal protein
Copper	Formation of hemoglobin; part of cytochrome enzyme system for energy production; metalloprotein of enzymes	Whole grains; legumes; shellfish; meats. Food content reflects soil content.
Fluoride	Formation of bones and teeth; enhances resistance to tooth decay	Drinking water if naturally fluoride-containing; fluoridated water; marine fish; tea
Iodine	A component of thyroxine; regulates basal metabolism, growth, development	Iodized salt; seafood; seaweed; dairy products. Food content reflects soil content.
Iron	Constituent of enzymes, hemoglobin, myoglobin; transport of oxygen and carbon dioxide; cellular oxidation (cytochrome compounds)	Meats, organ meats; shellfish; poultry; eggs; enriched and whole-grain cereals; dark green vegetables; dried fruits; legumes; nuts (from cookware)
Magnesium	Constituent of bones and teeth; catalyst in the conversion between ATP and ADP; protein synthesis; cation in intracellular fluid; neuromuscular irritability	Wheat bran, whole grains; meat; milk; nuts; leafy green vegetables; beans; seafood
Manganese	Component of enzymes in metabolic reactions involving protein, carbohydrate, and fat metabolism	Legumes; whole grains; nuts; fruits; vegetables; tea; cocoa powder; instant coffee
Molybdenum	Constituent of enzymes; xanthine oxidase, aldehyde oxidase, sulfite oxidase	Milk; whole grains; liver; legumes; leafy vegetables. Food content reflects soil content.
Phosphorus	Component of bones and teeth; organic compounds including proteins, lipids and nucleic acids; glucose absorption; buffer system; energy metabolism	Almost all foods, especially meat, fish, poultry; dairy products; eggs; legumes; whole grains; soft drinks; nuts
Potassium	Major cation in intracellular fluid; fluid, acid-base balance; muscle contraction; protein synthesis; glycogen formation	Most foods, especially vegetables; dried fruits; orange juice; bananas; whole grains; legumes; milk
Selenium	Component of enzymes: glutathione peroxidase; antioxidant with vitamin E	Seafood; whole grains; legumes; red meat; dairy products. Food content reflects soil content.
Sodium	Major cation in extracellular fluid; fluid, acid-base balance; cell membrane permeability, glucose absorption	Table salt, salt added to processed foods; baking soda, baking powder, seasonings; moderate amounts in meat, fish, poultry, vegetables, grains
Zinc	Component of over 70 metalloenzymes; functions in protein digestion; acid-base balance; anaerobic carbohydrate metabolism; wound healing; taste and smell	Meat; seafood; poultry; eggs; cheese; milk; whole grains; beans

FUTURE DIETARY STANDARDS

Historically, the RDAs have been determined on the basis of "essentiality," e.g., levels required to prevent deficiency symptoms. Today nutrient deficiency diseases are rare in industrialized societies, and the criteria of essentiality may be too narrow for the current state of nutrition. Dietary standards must respond to population needs as well as evolving scientific knowledge (Food and Nutrition Board, 1994; American Dietetic Association, 1993). The challenge to the Food and Nutrition Board is to develop a revision process of the RDA that continues to define and expand recommendations for nutrient requirements while encompassing the application of the concepts of reduction of the risk of chronic diseases.

Revision of the current RDA is the task of The Committee on the Scientific Evaluation of Dietary Reference Intakes (DRI Committee), which includes members of the Food and Nutrition Board and scientists from the United States and Canada. This DRI Committee will guide the work of nine individual subcommittees, seven of which will evaluate groups of related nutrients such as antioxidants or trace elements. Two additional subcommittees will interact with these subcommittees in addressing issues of establishment of maximum upper levels of intake and appropriate applications for reference intakes.

The new recommendations are tentatively designated the Dietary Reference Intakes (DRIs), an umbrella name to encompass the three specific types of reference intakes: Estimated Average Requirements, RDAs, and Maximum Upper Levels. Such an approach will extend the concept of nutrient to consider how the risk of chronic disease can be related quantitatively to nutrient intakes and dietary patterns (Monson, 1996). For instance, the new DRIs will address the relationship between calcium and osteoporosis. In addition, nonessential but valuable components of

TABLE 1–3 Vitamins in Human Nutrition

Vitamin	Major Functions	Significant Food Sources
Vitamin A retinol	Maintenance of epithelial cells and mucous membranes; growth; reproduction; formation of other light-receptor pigments	*Vitamin A:* fortified margarine, butter fat, liver, egg yolk; *Carotenoids:* dark green and yellow vegetables, yellow fruits
Vitamin D ergocholecalciferol (D_2), cholecalciferol (D_3)	Regulates calcium and phosporus absorption and metabolism	Fortified milk; fish oils; synthesis from dehydrocholesterol by exposure to sunlight
Vitamin E tocopherols	Antioxidant; protects polyunsaturated fatty acids, vitamin A and ascorbic acid, and cell membranes; shares action with selenium	Plant oils; leafy green vegetables; wheat germ; whole grains
Vitamin K phylloquinone (K_1), menaquinone (K_2)	Activation (carboxylation) of proteins required for blood coagulation; protein in bone	Green, leafy vegetables; liver; egg yolks; synthesis by intestinal bacteria
Thiamin	Coenzyme (TPP) to release energy from carbohydrates, fats and proteins; formation of ribose for DNA and RNA	Occurs in most foods in moderate amounts; pork, liver; whole or enriched grains; legumes
Riboflavin	Coenzymes (FMN and FAD) in energy metabolism; conversion of tryptophan to niacin	Milk and milk products; liver; meat, fish, poultry, eggs; whole-grain and enriched breads and cereals
Niacin nicotinic acid nicotinamide	Coenzymes (NAD & NADP) in energy metabolism; fatty acid synthesis	Meats, poultry, fish; whole-grain and enriched breads and cereals (milk and eggs are sources of tryptophan, which is converted to niacin)
Vitamin B_6 pyridoxine pyridoxal pyridoxamine	Coenzyme (PLP) in amino acid and fatty acid metabolism; conversion of tryptophan to niacin; production of antibodies; hemoglobin synthesis; glucogen degradation	Meats, fish, poultry; legumes; green, leafy vegetables; whole-grain breads and cereals
Pantothenic acid	Component of coenzyme A; release of energy from carbohydrates, fats and proteins; synthesis of cholesterol, fatty acids, hemoglobin	Organ meats; whole-grain cereals; most foods
Biotin	Coenzyme in carboxylation; release of energy from carbohydrates, fats, amino acids; amino acid, fatty acid, purine synthesis	Egg yolks; milk; organ meats; legumes, synthesis by intestinal microorganisms
Folate	Forms coenzymes for single carbon transfers in formation of nucleotides, heme	Dark green leafy vegetables; seeds; liver; kidney; fruits
Vitamin B_{12} cobalamin	Coenzyme in synthesis of amino acids, activation of folate coenzymes	Liver; meat; milk; eggs; cheese
Vitamin C ascorbic acid	Antioxidant; collagen synthesis; facilitate iron absorption, incorporation into hemoglobin; amino acid metabolism; activation of folate	Fruits, especially citrus; tomatoes, cabbage, peppers, broccoli, spinach, potatoes

TABLE 1–4 Median Heights and Weights and Recommended Energy Intake

Category	Age (years) or Condition	Weight (kg)	Weight (lb)	Height (cm)	Height (in)	FEE* (kcal/day)	Average Energy Allowance (kcal)[†] Multiples of REE	Per kg	Per Day[††]
Infants	0.0–0.5	6	13	60	24	320		108	650
	0.5–1.0	9	20	71	28	500		98	850
Children	1–3	13	29	90	35	740		102	1300
	4–6	20	44	112	44	950		90	1800
	7–10	28	62	132	52	1130		70	2000
Males	11–14	45	99	157	62	1440	1.70	55	2500
	15–18	66	145	176	69	1760	1.67	45	3000
	19–24	72	160	177	70	1780	1.67	40	2900
	25–50	79	174	176	70	1800	1.60	37	2900
	51+	77	170	173	68	1530	1.50	30	2300
Females	11–14	46	101	157	62	1310	1.67	47	2200
	15–18	55	120	163	64	1370	1.60	40	2200
	19–24	58	128	164	65	1350	1.60	38	2200
	25–50	63	138	163	64	1380	1.55	36	2200
	51+	65	143	160	63	1280	1.50	30	1900
Pregnant	1st Trimester								+0
	2nd Trimester								+300
	3rd Trimester								+300
Lactating	1st 6 months								+500
	2nd 6 months								+500

* Resting energy expenditure (REE); calculation based on FAO equations, then rounded.

[†] In the range of light to moderate activity, the coefficient of variation is ±20%.

[††] Figure is rounded.

Reprinted with permission from Recommended Dietary Allowances, 10th ed. Copyright 1989 by the National Academy of Sciences. Courtesy of the National Academy Press, Washington, D.C.

food such as dietary fiber, carotenoids, and phytoestrogens will be evaluated.

Each Estimated Average Requirement will be determined from the mean requirement for a specific nutrient based on the most appropriate criteria for adequacy for specific age-gender categories. The RDAs will be similar to current levels in that they will be derived from requirements plus two standard deviations, anticipating that the RDAs will meet the biological needs of 97.5% of the reference population. The Maximum Upper, or "safe," Level will be defined as the upper limit of intake known or predicted to be associated with a low risk of adverse effects in almost all members of the population group for which the recommendation is developed.

As work of the DRI Committee and subcommittees progresses, summaries will be disseminated. The first report on calcium, phosphorus, vitamin D, magnesium, and fluoride is expected to be published in 1997, and subsequent reports will be issued over a period of four to five years.

GUIDES FOR FOOD INTAKE

■ What tools are available to assist consumers in selecting nutritious, healthy diets?

■ Describe the Dietary Guidelines designed to promote long-term health for Americans.

Dietary Guidelines for Americans

Guidance to help Americans make healthy food choices is believed to be important in preventing or retarding the progression of some chronic diseases. A tool to assist in making food choices for healthy individuals aged 2 years or more is the 1995 Dietary Guidelines for Americans from the U.S. Departments of Agriculture and Health and Human Services (Fig. 1–1). To meet these guidelines individuals must choose a diet in which most of the calories

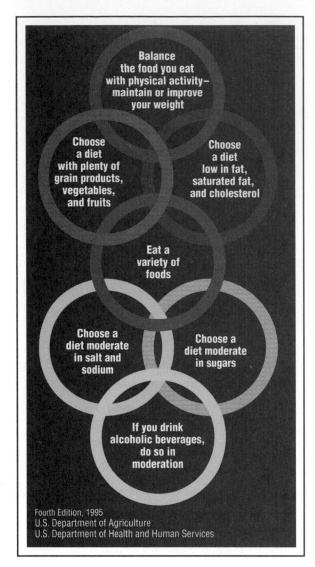

FIGURE 1–1. Dietary guidelines for Americans. (From Nutrition and Health: Dietary Guidelines for Americans. U.S. Dept. of Health and Human Services, 4th ed., Washington, DC: U.S. Government Printing Office, 1995.)

and sugar; and to increase intake of complex carbohydrates and fiber. If an individual consumes alcoholic beverages, moderation is important. Each of these recommendations is supported by a research base of established health benefits.

It is important for the total dietary intake to be balanced. Compliance with the Dietary Guidelines depends on the content of the total diet. The way in which a particular food fits into the diet depends on which other foods are consumed that day. For example, if most of the foods chosen are low in total and saturated fat, cholesterol, sugar, and sodium, some foods containing moderate amounts of these substances can be included. The reverse is also true. If one or more foods chosen are relatively high in total and saturated fat and cholesterol, other foods selected that day should be lower in these components. The Dietary Guidelines are designed to be a flexible guide to balance intake over a period of several days.

The Committee on Diet and Health, Food and Nutrition Board, Institute of Medicine of the National Academy of Sciences has also formulated guidelines to reduce the risk of chronic disease (Woteki and Thomas, 1992). These nine guidelines (Table 1–5) are similar to the Dietary Guidelines for Americans but also include recommendations regarding calcium, fluoride, and dietary supplements.

come from grain products, vegetables, fruits, lowfat milk products, lean meats, fish, poultry, and beans while choosing fewer kilocalories from fats and sweets. Nutrition experts believe following these seven principles will lead to improved health status and reduced risk of certain chronic diseases, such as coronary artery disease, stroke, diabetes mellitus, and some forms of cancer. The 1995 Dietary Guidelines emphasize the importance of eating a variety of foods and balancing food intake with physical activity to maintain or improve weight. A chart that accompanies the guidelines suggests healthy weight for height levels for adults of all ages (Fig. 1–2). Other guidelines incorporate recommendations to reduce consumption of fat, saturated fat, and cholesterol; to moderate consumption of sodium

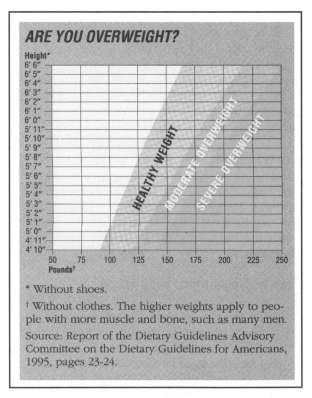

FIGURE 1–2. Healthy weights for Americans. (Report of the Dietary Guidelines Advisory Committee on the Dietary Guidelines for Americans, 1995, pp. 23–24.)

TABLE 1–5 The Nine Dietary Guidelines

1. Reduce total fat intake to 30% of your total calorie consumption. Reduce saturated fatty acid intake to less than 10% of calories. Reduce cholesterol intake to less than 300 mg daily.

2. Eat five or more servings of a combination of vegetables and fruits daily, especially green and yellow vegetables and citrus fruits. Also, increase your intake of starches and other complex carbohydrates by eating six or more daily servings of a combination of breads, cereals, and legumes.

3. Eat a reasonable amount of protein, maintaining your protein consumption at moderate levels.

4. Balance the amount of food you eat with the amount of exercise you get to maintain appropriate body weight.

5. It is not recommended that you drink alcohol. If you do drink alcoholic beverages, limit the amount you drink in a single day to no more than two cans of beer, two small glasses of wine, or two average cocktails. Pregnant women should avoid alcoholic beverages.

6. Limit the amount of salt (sodium chloride) that you eat to 6 g (slightly more than 1 teaspoon of salt) per day or less. Limit the use of salt in cooking and avoid adding it to food at the table. Salty foods, including highly processed salty foods, salt-preserved foods, and salt-pickled foods, should be eaten sparingly, if at all.

7. Maintain adequate calcium intake.

8. Avoid taking dietary supplements in excess of the U.S. RDA in any one day.

9. Maintain an optimal level of fluoride in your diet and particularly in the diets of your children when their baby and adult teeth are forming.

Reprinted with permission from Eat for Life. Copyright 1992 by the National Academy of Sciences. Courtesy of the National Academy Press, Washington, D.C.

Food Guide Pyramid

The Food Guide Pyramid is a practical and flexible tool developed to help consumers make healthy food choices. Because it incorporates the seven basic principles in the Dietary Guidelines for Americans, it is also an important tool in making food choices to reduce the risk of chronic disease. The pyramid is based on five food groups which, when the recommended number of servings from each group are consumed daily, form the foundation of a nutritionally adequate diet (Fig. 1–3). Typical serving sizes for each group are outlined in Table 1–6. The number of servings appropriate for an individual depends on the caloric level he or she requires. Table 1–7 indicates the number of servings appropriate for diets containing approximately 1600, 2200, and 2800 kilocalories. Caloric needs and the number of servings vary with age, gender, body size, and activity level. For most individuals, a diet that provides the recommended levels of nutrients will require at least the minimum number of servings recommended in Table 1–7.

The Dietary Guidelines recommend that foods from the grain products group, along with fruits and vegetables, form the foundation of healthful diets. Such foods tend to be low in fat, saturated fat, cholesterol, added sugar, and sodium. These foods should be accompanied by lean and low-fat choices from the third tier. Foods at the tip of the pyramid (fats, oils, and sweets) should be used sparingly. These foods, such as oil, butter, margarine, salad dressings, sugar, sodas, candy, and sweet desserts, are concentrated sources of fats and sugars that provide energy but few nutrients.

NUTRITION LABELING

◼ Describe the information available to consumers from the nutrition label.

◼ What are the uses of Daily Reference Values (DRV) and Recommended Dietary Intake (RDI)?

◼ What are the advantages of having regulations for nutrient claims and health claims on food products?

In this era of health consciousness, Americans are actively interested in what they eat. Unfortunately, in spite of the vast quantity of nutrition information available, it is difficult for consumers to make informed food choices. In response to the need for reliable, consistent, useful information, the Nutrition Labeling and Education Act of 1990 mandated new food labels and established regulations

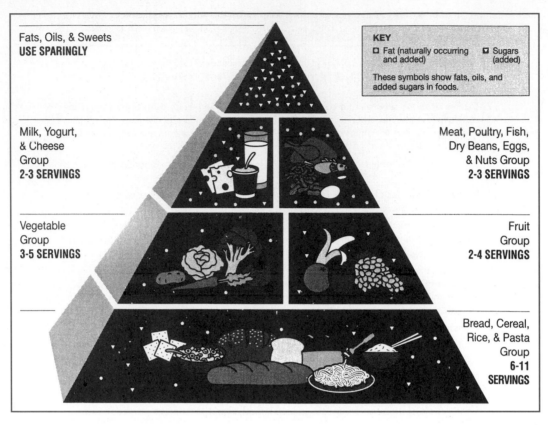

FIGURE 1–3. Food guide pyramid.

TABLE 1–6 The Daily Food Guide: Sample Serving Sizes

A TYPICAL SERVING FOR FOODS IN EACH GROUP FORMS THE BASIS FOR RECOMMENDED NUMBER OF SERVINGS

BREADS, CEREALS, RICE, AND PASTA
1 slice of bread
$\frac{1}{2}$ cup of cooked rice or pasta
$\frac{1}{2}$ cup of cooked cereal
1 ounce of ready-to-eat cereal

The amount of a food eaten may be more than one serving. For example, a dinner portion of spaghetti would count as two or three servings of pasta.

VEGETABLES
$\frac{1}{2}$ cup of chopped raw or cooked vegetables
1 cup of leafy raw vegetables

FRUITS
1 piece of fruit or melon wedge
$\frac{3}{4}$ cup of juice
$\frac{1}{2}$ cup of canned fruit
$\frac{1}{4}$ cup of dried fruit

MILK, YOGURT, AND CHEESE
1 cup of milk or yogurt
$1\frac{1}{2}$ to 2 ounces of cheese

MEAT, POULTRY, FISH, DRY BEANS, EGGS, AND NUTS
$2\frac{1}{2}$ to 3 ounces of cooked lean meat, poultry, or fish

Count $\frac{1}{2}$ cup of cooked beans, 1 egg, or 2 tablespoons of peanut butter as 1 ounce of lean meat (about $\frac{1}{3}$ serving)

FATS, OILS, AND SWEETS
LIMIT CALORIES FROM THESE especially if you need to lose weight

From Food and Drug Administration. Rockville, MD, 1993.

TABLE 1–7 Number of Servings from the Groups in the Food Guide Pyramid at Various Calorie Levels*

Food Group	About 1600	Calorie Level About 2200	About 2800
Bread	6	9	11
Vegetable	3	4	5
Fruit	2	3	4
Milk	2–3†	2–3†	2–3†
Meat	total of 5 oz	total of 6 oz	total of 7 oz

* The number of servings are appropriate for the calorie levels if lowfat, lean foods are chosen from the five major food groups and fats, oils, and sweets are used sparingly.

† Women who are pregnant or breastfeeding, teenagers, and young adults to age 24 need 3 servings.

From Food and Drug Administration. Rockville, MD, 1993.

governing nutrient and health claims for foods. Food labels are designed as a tool to help consumers select a healthy diet within the framework of the Food Guide Pyramid. Nutrition information on the label of most foods uses serving sizes that reflect portions of food usually eaten. These labels provide information on how the food fits in an overall daily diet.

Nutrition Facts Panel

The nutrition label shown in Figure 1–4 illustrates the required format and content for nutrition labels. This "Nutrition Facts" panel contains information to help consumers fit the food into their overall daily diet. The nutrient content of the food is listed as a percentage of a standard amount referred to as the daily values (DV). The DVs give only one standard for all individuals over the age of 4 years, except pregnant and lactating women. They consist of two separate sets of reference values: Daily Reference Value (DRV) for macronutrients—carbohydrate, fat, protein, saturated fat, cholesterol, fiber, sodium and potassium, and Recommended Dietary Intake (RDI) for vitamins, other minerals, and protein for certain age groups (Table 1–8). Thus, the DVs are a simpler set of standards than the RDA.

Since 1973, food labels have used the U.S. Recommended Daily Allowances (USRDA) established by the FDA for vitamins and minerals, but the RDIs have now replaced the USRDA. They are based on the highest RDA value from among the various gender and age groups listed in RDA tables published in 1968.

Percent Daily Value (%DV) shows how a food fits into the overall daily diet. Higher percentages reflect greater concentrations, and greater amounts, of nutrients. For most people the goal is to choose foods that add up to about 100% DV or more for total carbohydrate, dietary fiber, and vitamins and minerals, and 100% DV or less for total fat, saturated fat, cholesterol, and sodium. Defining nutrients as a percent of the Daily Value is intended to help consumers understand the role of individual foods in the context of the total daily diet.

The Daily Values for certain nutrients appear on package labels for both a 2000- and a 2500-calorie diet. While the 2000 calorie diet is assumed to be appropriate for many women, teenage girls, and less active men and the 2500 calorie diet for many men, teenage boys, and very active women, the actual range of energy intakes is very wide and must be adjusted accordingly. For example, the 65 g of fat listed for a 2000-calorie diet represents 30% of total kcal; however, a woman whose habitual intake is 1600 kilocalories who consumes 65 g of fat will be getting 36% of her energy from fat rather than the 30% or 53 g considered desirable.

Ingredient Labeling

Current labeling regulations require complete ingredient labeling on all processed, packaged foods, including standardized foods such as mayonnaise, macaroni, and bread, which previously were exempt. Ingredients are listed in the order of prevalence by weight so that the consumer knows which ingredients are dominant. The list assists people who may need to omit or limit certain ingredients from their diets due to allergies or intolerances.

Nutrient Content Claims

Certain terms defined by the FDA and the U.S. Department of Agriculture (USDA) can be used on the label to describe a food's nutrient content. Any term used to describe the nutrient content of a food means the same thing on every product on which it appears. Samples of such nutrient content claims are illustrated in Figure 1–5. The terms that can be used are "free," "low," "fewer," "light" (or "lite"), "reduced," "less," "more," and "high." "Lean" and "extra lean" also have been defined and apply specifically to the fat content of meat, poultry, and fish. The definitions of these terms in regard to sugar, calories, fat, cholesterol, sodium, and fiber content appear in Table 1–9.

Health Claims

Under certain circumstances, health claims linking a nutrient or a food to the risk of a disease or health-related condition are allowed on FDA-regulated products. The FDA has strict requirements about when and how these

A number of consumer studies conducted by FDA, as well as outside groups, enabled FDA and the Food Safety and Inspection Service of the U.S. Department of Agriculture to agree on a new nutrition label. The new label is seen as offering the best opportunity to help consumers make informed food choices and to understand how a particular food fits into the total daily diet.

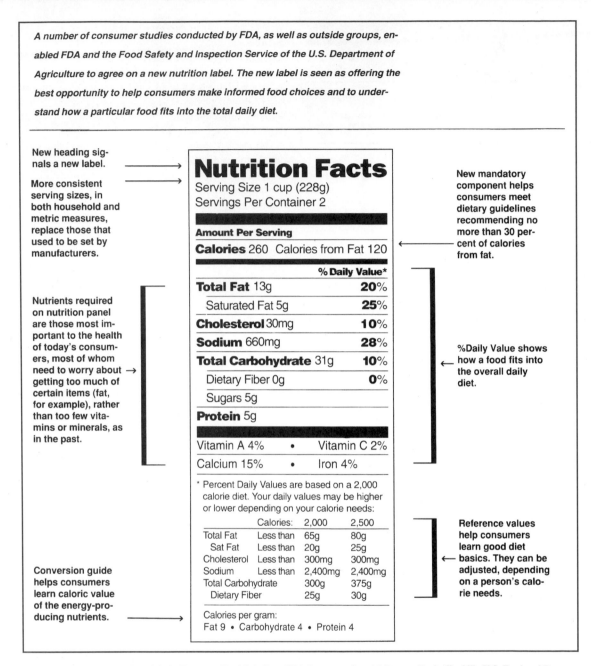

New heading signals a new label.

More consistent serving sizes, in both household and metric measures, replace those that used to be set by manufacturers.

Nutrients required on nutrition panel are those most important to the health of today's consumers, most of whom need to worry about getting too much of certain items (fat, for example), rather than too few vitamins or minerals, as in the past.

Conversion guide helps consumers learn caloric value of the energy-producing nutrients.

New mandatory component helps consumers meet dietary guidelines recommending no more than 30 percent of calories from fat.

%Daily Value shows how a food fits into the overall daily diet.

Reference values help consumers learn good diet basics. They can be adjusted, depending on a person's calorie needs.

Nutrition Facts
Serving Size 1 cup (228g)
Servings Per Container 2

Amount Per Serving
Calories 260 Calories from Fat 120

% Daily Value*

Total Fat 13g **20**%
Saturated Fat 5g **25**%
Cholesterol 30mg **10**%
Sodium 660mg **28**%
Total Carbohydrate 31g **10**%
Dietary Fiber 0g **0**%
Sugars 5g
Protein 5g

Vitamin A 4% • Vitamin C 2%
Calcium 15% • Iron 4%

* Percent Daily Values are based on a 2,000 calorie diet. Your daily values may be higher or lower depending on your calorie needs:

		Calories:	2,000	2,500
Total Fat	Less than		65g	80g
Sat Fat	Less than		20g	25g
Cholesterol	Less than		300mg	300mg
Sodium	Less than		2,400mg	2,400mg
Total Carbohydrate			300g	375g
Dietary Fiber			25g	30g

Calories per gram:
Fat 9 • Carbohydrate 4 • Protein 4

FIGURE 1–4. Nutrition facts label. (Focus on Food Labeling. FDA Consumer Special Report. Rockville, MD: U.S. Food and Drug Administration, May 1993.)

claims can be used, however. Health claims may use only the terms "may" or "might" in discussing the relationship of a food to a disease, may not state the degree of risk, may state that other foods play a role in that disease, and must phrase the claim so that the consumer can understand the nutrient and the disease and the nutrient's importance in a daily diet. Currently, the FDA allows statements about the relationships between a specific food or nutrient and the eight health claims listed in Table 1–10.

Model statements for labeling of products for these relationships also appear in Table 1–10.

Promoting Use of Food Labels

For food labeling to be effective, consumers must understand and use the labels on a regular basis. To facilitate this, the FDA and the USDA have embarked on a multi-

TABLE I–8 References for Daily Values on Nutrition Labels

REFERENCE DAILY INTAKES (RDI)*		DAILY REFERENCE VALUES (DRV)	
Nutrient	**Amount**	**Food Component**	**Basis for DRV**
Protein		Total fat	30% of calories
children 1–4 years	16 g	Saturated fatty acids	10% of calories
infants <1 year	14 g	Cholesterol	300 mg
pregnant women	60 g	Total carbohydrate	60% of calories
nursing mothers	65 g	Protein	10% of calories
Vitamin A	5000 IU	Dietary fiber	11.5 g/1000 calories
Vitamin C	60 mg	Sodium	2400 mg
Thiamin	1.5 mg	Potassium	3500 mg
Riboflavin	1.7 mg		
Niacin	20 mg		

REFERENCE DAILY INTAKES (RDI)*		Food Component	2000-Calorie Diet	2500-Calorie Diet
Calcium	1.0 g			
Iron	18 mg			
Vitamin D	400 IU	Total fat	65 g	80 g
Vitamin E	30 IU	Saturated fat	20 g	25 g
Vitamin B_6	2.0 mg	Cholesterol	300 mg	300 mg
Folic acid	0.4 mg	Total carbohydrate	300 g	300 mg
Vitamin B_{12}	6 μg	Protein	50 g	65 g
Phosphorus	1.0 g	Sodium	2400 mg	2400 mg
Iodine	150 μg	Potassium	3500 mg	3500 mg
Magnesium	400 mg			
Zinc	15 mg			
Copper	2 mg			
Biotin	0.3 mg			
Pantothenic acid	10 mg			

*Based on the 1968 Recommended Dietary Allowances.
From Food and Drug Administration, Rockville, MD, 1993.

year campaign to educate the public about the new food label. The FDA and the USDA and other government agencies will lead the campaign, but other participants include consumer, trade, and health groups. The goal of this educational campaign is to increase consumers' knowledge and effective use of the food label to allow them to make accurate and sound dietary choices.

Dietary Supplements

Since passage of the Nutrition Labeling and Education Act in 1990, there has been much controversy about the regulation of dietary supplements. Concerns have focused primarily on nutrition labeling, nutrient content, and the regulation of health claims. While the FDA supported reg-

ulating dietary supplements under the same rules as those established for conventional foods, the multibillion-dollar health food and supplements industries lobbied for a different and less restrictive network (Special Report, 1995).

The Dietary Supplement Health and Education Act passed in 1994 represented a compromise between the positions of the supplement industry and the FDA. The new law defines a dietary supplement as a new category of food containing one or more of the following: a vitamin; a mineral; an herb or other botanical ingredient; an amino acid; a dietary substance used to supplement the diet by increasing total dietary intake; and a concentrate, metabolite, constituent, or extract of any of the aforementioned ingredients.

Under the Act, labels on supplements are permitted to carry statements that describe how the intended nutrient

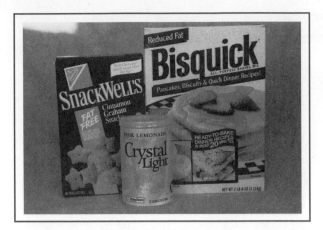

FIGURE 1–5. Examples of nutrient claims. (Courtesy of Kraft Foods, General Mills, and Nabisco.)

or dietary supplement may affect physiologic structure or function in human beings, such as "Vitamin D is required for proper bone development," but the label must also carry the declaration "This statement has not been evaluated by the U.S. Food and Drug Administration. This product is not intended to diagnose, treat, cure, or prevent any disease."

Health claims such as the claim that a supplement reduces the risk of a specific disease must meet the standard of "significant scientific agreement" and are subject to FDA oversight. Companies have 30 days after they begin marketing a dietary supplements to file their health claims and substantiating evidence with the FDA.

Provisions to protect public health allow the FDA to prove a product is unsafe for human consumption by evaluating whether the product poses a "significant or unreasonable risk." The FDA can prohibit marketing of a product if it is deemed unsafe or if it has been adulterated. Supplement manufacturers are required to notify the FDA at least 75 days before marketing a non-food product for which history of use or evidence of safety does not exist. Manufacturers must establish that the dietary ingredients or products are reasonably safe when used under the conditions recommended or suggested on the product label.

The FDA is responsible for drafting regulations to implement the new law.

NATIONAL HEALTH PROMOTION AND DISEASE PREVENTION

■ Describe the overall thrust of nutrition objectives of Healthy People 2000.

■ How is progress toward these objectives measured?

In the United States almost 12% of the economy is connected to health care. This expenditure, greater than that of most other nations, should be rewarded with the best health outcomes in the world; in fact, however, many of our health statistics indicate poor outcomes. There are a number of explanations or excuses for such results, including geographic size, ethnic diversity, socioeconomic heterogeneity, and individual choices.

National objectives for health promotion and disease prevention were first established in 1979. *Healthy People: The Surgeon General's Report on Health Promotion and Disease Prevention* focused on environmental and behavioral changes that Americans could make to reduce risks for mortality and morbidity. Specific national health objectives to reduce risks and prevent illness and death targeted improvements in public health by 1990.

Healthy People 2000

In 1990, the U.S. Department of Health and Human Services (HHS) released *Healthy People 2000: National Health Promotion and Disease Prevention Objectives*. This report continues and expands the efforts of the Healthy People Report of 1980. It seeks to improve the health of all Americans through reducing environmental and occupational hazards and encouraging people to make healthy lifestyle changes. The report outlined three broad public health goals for Americans during the 1990s:

- To increase the span of healthy life
- To reduce health disparities among population groups
- To achieve access to preventative services for everyone

Healthy People 2000 identifies 22 priority areas of health concern and specifies objectives or targets to be reached by the year 2000. Of the 300 objectives, 21 are nutrition objectives that identify national goals for fostering the dietary changes needed to reduce the risk of chronic disease and improve health status. These 21 objectives, listed in Table 1–11, address health status, risk reduction and interventions, and services designed to help the general population or specific populations meet specific targets. Baseline data were used to formulate each objective (e.g., the incidence of growth retardation in low-income children) and targets to be reached by the year 2000 (e.g., to reduce the prevalence of growth retardation to 10%). Recommendations are varied and include increasing the nutrition labeling of food products (see the section on Nutrition Labeling) and increasing the availability of reduced fat or low-fat food choices in supermarkets and in restaurants, as well as targeting specific populations through interventions and services in schools, worksites, and households.

Nutrition objectives address health promotion behaviors such as breast-feeding and improvement of the health status of children and other groups through reducing the prevalence of iron deficiency and growth retardation. Barriers to and strategies for achieving many of these objec-

TABLE 1–9 Approved Terms for Specific Nutrient Content Claims on Food Labels		
Calories	**Sugar**	**Fat**
Low calorie: 40 calories or less per serving. If the serving is 30 g or less or 2 tablespoons or less, per 50 g of the food. **Reduced or fewer calories:** at least 25% fewer calories per serving than reference food **Calorie free:** <5 calories per serving	**Sugar free:** <0.5 g per serving **No added sugar, without added sugar, no sugar added:** No sugars added during processing or packing, including ingredients that contain sugars (for example, fruit juices, applesauce, or dried fruit). Processing does not increase the sugar content above the amount naturally present in the ingredients. The food that it resembles and for which it substitutes normally contains added sugars If the food does not meet the requirements for a low- or reduced-calorie food, the product bears a statement that the food is not low-calorie or calorie-reduced and directs consumers' attention to the nutrition panel for further information on sugars and calorie content. **Reduced sugar:** at least 25% less sugar than reference food	**Fat free:** less than 0.5 g of fat per serving **Saturated fat free:** less than 0.5 g per serving and the level of trans-fatty acids does not exceed 1% of total fat **Low fat:** 3 g or less per serving. If the serving is 30 g or less or 2 tablespoons or less, per 50 g of the food **Low saturated fat:** 1 g or less per serving and not more than 15% of calories from saturated fatty acids **Reduced or Less fat:** at least 25% less per serving than reference food **Reduced or less saturated fat:** at least 25% less per serving than reference food **FAT CONTENT OF MEAT, POULTRY, FISH** *Lean:* <10 g fat, 4 g saturated fat, and <95 mg cholesterol per serving and per 100 g. *Extra lean:* <5 g fat, 2 g saturated fat, and <95 mg cholesterol per serving and per 100 g.
Cholesterol	**Sodium**	**Fiber**
Cholesterol free: <2 mg of cholesterol and ≤2 g of saturated fat per serving **Low cholesterol:** ≤20 mg and ≤2 g of saturated fat per serving and, if the serving is ≤30 g or ≤2 tablespoons or less, per 50 g of the food **Reduced or less cholesterol:** at least 25% less and 2 g or less of saturated fat per serving than reference food	**Sodium free:** <5 mg per serving **Low sodium:** ≤140 mg per serving and, if the serving is 30 g or less or 2 tablespoons or less, per 50 g of the food **Very low sodium:** ≤35 mg per serving and, if the serving is 30 g or less or 2 tablespoons or less, per 50 g of the food **Reduced or less sodium:** at least 25% less per serving than reference food	**High fiber:** ≥5 g per serving. (Foods making high-fiber claims must meet the definition for low fat, or the level of total fat must appear next to the high-fiber claim.) **Good source of fiber:** 2.5 g to 4.9 g per serving. **More or added fiber:** ≥2.5 g more per serving than reference food

From Food and Drug Administration, Rockville, MD, 1993.

tives may overlap, and progress toward achievement of one objective may affect progression toward others.

Progress Toward Healthy People 2000 Objectives

Baseline data, used initially to establish targets for each objective, can be updated and expanded to monitor progress toward the target as we approach the year 2000. The Healthy People 2000 Objectives Work Group recently evaluated the progress that has been made toward achieving the nutrition goals of Healthy People 2000 (Lewis, 1994). Sources of data used for the update varied with the objective, but included vital statistics, food consumption surveys from the USDA, the National Health and Nutrition Examination Surveys (NHANES) con-

TABLE 1–10 Approved Health Claims for Use on Food Labels

Nutrient/Food	Food Requirements	Model of Statement on Label
Calcium and osteoporosis	High in calcium; assimilable (bioavailable). Supplements must disintegrate and dissolve; phosphorus content cannot exceed calcium content.	Regular exercise and a healthy diet with enough calcium helps teens and young adult white and Asian women maintain good bone health and may reduce their high risk of osteoporosis later in life.
Sodium and hypertension	Low sodium	Diets low in sodium may reduce the risk of high blood pressure, a disease associated with many factors.
Dietary fat and cancer	Low fat; fish and game meats must be "extra lean"	Development of cancer depends on many factors. A diet low in total fat may reduce the risk of some cancers.
Saturated fat and cholesterol/coronary heart disease	Low saturated fat Low cholesterol Low fat Fish and game meats must be "extra lean"	While many factors affect heart disease, diets low in saturated fat and cholesterol may reduce the risk of this disease.
Fiber-containing grain products, fruits and vegetables and cancer	Dietary fiber Low fat Good source of dietary fiber (without fortification)	Low-fat diets rich in fiber-containing grain products, fruits, and vegetables may reduce the risk of some types of cancer, a disease associated with many factors.
Fruits, vegetables, and grain products that contain fiber, particularly soluble fiber and heart disease	Low saturated fat Low cholesterol Low fat At least 0.6 g of soluble fiber per reference amount (without fortification)	Diets low in saturated fat and cholesterol and rich in fruits, vegetables and grain products that contain some types of dietary fiber may reduce the risk of heart disease, a disease associated with many factors.
Fruits and vegetables	Low fat Good source (without fortification) of at least one of the following: vitamin A, vitamin C, or dietary fiber	Low-fat diets rich in fruits and vegetables (foods that are low in fat and contain dietary fiber, vitamin A, or vitamin C) may reduce the risk of some types of cancer, a disease associated with many factors. Broccoli is high in vitamins A and C, and is a good source of dietary fiber.
Folate and neural tube defects	Good source of folate	Women who consume adequate amounts of folate throughout their childbearing years may reduce their risk of having a child with NTD. Such birth defects, although uncommon, are serious. Fruits, dark green leafy vegetables, legumes, enriched grain products, fortified cereals, and supplements are good folate sources. Mothers of children with spinal cord birth defect should consult a physician before becoming pregnant again. Folate intake should be limited to 1000 μg/day.

From U.S. Food and Drug Administration, Rockville, MD, 1993.

ducted by the National Center of Health Statistics (NCHS), and specialized surveys such as the FDA's Food Label and Package Survey and the National Restaurant Association's Survey of Chain Operators.

For several objectives, progress could not be ascertained because newer data are not yet available, or because insufficient time had elapsed since a baseline was established.

The group concluded that progress has been made toward the targets for seven objectives. Deaths due to coronary heart disease (2.1) and cancer deaths (2.2) have declined. Growth retardation (2.4) has decreased for low-income children and most of the high-risk subpopulations.

The target for objective 2.5 is to reduce dietary fat and saturated fat intake to an average of 30% and 10%, respectively, from baseline data of 36% for total fat and 13% for saturated fat. Data collected in the 1988 to 1991 NHANES indicate that current intake of total fat and saturated fat has declined on average to 34% and 12% of calories respectively.

TABLE 1–11 Healthy People 2000: Nutrition Objectives

2.1 Reduce coronary disease death to no more than 100 per 100,000 (Age-adjusted baseline: 135 per 100,000 in 1987)

2.2 Reverse the rise in cancer deaths to achieve a rate of no more than 130 per 100,000 (Age-adjusted baseline: 133 per 100,000 in 1987)

2.3 Reduce overweight to a prevalence of no more than 20% among people age 20 years and older and maintain prevalence at no more than 15% among adolescents aged 12 through 19 years. (Baseline: 26% for people aged 20 through 74 years in 1976–1980, 24% for men and 27% for women; 15% for adolescents aged 12 through 19 years in 1976–1980)

2.4 Reduce growth retardation among low-income children aged 5 years and younger to less than 10%. (Baseline: up to 16% among low-income children in 1988, depending on age and race/ethnicity)

2.5 Reduce dietary fat intake to an average of 30% of energy or less and average saturated fat intake to less than 10% of energy among people aged 2 years and older. (Baseline: 36% of energy from total fat and 13% from saturated fat for people aged 20 through 74 in 1976–1980; 36% and 13% for women aged 19 through 50 in 1985

2.6 Increase complex carbohydrate and fiber-containing foods in the diets of adults to five or more daily servings for vegetables (including legumes) and fruits, and to six or more daily servings for grain products. (Baseline: two and a half servings of vegetables and fruits and three servings for grain products for women aged 19 through 50 in 1985)

2.7 Increase to at least 50% the proportion of overweight people aged 12 years and older who have adopted sound dietary practices combined with regular physical activity to attain an appropriate body weight. (Baseline: 30% of overweight women and 25% of overweight men for people aged 18 and older in 1985)

2.8 Increase calcium intake so at least 50% of youth aged 12 through 24 years and at least 50% of pregnant and lactating women consume three or more servings daily. (Baseline: 7% of women and 14% of men aged 19 through 24 and 24% of pregnant and lactating women consumed three or more servings, and 15% of women and 23% of men aged 25 through 50 consumed two or more servings in 1985–1986)

2.9 Decrease salt and sodium intake so at least 65% of home meal preparers prepare foods without adding salt, at least 80% of people avoid using salt at the table, and at least 40% of adults regularly purchase foods modified or lower in sodium. (Baseline: 54% of women aged 19 through 50 years who served as the main meal preparer did not use salt in food preparation, and 68% of women aged 19 through 50 did not use salt at the table in 1985; 20% of all people aged 18 and older regularly purchased foods with reduced salt and sodium content in 1988)

2.10 Reduce iron deficiency to less than 3% among children aged 1 through 4 years and among women of childbearing age. (Baseline: 9% of children aged 1 through 2 years, and 4% for children aged 3 through 4 years, and 5% for women aged 20 through 44 years in 1976–1980)

2.11 Increase to at least 75% the proportion of mothers who breast-feed their babies in the early postpartum period, and to at least 50% the proportion who continue breastfeeding until their babies are 5 to 6 months old. (Baseline: 54% at discharge from birth site and 21% at 5 to 6 months in 1988)

2.12 Increase to at least 75% the proportion of parents and caregivers who use feeding practices that prevent baby bottle tooth decay. For parents and caregivers with less than a high school education and for American Indian/Alaska native parents and caregivers, there is a special population target of 65%. (Baseline data available in 1991)

2.13 Increase to at least 85% the proportion of people aged 18 and older who use food labels to make nutritious food selections. (Baseline: 74% used labels to make food selections in 1988)

2.14 Achieve useful and informative nutrition labeling for virtually all processed foods and at least 40% of fresh meats, poultry, fish, fruits, vegetables, baked goods, and ready-to-eat carry-away foods. (Baseline: 60% of sales of processed foods regulated by FDA had nutrition labeling in 1988; baseline data on fresh and carry-away foods unavailable)

2.15 Increase to at least 5000 brand items the availability of processed food products that are reduced in fat and saturated fat. (Baseline: 2500 items reduced in fat in 1986)

2.16 Increase to at least 90% the proportion of restaurants and institutional food service operators that offer identifiable low-fat, low-calorie food choices, consistent with the *Dietary Guidelines for Americans*. (Baseline: About 70% of fast food and family restaurant chains with 350 or more units had at least one low-fat, low-calorie item on their menu in 1989)

2.17 Increase to at least 90% the proportion of school lunch and breakfast services and at least 50% of child care food services with menus that are consistent with the nutrition principles in *Dietary Guidelines for Americans*. (Baseline data available in 1993)

2.18 Increase to at least 80% the receipt of home food services by people aged 65 and older who have difficulty in preparing their own meals or are otherwise in need of home-delivered meals. (Baseline data available in 1991)

2.19 Increase to at least 75% the proportion of the nation's schools that provide nutrition education from preschool through grade 12, preferably as part of quality school health education. (Baseline data available in 1991)

2.20 Increase to at least 50% the proportion of work sites with 50 or more employees that offer nutrition education and/or weight management programs for employees. (Baseline: 17% offered nutrition education activities and 15% offered weight control activities in 1985)

2.21 Increase to at least 75% the proportion of primary care providers who provide nutrition assessment and counseling and/or referral to qualified nutritionists or dietitians. (Baseline: Physicians provided diet counseling for an estimated 40% to 50% of patients in 1988)

From Healthy People 2000: National Health Promotion and Disease Prevention Objectives. Washington, DC: U.S. Department of Health and Human Services, 1990.

The availability of reduced-fat processed foods (2.15) has increased, more processed foods have informative nutrition labeling (2.14), and more restaurants appear to be offering low-fat and low-calorie selections (2.16). The proportion of worksites that offer nutrition education or weight management programs for employees has increased (20.20). In spite of that change, however, the proportion of the population that is overweight (2.3) has actually increased from a baseline of 26% to 34%, and the percentage of overweight people engaging in appropriate weight-loss practices (2.7) has declined.

NUTRITION MONITORING

■ How are data collected and used for nutrition monitoring?

The National Nutrition Monitoring and Related Research Act of 1990 requires the federal government to develop a Ten-Year Comprehensive Plan for Nutrition Monitoring and Related Research. The plan, formulated by a Joint USDA-DHHS Working Group, serves as the basis for planning and coordinating the activities of federal and state agencies that provide information about dietary and nutrition status of the U.S. population, conditions existing in the United States that affect the dietary and nutrition status of individuals, and the relationship between diet and health. The primary purpose of the ten-year plan is coordination to ensure that methods of collection and reporting data are comparable for all participating agencies.

The major measurement components of nutrition monitoring are nutrition and health-related measurements, food and nutrient composition, knowledge, attitudes and behavior assessments, food composition and nutrient data bases, and food supply determinations.

The information accumulated for nutrition monitoring becomes part of data bases used for public policy decisions regarding nutrition education, public health nutrition programs, food assistance programs, regulation of food enrichment and fortification, labeling of the food products, food production, safety, and marketing. Such data have been the basis of Healthy People 2000, and also have been used in formulating the Dietary Guidelines for Americans, food plans for Welfare and Food Stamp Programs, and regulations governing food programs. Nutrition monitoring will continue to provide data essential for making future decisions regarding all aspects of public policy.

Most of the available information on the dietary intake or nutrition status of the American population has been accumulated from government surveys. Two of the most significant are the National Food Consumption Survey conducted by the U.S. Department of Agriculture (USDA) and the National Health and Nutrition Examination Surveys of the National Center for Health Statistics (NCHS). Because data from these surveys is cited throughout this text, a brief introduction is provided here.

The National Food Consumption Survey (NFCS) is conducted every 10 years, allowing comparison of food intake of the American population across several decades. The most recent, the 1987–1988 survey, collected demographic and three-day food consumption (at home or outside the home) data from about 8000 individuals. The information obtained from NFCS has been compared to various age- and gender-appropriate RDAs to assess adequacy of intake. The information also has been used to explore the relationship of nutrition to socioeconomic factors such as income, education, size of household, and geographic location. In 1985 the USDA initiated The Continuing Survey of Food Intake of Individuals (CSFI), a continuous survey of the food intake of women aged 23 through 50 and their children 1 through 5 years of age. The CSFI is performed annually except for the years in which the regular 10-year survey of household and individuals is performed.

The National Health and Nutrition Examination Survey (NHANES) is a series of national examination studies conducted approximately every 5 years on a random sample of the American population. The NHANES are designed to produce nationally representative data regarding the civilian, noninstitutionalized U.S. population. It gathers periodic information on diet, nutrition status, and health outcomes through interviews, standardized examinations, analyses of blood and urine samples, and anthropometric measurements. The information on food intake is gathered using a 24-hour dietary recall. These data allow an assessment of the status of the population and an investigation of possible relationships between dietary habits and specific heath problems.

The NHANES II survey was conducted between 1976 and 1980. A probability design was used to obtain a representative sample of the population ages 6 months to 74 years. From 1982 to 1984 the NCHS also conducted a survey of food intake among the Spanish-speaking populations, now referred to as the Hispanic NHANES.

NHANES III covers a 6-year period (1988–1994) and includes dietary information and physiologic measurements on about 40,000 individuals from households in 81 counties across the United States. The upper age limited for inclusion of subjects in NHANES II was 74 years, but NHANES III included all individuals aged 2 months or older. Also, NHANES III was designed to produce national data for African Americans, Mexican-Americans, children, and older adults (Brietel, 1994). Individuals who participated in the NHANES III will be followed over time for longitudinal information on health status.

The food intake data from the 1987 NFCS and the CSFI and the nutrition assessment data from the NHANES are coupled with data from vital statistics and epidemiologic studies conducted by the National Institutes of Health and various academic institutions to provide the basis for nutrition monitoring.

NUTRITION ACROSS THE LIFE SPAN

■ How do differentiation, growth, development, maturation and, aging progress across the life span?

■ What are the nutrition-related characteristics of these stages?

The continuum of life encompasses growth, development, maturation, and aging. With the exception of the brain and the nervous system, the cells of the body constantly form, function, age, and die only to be replaced by new cells. Throughout life, the body as a whole and its individual systems, organs, tissues, and cells grow, develop, function, and decline in this pattern. Across this sequence of life span events there are changes in body size, proportion, and composition.

In the first two decades of life, cell formation, **differentiation**, growth, and **development** predominate. Growth of an individual is a composite of many tissues and organs growing at different rates. The early stages of the life span are characterized by rapid growth and development, which proceed in an orderly and predictable sequence. Overall, growth is characterized by a period of **hyperplasia** and rapid cell differentiation. During this period, the tissue, organ, or individual is particularly susceptible to physical and environmental influences. For example, an infant who has inadequate food intake during this critical period in brain growth may in the long run have fewer brain cells and compromised intellectual development. As growth progresses, hyperplasia is accompanied by **hypertrophy**, and eventually hypertrophy predominates. A normal healthy infant, child, or adolescent grows and develops at a genetically predetermined rate that can be compromised or accelerated by environmental factors including undernutrition, imbalanced nutrient intake, or overnutrition.

Growth and development gradually decline as the individual moves into early adulthood. Some growth, such as that of bone, extends well into the third decade. After growth ceases and maturation is complete the process of cell turnover becomes static, with formation and breakdown in a general state of equilibrium. Gradually, with age, there is a net decrease in some body tissues and organs, resulting in a decline in functional cells. Aging is the regression of physiologic function accompanied by advancement of age. Although aging is a problem of the whole body, each organ independently loses its function, and as a result, the body becomes **senescent**. Individuals age at varying rates. The process is governed by genetics, race, and gender, but is influenced by early life events, social and behavioral factors, activity, substance use habits, and the accompanying pathology.

Although all humans have essentially the same nutritional needs, the concentration and balance may differ at various points in the life span. The stages of the life span and their nutrition-related characteristics are illustrated in Table 1–12. The rapid growth and development of the embryo and fetus depend on the maternal diet and reserves. Because of rapid growth and cell differentiation, the embryonic and fetal stages are vulnerable to undernutrition and toxic substances such as alcohol and drugs.

The neonatal period (the first 30 days after birth) is a time of critical adjustments to the extrauterine environment. Energy and nutrient needs are high to maintain basal metabolism and support growth. Compared to in-utero growth, the changes of infancy are slow, but they are still demanding, as body weight increases threefold in the first year of life. This is a period of high nutritional demand during which energy and nutrient requirements per unit of body weight are two to three times those of adults.

In terms of nutritional needs, infants and children are not simply small adults. Every stage of growth is thought to be influenced by nutrition. Although progress in growth is most often measured as physical growth (gains in stature and weight of individual infants, children, or adolescents), such measurements do not reflect changes in all of the components of growth. While growth of skeletal muscle approximates that of the whole body, growth of many other tissues, such as reproductive organs, brain, and adipose tissue follows very different patterns. After infancy, a relatively slower but steady rate of growth and development prevails through childhood. The amounts of nutrients children require to sustain normal growth and development often exceed those required by adults. For example, children need 50% more total calcium than adults to promote adequate bone formation.

 K E Y T E R M S

differentiation: process of acquiring individual characteristics or functions; progressive diversification

development: the acquisition of function or progression to a more advanced stage of complexity for greater facility in function

hyperplasia: increase in the number of cells

hypertrophy: enlargement due to an increase in cell size

senescent: exhibiting signs of the process of growing old

TABLE 1-12 Periods of the Life Span

Period	Approximate Ages or Time	Nutrition-Related Characteristics
Embryonic	8 weeks after conception	Rapid cell differentiation; development of specific tissues, organs, and systems
Fetal	Last 7 months of in-utero growth	Rapid growth; elaboration of tissues, organs; early functional activities of body systems
Neonatal	First month of postnatal life	Adjustments to postnatal environment; initiation of respiration; maintenance of body temperature and other functions; initial oral feeding
Infancy	Neonatal to 1 year	Rapid growth and development; maturation of functions
Late Infancy	1–2 years	Decelerating growth rate; increased development, especially of motor skills; increased independence, including in eating
Childhood Preschool	2–6 years	Slow, steady growth; increased physical activity and coordination of motor functions; rapid cognitive development
School	Girls: 6–10 years Boys: 6–12 years	Steady growth; continued physical and cognitive development; increasing responsibility for own food habits
Adolescence Prepubertal	Girls: 10–12 years Boys: 12–14 years	Accelerated growth rate; rapid gains in weight and height; changes in hormone levels, reproductive organs
Pubertal	Girls: 12–14 years Boys: 14–16 years	Development of secondary sex characteristics; changes in body composition; increased need for independence
Postpubertal	Girls: 14–18 years Boys: 16–20 years	Maximum gains in height; continuing increases in bone mass; cognitive development; increased independence
Early adult	20–45 years	Growth and skeletal development; completed gradual decrease in energy expenditure
Middle age	45–65 years	Tendency to increased body weight; decreased physical activity; energy needs stabilize
Older adults	65+ years	Decreased physical activity and mobility over time; increased chronic disease, often multiple; increased use of medication

Adolescence is a period of very rapid growth. The total nutritional requirements of adolescents are greater than those of adults except during pregnancy and lactation, yet meeting nutritional needs of adolescents is complicated. Changes in physiologic, psychological, and social development may compromise food habits. As a result, this group is particularly vulnerable to poor nutrient intake and disordered eating.

Nutritional needs tend to stabilize in early adulthood. It is difficult to define stages of adulthood. It begins in the early twenties, but the transition to middle and old age has relatively few markers and there is wide variability between individuals. Middle age traditionally was said to begin around age 40, but the generation of baby boomers who are now approaching 50 have stretched that definition. Similarly, the definition of an older adult is arbitrary. Due to the heterogeneous nature of the elderly population, it is difficult to define "old age" as a chronological milepost. In fact, with increased longevity and population trends, this is a rapidly growing segment of the American population.

Across the period of adulthood, decreases in energy expenditure with no corresponding decrease in dietary intake contribute to accelerated weight gain. This is a time when clinical signs of the slow insidious processes of chronic disease begin to appear. For many adults these disorders may require substantial changes in diet or lifestyle. For many, the associated medical care and medication may diminish resources needed to obtain an adequate diet. Nutritional status may also be compromised by interactions between medications and diet.

TEXT OVERVIEW

This text explores each stage across the life span in the context of physiologic, social, psychological, and cognitive development, which influence nutrition needs and food-related behaviors and practices. Unique characteristics and nutrition-related concerns are emphasized. This chapter addresses some of the basic information and skills needed to apply nutrition principles. The next two chapters discuss techniques for measuring and evaluating nutrition status and planning and counseling for changing food-related behavior and improving nutrition status.

Chapters 4 through 7 begin with infancy and follow the chronological progression through adolescence. In each chapter interrelationships among physiologic, biochemical, and sociological factors and their impact on nutrient recommendations and food behaviors are explored. Chapters 8, 9, and 10 address the special needs and concerns of the reproductive period. Maintenance of nutrition status and promotion of health through maturity and aging are stressed in Chapters 11 and 12. Areas of nutrition that are common to many stages of the life span—eating dilemmas and physical activity and fitness—are discussed in separate chapters. Concerns such as dental health, smoking, and alcohol and other substance use are incorporated in individual chapters or sections. The Application sections following each chapter emphasize application of principles or expand on nutrition care, and illustrate how nutrition influences each stage of the life span.

CONCEPTS TO REMEMBER

▶ Nutrition is important to health and well-being at every stage of the life span.

▶ Food provides energy and nutrient needs that are essential for sustenance and health.

▶ Food consumption patterns are factors in the development and progression of some chronic diseases.

▶ Dietary Standards define nutritional needs and serve as a basis for development of food guides, food standards, food products and services, menu plans, nutritional counseling, and educational materials.

▶ Food guides for promoting nutritional adequacy and long-term health include the Dietary Guidelines for Americans and the Food Guide Pyramid.

▶ Current nutrition labeling regulations mandate a label format that provides consumers with a tool for selecting a healthy diet.

▶ The Dietary Supplement Health and Education Act of 1994 defines a dietary supplement and outlines specific statements that may appear on product labels.

▶ Healthy People 2000 is a report that identifies 22 areas of priority health concerns and specific public health objectives or targets to be met by the year 2000. Success in meeting the 21 nutrition objectives is tracked by a National Nutrition Monitoring program that includes the National Health and Nutrition Examination Surveys.

▶ All people have the same nutritional needs, but specific amounts vary at different stages of the life span.

▶ Across the life span, physiologic, psychological, cognitive, and social development influence nutrition needs and food-related behaviors.

References

American Dietetic Association. ADA testifies on need for revised RDAs. J Am Diet Assoc 1993;93:864.

Berdanier CD. Omega-3 fatty acids: a panacea? Nutr Today 1994;29:28.

Brietel RR. Assessment of the U.S. diet in national surveys: national collaborative efforts and NHANES. Am J Clin Nutr 1994;59 (Suppl):164S.

Food and Nutrition Board. How should the recommended dietary allowances be revised? A concept paper from the Food and Nutrition Board. Nutr Rev 1994;52:216.

Gibbons A. Gerontology research comes of age. Science 1990;250:622.

Lewis CJ, et al. Healthy People 2000. Report on the 1994 Nutrition Progress Review. Nutr Today 1994;29:6.

Monson E. New dietary reference intakes proposed to replace the Recommended Dietary Allowances. J Am Diet Assoc 1996;96:754.

National Research Council. Recommended dietary allowances. 10th ed. Washington, DC: National Academy of Sciences, 1989.

Schaefer EJ. New recommendations for diagnosis and treatment of plasma lipid abnormalities. Nutr Rev 1993;51:246.

Special Report. Dietary supplements: recent chronology and legislation. Nutr Rev 1995;53:31.

U.S. Departments of Agriculture and Health and Human Services. Dietary Guidelines for Americans. Home and Garden Bulletin No. 232, 1995. Washington, DC: 1995.

Willett WC, et al. Relation of meat, fat, and fiber intake to the risk of colon cancer in a prospective study among women. N Engl J Med 1990;323:1664.

Woteki CE, Thomas PR. Eat for life. Washington, DC: National Academy Press, 1992.

Additional Resources

Dietary Standards

Achterbery C, et al. How to put the Food Guide Pyramid into practice. J Am Diet Assoc 1994;94:1030.

Dairy Council Digest. Dietary guidance: Philosophies and Issues. Vol 66, No 2. Rosemont, IL: National Dairy Council, 1995.

Lachance P, Langseth L. The RDA concept: Time for a change? Nutr Rev 1994;52:266.

Food Labeling

Focus on Food Labeling. FDA Consumer. Special Report. Rockville, MD: Food and Drug Administration, 1993.

APPLICATION: Assessing and Interpreting Nutrition Research

Eating fruits and vegetables reduces the risk of cancer!
Folic acid supplements during pregnancy prevent neural tube defects in infants.
Vitamin E found to cut heart attack risk!
Too much supplemental vitamin A can cause birth defects.

Such are the headlines or lead-ins for reports about nutrition research that reach the public almost daily. They arrive via print, radio, and television, all of which have a powerful role in disseminating information and providing dietary recommendations to consumers (American Dietetic Association, 1994).

A brief report of the most recently published study is likely to be aired on the morning news, often before the journal containing the research article is in the hands of the subscribers. A follow-up of the news report might be a feature on the evening news or a more in-depth health report. Expanded coverage of the potential implications of the study for health and diet may occur in interviews or on talk shows. In a few days, though, there is another study to report and yesterday's news topic is shelved awaiting another study, which may confirm or refute its results.

Newspapers also rush to report nutrition news. News stories summarizing the latest study usually are published the day after initial reports on radio and television. Within days there may be in-depth coverage in the newspaper's feature section. Over the next few weeks "fillers" prepared by the news services may appear in various sections of the paper.

Weekly news magazines also report nutrition research. Other weekly and monthly publications may feature articles that build on research reports. They tend to include suggestions for improving health such as diet and exercise programs, menu and recipe ideas, and tips to implement change. According to the American Council on Science and Health (1989), most publications provide accurate and useful information. However, the variations in how research is interpreted and the applications conveyed in all these sources may send mixed signals that confuse the consumer and frustrate efforts to implement nutrition advice.

In addition, throughout print and electronic media coverage, there are advertisements promoting foods, products, and services that might promote or refute nutrition-health messages being conveyed in the news.

Interest in nutrition and health has never been greater among Americans than it is now. In a telephone survey conducted by the Food Marketing Institute (1994), the majority of consumers (62%) indicated that they are concerned about the nutritional content of their diets, and 84% indicated that they were concerned about the effects of their food choices on future health. Never have consumers had greater access to nutrition information. Individuals concerned about nutrition and health are eager recipients of information about diet and nutrition information the media provides.

A recent survey of a nationally representative sample of 2000 American households, however, found that one-third of the respondents agreed with the statement that "trying to eat healthy is too complicated and confusing" (National Live Stock and Meat Board, 1994). In many instances, rather than incorporating new research information into a coherent picture of what constitutes a healthful diet, much of the public is burdened with a collection of fragmented facts and a perception that foods can be concisely classified as "good" or "bad" (Goldberg, 1992).

Many obstacles may impair the consumer's ability to use new nutrition research information to make long term improvements in health. They are discussed in the following paragraphs.

fillers: news pieces of consumer interest that are prepared to be used to fill empty spaces in page makeup

nationally representative sample: selection of study subjects whose demographic characteristics reflect those of the American population

Understanding of Nutrition and Diet Recommendations Change over Time

As understanding of nutrition and its relationship to health evolves, advice regarding food intake will also evolve. For nutrition researchers, practitioners, and policy makers this is a reasonable and inevitable consequence of progress in nutrition research. The lay public, on the other hand, tends to view alterations in dietary recommendations as an indication of indecision on the part of the scientific community, which may become yet another source of confusion about what to eat to follow a healthful diet (FDA, 1988).

The Nutrition-Health Message Is Complex

Some dietary recommendations are relatively easy to understand and implement. For example, Americans have been encouraged to limit their fat intake to no more than 30% of total calories. This recommendation has been incorporated into the Dietary Guidelines for Americans and many other "health messages" to the public. Its effectiveness is reflected in the decline in fat consumption in the United States over the last two decades.

On the other hand, Americans are also being advised that the dietary fat they eat should be divided somewhat equally among saturated, monounsaturated, and polyunsaturated fats. This concept may be too complicated for many laymen to implement. It has become even more complicated in recent years, with research reports suggesting that consumption of omega-3 fatty acids may reduce the risk of cardiovascular disease or that margarines and solid fats, produced by hydrogenation of vegetable oils, may be more atherogenic because of the formation of trans fatty acids.

Nutrition Research Is Subject to Interpretation

Participants in the promotion of nutrition information include government agencies, health professionals, advocacy groups, and producers of food, diet and health products. Interpretation of nutrition research and its implications for diet and health may be influenced by the goals, agenda, and bias of the groups who attempt to influence eating behavior.

As discussed in this chapter, government agencies play a key role in nutrition. Their roles include research, food safety, food labeling, nutrition monitoring and administration of food, and nutrition and health programs, as well as dissemination of reliable information. The Food Guide Pyramid and the Dietary Guidelines for Americans are prominent among the educational tools from federal agencies. They are updated as the preponderance of scientific evidence dictates changes are appropriate. However, it has been suggested that their diet-health message, while accurate and useful, is often so general that consumers may not readily understand how to act on them (Goldberg, 1992).

Health professionals, especially dietitians, provide nutrition information through advice, education, and counseling (see Chapter 3). In these roles, they may help consumers interpret and use nutrition information. Health-related volunteer organizations, whose overall goals often parallel those of government agencies, also have recommendations that may differ, if only slightly, from government agencies. Often, however, such differences may be a source of confusion to the consumer.

Some of the most distracting signals or information comes from the food industry. A food producer emphasizes the nutritional attributes of the products it markets when it furthers the goal of selling its product. When products to be sold are contrary to recommended nutrition practices, other features are promoted, in apparent lack of concern for nutrition.

Special interest groups may distort the nutrition message for their own purposes. Their agenda or perspective frequently is dominated by the desire to sell products or materials or to support their point of view. They are very good at using scientific facts to build

---

fish and marine oils are rich in omega-3 fatty acids

---

hydrogenation: a process that converts vegetable oil to fats with higher melting points and greater stability (longer shelf life). This process creates partially saturated fat by breaking the double bonds of polyunsaturated fatty acids. There is also rapid breaking and reforming of double bonds in monounsaturated fatty acids. The initial double bond is "cis" and the new bond formed in this process is "trans"

---

atherogenic: promotes the development of atherosclerosis

---

trans fatty acid: fatty acid with a double bond formed in hydrogenation. The normal, *cis*, fatty acid is saturated and a new double bond, *trans*, is formed, which has a different relationship to the carbon chain (R).

cis

trans

a case (sometimes fictional) for their cause. They add to the confusion and may actually mislead the consumer. The average consumer cannot be expected to understand the agendas and bias of these diverse groups.

To assist individuals in interpreting nutrition research information, a coalition of food and nutrition professionals, Food and Nutrition Science Alliance, encourages consumers to question the accuracy of nutritional statements marked by any combination of the following characteristics:

1. Recommendations that promise a quick fix.
2. Dire warnings of danger from a single product or regimen.
3. Claims that sound too good to be true.
4. Simplistic conclusions drawn from a complex study.
5. Recommendations based on a single study.
6. Dramatic statements that are refuted by reputable scientific organizations.
7. Lists of "good" and "bad" foods.
8. Recommendations made to help sell a product.
9. Recommendations based on studies published without peer review.
10. Recommendations from studies that ignore differences among individuals or groups.

peer review: the research design and results have been reviewed by experienced researchers knowledgeable in the area of the research.

The Time Between a Report of a Research Study and Dietary Recommendations Can Be Long

The current need for researchers to publish results as quickly as possible is motivated by a technology that operates on instant access to information and the need of researchers to publish and gain recognition in order to secure or maintain funding or, in university settings, achieve promotion and tenure. For the media, the perceived need to present the findings of major articles from scientific literature the day they are released reflects the race to be first with the facts. The payoff is increased circulation and more viewers and listeners, which translate into enhanced revenues from advertisers.

replicate: to repeat the research to demonstrate that the results can be reproduced.

clinical trials: studies in which the application of the reported findings is studied in intervention studies with humans using a control group and an experimental group for comparison.

However, the results of a single research study rarely provide sufficient evidence to serve a basis for recommending dietary changes. Too often it is the provocative nature of the findings rather than their scientific significance that determines which study will be headline news (Goldberg, 1992). It will be months and more likely years until research is replicated by other researchers and in clinical trials. Unfortunately, dramatic headlines may do more to alarm than to inform. When that happens, the damage done to public confidence in the nutrition-health messages can be devastating.

Nutrition Research May Be Specific But Diets Are Not

postulated nutrient disease relationships:
osteoporosis: calcium
cancer: beta carotene, total fat
cardiovascular disease: total fat, saturated fat, vitamin E, sodium

Understanding and using the nutrition research information is compounded by the relatively specific nature of relationships between nutrition and health and the complexity of diets. Examples of postulated relationships between certain nutrients and disease appear in the margin. In most instances evidence for these relationships is associated with long-term consumption patterns. Identification of nutrients related to specific diseases logically leads to the development of recommendations which focus on prevention of that disease. However, people do not eat one diet to reduce the risk for cardiovascular disease and another to prevent cancer. They eat meals and snacks. The challenge is to incorporate changes that may reduce the risk of disease into a diet that is nutritionally adequate and fits the lifestyle of the individual.

There is ample evidence that the public responds to nutrition and health information reported by the media (Belicha and McGrath, 1990). The tendency of the electronic and print media to share the most provocative results of research studies creates the potential for misinformation, misunderstanding, and disbelief. This is compounded by the fact that not all studies have similar results. One study does not refute an entire body of evidence but many, sometimes hundreds, may provide the basis for recommendations regarding dietary change.

The conflicting agendas of media interests, many groups that promote nutrition information, and persuasive advertising compete with personal concerns and reliable information about nutrition and health. Consumers are confused by conflicting views on nutrition issues that appear in the popular media. Increasing recognition of the effect of nutrition on lifetime health and well-being has led to more attention to promotion of reliable nutrition information and nutrition education by community health agencies, government agencies, the food industry, and a variety of health professions. Nutrition education and counseling are emerging as important professional focus points for the future.

REFERENCES

American Council on Science and Health Special Report. The 1986–1988 ACSH survey on nutritional accuracy in American magazines. New York: Council on Science and Health, March, 1989.

The American Dietetic Association and International Food Information Council. How are Americans making food choices? 1994 Update. Prepared by The Gallup Organization, April, 1994.

Belicha T, McGrath J. Mass media approaches to reducing cardiovascular disease risk. Public Health Rep 1990;105:245.

Food and Drug Administration. 1988 health and diet survey. Washington, DC: Center for Food Safety and Applied Nutrition, Consumer Health Study Section, 1988.

Committee on Diet and Health. Diet and health: implications for reducing chronic disease risk. Food and Nutrition Board, Commission on Life Sciences, National Research Council, National Academy of Sciences. Washington, DC: National Academy Press, 1989:678.

Food Marketing Institute. Trends in the United States. Consumer attitudes and the supermarket 1994. Conducted for Food Marketing Institute by Opinion Research Corporation. Washington, DC: 1994.

Goldberg JP. Nutrition and health communication: the message and the media over half a century. Nutr Rev 1992;50:71.

National Live Stock and Meat Board. Eating in America today. A dietary pattern and intake report. 2nd ed. Chicago: National Livestock and Meat Board, 1994.

CHAPTER 2

NUTRITION ASSESSMENT

The health and productivity of an individual or a population are related to nutritional well-being. Knowledge of nutrition status provides the basis for formulating individual nutrition care as well as community-based nutrition intervention and education programs.

    Students of nutrition are familiar with large surveys such as the National Health and Nutrition Examination Survey (NHANES), part of the continuing nutrition surveillance system of the United States population. The same general techniques employed in such surveys are applied across all stages of the life cycle to identify individuals at nutritional risk and to plan nutrition intervention for improvement of nutrition status, e.g., health of the body as it relates to energy and nutrients.

THE NUTRITION CARE PROCESS

■ What is the role of nutrition assessment in the nutrition care process?

Nutrition assessment initiates the nutrition care process, an organized series of activities that identifies nutrition risk and implements a plan of intervention. The nutrition care process includes analysis of nutrition risk, development of a care plan, implementation of that plan, and evaluation of the effectiveness of the intervention (Fig. 2–1; American Dietetic Association, 1994). Documentation of assessment, care, and evaluation occurs at each stage of the process.

OVERVIEW OF NUTRITION ASSESSMENT

■ Describe commonly used assessment techniques and the body compartments they estimate.

■ Which assessment tools are important in identifying nutrition risk?

■ Which assessment techniques are useful in documenting nutrition deficiency?

■ How does nutrition screening differ from nutrition assessment?

Nutrition assessment is a process or series of measurements that define nutrition status. It is designed to identify individuals who, without change or intervention, will develop malnutrition. Malnutrition can refer to undernutrition (such as underweight, poor protein status, or a vitamin deficiency) or overnutrition (such as obesity, hyperlipidemia, or vitamin toxicity). Nutrition screening uses some simple assessment techniques to identify characteristics known to be associated with nutrition problems and clients who may benefit from assessment and intervention. It may be completed in many settings by a member of the healthcare team: dietitian, dietetic technician, nurse, physician, or other healthcare professional.

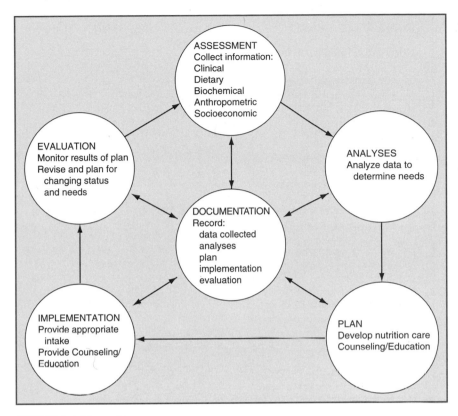

FIGURE 2–1. The nutrition care process.

Development of a Nutrient Deficiency

A sequence of events in the development of a nutrient deficiency might be as follows (Fig. 2–2): The dietary intake of a certain nutrient is low. If low intake continues over time, body tissue levels of that nutrient will decline. Continued low intakes will cause impairment of certain body functions and, eventually, the lack of the nutrient will result in physical signs and symptoms of a deficiency. Nutrition assessment techniques can be used to identify stages of this process. For example, a dietary interview with a client reveals a low intake of thiamin, which could lead to a deficiency disease known as beriberi. An inadequate intake initially causes low tissue levels, which can be measured by blood or urine levels of the vitamin. Even lower tissue levels result in a decrease in the activity of thiamin-dependent enzymes such as transketolase. As the deficiency progresses, pyruvate (an intermediary product of glucose breakdown), which requires a thiamin-containing coenzyme for metabolism, increases in the blood. Eventually symptoms of beriberi, such as anorexia, depression, and changes in the function of the central nervous system, are observed.

A nutrient deficiency due to inadequate dietary intake, such as the one just described, is called a primary defi-

ciency. Progression to a deficiency state may also occur when dietary intake appears to be adequate if requirements for the nutrient increase, if absorption or utilization of the nutrient is severely curtailed, or if nutrient excretion increases. Such a deficiency is referred to as a secondary nutrient deficiency.

Nutrition Assessment Techniques

Nutrition assessment may be performed in the hospital, an extended care facility, a physician's office, or an outpatient or community clinic. Nutrition assessment is based not on a single determination but on a group or series of measurements and observations that provide an estimate of nutritional status. Techniques used for nutrition assessment must reflect nutrition status, be readily available in that particular healthcare setting, and be of reasonable cost. Another important criterion for selecting an assessment parameter is that it must be repeatable so that the impact of intervention can be monitored. Data collected for nutrition assessment, often categorized as anthropometric, laboratory or biochemical, clinical, and dietary, are combined to provide a picture of nutrition status.

Deficiencies of specific vitamins or minerals occur in-

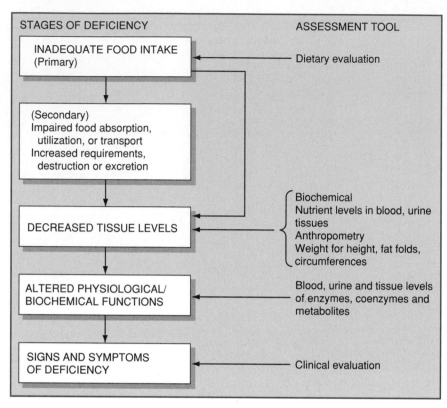

FIGURE 2–2. Sequence of events in prolonged nutrition inadequacy and appropriate assessment techniques.

frequently in people in developed countries. General malnutrition, which is associated with inadequate food intake or impaired utilization of food sources, is more common and involves several nutrients. Therefore, nutrition assessment of individuals centers on their macronutrient status, particularly energy and protein status. Because iron deficiency is a concern for many age groups, iron status is often part of the nutrition assessment.

Body Macronutrient Components

The major body components are water, protein, fat, and mineral. From an assessment point of view, macronutrients in the body can be divided into two compartments, body fat and fat-free mass. Fat, the major energy reserve, is the most variable component of the body. Body fat mass can be estimated from fatfold(skinfold) measurements at a variety of body sites, the most common of which is the triceps fatfold. Body fat is sensitive to acute malnutrition and can be used as an indirect estimate of energy balance.

The fat-free components of the body include bone, skeletal muscle mass and nonskeletal soft tissue (Fig. 2–3). **Somatic** and **visceral** proteins are considered metabolically active because they can be drawn upon to meet body

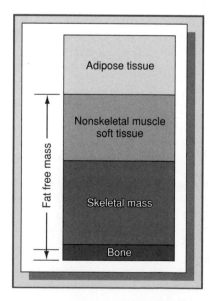

FIGURE 2–3. A tissue system model of body composition. (From Wang Z-M, Pierson RN, Heymsfield SB. The five-level model: a new approach to organizing body-composition research. Am J Clin Nutr 1992;56:19. © Am J Clin Nutr. American Society for Clinical Nutrition.)

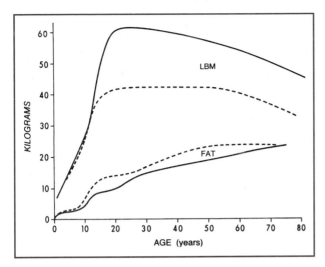

FIGURE 2–4. Average values for lean body mass (LBM) and fat across the life span. Solid lines represent males; and broken lines represent females. (Adapted from Forbes GB. Body composition: influence of nutrition, disease, growth and aging. In Shils ME, et al. Modern nutrition in health and disease. Philadelphia: Lea & Febiger, 1994.)

TABLE 2–1 Parameters for Evaluation of Nutrition Status	
Body Compartment	**Parameter**
Adipose tissue	Weight for height
	Body mass index (BMI)
	Fatfolds
	Triceps (TFF)
	Subscapular (SSFF)
Visceral protein	Serum proteins
	Albumin
	Transferrin
	Pre-albumin (PA)
	Retinol-binding protein (RBP)
	Immune proteins
	Total lymphocyte count (TLC)
Somatic protein	Midarm muscle circumference (MAMC)
	Midarm muscle area (MAMA)
	Creatinine height index (CHI)
Iron	Hemoglobin, hematocrit (hgb, hct)
	Total iron binding capacity (TIBC)
	Serum ferritin
	Free erythrocyte protoporphyrin

needs. The status of these proteins is assessed by different methods. Because the human body does not store protein as it does fat, decreases in body protein result in loss of structural units such as skeletal protein as well as visceral proteins such as serum albumin. Nutrition assessment measurements must reflect these body compartments. Because the amount and proportion of lean body mass and body fat change across the life span (Fig. 2–4), data related to these compartments are interpreted using gender- and age-specific standards.

Somatic protein may be evaluated from anthropometric measurements and from the determination of the amount of creatinine, a metabolite of muscle metabolism, excreted in the urine. Visceral protein status is assessed by biochemical analyses of serum proteins and immune proteins, most often the total lymphocyte count (TLC). Table 2–1 lists representative measurements of major body compartments used in nutrition assessment, which will be discussed in this chapter.

Application of Nutrition Assessment

The level at which assessment techniques are applied varies. A dietary interview in a health clinic or private practice setting may be used to develop counseling plans to adjust the patient's nutrient intake. A young child may be evaluated for eligibility for the Women, Infants, and Children (WIC) supplemental food program by using anthropometry (weight and height measurements), dietary intake, and a simple blood test. At another level, the hospitalized patient who is receiving total parenteral nutrition (delivery of nutrients directly into the bloodstream) may

be assessed using all of the above plus a series of laboratory tests.

Nutrition assessment is the first step in the nutrition care process. It is a multifactorial approach in which several kinds of information are collected and used to evaluate an individual's nutrition status. In this introduction to nutrition assessment, anthropometric, biochemical, clinical, and dietary measurements are described, and examples for use and interpretation are discussed.

ANTHROPOMETRY

■ What are the advantages and limitations of using anthropometric measurements for nutrition assessment?

■ Which anthropometric measurements are commonly used, and how are they interpreted?

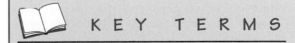

K E Y   T E R M S

somatic: protein within skeletal muscle
visceral: proteins of the organs (viscera) and circulation

Anthropometry is the measurement of physical dimensions of the human body. In the hands of an experienced practitioner, anthropometry is a useful technique for estimation of body composition. Several parameters can be used to estimate body fat (energy) and somatic protein status. In undernutrition, skeletal muscle and fat stores are depleted earlier than proteins of organs; therefore, low levels in these compartments can be an early indicator of nutritional depletion. The reliability of anthropometric measurements in estimating body fat and protein has been validated using densitometry (underwater weighing) (Gray et al, 1990; Durnin and Womersley, 1974; Jackson and Pollock, 1985).

Anthropometric techniques are rapid and repeatable. The required equipment (scales, tape measures, and calipers) is readily available, inexpensive, and portable. However, accurate and reliable anthropometric measurements require a skilled, careful measurer and quality equipment that is calibrated regularly. Standard techniques for anthropometry have been established. Those used most frequently are described briefly in this chapter. Keys to successful anthropometry are the **accuracy** and **reliability** of each measurement. Measurements should be repeated and recorded immediately to reduce the chance of error. If the two measurements are substantially different, a third reading should be made.

There are dozens of anthropometric measurements that can be used (Lohman et al, 1988). This introductory discussion includes only stature (height), weight, upper arm circumference, and triceps and subscapular fatfolds.

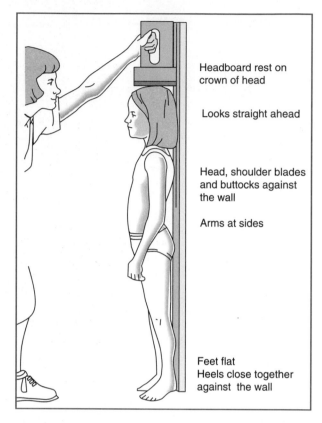

Headboard rest on crown of head

Looks straight ahead

Head, shoulder blades and buttocks against the wall

Arms at sides

Feet flat
Heels close together against the wall

FIGURE 2–5. Accurate determination of height requires careful positioning of the subject.

Weight for Height

The most common anthropometric measurements, stature and weight, can be useful for preliminary assessment of energy and protein stores.

HEIGHT Stature is a major component of body size and is important for evaluation of growth in children and weight status in adults. Accurate measurement of standing height requires a nonstretchable tape or measuring stick attached to a vertical surface and a moveable horizontal or right-angle headboard for reading. For measurement, the subject stands erect, without shoes, with weight equally distributed on both feet and heels together and touching the vertical board (Fig. 2–5). Arms hang freely at the sides of the trunk with palms facing the thighs. Looking straight ahead so that the line of vision is perpendicular to the body, the subject takes a deep breath and holds that position while the horizontal headboard is brought down firmly on the top of the head. Stature is recorded to the nearest 0.1 cm or ¼ inch.

WEIGHT Body weight is a composite measure of total body size. It is important in screening for unusual growth, obesity, or undernutrition and is a component in equations that predict energy needs and body composition. Weight is measured on a leveled platform scale with a beam and moveable weights. The subject, in minimal clothing and without shoes, stands with weight evenly distributed on both feet. Weight is recorded to the nearest 0.1 kg or ¼ lb.

Measurements of stature and weight are interpreted by comparison to tables derived from a reference population or to the individual's former or usual weight. Gains in stature and weight in infants and children are important indicators of growth status and are discussed in the chapters on growth.

Usual Weight In the healthcare setting recent changes in body weight can be an important indicator of nutrition status. Changes may be reported as percentage of body weight lost or of previous or usual body weight using the following calculations:

% weight loss =
   [(usual weight − current weight)/usual weight] × 100

% usual weight = (current weight/usual weight) × 100

Height–Weight Tables For adults, body weight for height can be assessed through the use of height–weight tables. Height–weight tables have been generated from data from the insurance industry, studies on build and blood pressure, the American Cancer Society study, and the NHANES data. Most tables reflect average weights, but these weights are not necessarily those at which people feel, look, or perform their best. Therefore, terms such as "desirable" or "ideal" weight are inappropriate; the terms "reference weight" or "relative weight" are more accurate. The most frequently used reference tables, the 1983 Height and Weight Tables from the Metropolitan Life Insurance Company (Metropolitan, 1983), are located inside the back cover of this text. These tables provide weight ranges for height based on the 1979 Build Study, which included approximately 4 million policy holders of 25 insurance companies. Data from adults with significant disease were omitted. Weights for a given stature are those associated with the greatest longevity. The 1983 tables include weight ranges for small, medium, and large frame for each height. Interpretation of body weight for height can be enhanced by use of the appropriate frame size designation, especially in distinguishing between individuals who have large fat-free mass and those who have high body weights due to excess fat.

Frame size is a skeletal concept. Determinants of size should be based on skeletal dimensions, which reflect body build but are not influenced by the degree of body fat. A variety of body breadth and diameter measurements, including ankle, elbow, wrist, shoulder, and hip, have been suggested to represent body frame size (Himes and Bouchard, 1985; Mitchell, 1993). The frame measure for which reference data from a large population are available is elbow breadth. Elbow breadth is measured with a broad-faced sliding anthropometer while the right arm is extended and the forearm bent upward at a 90-degree angle with the wrist toward the body (Fig. 2–6). Measurement is made between the two prominent bones on either side of the elbow. Pressure is exerted to compress soft tissues and record the breadth to the nearest 1 mm. Elbow breadth correlates with fat-free body mass (Frisancho, 1990). Frame size was not measured on the insured population that is the basis for the 1983 Metropolitan Tables. Categories for frame size were determined from elbow breadth measurements of the subjects in NHANES I and II (see Chapter 1). The frame size designations that accompany the 1983 Height and Weight Tables were formulated by dividing the elbow breadth measurements into quartiles. Medium frame corresponds to elbow breadths between the 25th and 75th percentiles in each height category. Values above the 75th percentile and below the 25th percentile were designated as large and small frame, respectively (Frisancho and Flegel, 1983).

Relative Weight Relative weight is the individual's actual weight expressed as a percentage of the reference weight. The Metropolitan Height–Weight Tables are used

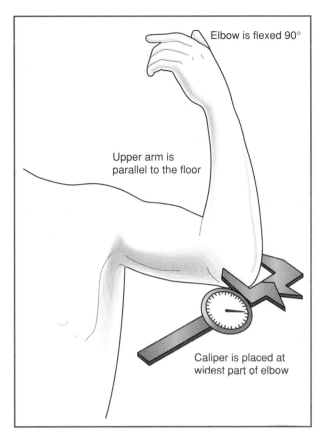

FIGURE 2–6. Elbow breadth is measured between the two prominent bones on either side of the elbow.

by selecting the appropriate frame size based on elbow breadth. Reference weight is a range for the individual's gender, height, and frame size. Usually, the midpoint of this weight range is used to calculate the Metropolitan relative weight (MRW), as follows:

$$MRW = (\text{Current weight/reference weight}) \times 100$$

It should be noted that the Metropolitan Height–Weight Tables contain values for measurements made with the subject wearing 1-inch heels and clothing weighing approximately 5 pounds for men and 3 pounds for women. These values must be added when using the tables if barefoot height and nude weights are used.

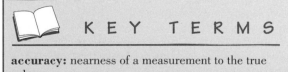

K E Y   T E R M S

accuracy: nearness of a measurement to the true value
reliability: the extent to which the same measurement is obtained on repeated trials

TABLE 2–2 Underweight, Acceptable Weight, Overweight, and Obesity Based on Body Mass Index (BMI)

Category	BMI	
	Males	Females
Underweight	<20.7	<19.1
Acceptable weight	20.7–26.4	19.1–25.8
Marginal overweight	26.4–27.8	25.8–27.3
Overweight	27.8–31.1	27.3–32.3
Severe overweight	31.1–45.4	32.3–44.8
Morbid obesity	>45.4	>44.8

Used with permission of Ross Products Division, Abbott Laboratories, Columbus, Ohio. From ML Rowland, A nomogram for computing body mass index, using the nomogram. *Dietetic Currents,* 1989;16(2):6–7.

For a 35-year-old man who is 72 in (183 cm) in stature with a medium frame and weighs 150 lb (68 kg), the reference weight range would be 157 to 170 lb (71.3 to 77.2 kg). Using the midpoint of the range of weight for stature, his MRW would be:

$$\text{MRW} = 68 \text{ kg}/74.3 \times 100 = 92 \text{ or } 92\%$$

Body Mass Index A variety of other height/weight indices have been used to assess body weight for height in adults. The body mass index (BMI) estimates total body mass. Because BMI is highly correlated with total body fat (Micozzi et al, 1986; Revicki and Israel, 1986), it is considered a general indicator of body fatness. BMI can be determined using this calculation:

$$\text{BMI} = \text{weight (kg)/height (m}^2)$$

For a 35-year-old man who is 183 cm tall and weighs 68 kg, the BMI would be:

$$\text{BMI} = 68 \text{ kg}/1.83^2 = 20.2$$

Using the definitions of BMI in Table 2–2 for underweight, acceptable weight, overweight, and obese, he would be slightly underweight.

BMI does not distinguish excess fat from muscularity as the source of excessive body weight (Frisancho and Flegel, 1983; Smalley et al, 1990). A more direct indicator of obesity is body fatfolds, discussed in the following section.

Fatfolds

Fatfolds, sometimes called skinfolds, are indicators of body fat and, therefore, of energy reserves. They can be made on almost any site of the body where subcutaneous fat is present, but the most frequently measured fatfolds are those of the triceps, biceps, subscapular, suprailiac, abdomen, and thigh. A fatfold is actually the thickness of a double fold of skin and subcutaneous adipose tissue (Fig. 2–7). Calipers calibrated to exert standardized pressure per unit of jaw surface are used for the measurement. The fatfolds that are most readily measured and for which there are therefore reference data from large population studies are the triceps and subscapular.

TRICEPS FATFOLD The triceps fatfold (TFF) is measured in the midline at the back of the arm, over the triceps muscle, at a point midway between the lateral projection of the shoulder and the elbow (Fig. 2–8). The measurement is taken with the subject's right arm hanging loosely and comfortably at the side. The caliper is held in the measurer's right hand. Standing behind the subject, the measurer picks up the triceps skinfold approximately 1 cm above the marked midpoint. The tips of the calipers are applied to the fatfold at the marked level, and the fold is measured to the nearest 0.1 mm.

SUBSCAPULAR FATFOLD Figure 2–9 illustrates measurement of the subscapular fatfold (SSFF). The subject stands with the arm relaxed to the side. The calipers are applied at the site along the axis of the inferior angle of the scapula and the fatfold is measured to the nearest 0.1 mm.

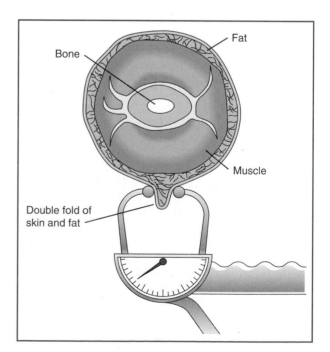

FIGURE 2–7. The fatfold measurement is a double thickness of fat and skin.

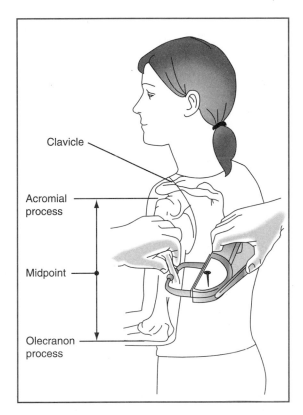

FIGURE 2–8. The triceps fatfold is measured at the midpoint between the acromial process and the olecranon process.

INTERPRETATION OF FATFOLD MEASURE-MENTS Fatfold measurements for a given individual are evaluated by comparison with age- and gender-specific percentile distribution of a reference population, in most instances using the data from the NHANES survey. Reference tables for triceps fatfold and subscapular fatfold are in Appendices 3A and 3B. If a 35-year-old man has a TFF of 9.0 mm and an SSFF of 16 mm, consulting Appendices 3A and 3B would reveal that 9.0 mm is equal to the 25th percentile for TFF and 16 mm is just below the 50th percentile for SSFF. This indicates that, compared to a reference population, this man's TFF is lower than 75% and higher than 24% of the reference population and his SSFF is almost at the midpoint for the reference population. It can be readily seen that values below the 10th percentile or above the 90th percentile suggest very low or very high fat reserve and, therefore, increased risk of malnutrition or obesity, respectively. Sometimes measurements fall between the percentiles shown on the tables and must be estimated from the data available. For a man of the same age, a triceps fatfold of 7.9 mm falls between the 15th and 25th percentiles, or at approximately the 20th percentile. Many clinicians believe that a more accurate representation of total body fat can be obtained by taking an average of two or more fatfolds, including peripheral and central fat reserves such as the triceps fatfold and the subscapular or suprailiac fatfolds.

Body fatness is of interest for two reasons. Too little fat is associated with undernutrition, and too much with increased risk of chronic disease. Excess body fat is a specific risk factor for many diseases, including cardiovascular disease, diabetes, and certain cancers. Measurement of fatfold thicknesses at different body sites can characterize the distribution of subcutaneous adipose tissue, which may be significant in predicting risk for certain diseases. Long-term research studies indicate that the site of fat storage, specifically abdominal as opposed to gluteal (hip) fat storage, is a major risk factor for mortality from cardiovascular diseases (Kannel et al, 1991) and endometrial cancer (Schapira et al, 1991).

Midarm Circumference

The triceps fatfold, an independent measure of body fat, is also used with the midarm circumference (MAC) to calculate two estimators of somatic protein status: midarm muscle circumference (MAMC) and midarm muscle area (MAMA) (Heymsfield et al, 1982). Midarm circumference is measured at the same site as the triceps skinfold.

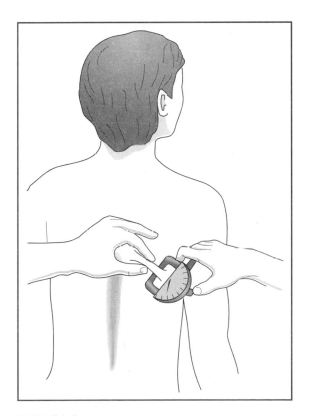

FIGURE 2–9. Measurement of the subscapular fatfold.

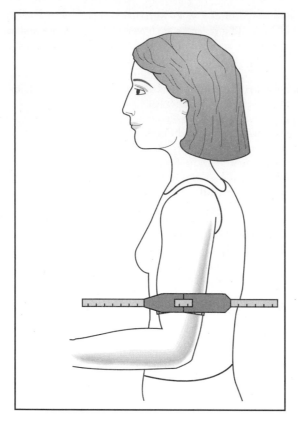

FIGURE 2–10. Midarm circumference is measured at the midpoint of the upper arm, the same site as the triceps fatfold.

The subject stands erect with the arm hanging freely at the side of the trunk, palm facing the thigh. A flexible, nonstretchable tape is placed around the arm so that it is touching the skin but not compressing the soft tissues (Fig. 2–10). The circumference is recorded to the nearest millimeter.

MIDARM MUSCLE CIRCUMFERENCE Midarm muscle circumference is calculated using the following formula:

$$MAMC = MAC - (\pi \times TFF)$$

with MAC and TFF given in cm. The MAMC for a 35-year-old man with a MAC of 30.4 cm and a TFF of 8.5 (.85 cm) would be calculated as follows:

$$MAMC = 30.4 - (3.14 \times .9)$$

$$MAMC = 27.5 \text{ cm, or } 275 \text{ mm}$$

Midarm muscle area is calculated from the circumference of the upper arm and the triceps fatfold values using the following formulas:

$$MAMA \text{ for females} = \frac{[MAC (\pi \times TFF)]^2}{4\pi} - 6.5$$

$$MAMA \text{ for males} = \frac{[MAC (\pi \times TSF)]^2}{4\pi} - 10$$

In these equations, π equals 3.14, MAC is midarm circumference in cm, and TFF is triceps fatfold in cm. The constants (6.5 and 10) that are subtracted at the end of the calculation account for the presence of bone, nerves, and vascular tissue in the upper arm (Heymsfield et al, 1982). The MAMA for the man used in the previous example above would be calculated as follows:

$$MAMA = \frac{[30.4 - (.9 \times 3.14)]^2}{4 \times 3.14} - 10$$

$$= 27.57^2/12.56 - 10$$

$$= 760.2/12.5$$

$$= 60.52 \text{ cm}^2 \text{ or } 605.2 \text{ mm}^2$$

The MAMC and MAMA are interpreted using the percentile distribution of the NHANES data in Appendices 3C and 3D. Consulting Appendix 3C would reveal that a MAMC value of 27.5 is just above the 25th percentile. Appendix 3D indicates that a MAMA of 60.52 cm² is slightly below the 10th percentile.

BIOCHEMICAL MEASUREMENTS

■ What are the advantages and limitations of biochemical measurements for nutritional assessment?

■ Describe three measures of visceral protein status and are significance of decreases in these measurements.

■ What does a decreased level of serum ferritin, hemoglobin, or hematocrit tell you about iron status?

Biochemical tests for assessment must reflect body levels of the specific nutrient and be sensitive to a depletion of body stores. They may be measurements of nutrients or their metabolites (products of the metabolism of the nutrient), substances that contain the nutrient (such as hemoglobin for iron), enzymes that require the nutrient (such as transketolase for thiamin), or substances that result from abnormal metabolism due to a deficiency of the nutrient (such as elevated pyruvate levels in thiamin deficiency). Laboratory tests are performed on available body tissues, usually blood or urine. Biochemical tests are the most objective and quantitative measures of nutritional status. They can detect nutrient deficits long before alterations in anthropometric measures or clinical signs or symptoms appear. Because biochemical tests may be in-

TABLE 2–3 Biochemical Tests for Assessment of Nutritional Status

Nutrient	Laboratory Test
PROTEIN	Serum albumin, transferrin prealbumin, retinol-binding protein, total lymphocyte count (TLC), creatinine excretion
FAT-SOLUBLE VITAMINS	
Vitamin A	Serum carotene, retinol-binding protein, retinol, conjunctival impression cytology, dark adaptation
Vitamin D	Serum 25-OH vitamin D_3 Serum alkaline phosphatase
Vitamin E	Serum tocopherol, erythrocyte hemolysis test
Vitamin K	Prothrombin time, plasma vitamin K, clotting factors
WATER-SOLUBLE VITAMINS	
Vitamin C	Serum vitamin C, leukocyte vitamin C
Thiamin	Transketolate activity in RBC with and without TPP Urinary thiamin
Riboflavin	Glutathione reductase activity in RBC with and without FAD, plasma riboflavin Urinary riboflavin
Niacin	Urinary metabolites of niacin (N_1-methylnicotinamide and 2-pyridone)
Vitamin B_6	Plasma and erythrocyte pyridoxal-5-phosphate, plasma pyridoxal, transaminase activity in RBC, plasma and urinary vitamin B_6 and 4-pyridoxic acid, urinary xanthurenic acid after tryptophan load
Folate	Serum folate, folate in RBC
Vitamin B_{12}	Serum vitamin B_{12}, vitamin B_{12} in RBC, increased urinary methylmalonic acid
Biotin	Serum biotin, urinary biotin
MINERALS	
Calcium	Bone mineral content
Copper	Serum copper
Iodine	Serum protein-bound iodine (PBI), uptake of radioiodine (^{131}I)
Iron	Serum ferritin, serum iron, total iron binding capacity (TIBC) or transferrin saturation, free protoporphyrin in RBC, hemoglobin, hematocrit, mean corpuscular volume, mean corpuscular hemoglobin
Magnesium	Serum magnesium, magnesium in RBC
Potassium	Serum potassium
Zinc	No specific sensitive biochemical indicator, serum zinc, urinary zinc, hair zinc

fluenced by non-nutrition factors such as diseases or medication use, they are used with other parameters for assessment.

Measurements on Blood

NUTRIENTS Nutrients in blood may be measured in **plasma** or **serum** as well as in specific cellular components such as red blood cells (RBC) or white blood cells (WBC). In most cases serum and plasma concentrations are similar. The potential effect of recent dietary intake on nutrient levels can be reduced by collecting fasting blood samples. Measurements of nutrients or products in blood are reported per unit of blood, i.e., g, mg, or μg per deciliter (dL) or liter (L). Body hydration status may influence actual values reported. For example, an individual who is dehydrated may appear to have high nutrient levels, but when body fluids are returned to normal, the values may drop to normal or below normal levels. Laboratory tests have been developed for assessment of many nutrients (Table 2–3). For some nutrients, blood tests may not be sensitive indicators of nutrition status because of large body stores (e.g., fat-soluble vitamins), or because blood levels are regulated by hormones (e.g., calcium).

METABOLITES Vitamins often function as coenzymes in the metabolism of carbohydrate, protein, or fat. The absence of a vitamin to synthesize a coenzyme may block a normal series of reactions, resulting in an increase of an intermediary product or byproduct in the blood. For instance, citing the example used earlier, an increase in pyruvate in the blood occurs when there is insufficient thiamin for carbohydrate metabolism to proceed normally. The presence of abnormal metabolic substances or abnormal amounts of certain products can be an indicator of an inadequacy.

ENZYMES Many nutrients are parts of enzyme systems, and nutrient status may be assessed by measuring a coenzyme or the activity of an enzyme that requires the nutrient. To return to the initial example of a thiamin deficiency, the enzyme transketolase requires thiamin. If thiamin is deficient, enzyme activity is reduced. A reduced level of transketolase activity in red blood cells may,

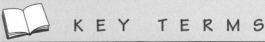

K E Y   T E R M S

plasma: whole blood from which blood cells have been removed
serum: whole blood that remains after cells and clotting factors have been removed

therefore, indicate a deficiency of thiamin before metabolic changes or deficiency symptoms occur.

FUNCTIONAL TESTS Functional tests of nutrition status measure one or more physiologic processes that rely on a nutrient. Examples include determination of dark adaptation for vitamin A status or response to an injected antigen for protein status. Some functional tests are nonspecific, such as immune response; these, therefore, may indicate general nutrition status but do not allow identification of specific nutrient deficiencies.

Urine

The presence of nutrients or their metabolites in urine may be useful in assessing nutrition status. Urinary levels of many nutrients reflect dietary intakes. For example, if an individual has adequate tissue levels of water-soluble vitamins, any intake in excess of the amount required for body turnover is excreted in the urine. If tissue levels are low, a larger portion of dietary intake is retained in the body and urinary excretion is proportionately less, suggesting a potential deficiency.

The presence of substances not normally excreted in the urine can be an indicator of decreasing levels of the nutrient in the body. For example, in the absence of folate-containing coenzymes, the metabolism of the amino acid histidine is blocked, resulting in excretion of a metabolite of folate (formimino glutamic acid) not normally found in urine. Its presence, therefore, is indicative of a folate deficiency.

Somatic Protein

CREATININE HEIGHT INDEX (CHI) Creatinine is the urinary metabolite of the catabolism of creatine phosphate, a compound in muscle that stores high-energy phosphate for muscle contraction. The amount of creatinine excreted by a healthy adult in a 24-hour period is a relatively constant proportion of muscle mass (Keshaviah et al, 1994). Lean body mass can be estimated by measuring the amount of creatinine excreted and comparing that amount to a population-based standard. Table 2–4 gives creatinine excretion levels by height, frame size, and reference weight for males and females. Urinary creatinine excretion is expressed as the creatinine height index (CHI), which is a percentage of the standard.

It is calculated as follows:

% CHI = actual urinary creatinine/reference urinary creatinine ×100

A CHI of 60% to 80% is considered a moderate; less than 60% is considered a severe deficit of body muscle mass

(Blackburn, 1977). As will all tests, however, the results must be interpreted carefully, because urinary creatinine can be influenced by diet, exercise, drugs, stress, and kidney function.

Visceral Protein

Visceral proteins are proteins in the circulation (erythrocytes, lymphocytes, and serum proteins) and those in body organs (liver, kidney, heart, pancreas, and other organs). Several measurements of proteins in the blood are considered reliable indicators of visceral protein status. These proteins have many functions, however, including transport or storage of nutrients, fluid and acid-base balance, and immune responses. Therefore, laboratory tests have some limitations, and their interpretation must be considered in the context of an individual's overall health status. Several serum proteins and a measure of immunocompetence, the total lymphocyte count (TLC), are discussed in this section.

SERUM PROTEINS Serum proteins that are used to monitor nutrition status are selected because they reflect protein status, have a rapid rate of synthesis and a constant catabolic rate (Spiekerman, 1993), and are responsive to protein and energy restriction and repletion (Young et al, 1990). The liver is the major site for synthesis of serum proteins and one of the first organs to be affected by protein undernutrition.

Approximately 50% to 60% of the serum protein is albumin. Low concentrations of serum albumin are associated with increased risk of morbidity and mortality in hospitalized patients (Herrman et al, 1992). The level of serum albumin is an indicator of visceral protein status. Because it has a **half-life** of about 20 days, it is not very sensitive to short-term changes in protein status.

Several other circulating proteins synthesized by the liver have a shorter half-life and are useful for nutrition assessment, including serum transferrin, prealbumin, and retinol-binding protein. Table 2–5 shows the normal range of serum protein levels for adults. Lower levels are associated with protein deficiency. Interpretation of serum protein values requires knowledge of the diagnosis and general condition of the client, because serum protein levels can be influenced by many factors, including liver disease, medication, stress, exercise, and infection.

IMMUNE PROTEINS The relationship between nutrition and immune function is complex. Undernutrition can lead to impaired immunocompetence and infection. Because changes in immune response occur early in nutritional deficiency, tests of immune function can be indicators for assessment of nutrition status and an index of response to nutrition intervention. The most common laboratory test is a complete blood count (CBC). It counts

TABLE 2–4 Standards for Creatinine Height Index

MEN

| Height | | Small Frame | | Medium Frame | | Large Frame | |
in	cm	Reference Weight (kg)	Creatinine (mg/24 h)	Reference Weight (kg)	Creatinine (mg/24 h)	Reference Weight (kg)	Creatinine (mg/24 h)
61	154.9	52.7	1,212	56.1	1,290	60.7	1,396
62	157.5	54.1	1,244	57.7	1,327	62.0	1,426
63	160.0	55.4	1,274	59.1	1,359	63.6	1,463
64	162.5	56.8	1,306	60.4	1,389	65.2	1,500
65	165.1	58.4	1,343	62.0	1,426	66.8	1,536
66	167.6	60.2	1,385	63.9	1,470	68.9	1,585
67	170.2	62.0	1,426	65.9	1,516	71.1	1,635
68	172.7	63.9	1,470	67.7	1,557	72.9	1,677
69	175.3	65.9	1,516	69.5	1,598	74.8	1,720
70	177.8	67.7	1,557	71.6	1,647	76.8	1,766
71	180.3	69.5	1,599	73.6	1,693	79.1	1,819
72	182.9	71.4	1,642	75.7	1,741	81.1	1,865
73	185.4	73.4	1,688	77.7	1,787	83.4	1,918
74	187.9	75.2	1,730	80.0	1,846	85.7	1,971
75	190.5	77.0	1,771	82.3	1,893	87.7	2,017

WOMEN

| Height | | Small Frame | | Medium Frame | | Large Frame | |
in	cm	Reference Weight (kg)	Creatinine (mg/24 h)	Reference Weight (kg)	Creatinine (mg/24 h)	Reference Weight (kg)	Creatinine (mg/24 h)
56	142.2	43.2	778	46.1	830	50.7	913
57	144.8	44.3	797	47.3	851	51.8	932
58	147.3	45.4	817	48.6	875	53.2	958
59	149.8	46.8	842	50.0	900	54.5	981
60	152.4	48.2	868	51.4	925	55.9	1,006
61	154.9	49.5	891	52.7	949	57.3	1,031
62	157.5	50.9	916	54.3	977	58.9	1,060
63	160.0	52.3	941	55.9	1,006	60.6	1,091
64	162.5	53.9	970	57.9	1,042	62.5	1,125
65	165.1	55.7	1,003	59.8	1,076	64.3	1,157
66	167.6	57.5	1,035	61.6	1,109	66.1	1,190
67	170.2	59.3	1,067	63.4	1,141	67.9	1,222
68	172.7	61.4	1,105	65.2	1,174	70.0	1,260
69	175.2	63.2	1,138	67.0	1,206	72.0	1,296
70	177.8	65.0	1,170	68.9	1,240	74.1	1,334

From Grant A, DeHoog S. Nutritional assessment and support. 4th ed, 1991. Northgate Station, Seattle, WA 98125. Reprinted with permission.

erythrocytes and leukocytes (white cells) and platelets. A differential (the normal differential for WBC is: lymphocytes 20–40%, neutrophils 50–70%, eosinophils 1–4%, basophils 0–4%, and monocytes 2–8%) count gives the percentage of different types of white blood cells (WBC) in the sample. Lymphocytes have a relatively short half-life and can, therefore, reflect short-term changes in protein

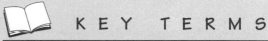

K E Y   T E R M S

half-life: the time in which half the concentration of a substance in the plasma is turned over

status. The total lymphocyte count (TLC) can be calculated using the total WBC count and differential by applying the following equation:

$$TLC = \frac{Total\ WBC \times \%\ lymphocytes}{100}$$

Normal values for TLC are found in Table 2–5. Such data must be interpreted with caution because TLC can be influenced by radiotherapy, surgery, and immunosuppressive medication as well as viral infections and some medications.

Iron Status

Iron deficiency is the most frequent nutritional deficiency worldwide and the most common cause of anemia. Early stages are characterized by progressive reduction in the amount of stored iron as measured by serum ferritin. With iron depletion, iron stores decline, resulting in a reduced iron supply to cells and a decreased concentration of iron carried in transferrin (decreased transferrin satura-

tion). The **total iron binding capacity** (TIBC) increases. Concentrations of protoporphyrin, a precursor of heme, increase in erythrocytes when the iron supply is inadequate for normal hemoglobin synthesis. The final stage, iron deficiency anemia, occurs with depletion of iron stores and declining levels of circulating iron. It is characterized by reduced concentration of hemoglobin, which impairs the ability of erythrocytes to carry oxygen to body cells. Laboratory tests used to assess iron status are described in Table 2–6.

Hemoglobin is probably the most widely used screening test for iron deficiency anemia, but the hemoglobin level does not decline until iron reserves are exhausted. Hence, hemoglobin is diagnostic of deficiency but not predictive of impending deficiency. Interpretation of hemoglobin levels is limited by variations in age, gender, race, and cigarette smoking. Decreased levels occur with deficiencies of Vitamin B_{12} and folate as well as protein energy malnutrition. Levels also decline in response to chronic infection, inflammation, and hemorrhage. Changes in hematocrit levels in iron deficiency tend to parallel those of hemoglobin.

TABLE 2–5 Visceral Proteins For Nutrition Assessment

	Normal Value (range)	Half-Life (days)	Function	Nutritional Significance
Albumin	35–55 g/L	18–20	Maintains plasma oncotic pressure; carrier for small molecules	Large body pool is 4–5 g/kg body weight. Indicator of long-term protein status and decreased protein intake.
Transferrin	2.0–4.0 g/L	8–10	Binds and transports iron in plasma; accepts iron from sites of hemoglobin destruction, storage sites, and iron absorbed from intestine.	Body pool is <0.1 g/kg body weight. Compared to albumin, smaller body pool and shorter half life; better index of changes in protein status. Levels increase with iron deficiency, pregnancy and estrogen therapy.
Prealbumin	200–400 mg/L	2–3	Binds thryroxine; carrier for retinol-binding protein (also referred to as thyroxine-binding prealbumin)	Body pool is 0.01 g/kg body weight. Better indicator of recent dietary intake than overall nutrition status.
Retinol-binding protein (RBP)	3–6 mg/L	8–12 h	Liver protein; transports vitamin A in plasma; binds to prealbumin.	Body pool is 0.002 g/kg body weight. Responds quickly to protein energy deprivation and nutrition intervention; better indicator of recent dietary intake than overall nutrition status.
Total lymphocyte count (TLC)	1500–4000 cells/mm^3	4–6	20–40% of total white blood cells. Part of antigen-specific defenses of the immune system.	Good indicator of general malnutrition. Declines early in protein energy deficiency. Responds to nutrition intervention.

TABLE 2–6 Laboratory Tests of Iron Status

Laboratory Measurement	Normal Value	Nutritional Significance
Hemoglobin Males Females	 140–180 g/L 120–160 g/L	Index of the blood's oxygen carrying capacity; does not become abnormal until late stages of iron deficiency.
Hematocrit (packed cell volume) Males Females	 40–54% 38–46%	Percentage of red blood cells (RBC) that make up entire volume of blood; largely dependent on the number of RBC.
Serum iron Males Females	 70–150 μg/dL 80–150 μg/dL	Measures total iron in the blood, including that bound to transferrin.
Serum ferritin Males Females	 20–30 μg/L 20–120 μg/L	Found primarily in liver, spleen, and bone marrow. Ferritin declines as iron stores become depleted. Sensitive test for detecting iron deficiency before changes in cells are seen.
Transferrin saturation and total iron binding capacity (TIBC)	About 30% of available iron-binding sites are occupied or saturated.	TIBC measures the amount of iron capable of being bound in the blood. In uncomplicated iron deficiency, TIBC increases as transferrin saturation decreases.
Free erythrocyte protoporphyrin	>1.24 μmol/L RBC	A precursor of heme, protoporphyrin accumulates in RBC when the amount of heme formed is limited by iron deficiency; it may increase twofold over normal values; levels also increase in lead poisoning.
Mean corpuscular volume (MCV)	76–100 μg/m^3	Indicates size of red blood cell. Increases in megaloblasic anemia (vitamin B_{12} or folate) and decreases in microcytic anemia (Iron)
Mean corpuscular hemoglobin concentration (MCHC)	33–37 g/dL	Indicates hemoglobin content per volume of RBC. Value low when hemoglobin is decreased.

In some settings, the only blood test available may be the hemoglobin or hematocrit. In a WIC clinic, a hematocrit or hemoglobin level for a child can be determined from a few drops of blood obtained from a fingerstick. To obtain a hematocrit, a small amount of blood is centrifuged in a small tube to separate cellular components from the fluid portion. The cellular part that settles to the bottom is referred to as the packed cell volume, or hematocrit (Fig. 2–11). Hematocrit is reported as a percentage of the total, i.e., packed cell volume, or percentage of total blood volume.

CLINICAL ASSESSMENT

■ At what stage are clinical signs appropriate for nutrition assessment?

■ What are the limitations of using clinical observations in nutrition assessment?

Clinical evaluation consists of a medical history and a physical examination for possible evidence of malnutri-

tion. The physical examination is incorporated into population-based nutrition surveys such as NHANES. It is also used for individual nutrition assessment in hospitals and clinics. Clinical observation is useful only for the overt signs of the most advanced stages of malnutrition, after depletion of body stores. Consequently, its usefulness is limited in identifying impending nutritional problems.

Accurate clinical assessment requires a skilled observer to detect physical signs and interpret symptoms reported by the client that are indicative of malnutrition. Physical signs of malnutrition appear most quickly in tissues that are replaced rapidly, such as skin and the tissues of the digestive tract. The most commonly observed tissues are su-

K E Y T E R M S

total iron binding capacity: the amount of iron capable of being bound to serum proteins, particularly transferrin

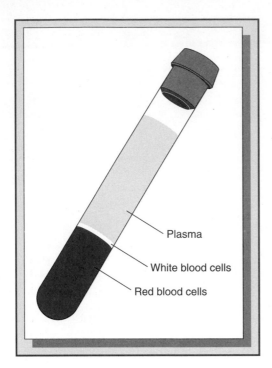

FIGURE 2–11. When centrifuged, normal blood separates into plasma (60%), red blood cells (40%), and white blood cells (<0.1%). The red cell component is known as the hematocrit or packed cell volume.

perficial epithelial tissues, especially skin, eyes, hair, mucous membranes, teeth, and tongue. Attention is given to loss of fat and muscle, but these changes can be quantified by anthropometry using the triceps fatfold and upper arm muscle area.

Clinical assessment is the most subjective of the nutrition assessment measures. Interpretation of clinical data depends on examiner experience and bias. Bias can be minimized by standardizing the criteria used to define physical signs and by training examiners. Interpretation is also complicated because deficiencies of several nutrients often occur simultaneously and clinical symptoms may reflect a lack of more than one nutrient. Critical physical signs and symptoms of malnutrition are nonspecific, and, therefore, must be interpreted in conjunction with laboratory, anthropometric, and dietary data before specific nutrient deficiencies can be identified. The physical signs of malnutrition are summarized in Table 2–7.

DIETARY INTAKE

■ Describe the techniques that can be used to estimate current or typical dietary intake.

■ How is information regarding dietary intake interpreted and used?

■ What are its limitations?

Knowledge about energy and nutrient intake is important in making an accurate nutrition assessment. As illustrated in the earlier description of the development of a thiamin deficiency, knowing how much of a nutrient the subject has eaten can contribute to identifying the potential for a deficiency. In advanced stages of deficiency, knowing the person's dietary intake can suggest or confirm the cause of biochemical abnormalities or physical changes. It also serves as a base for planning nutrition care, counseling, and education. Assessing the adequacy of energy and nutrient levels involves careful and complete collection of dietary intake data and an evaluation of the nutrient content using food group systems or tables of food composition or computerized nutrient analysis programs.

Collecting Dietary Information

Information about food intake of groups or individuals can be obtained using one of several basic methods (Block, 1994; Medlin, 1988; Morgan, 1987). Selection of an appropriate technique is guided by the purpose of the assessment and available resources, including time, personnel, and funds. Information may be confirmed or expanded using more than one tool or combination of tools. All methods are limited by the individual's willingness and ability to report food intake honestly and completely. Commonly used dietary evaluation techniques are described here. (The use of some of these techniques in nutrition counseling is discussed in Chapter 3.)

DIETARY HISTORY Information about a person's food habits may be obtained from a comprehensive interview conducted by a dietitian. Information gathered in the diet or nutrition history includes not only the types and amounts of foods typically consumed but also patterns of intake, use of supplements and alcohol, and relevant information about personal, psychosocial, and economic factors that influence food intake. Although the dietary interview is time-consuming and requires a skilled professional to obtain accurate information, it provides information about usual intake patterns that is essential in planning dietary changes. The process can be expedited by having the client complete a food frequency questionnaire or 24-hour dietary recall in advance of the personal interview.

TWENTY-FOUR HOUR RECALL The 24-hour dietary recall is more rapid and less expensive than the diet history. Clients are asked to recall the specific foods and amounts they have consumed during the previous 24-hour period. Forms or questions may be structured to obtain a complete description of intake. Photographs, food models, and measuring utensils can help the client judge the amounts of foods consumed. This method is not suitable for individuals who have difficulty remembering or estimating portion sizes.

TABLE 2–7 Clinical Signs Associated with Malnutrition

Body System/Normal Appearance	Clinical Finding	Possible Deficiency
HAIR Shiny; firm in the scalp	Lack of natural shine; dull and dry; sparse; loss of color; pluckable	Protein-energy malnutrition (PEM)
FACE Skin color uniform; smooth, healthy appearance	Pallor; dark skin over cheeks and under eyes; flakiness of skin of nose and mouth; swollen face; enlarged parotid glands; flaky dermatitis	PEM, vitamin A, vitamin B_{12}, iron folate
EYES Bright, clear, shiny; no sores at corners; membrane pink and moist.	Membranes pale; night blindness; Bitot's spots (dull, dry lesions on conjunctiva); redness and fissuring of eyelid corners; dryness of eye membranes; cornea is dull and soft	Iron, vitamin A, riboflavin, vitamin B_6
LIPS Smooth, not chapped or swollen	Swelling of mouth or lips; lesions at corners of the mouth (cheilosis)	Niacin, riboflavin, protein, vitamin B_6, iron
TONGUE Deep reddish in appearance; surface papillae present	Swelling; scarlet and raw; purplish color; smooth; swollen sores	Vitamin B_6, niacin, iron, vitamin B_{12}, folate, riboflavin
TEETH No cavities; no pain	Missing teeth; gray or black spots (fluorosis); decay; unfilled cavities	Fluoride, poor dietary habits, poor oral hygiene (excess fluoride)
GUMS Healthy, red; do not bleed; not swollen	"Spongy," pale, bleed easily; receding	Vitamin C
SKIN Smooth, firm; no rashes or spots	Dry, rough (xerosis); flakiness; sores; red swollen pigmentation of light-exposed areas; black and blue marks due to skin bleeding; scaling	Essential fatty acid, vitamin A, protein, vitamin C, vitamin K., niacin
NAILS Firm, pink	Nails are spoon-shaped (koilonychia); brittle, ridged	Iron
GLANDS Face and neck not swollen	Thyroid enlargement; parotid enlargement	Iodine, PEM, bulimia
MUSCLE Good muscle tone and posture	Muscle wasting; pain; weakness; twitching; cramps	Potassium, sodium PEM, vitamin B_6, magnesium, thiamin
BONES AND JOINTS Bone development appropriate for age	Epiphyseal thickening; deformities; bone pain	Calcium, vitamin D, vitamin C
CARDIOVASCULAR Normal heart rate and rhythms, normal blood pressure for age	Rapid heart rate, enlarged heart; abnormal rhythm	PEM, potassium, thiamin, magnesium
GASTROINTESTINAL No palpable organs; normal digestion	Liver enlarged; enlargement of spleen; abnormal digestion; wasting	PEM, iron, niacin
NERVOUS Psychologically stable; normal reflexes	Mental irritability, disorientation; burning and tingling of hands and feet; loss of position and vibratory sense; weakness and tenderness of muscles; loss of ankle and knee reflexes	Thiamin, vitamin B_6, vitamin B_{12}, niacin

Adapted from Walker WW, Hendricks KM. Manual of Pediatric Nutrition. Philadelphia: WB Saunders, 1985.

FOOD RECORDS Carefully completed food records provide sufficiently detailed information for an analysis of energy and nutrient intake. The client is instructed in how to measure and record the food items he or she has eaten. Food records are usually kept for 2 to 7 days. The number of days needed to provide reliable information for nutrient analysis varies with the nutrient studied, but a minimum appears to be 3 days (Schlundt, 1988; Basiotis et al, 1987).

FOOD FREQUENCY QUESTIONNAIRE The food frequency questionnaire can provide information about an individual's food intake over a specified length of time. It consists of a list of foods and a scale indicating the frequency of consumption of that food over a given period of time such as a week or month. An abbreviated food frequency checklist is given in Appendix 3E. A food frequency report is particularly useful when specific food items or groups that provide the nutrient of interest, such as fat, calcium, or vitamin A, can be identified (Briefel et al, 1992). The food frequency questionnaire has been used extensively in epidemiologic surveys to investigate potential relationships between specific nutrients and disease incidence or risk (Roidt et al, 1988).

Interpretation of Dietary Information

Data obtained using the dietary methods described can be very useful in assessing nutrition status and planning nutrition care. The information they provide about food intake can be interpreted using several guides or standards, including food groups, the Dietary Guidelines, or dietary standards such as the RDA. A quick, general evaluation of food intake data can be made by comparing the foods and number of servings to a food group plan. Several food group plans are available. The simplest and most frequently used system is the five groups of the food guide pyramid (Table 2–8). A comparison of dietary intake to recommended amounts in food groups can identify potential inadequacies of protein, iron, calcium, riboflavin, and vitamins A and C but is limited in estimating energy and other nutrients.

A similarly rapid evaluation using the exchange system allows the practitioner to estimate energy, protein, fat, and carbohydrate intake as well as some of the same vitamins and minerals as the Food Guide Pyramid. The exchange system, originally developed for diet planning for individuals with diabetes, has been used extensively for diets that require controlled intake of kilocalories or macronutrients. Comparison of food intake with the Dietary Guidelines can identify dietary inadequacies or excesses that may contribute to decreased or increased risk of certain chronic diseases.

Assuming the information provided regarding dietary intake is complete and accurate, a more precise evaluation can be made by determining the quantities of nutrients in the food consumed. Energy and nutrient levels can be calculated using tables of food composition. Calculations may be done by hand, but over the past few years computerized nutrient analysis programs have become widely used. (A sample printout of a nutrient analysis appears in Application 2 at the end of this chapter.) The traditional source of nutrient data is Agriculture Handbook No. 8, the United States Department of Agriculture's (USDA) standard reference publication. Additional data may be obtained from universities, food manufacturers, and independent laboratories. A well-maintained nutrient data base includes all available data and is updated as new information becomes available. Calculations of nutrients from dietary intake data can give a reasonable approximation of actual intake based on analyzed values.

STANDARDS FOR EVALUATION OF NUTRIENT INTAKE One of the stated purposes for the Recommended Dietary Allowances (RDA) is assessing the nutritional adequacy of diets consumed by specific population groups. Use of this standard is complicated by the fact that many RDAs are based on the average requirement (the level of intake below which a deficiency would occur) plus a margin of sufficiency or a safety factor. Therefore, diets below the RDA are not necessarily "deficient." A number of large population studies have used levels below 70%, or two-thirds, of the RDA to designate inadequate intakes. The RDAs are not designed to assess the intakes of individuals but, because there is no other standard that permits comparison, they are often used to do so. Such a comparison must be interpreted with discretion. It is important to recognize that intake levels below the RDA or even below 70% of the RDA are not automatic indicators of nutrient deficiency. At best, they are suggestive of nutritional risk, the extent of which can be evaluated only by biochemical and clinical assessment. In addition the RDAs are formulated for most healthy individuals and may not be appropriate in stress, disease, or illness.

The RDAs for energy and protein are based on body size. In assessment of dietary intakes, energy and protein adequacy should be evaluated on the basis of actual body weight, if it is within acceptable limits, or reference weight. This is particularly important for both over- and underweight adults and for children, who, at any particular age, may vary widely in size and in energy and protein needs.

NUTRITION ASSESSMENT ACROSS THE LIFE SPAN

Throughout this chapter nutrition screening and assessment have been discussed in relation to adult needs. Standards for comparison are based on adult populations, and the same techniques and principles are applied across the

TABLE 2–8 Food Group Evaluation Chart Using Food Guide Pyramid

Food Consumed (Mixed foods will count in more than 1 group)	Food Group				
	Milk	Meat	Vegetables	Fruit	Grains
Total servings					
Minimum recommended servings	2	2	3	2	6
Assessment:					

life span. Their application in growth and development, reproduction, and aging are discussed in individual chapters, along with age and gender-specific standards for evaluation.

Nutrition screening and assessment are important in formulating and providing nutrition guidance and care to all age groups, from infancy to old age. Each stage presents unique physiologic demands and social and psychological factors, as well as health concerns, that impact on nutrition status. Some general characteristics of various stages of the life span and the measurements recommended for nutrition screening appear in Table 2–9. The goal of nutrition screening is to identify individuals who will benefit from nutrition assessment and intervention.

TABLE 2–9 Appropriate Measurements for Nutrition Screening Across the Life Span

Stage	Characteristics	Anthropometry	Biochemical	Clinical	Dietary
Infancy	Birth weight, rapid growth and development	Weight/length, head circumference	Hemoglobin, hematocrit	Color; response to stimuli; overall growth rate	Bottle or breast-feeding, supplemental feedings; sources of iron, fluoride, vitamin D
Childhood	Slow, steady growth; increased physical activity; development of food habits; increased social interaction; skill development	Weight/height, arm circumference fatfolds	Hemoglobin, hematocrit	Skin color, texture, musculature; subcutaneous fat; oral cavity; overall growth rate	Food intake, appetite, feeding/snacking patterns, food jags, pica; food/nutrient supplements
Adolescence	Rapid growth and development, sexual maturation; increasing independence	Weight/height, changes in body composition, fatfolds	Hemoglobin, hematocrit	General appearance: hair, skin, eyes, musculature, body fat/patterns; oral cavity; secondary sex characteristics	Food intake, where and with whom; fad diets; snacking; nutrient supplements; substance use/abuse
Pregnancy	Weight gain/fetal growth and development; maternal physiologic changes	Prepregnancy weight, gestational weight gain	Hemoglobin, hematocrit, glucose tolerance test, protein in urine	General appearance; blood pressure; pattern of weight gain; edema	Appetite, food intake, pica, iron/folate intake; nausea, vomiting, heartburn, constipation; smoking, alcohol intake
Lactation	Milk production; maternal–infant bonding, weight loss, changes in body composition	Gestational weight gain, postpartum weight loss, current weight status	Hemoglobin, hematocrit	Appearance, hair, skin, eyes, muscle tone; weight changes	Energy and nutrient intake; breast-feeding/supplemental feedings; feeding difficulties
Adult	Stable weight or weight gain; decreased physical activity; increased risk for chronic disease; tendency to increase body fat	Weight for height; recent weight changes; fatfolds, abdominal/gluteal circumference ratio	Hemoglobin, hematocrit, blood glucose, blood lipid levels	General appearance, hair, skin, and eyes; blood pressure; dental health; weight history	Food intake, especially fat, saturated fat, and sugar, fiber, calcium; snacking habits; nutrient supplements; alcohol intake; dieting patterns
Older Adults	Tendency to lose muscle mass, increase body fat; age-related physical changes; concerns about income/health care costs; increased incidence of chronic diseases and medication use	Weight for height, recent weight change, fatfolds	Hemoglobin, hematocrit, blood glucose, blood lipid levels	Skin color, pallor; dentition; blood pressure; physical changes	Food intake and patterns; nutrient supplements; ability to purchase/prepare food; changes in food habits; dietary restrictions

Adapted from Davis J, Sherer K. Applied nutrition and diet therapy for nurses, 2nd ed. Philadelphia: WB Saunders, 1994.

CONCEPTS TO REMEMBER

▶ Nutrition assessment is a process or series of measurements used to identify individuals at nutritional risk.

▶ Nutrition assessment, the first step in the nutrition care process, forms the basis for planning and implementing nutrition care, counseling and education, and evaluating the effectiveness of intervention.

▶ Measurements selected for nutrition assessment must reflect body status and must be readily available at a cost that allows them to be repeated for monitoring the impact of intervention.

▶ Data used for nutrition assessment are based on anthropometric and biochemical measurements, clinical evaluation, and assessment of dietary intake and food patterns.

▶ Most individuals who are at nutritional risk have compromised energy and protein status. Nutrition assessment focuses on determination of the adequacy of energy and somatic and visceral protein status but can be expanded to include other vitamins and minerals, especially iron.

▶ The goal of nutrition screening is to identify individuals who may benefit from assessment and intervention.

References

American Dietetic Association. ADA's definitions for nutrition screening and nutrition assessment. J Am Diet Assoc 1994;94:838.

Basiotis PP, et al. Number of days of food intake records required to estimate individual and group nutrient intakes with defined confidence. J Nutr 1987;117:1138.

Blackburn GL, et al. Nutritional and metabolic assessment of the hospitalized patient. JEPN 1977;1:11.

Block G, et al. Validation study of two food frequency questionnaires with WIC women and children. Am J Publ Health 1994;84:53.

Briefel RR, et al. Assessing the nation's diet: limitations of the food frequency questionnaire. J Am Diet Assoc 1992;92:959.

Durnin JVGA, Womersley J. Body fat assessed from total body density and its estimation from skinfold thickness: measurements on 481 men and women aged from 16 to 72 years. Br J Nutr 1974;32:77.

Frisancho AR, Flegel PN. Elbow breadth as a measure of frame size for U.S. males and females. Am J Clin Nutr 1983;37:311.

Frisancho AR. Anthropometric standards for the assessment of growth and nutritional status. Ann Arbor: University of Michigan Press, 1990.

Gray DS, et al. Skinfold thickness measurements in obese subjects. Am J Clin Nutr 1990;51:571.

Herrman FR, et al. Serum albumin level on admission as a predictor of death, length of stay and readmission. Arch Intern Med 1992;152:125.

Heymsfield SB, et al. Anthropometric measurement of muscle mass: revised equations for calculating bone-free arm muscle area. Am J Clin Nutr 1982;36:680.

Himes JH, Bouchard C. Do the new Metropolitan Life Insurance weight–height tables correctly assess body from and body fat relationships? Am J Public Health 1985;75:1067.

Jackson AS, Pollock MI. Practical assessment of body composition. Physician Sportsmed 1985;13:76.

Kannel WB, et al. Regional obesity and risk of cardiovascular disease: the Framingham study. J Clin Epidemiol 1991;44:183.

Keshaviah PR, et al. Lean body mass estimation by creatinine kinetics. J Am Soc Nephrol 1994;4:1475.

Lohman TG, et al. Anthropometric standardization reference manual. Champaign, IL: Human Kinetics Books, 1988.

Medlin C, Skinner JD. Individual dietary intake methodology: a 50-year review of progress. J Am Diet Assoc 1988;88:1250.

Metropolitan Height and Weight Tables. Statistical Bulletin of the Metropolitan Life Insurance Company 1983;64 (Jan–Jun):3.

Micozzi MS, et al. Correlations of body mass indices with weight, stature, and body composition in men and women in NHANES I and II. Am J Clin Nutr 1986;44:725.

Mitchell MC. Frame size in older adults: a comparison of four measurements. J Am Diet Assoc 1993;93:53.

Morgan KJ, et al. Collection of food intake data: an evaluation of methods. J Am Diet Assoc 1987;87:888.

Revicki DA, Israel RG. Relationship between body mass indices and measures of body adiposity. Am J Clin Nutr 1986;76:992.

Roidt L, et al. Association of food frequency questionnaire estimates of vitamin A intake with serum vitamin A levels. Am J Epidemiol 1988;128:645.

Schapira DV, et al. Upper-body fat distribution and endometrial cancer risk. JAMA 1991;266:1808.

Schlundt DG. Accuracy and reliability of nutrient intake estimates. J Nutr 1988;118:1432.

Smalley KJ, et al. Reassessment of body mass indices. Am J Clin Nutr 1990;52:405.

Spiekerman AM. Proteins used in nutritional assessment. Clin Lab Med 1993;13:353.

Young VR, et al. Assessment of protein nutritional status. J Nutr 1990; 120:1469.

Additional Resources

Gibson RS. Principles of Nutritional Assessment. New York: Oxford University Press, 1990.

Lee RD, Nieman DC. Nutritional Assessment. St. Louis: Mosby, 1996.

Simko MD et al. Nutrition Assessment. A Comprehensive Guide for Planning Intervention. 2nd ed. Gaithersburg MD: Aspen Publishers Inc, 1995.

APPLICATION: A Case for Nutrition Assessment

Information from anthropometric, biochemical, clinical, and dietary measurements or observations described in this chapter can be used to develop a profile of the nutritional status of an individual. This application is designed to demonstrate:

- The use of anthropometric, biochemical, clinical, and dietary information to evaluate the nutritional status of an individual
- The use of the nutritional assessment, as a basis for recommendations to improve nutritional status.

The Case

Katherine is a 22-year-old graduate student who was admitted to the hospital following a skiing accident. She was alert and in some pain, but her only obvious injury was a broken ankle. Her ankle was placed in a cast and she was given some medication for pain prior to discharge. Because of her general appearance and low body weight, an appointment was made for a nutritional evaluation in the outpatient clinic the following week. She was told not to eat before coming to the appointment and was instructed to bring a 24-hour urine sample.

When Katherine arrived in the clinic, a blood sample was drawn and sent to the laboratory for analyses, she was weighed and measured, a physician completed a physical examination, and the dietitian conducted a dietary interview.

A summary of the anthropometric and laboratory data recorded in her clinic medical record appears in the margin.

Clinical Evaluation

Katherine's medical history revealed that she had a broken arm at age 10, and an appendectomy at age 15. Her mother has diabetes mellitus. A summary of Katherine's physical examination follows: Patient appears to be pale, underweight with limited musculature and fat. Her hair is dull and skin dry, scaling and rough. All other parameters appear to be normal.

Dietary Intake

The dietary history completed by the dietitian revealed the following facts. Katherine lives with a roommate in a small apartment off campus. Her basic income is a monthly stipend as a graduate teaching associate, but she earns a small amount tutoring parttime. She maintains that she doesn't have enough money to purchase an adequate diet and that she is too busy to eat. She does not like to cook and is not particularly interested in food. A typical weekday intake, which is usually obtained from a cafeteria on campus or a nearby fast-food restaurant, appears in the margin.

Weekends are different in that Katherine sleeps in and does not eat until noon. Lunch often is a sandwich, as indicated, or a very late breakfast with sausage, eggs, and toast or bacon and waffles. She denies consuming alcoholic beverages and takes no medication except an occasional aspirin. She denies taking any vitamin or mineral supplements. Her food preferences are for sandwiches with mustard only—no lettuce or tomato. She will eat green salads but does not drink milk and maintains that she cannot afford fruit or fruit juices.

Assessment

Because the results from laboratory data are not usually available immediately, assessment, planning, and intervention counseling are likely to involve two or more sessions. A counseling session in which the dietitian uses dietary information and other assessment data as the bases for planning and implementing intervention is illustrated in Application 3. In this application, the anthropometric, biochemical, clinical, and dietary

---

Anthropometry:
Height: 168 cm (5'6")
Weight 47.7 kg (105 lb)
(weight 6 months ago was 59.1 kg)
Mid-arm circumference: 21.2 cm
Triceps fatfold: 10.5 mm (1.05 cm)
Subscapular fatfold 7.4 mm (.59 cm)
Elbow breadth: 69.9 mm (2¾ in)]
Biochemical (Laboratory Findings):
Hemoglobin: 100 g/L
Hematocrit: .32 or 32%
Serum albumin: 2.2 g/dL
Serum transferrin: 155 mg/dL
Urinary creatinine 725 mg/24 hr
White blood cells 4000 mm^3
Differential: lymphocytes 25%

---

7 a.m.: Black coffee
10 a.m.: Black coffee, donut or muffin
Noon: Sandwich (ham or hamburger)
French fries or potato chips
Diet cola or iced tea
Afternoon: coffee
6 p.m.: Mixed green salad of lettuce, spinach, and endive—2 cups
1 oz cheese, 1 hard-cooked egg
Low-calorie, low-fat dressing
6–8 saltine crackers or a roll
No margarine or butter
11 p.m.: Several diet colas

information obtained from Katherine are used to evaluate energy, visceral, and somatic protein status as well as to consider vitamin and mineral status.

A reminder: The following information is available related to the compartments to be studied:

Energy reserves: indirectly, weight for height, fatfolds

Visceral protein: serum albumin, serum, transferrin, total lymphocyte count

Somatic protein: mid-arm circumference with TFF to estimate mid-arm muscle circumference and mid-arm muscle area, urinary creatinine

Iron status: serum transferrin, hemoglobin, hematocrit

Confirming and supporting information provided by dietary intake data and clinical signs

Body Energy Reserves

Body energy reserves can be assessed indirectly using body weight or weight for height, in this case, percent of usual body weight Metropolitan Relative Weight or body mass index. To use the Metropolitan Height–Weight Table (inside the back cover), frame size must be determined. An elbow breadth of 69.6 mm (2¾ in) indicates a "large" frame size. For a woman of large frame size who is 168 cm (5′6″ or 5′7″ with the 1-inch heels assumed in the chart), a reference weight range is 133–147 lb. Using the midpoint of that range, the MRW would be calculated.

Calculation of the BMI reveals that Katherine would be categorized as underweight.

% Usual Body Weight = current weight/ previous weight = 105/130 lb = **81%** of usual weight—6 months ago

$$MRW = 105/140 = 75 \text{ or } 75\%$$

$$BMI = \frac{47.7}{1.68^2} = 16.9$$

FATFOLDS

Body fat reserves can be assessed by comparing Katherine's fatfold values to those from a reference population. Consulting Appendices 3A and 3B reveals that Katherine's **TFF** of 10.5 mm is equal to the 5th percentile value. Her subscapular fatfold (**SSFF**) is 7.4, which is below the 10th percentile value of 6.5 mm.

ENERGY INTAKE

A typical daily intake determined from Katherine's dietary history can be used to estimate caloric intake. The dietitian's quick estimation was that Katherine's energy intake ranged from 1000 to 1400 kcal. For their next session she will have a printout of the computerized diet analysis to share with Katherine. The computer printout reveals that for a typical day, Katherine consumed 1008 kcal, a level well below the RDA (Table A2–1).

Somatic Protein

Katherine excreted 725 mg of creatinine in a 24-hour period. Table 2–4 reveals that the reference level for a female of Katherine's height and frame size is 1,190 mg. From this the **creatinine height index** can be calculated.

Katherine's midarm circumference (21.2) and TFF (1.05 cm) are used to determine **midarm muscle circumference.** A comparison of 17.9 cm to reference values from NHANES data given in Appendix 3C reveals that her value is equal to the 5th percentile for her age and gender.

Midarm muscle area is calculated from the midarm circumference and the triceps fatfold. The calculations using Katherine's measurements are found in the margin. Comparison of this value with Appendix 3D reveals that Katherine's MAMA is well below the 5th percentile level, suggesting low somatic protein status.

Creatinine height index = actual creatinine/reference value $\times$ 100

CHI = 725/1190 = **60.9%**

MAMC–MAC–($\pi \times$ TFF)

MAMC = 17.9 cm

$$\begin{aligned} \textbf{MAMA} &= 21.2 - [1.05 \times 3.14]^2/12.56 \\ &= [21.2 - 3.297]^2/12.56 \\ &= 285.6/12.56 - 6.5 \\ &= \textbf{19.0 cm}^2 \end{aligned}$$

Visceral Protein

Comparison of Katherine's levels of 22 g/L for **serum albumin,** and 1.55 g/L for **serum transferrin** to values shown in Table 2–5 indicates levels below the normal range, suggesting moderate depletion of visceral protein. Another indicator, the **total lympho-**

TABLE A2-I **Computerized Summary of Calories and Nutrients in a Typical Diet for Katherine**

Analysis: Katherine	Female Height: 66 in		Age: 22 Weight: 105 lb		

Nutrient		%RDA	Nutrient		%RDA
Calories	1008	56%	Folate	196 mcg	109%
Protein	37.2 g	98%	Pantothenic	2.14 mg	31%
Carbohydrates	113 g	43%	Vitamin C	20.8 mg	35%
Fat: Total	46.3 g	77%	Vitamin D	.927 mcg	9%
Saturated Fat	16.1 g	80%	Vit E-Alpha E	3.91 mg	49%
Mono Fat	14 g	70%	Calcium	488 mg	41%
Poly Fat	12.3 g	61%	Copper	.536 mg	21%
Omega 3 FA	.969 g	—	Iron	8.06 mg	54%
Omega 6 FA	11.3 g	—	Magnesium	154 mg	55%
Cholesterol	306 mg	102%	Manganese	2.09 mg	60%
Dietary Fiber	5.54 g	31%	Phosphorus	723 mg	60%
Total Vit A	453 RE	57%	Potassium	1971 mg	99%
A-Retinol	184 RE	—	Selenium	55.9 mcg	102%
A-Carotenoid	269 RE	—	Sodium	2201 mg	92%
Thiamin-B1	.725 mg	80%	Zinc	4.98 mg	42%
Riboflavin-B2	1.04 mg	95%	Complex Carbs	79 g	—
Niacin-B3	11.5 mg	96%	Sugars	28.7 g	—
Niacin Equiv.	11.5 mg	96%	Alcohol	0 g	—
Vitamin B6	.463 mg	29%	Caffeine	604 mg	—
Vitamin B12	1.69 mcg	84%	Water	2936 g	—

TLC = WBC × % lymphocytes/100
4000 × 25/100 = 1000

cyte count (TLC), can be determined from the total white cell count and the percentage of lymphocytes. According to Table 2–5, such a level is below normal values, suggesting malnutrition. Katherine's typical daily intake of protein is near or only slightly below the RDA.

Vitamin and Mineral Status

Katherine's levels of **hemoglobin** (100 g/L) and **hematocrit** (32%) are in the deficient range. While she does consume beef or pork and an egg on a regular basis, as well as some dark green leafy vegetables, the actual amount of iron consumed in the absence of other dietary sources is low. Evaluation of the dietary intake in comparison to the **Food Guide Pyramid** (see Table 2–8) reveals other potential low intakes of nutrients such as calcium, riboflavin and zinc, which may not be apparent in the other assessment parameters. The printout from a computerized diet program shows the comparison of Katherine's nutrient intake to the RDA (Table A2–2).

Clinical Evaluation

The clinical signs observed for Katherine must be interpreted with caution because they are subjective and also can indicate a number of situations or conditions other than malnutrition. In this case, pallor is consistent with iron deficiency anemia, and the general condition of the hair and skin indicates a possibility of inadequate protein intake as well as deficiencies of other nutrients.

Summary of Nutrition Assessment

The following might represent a summary of the calculation and data that can be used for nutritional assessment in this case. It should be pointed out that, in order to explore many kinds of data, several tests or measurements have been reported for each body compartment in this case. In an actual situation, it is unlikely that all of this information would be available for one individual.

A summary statement might be fashioned as follows:

Katherine appears to be at nutrition risk. Her energy reserves are compromised, as evidenced by a loss of body weight of almost 20% in the last 6 months and an MRW of 75. The triceps and subscapular fatfold values are below the 10th percentile. The dietary history confirms a low energy intake. A persistent intake at this level would be a major contributor to continued weight loss.

Measures of somatic protein status suggest low reserves. The MAC (20.2 cm) is below the 5th percentile and MAMA (22.7 cm^2) below the 15th percentile. The creatinine height index is 61% of the reference value, suggesting depletion of somatic protein. Visceral protein levels of serum albumin (22 g/L or 2.2 g/dL), serum transferrin (1.55 mg/L or 155 mg/dL), and TLC (1000) are below normal values and suggest moderate deficit.

TABLE A2–2 Graphic Comparison of Dietary Intake to the RDA from a Typical Diet for Katherine

NUTRIENT	VALUES	Goal%	|------- 25 ------- 50 ------- 75 ------- 100 -------- >
Calories	1008	56%	###############
Protein	37.2 g	98%	#############################
Carbohydrates	113 g	43%	###########
Fat Total	46.3 g	77%	#####################
Saturated Fat	16.1 g	80%	########################
Mono Fat	14 g	70%	###################
Poly Fat	12.3 g	61%	#################
Omega 3 FA	.969 g	—	
Omega 6 FA	11.3 g	—	
Cholesterol	306 mg	102%	##############################
Dietary Fiber	5.54 g	31%	#########
Total Vit A	453 RE	57%	#################
A–Retinol	184 RE	—	
A–Carotenoid	269 RE	—	
Thiamin-B1	.725 mg	80%	#######################
Riboflavin-B2	1.04 mg	95%	###########################
Niacin-B3	11.5 mg	96%	############################
Niacin Equiv.	11.5 mg	96%	############################
Vitamin B6	.463 mg	29%	##########
Vitamin B12	1.69 mcg	84%	########################
Folate	196 mcg	109%	############################# ###
Pantothenic	2.14 mg	31%	#########
Vitamin C	20.8 mg	35%	###########
Vitamin D	.927 mcg	9%	####
Vit E-Alpha E	3.91 mg	49%	#############
Calcium	488 mg	41%	###########
Copper	.536 mg	21%	######
Iron	8.06 mg	54%	##############
Magnesium	154 mg	55%	##############
Manganese	2.09 mg	60%	###############
Phosphorus	723 mg	60%	###############
Potassium	1971 mg	99%	#############################
Selenium	55.9 mcg	102%	#############################
Sodium	2201 mg	92%	###########################
Zinc	4.98 mg	42%	###########
Complex Carbs	79 g	—	
Sugars	28.7 g	—	
Alcohol	0 g	—	
Caffeine	604 mg	—	
Water	2936 g	—	

The dietary history suggests that daily protein intake is near or only slightly below the RDA. However, that level would not be sufficient to meet the needs of an individual who is in negative energy balance and who continues to lose weight. Therefore, it would be reasonable to assume that protein intake is inadequate relative to her current need. Hemoglobin and hematocrit levels (100 g/L or 10 g/dL and 32% respectively) are indicative of iron deficiency. This is supported by dietary intakes below the RDA. Intake levels of several other nutrients, including calcium, riboflavin, and zinc, are below the RDA.

Nutrition Care Plan

Katherine needs to improve her dietary intake to avoid progressive malnutrition. There is no question that nutrition intervention is appropriate. She needs to increase her total food consumption to provide sufficient kilocalories to prevent continued weight loss and nutrient deficiencies. Her increased intake should include 2 servings of dairy products, 3 to 4 servings of whole grain breads and cereals, 3 to 4 servings of fruits and vegetables, and one serving of lean meat, fish, poultry, or meat alternative per day.

If other causes of iron deficiency are ruled out, Katherine needs a supplement of ferrous iron until her hemoglobin and hematocrit levels return to normal values.

Implementation

If Katherine were admitted to the hospital, part of the nutrition care plan would be to provide a balanced diet and encourage its consumption. Since the assessment occurred in an outpatient setting, the nutrition care plan will concentrate on recommendations for dietary improvement using nutrition education and counseling. Nutrition counseling for Katherine will be the focus of Application 3 at the end of the next chapter.

Evaluation

The effectiveness of the nutrition care and counseling of Katherine will be evaluated in two ways. First, the effectiveness of the counseling will be judged on the changes she makes in her dietary intake. These, in turn, should be reflected in improvement in the nutritional assessment parameters measured in the initial assessment, i.e. anthropometry and biochemical indices.

Documentation

A summary of the assessment of Katherine's nutritional status and the nutrition care plan will be recorded in her chart in the clinic. When she returns for follow-up visits, her progress will be evaluated and documented in the medical record.

CHAPTER 3

PROMOTING DIETARY CHANGE: NUTRITION COUNSELING

Nutrition needs and dietary patterns change across the life span. An individual's relationship with food changes and evolves throughout the processes of growth and development, maturation, reproduction, and aging. The infant is totally dependent on his parents for a consistent source of nutrients and a positive feeding relationship. Parents also guide their children through new experiences with food and, hopefully, assist them in making healthy food choices. Adolescence is characterized by greater independence in food choices and development of dietary and health behaviors that may last a lifetime. The increased energy and nutrient needs of pregnancy and lactation require judicious dietary changes to support fetal and maternal growth and milk production. With maturation and aging, changes in food behaviors may be required to meet nutritional needs, promote optimum health, or adapt to changes required for specific nutrition-related problems.

Individuals of all ages often require assistance to establish or modified dietary habits. Nutrition counseling is an important tool to support individuals and families in the process of changing food behaviors to optimize health. The purpose of this chapter is not to teach the student to be a nutrition counselor but to offer an overview of fundamental approaches to assist individuals in changing food-related behaviors.

THE CHALLENGES OF NUTRITION COUNSELING

■ Who does nutrition counseling?

■ What are the general characteristics of nutrition counseling?

■ What are the unique challenges to the nutrition counselor and dietitian?

Nearly every health care professional has the opportunity to interact with individuals at various stages of the life span and to influence their food choices. For example, a

pharmacist may offer tips on healthy eating as she answers an individual's questions about the proper way to take a medication. A nurse may provide some nutrition guidance while teaching a newly diagnosed diabetic how to administer insulin or while providing care to a home-bound client. However, as shown in Figure 3–1, nutrition counseling is a client-centered, ongoing process that involves assessment, intervention, and communication (Monk et al, 1995). It bridges the gap between the science of nutrition and the art of helping others. Most frequently the nutrition counselor is a Registered Dietitian (R.D.) (Table 3–1).

Nutrition counseling is an integral part of the Nutrition Care Process discussed in Chapter 2. Several things must exist for effective nutrition counseling. There is a relation-

Contributed by Martha Orabella.

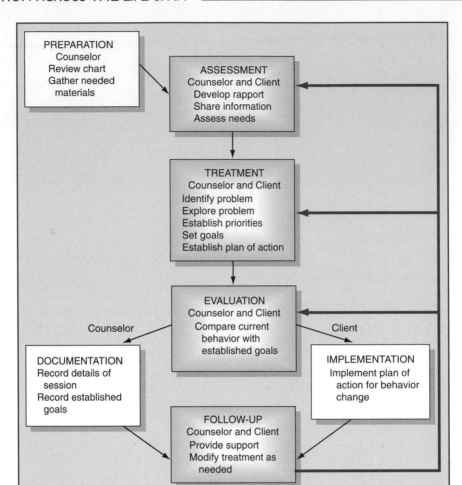

FIGURE 3–1. Components of nutrition counseling intervention.

TABLE 3–1 Definition of the Registered Dietitian by the Commission on Dietitic Registration

The Registered Dietitian is an individual who:

Has completed the minimum of a baccalaureate degree granted by a U.S. regionally accredited college or university

Has met current minimum academic requirements (Didactic Program in Dietetics) as approved by The American Dietetic Association

Has completed a preprofessional experience accredited/approved by The American Dietetic Association

Has successfully completed the Registration Examination for Dietitians

Has accrued 75 hours of approved continuing education every 5 years.

From The American Dietetic Association, Chicago, IL: 1994.

ship between the counselor and the client in which the nutrition counselor acts as the teacher or helper as well as the facilitator or negotiator. The client is the learner or help seeker, who actively participates in the counseling process. The counselor and clients work together in a process that focuses on **self-management training** for the client.

Making a change in eating behaviors provides a unique challenge to the client and the nutrition counselor. Obviously, everyone needs to eat. Unlike starting a new exercise program in which something new is added to a person's routine, changes in eating behavior must be built upon existing food habits. Food habits are influenced by a multitude of factors, including culture, religion, education, socioeconomic status, and physical and mental abilities. The nutrition counselor's challenge is to understand these influences and to assist the client in adapting his diet to meet the needs in the world in which he lives.

Successful nutrition counseling is based on a two-way

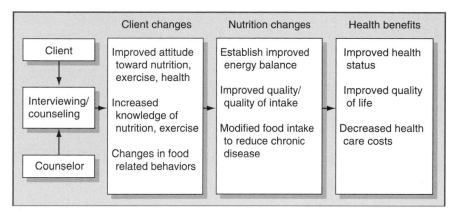

FIGURE 3–2. The relationship of nutrition counseling to improved health benefits and costs.

exchange of information. All activities are based on the client's condition and information provided by the client. The counselor provides information but, more importantly, he or she helps the client in problem solving to effect change in usual behavior and to anticipate or prepare for special occasions and times of stress when compliance becomes more difficult (Hodges and Vickery, 1989). Nutrition counseling is of great importance to overall health and well-being. Successful dietary changes that improve the quality of the diet reap benefits in improved health status, control of disease or medical conditions, a reduction in the cost of health care, and an improved quality of life (Fig. 3–2) (Danish, 1986).

SETTINGS FOR NUTRITION COUNSELING

■ What are the settings in which nutrition counseling occurs?

■ What are the differences between inpatient and outpatient counseling in terms of needs of the patient/client and expected outcomes?

Counseling in the Hospital

The length of most hospital stays has been reduced significantly in recent years. Most hospitalized patients are acutely ill. Such circumstances make it impossible to provide adequate information or develop the skills needed by patients for lasting changes in dietary intake. Therefore, the nutrition counselor in a hospital setting focuses on "survival skills"—those basic principles the patient and his family must know to avoid further problems after discharge. Survival skills may include, but are not limited to, basic types of foods to chose, the timing of meals, and portion sizes. Such information is designed to allow the patient to function until follow-up counseling can be initiated.

Community-Based Counseling

Recent changes in health care have resulted in growing emphasis on the provision of health care outside the hospital environment. Nutrition counseling can be very successful in community-based settings. Usually, the client's medical condition is more stable and she is better able to focus on making changes needed to meet nutrition needs. The emphasis of nutrition counseling is client self-management. The framework for self-management is best established in a setting where the dietitian and client can work together to solve problems as they arise. With ongoing nutrition counseling, the client is able to focus on the "whys" and "hows" of eating behaviors. Time between counseling sessions allows the client to experiment with different food products and problem-solving techniques.

Nutrition counseling takes place in many settings, such as hospital-affiliated outpatient clinics, physicians' offices, community health clinics, and government programs or agencies. In some settings, health care, including nutrition counseling, may be provided for specific groups such as members of a health maintenance organization or employees of a corporation. In some situations, the nutrition counselor has limited office space and counseling sessions must be held in temporary locations such as a corner of the activity room, the cafeteria, or a borrowed examining room. In such circumstances the nutrition counselor must assure the client of his undivided attention.

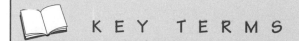

K E Y   T E R M S

Self-management training: Interactive individualized education and counseling that assists a client in developing skills and habits to change behaviors and thus improve health status, control disease or medical condition, and improve quality of life.

INTERPERSONAL COMMUNICATION

■ What are the characteristics of interpersonal communication?

■ What factors may interfere with interpersonal communication?

■ How do listening skills promote the success of nutrition counseling?

Interpersonal communication coordinates the exchange of information in a counseling session. To appreciate the complexity of the interactions between counselor and client, an overview of interpersonal communication is included here.

Sender and Receiver

Whenever two people communicate, one person is acting as the sender of information and the other as the receiver of that information (Fig. 3–3). The roles of sender and receiver change constantly throughout any conversation. The message that is sent or received is subject to interpretation. Often a person is influenced by the message he receives and thus adapts subsequent messages he sends.

Verbal and Nonverbal Messages

An information exchange is composed of both verbal and nonverbal messages. Verbal communication involves the actual words that are written or spoken. Nonverbal communication is not what is said but how it is said and all the other things that are also part of a message, such as facial expression, tone of voice, eye contact, gesture, and touch (Holli, 1991).

The verbal and nonverbal messages in a conversation may reinforce or contradict one another. A client may say that he is interested in learning about how to lower the fat content of his diet. However, if during the counseling session, he does not maintain eye contact, taps his foot, and constantly glances at his watch, the nonverbal message he

sends is one of disinterest and impatience. His actions are speaking louder than his words. A nutrition counselor can use nonverbal communication effectively to reinforce a verbal message. A warm smile can help the client feel more comfortable. A simple nod of the head can reassure the client that the counselor is listening and interested in what he is saying.

Interference

Interference is any factor outside of the message being sent or received that can influence the message. Interference can be external factors in the environment such as temperature, lighting, or noise levels in the room. The counselor and client should be seated close enough to facilitate conversation while maintaining a nonthreatening neutral space. It is preferable for there to be no physical barrier, such as a desk, directly between the client and the counselor.

People can also act as sources of interference. A family member or the client's support person may, instead of helping, disrupt the relationship between the counselor and the client. For example, a domineering spouse may prevent the client from answering questions directed to him, or a young client may be intimidated by the presence of a parent and may not provide truthful answers for fear of later reprisals. Such situations require diplomacy from the counselor to facilitate change without insulting or alienating the person accompanying the client.

Internal factors, such as the physical, emotional, and psychological state of the counselor or client, may also be sources of interference. It is difficult to control for internal sources of interference, but the experienced counselor can minimize their effect by putting the client at ease. Interference also may come from language itself. Because of differing ethnic and cultural backgrounds, words have different meanings to different people. In a healthcare setting, terms and explanations used must be ones that the client will understand.

Listening

LISTENING SKILLS Because communication is a two-way process, effective listening is essential. In many instances, development of rapport with a client and promotion of a helping relationship is fostered only when a counselor listens attentively and nonjudgmentally (Samovar and Mills, 1992). Listening is an active process. It can be a highly subjective experience, with interpretation of what is heard varying from person to person. A counselor can become a better listener by concentrating on developing listening skills such as the following:

• Openness—be willing to explore new ideas without personal prejudices.

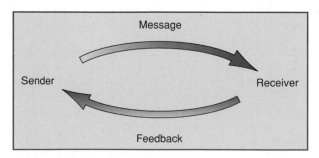

FIGURE 3–3. The roles of sender and receiver change constantly throughout the counseling session.

- Concentration—focus on what the speaker is saying; analyze the speaker's verbal and nonverbal messages.
- Attention—convey full attention to the client (maintain eye contact, empathetic facial expressions, and relaxed posture).
- Comprehension—interpret the client's meaning of the communication (Curry-Bartley, 1986).

Listening is a multi-step process that involves not only the ear receiving the sound waves but also the mind focusing on the sounds heard (Samovar and Mills, 1992). These sounds must be interpreted by the brain, remembered for later use, and evaluated for meaning. The final step in listening is responding to the message both verbally and nonverbally.

LISTENING RESPONSES Listening responses serve to increase the comfort level of the client and to build rapport. They are as important as the questions asked. An appropriate response lets the client know that the counselor is paying attention to what he or she is saying. It also facilitates the flow of the interview and bridges a series of questions and answers. Some of the most frequently encountered listening responses are those that serve to clarify, paraphrase, or summarize.

Clarifying Clarifying allows the counselor to gather more information after the client has provided a vague or unclear answer. A clarifying response helps the counselor make sure that he has interpreted a message as it was intended. For example:

MRS. JOHNSON: I guess I can cut back on my portions, it is just my husband . . . he loves to eat and says he loves to see me eat. He always insists I eat dessert with him. He says he doesn't want his friends thinking he can't afford for us to eat well.

AMY SMITH, R.D.: Are you saying you feel your husband is not supportive of your changing your eating behaviors?

This clarifying response serves to focus the client on her perceptions of her husband's support. It also keeps the client and the counseling session focused on making behavior changes.

Paraphrasing Paraphrasing involves restating or rephrasing what the client has said in the counselor's own words. This can clarify the content or the meaning of the message. It ensures that the client and counselor understand the words used as being the same. An example is:

MRS. ADAMS: I can do everything you say and avoid all sweets but I can't stop using sugar.

AMY SMITH, R.D.: Are you saying that you can avoid foods that contain sugar but not sugar itself?

or

Are you saying that your biggest problem in following this diet is the use of artificial sweeteners?

This paraphrasing response helps the counselor make sure that she and the client have a mutual understanding

of the words sugar, sweets, and artificial sweeteners and will make planning more effective.

Summarizing Summarizing is used to bring closure to the interview or a segment of the interview. It can help bring disjointed thoughts and feelings together, and ensure that the interview is focused on the needs of the client and that it is progressing in an appropriate direction.

Effective summarizing takes practice so that the concerns of the client are not minimized. The counselor must refer to the major topics of discussion as well as the emotions or feelings expressed by the client. Merely stating, "Well it seems you have your work cut out for you if you want to follow this low-sodium, low-fat diet," does not create a feeling of good will and would be rather discouraging, if not insulting, to the client.

A more appropriate response for the counselor would be: "I can appreciate that you have a number of changes to make in your eating habits. We have agreed on your trying ways you can prepare your meals at home and how to make choices in restaurants. These changes will lead you to a healthier ways of eating, with less fat and less salt, and will be a very important part of your recovery from the heart attack." This summarization reviews the major changes that a client has to make, and it focuses on the client's role in decision making and behavior change.

INTERVIEWING: AN ESSENTIAL PART OF COUNSELING

■ What are the purposes and components of the dietary interview?

■ Summarize the purposes of the various stages of the interview.

■ How does the interview relate to nutrition counseling?

An interview is an interaction between two or more people during which information is gathered. An interview can occur independently or as part of a nutrition counseling session. In a hospital setting, an initial interview, often compiled by a clerk or dietetic technician, may focus simply on the food and beverage preferences and identification of food intolerances. As the Nutrition Care Process develops, subsequent interviews elicit detailed information about a patient's dietary patterns and factors influencing food choices.

An interview is more than just a series of questions and answers; it is a guided communication process in which information is gathered and focus and direction established. It promotes rapport between counselor and client, puts the client at ease, and establishes an environment in which the client feels comfortable answering questions and revealing personal information about himself. An interview sets the stage for the counseling session.

A nutrition counseling session always includes an interview. An interview is composed of three parts: a beginning stage, a questioning stage, and an ending stage. The inter-

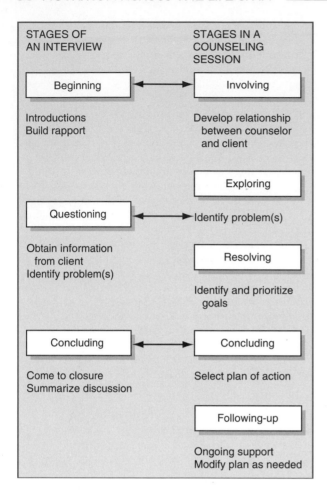

STAGES OF AN INTERVIEW	STAGES IN A COUNSELING SESSION
Beginning	**Involving**
Introductions Build rapport	Develop relationship between counselor and client
	Exploring
Questioning	Identify problem(s)
Obtain information from client Identify problem(s)	**Resolving**
	Identify and prioritize goals
Concluding	**Concluding**
Come to closure Summarize discussion	Select plan of action
	Following-up
	Ongoing support Modify plan as needed

FIGURE 3–4. The relationship between an interview and a nutrition counseling session.

view process can be incorporated into the counseling process (Fig. 3–4). The nutrition counselor is skilled in directing the interview to collect necessary information in a timely and concise manner.

Beginning Stage

The purpose in the beginning stage of an interview is to make introductions and to begin to establish rapport. When first meeting a client, the nutrition counselor must introduce herself and state her title or credentials. An initial contact may begin simply like this. The nutrition counselor asks, "Are you Mr. Brian Jones? I am Amy Smith, a Registered Dietitian. May I call you Mr. Jones? Or what name do you prefer?"

To set the stage for the interview and to build rapport, the counselor may begin by asking who referred the client for nutrition counseling. The client, in answering this question, may begin to reveal what his counseling needs are or what he hopes to gain from the counseling session.

Mr. Jones may state, "Dr. Johnson wants you to give me some list to help get these pounds off me. I've got too much fat in my blood and my heart is not working right." Such a response helps provide the counselor with insight as to Mr. Jones's expectations and his perception of his health problem. This response also reveals that he may not realize the wealth of information a dietitian can provide.

It is important to ask the client why he thinks he is there. A simple question such as "What do you hope to learn today?" helps the counselor focus on the needs and concerns of the client.

Questioning

Once introductions have been made and the needs of the client identified, the interview progresses to the questioning or exploring stage. During this part of the interview the counselor directs the client through a series of questions to determine dietary patterns and identify problems.

The questions are designed to obtain the greatest amount of information from the client in a reasonable amount of time. It is important that the client not feel rushed to answer questions, but it is also important to keep the interview focused on obtaining necessary information. The questioning stage of the interview may use several of the assessment tools discussed in Chapter 2. A dietary history, 24-hour recall, and food frequency analysis are all important ways to gather information and assess the dietary intake of a person.

The types of questions asked during an interview vary depending on the purpose but generally include a combination of open-ended, closed-ended, and follow-up questions.

OPEN-ENDED QUESTIONS Open-ended questions are probing questions that serve to gather the most information possible. They are usually used near the beginning of the interview and are phrased so they require more than a "yes" or "no" answer. These questions begin with "who," "what," "when," "where," "why," and "how." Examples of open-ended questions include: "Please tell me about yourself. What do you like to eat? Why do you feel you have gained weight?"

The advantage of open-ended questions is that they encourage the client to provide information about himself and express what he feels is important. This can help him feel more comfortable in the interview. Open-ended questions tend to be less threatening to the client and also convey the message that the counselor is interested in what the client is saying.

However, open-ended questions can be time consuming, and some of the information obtained can be irrelevant. Although it is interesting that a client has a new grandchild, this information does not help the dietitian to counsel the new grandmother more effectively on reducing her fat intake.

CLOSED-ENDED QUESTIONS Closed questions limit the answers a client is able to give. They are more directed and give the interviewer greater control over the flow of the conversation. They elicit quick answers, such as "yes" or "no." Examples of closed questions include: "Who prepares your meals for you? Do you have any food allergies? Have you ever tried to cook with egg substitutes? Do you salt your food at the table?"

The disadvantage of closed questions is that one may obtain incomplete answers. If the counselor asks, "Do you drink orange juice?", the client may respond "No." The client may, however, drink large quantities of grapefruit juice, which the interviewer would not know from the way the question was asked.

FOLLOW-UP QUESTIONS Follow-up questions help the counselor obtain specific information or direct the client's focus to a given topic. For example, during a 24-hour recall the client may state that she has coffee every morning. Appropriate follow-up questions may include, "What type of coffee do you drink, regular or decaffeinated?" and "Do you put anything in your coffee?"

LEADING QUESTIONS Leading questions are to be avoided because they may distort the client's response. A leading question may cause the client to answer in the way she thinks the interviewer wants to hear rather than providing the truthful information. Examples include, "You don't drink alcohol, do you?" and "What do you eat for breakfast?" The latter question implies that the client should eat breakfast. A more appropriate question would be, "What is the first thing you have to eat or drink in the day?" This does not imply that the client should eat breakfast or should eat first thing in the morning. A counselor is cautious not to reflect personal beliefs in the questions asked.

Closing the Interview

Although the conclusion takes the least amount of time, it is very important in bringing the interview to some type of closure. The conclusion summarizes the topics discussed, acknowledges the client's time and cooperation, and facilitates the transition to counseling.

NUTRITION COUNSELING

■ Describe the steps of the nutrition counseling process.

■ Why does successful counseling often require more than one session?

■ What are outcomes that can be expected from nutrition counseling?

Nutrition counseling is a dynamic process that builds from an interview (see Fig. 3–4). The beginning of an interview and the involving stage of a counseling session are the same if the interview is integrated into the counseling session. Both seek to build rapport between the counselor and the client, and both are used to obtain information. The counseling session builds from the responses given in the exploring stage and progresses to the resolving stage with identification of problems, self-management training, and establishment of mutually set goals. The conclusion of a counseling session serves to summarize and focus the client on the agreed-upon course of action. Follow-up is an essential component of counseling. It provides support and additional information to the client and the opportunity to modify behavioral goals as needed to meet the client's changing needs. Throughout the counseling process, the nutrition counselor gathers information to assess the short- and long-term effectiveness or outcomes of the session.

Preparation

Preparation for a counseling session involves reviewing all the pertinent information available about the client. The inpatient medical record includes the medical history, laboratory values, current body weight, a weight history, medications, and treatment plans. If psychosocial concerns have been addressed in the record, this can provide useful background information for counseling.

In an outpatient setting, information regarding the medical background, laboratory data, and medications may be limited. The counselor may have only a physician referral, the client's name, and the diagnosis or problem, such as excess weight gain. Sometimes it is only after beginning the interview that the counselor obtains essential information, such as that the weight gain occurred after the client began to take a certain medication.

A well-prepared nutrition counselor has skills to facilitate behavior change (Trudeau and Dube, 1995), and is familiar not only with current scientific literature but also with related "news" or reports in the popular media. Often a client refers to the latest article in the newspaper, a health magazine, or a feature story on a popular news show. It is also important for the counselor to be aware of new or specialty food products available in supermarkets and health food stores.

Assessment

Assessment in the counseling session uses data from the assessment techniques described in Chapter 2 augmented by information gathered in the interview. The skilled interviewer explores psychosocial, economic, and cultural issues, exercise patterns, and substance use and also assesses the client's knowledge and readiness to learn and change.

Intervention

Problems identified in the interview form the basis of problem-solving intervention in the nutrition counseling session. An in-depth discussion of treatment theories and behavior modification is beyond the scope of this text, but an overview of treatment techniques is presented, with emphasis on common problems and solutions encountered in a counseling setting. As the counseling session progresses from the involving to the exploring and resolving stages, the counselor and the client work together in problem identification and move to the resolving stage which, focuses on self-management training on identified behavior goals.

PROBLEM IDENTIFICATION   To assist in identifying and prioritizing nutritional problems, the counselor may begin by explaining the client's medical condition as it pertains to nutrition. For example, the treatment portion of a counseling session for a patient with high blood cholesterol levels could begin with the following conversation:

AMY SMITH, R.D.: Mr. Jones, the doctor said in the letter that your blood level of cholesterol is too high. He is particularly concerned about it because of your family history of heart disease. And you just told me you were worried because your brother had a heart attack when he was your age.

MR. JONES: I just don't want to end up in the hospital. Now how high was my cholesterol?

AMY SMITH, R.D.: The laboratory report said 274. The National Cholesterol Education Program has established below 200 as a goal for cholesterol for healthy Americans. Do you know what cholesterol is?

MR. JONES: I guess it's something I eat. Aren't potato chips and fries and greasy stuff full of it? I just know it can plug up my heart.

AMY SMITH, R.D.: Well, you are correct in that cholesterol is found in some foods that you eat. Cholesterol is a waxy substance that is made by animals. It is found only in animal products, but your body also makes it. Researchers have found that to control your blood cholesterol you need to limit both the amount of cholesterol you eat and the amount of total fat and saturated fat that you eat. The foods you mentioned—potatoes—and all fruits and vegetables do not naturally contain cholesterol. You need to be careful because when a potato is made into chips and fries, it is usually cooked in oil. How a food is prepared can increase its fat content. A good rule is, as you put it, stay away from that "greasy" stuff.

At this point the counselor has established a treatment goal with the client, to limit dietary intake of cholesterol, saturated fats, and fat. Her explanation of cholesterol can serve as a framework for problem and goal identification.

PROBLEM EXPLORATION   A dietary history is an effective way to begin to explore the client's typical or usual food habits. Such information serves to identify eating patterns and behaviors, which will become the focus of the counseling session. An additional advantage is that it allows the client to talk about himself, which facilitates a two-way exchange of information.

The counseling session between Amy Smith, R.D., and Mr. Jones may continue with Amy obtaining a 24-hour recall.

AMY: Mr. Jones, it would be helpful for you to tell me everything you ate or drank yesterday. What time did you get up?

MR. JONES: I got up about 6:30 in the morning.

AMY: What was the first thing you had to eat or drink?

MR. JONES: Well, I have to take my blood pressure medicine first thing in the morning so I usually take that with a small glass of juice.

AMY: What type of juice? How much?

MR. JONES: I usually drink orange juice, and I just have a small glass.

AMY: What did you have yesterday? I will be asking about what you usually eat and drink when we finish with what you ate yesterday.

MR. JONES: I had a small glass of orange juice.

Amy refers to the measuring cups and spoons and realistic food models she has displayed in her office to help Mr. Jones estimate portion sizes.

AMY: What is the next thing you ate or drank?

MR. JONES: I sat down with a cup of coffee.

AMY: Was it regular or decaffeinated? Do you usually put anything in your coffee?

MR. JONES: "I drink regular coffee and I put cream and sugar in it."

Amy questions him about the amount of cream and sugar he uses and also clarifies if he uses real cream, milk, or non-dairy creamer in his coffee. Special attention is also given to cooking methods and the use of fats such as cream, butter, margarine, or cooking oil when counseling for changes to lower serum cholesterol levels.

AMY: What is the next thing you ate yesterday?

MR. JONES: Well, my wife made scrambled eggs, sausage, and toast.

AMY: How many eggs did you have?

She allows him to answer and then continues to ascertain the quantity of food that he ate and how it was prepared.

AMY: How were your eggs fixed? Were they mixed with milk or anything else when they were scrambled? How many pieces of sausage did you have? Was it sausage patties or links?

Amy continues to direct the interview to complete the 24-hour recall. She pays special attention to between-meal snacks, beverages, portion sizes, preparation methods, and the use of condiments. After obtaining a 24-hour recall, the counselor can go back and review the client's reported intake to determine if it was typical.

ESTABLISHING PRIORITIES While obtaining dietary information, the counselor may become aware of food choices and eating habits that should be altered. The client and counselor examine behavior alternatives and begin to establish goals as the counseling session moves toward the resolving stage. To effect change, goals must be achievable and must be established mutually. Frequently goals must be prioritized so that the client is not overwhelmed by too many behavior changes.

In the resolving stage, the counselor and client may focus on changing current problem eating behaviors. In this example, food choices that are high in fat or cholesterol and food preparation methods that add fat to the diet are discussed. Amy has begun to discuss the fat content of Mr. Jones's current food choices so that he can decide what changes he is willing to make to limit his fat intake.

AMY: Mr. Jones, you said that you had a ham and cheese sandwich and potato chips for lunch. To lower your cholesterol below the current level of 274, you need to limit the amount of fat that you eat. Ham can be a low-fat choice depending on which type you buy.

Amy shows Mr. Jones some food labels from packages of lunchmeat so that he can learn how to read a food label.

AMY: By reading labels, you can decide which ham or lunchmeat is lower in fat at so that it will be a good choice for lunch. Turkey breast, tuna or chicken salad made with non-fat mayonnaise, reduced-fat peanut butter, and reduced-fat cheeses are some of the things that you could choose for lunch. Of the things that we have talked about, what do you think you would like to try?

Amy and Mr. Jones discuss lunch choices and make a list of things Mr. Jones is willing to try. Together, they review the list of his day's intake and list possible food choices and behavior changes. Mr. Jones and Amy prioritize changes they agree could or should be made. It is important for necessary changes to be limited and prioritized so that the client will not feel overwhelmed.

Mutually Established Goals

Once the client and counselor have explored problem behaviors and established treatment priorities, goals are set. Many people begin a counseling session with only a vague idea of what they hope to accomplish. They may wish to lose weight, get their blood sugar under control, or simply "eat better." The nutrition counselor assists the client in establishing treatment goals and also in understanding the implications of those goals.

Formulation of short-term goals makes problems seem more manageable. Goals established as part of a counseling session have several important purposes. They are specific and help the client focus on exactly what needs to be done. Goals can be great motivators. However, to serve as a motivator, a goal must be obtainable. Instead of a general goal of "lose weight," a more appropriate goal would be to "change specific food behaviors," which will decrease caloric intake and improve the quality of the diet. A goal of increasing the intake of fruits, vegetables, whole-grain cereals, and low-fat meat and dairy products will promote weight loss but removes the emphasis on weight loss, placing it on healthful food habits instead.

A client who embraces a new lifestyle that emphasizes exercise and a balance of low-fat food choices will enjoy much more success with long-term weight management and its health benefits than someone who merely follows a meal plan reduced in kilocalories until weight loss is accomplished. The role of the nutrition counselor is to facilitate behavioral changes that lead to effective self-management. Many people who have nutrition-related problems do not lack knowledge of nutrition. Instead, they lack the skills needed to transform the nutrition knowledge into changes in behavior.

Self-Management

The goal of any nutrition counselor is to help a client change his or her behavior by acquiring knowledge and developing skills needed to make behavior changes and to sustain those changes (Danish, 1986). A counselor encourages a client to function independently in any eating situation. A variety of tools and techniques can assist a client in dealing successfully with difficult eating situations.

A cornerstone of self-management is self-monitoring. Self-monitoring can take many forms and vary in complexity. Tools range from a detailed food and behavioral diary for recording every food item eaten and the situation surrounding the eating event to a simple food checklist on which the client merely places a check next to a food group when a food item is consumed. Such a checklist can assist a person in tracking the adequacy of the diet or monitoring energy intake.

A nutrition counselor encourages an individual to recognize his or her limits and seek help when faced with a difficult situation. For example, a client who is working to lose weight or maintain a lower body weight will experience fluctuations in body weight. She may define an acceptable weight range for these fluctuations and determine that the upper limit of that range is a "red-flag" weight. If she hits this "red-flag" weight, the client knows that she is having serious problems with eating behaviors and may seek additional counseling. For many individuals, weight control is a life-long struggle that requires ongoing treatment patterns, similar to those for chronic diseases. Treating the problem in a stepwise manner ensures that weight gain or problem eating habits do not get out of control.

Written goals and suggestions as well as printed handouts related to the specific information discussed in the counseling session are essential to help the client in initiating self-management techniques at home. The counseling session is concluded with a review of the goals that have been established to make certain that there is a mutual understanding of what is to be done.

Outcome Assessment

The final aspect of any counseling session is evaluation of success. Throughout each session the nutrition counselor evaluates the client's compliance potential and directs the session accordingly. "Compliance potential" refers to the client's commitment as well as his or her ability and readiness to use the information provided to make the needed behavioral changes.

To evaluate the client's progress effectively, a nutrition counselor keeps careful notes detailing a counseling session. Outcomes of a single counseling session or a series of sessions can be assessed in terms of behavioral, functional, and clinical outcomes (American Dietetic Association, 1996). Some examples of these outcomes appear in Table 3–2.

Behavioral outcomes are measures of change in the client's behavior as related to food selection and preparation and activity. These changes, if sustained, will ultimately result in improvements in clinical or functional outcomes. It is much easier to objectively evaluate a client's progress, document the effectiveness of counseling, and plan future counseling sessions when specific measurable behavioral goals have been established. The client's current behaviors can be evaluated by comparison with the goal behavior and with previous behaviors. Clients may not always achieve each goal established, and outcomes must be assessed instead in terms of how much progress has been made. For example, a client's nutritional plan includes a goal to eat six or more fruits and vegetables daily. An analysis of food records may reveal that the current level of consumption, three servings, while below the goal and levels recommended in the food guide pyramid, is well above the almost zero intake reported at the initial counseling session. Such a change can be viewed as success because there is improvement that can result in positive health benefits. Similar advantages can be accrued by an individual attempting to reduce body weight. If part of the excess weight is lost and that loss is maintained, even if the original goal is not achieved, overall health may improve (Goldstein, 1992).

TABLE 3–2 Examples of Assessment Outcomes for Nutrition Counseling Intervention

BEHAVIORAL OUTCOME
The Client Does:
Eat more fruits and vegetables
Limit intake of food high in fat
Consume intake of whole-grain products
Accurately read food labels
Participate in 30 minutes of aerobic activity 3 times a week
Walk for 30 minutes 4 times a week

FUNCTIONAL OUTCOMES
The Client Is Able to:
Shop for food using a riding supermarket cart
Use a fork and spoon to feed herself
Increase his level of physical activity
Prepare simple meals
Cook for himself

CLINICAL OUTCOMES
The Client Has:
Weight loss or gain
Increase/decrease in fatfolds
Increase in muscle circumference
Increase in serum albumin and transferrin values
Normal levels of hemoglobin and hematocrit
Improved appearance—pallor diminishes, color improves
Improved growth (child)

Functional outcomes measure physical capability, social functioning, and mental and emotional health and well-being. Improvement in health and nutrition status may contribute to increased functional ability and quality of life, including such functions as self-feeding or simple food preparation.

Clinical outcomes refer to anatomic and physiologic measures such as anthropometric and biochemical parameters and clinical signs and symptoms. Changes in anthropometric measurements such as body weight and fatfolds are useful, long-term indicators of success. In some instances, laboratory tests for serum proteins (see Chapter 2) or blood levels related to medical conditions such as glucose or lipids may be used to monitor progress. Such tests require interpretation in the context of the client's health status and her medication use (Bell, 1986).

Other measurable benefits may be the client's perception of the effectiveness of counseling and the behavior changes he or she has made. Hauchecorne and colleagues (1994) reported that clients of nutrition counseling cited such benefits as emotional support, fulfillment of interpersonal needs, and a greater sense of control over their conditions.

Follow-Up

Nutrition counseling is a multi-step process. The initial counseling session serves primarily to establish rapport between the counselor and the client. Goals for nutrition counseling may be discussed and nutritional or behavioral problems explored. It is, however, difficult to do much problem solving or use any type of behavior modification techniques in a single counseling session.

Follow-up counseling sessions are essential for problem solving and effecting behavior change. The time between counseling sessions can be used by the client to experiment with behavior change strategies. Careful record-keeping provides invaluable information about successes and shortcomings for the next counseling session. Follow-up counseling sessions also provide an opportunity for the client to re-evaluate and revise goals and strategies for behavior change.

Most clients require more frequent follow-up when making significant changes in eating behaviors. Initially, counseling sessions may be scheduled weekly, becoming less frequent as the client becomes more comfortable and confident with the behavior change. The client should feel free to contact the nutrition counselor with problems as they arise. A client with a chronic disease, multiple health problems, or obesity may need long-term nutrition coun-

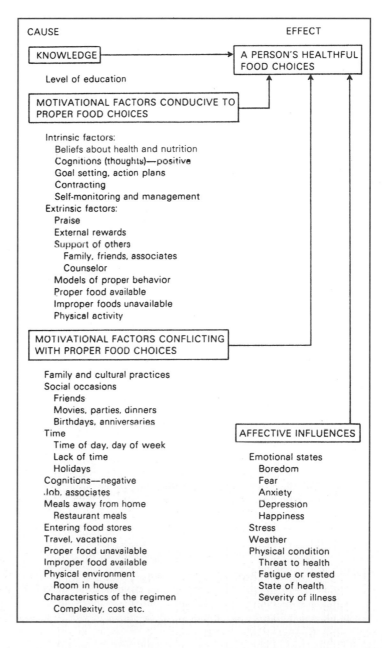

FIGURE 3–5. Variables motivating change in food-related behavior. (From Holli BB, Calabrese RJ. Communication and education skills: the dietitian's guide. 2nd ed. Philadelphia: Lea and Febiger, 1991.)

seling with intermittent follow-up sessions over a period of months or years (Perri, 1992).

Documentation

It is essential that the nutrition counseling process and its outcomes be documented. If counseling is taking place in a hospital or clinic setting, written documentation is entered in the patient's or client's medical record. In more informal settings, record keeping may be less systematic, but the content and outcome of each counseling session is documented. If a Registered Dietitian works independently, she is likely to maintain her own client records and will document the counseling through communication with the clinic, agency, or physician who referred the client.

MOTIVATION

■ What is the importance of motivation in behavior change?

■ What motivational factors promote or interfere with positive changes in food-related behavior?

Knowledge alone is not enough to cause behavior change. Motivation is the driving force that causes a person to act. For any lifestyle change to succeed, a person must be motivated. A multitude of personal and environmental factors can influence an individual's motivational levels. Motivational factors that promote and conflict with choices related to food and health are illustrated in Figure 3–5. The reader will readily recognize many of these factors and be able to identify how they relate to her own behaviors.

Motivational factors can have positive or negative influences in helping an individual select healthy food-related behaviors. The counselor can use his or her knowledge of motivational factors to identify those that are most relevant to an individual client. Acting as a facilitator, he or she can encourage the client to capitalize on the factors that are conducive to positive food choices and avoid or minimize those that conflict with desired eating behaviors. Motivators are unique to each person, and they can change over time and with different situations. The counselor assists the client in recognizing changes in motivating factors in order to use them for the greatest benefit.

CONCEPTS TO REMEMBER

➧ Nutrition counseling is a client-focused, interactive process in which the nutrition counselor assists individuals in developing knowledge, skills, and habits to change behaviors and thus improve health status.

➧ Nutrition counseling involves assessment, intervention, and communication.

➧ Successful nutrition counseling depends on the communication and listening skills of the counselor.

➧ Nutrition counseling is an important part of the nutrition care process that assists individuals in changing food-related behaviors.

➧ The components of the nutrition counseling session are preparation, assessment, treatment, evaluation, and follow-up.

➧ Assessment of counseling outcomes is essential to document progress and plan future counseling.

➧ Motivation is essential to successful outcomes of nutrition intervention.

➧ Motivational factors can both promote and conflict with choices to improve dietary patterns.

References

American Dietetic Association. Medical nutrition therapy across the continuum of care. Chicago, 1996.

Bell LR. Nutrition counseling: the critically and terminally ill patient. Top Clin Nutr 1986;1:1.

Curry-Bartley KR. The art and science of listening. Top Clin Nutr 1986;1:14.

Danish SL, et al. Nutrition counseling skills: continuing education for the dietitian. Top Clin Nutr 1986;1:25.

Goldstein DJ. Beneficial effects of modest weight loss. Int J Obes 1992;16:397.

Hauchecorne CM, et al. Evaluation of nutrition counseling in clinical settings: Do we make a difference. J Am Diet Assoc 1994;94:437.

Hodges PAM, Vickery CE. Effective counseling: strategies for dietary management. Rockville MD: Aspen, 1989.

Holli BB, Calabrese RJ. Communication and education skills: the dietitian's guide. 2nd ed. Philadelphia: Lea & Febiger, 1991.

Monk A, et al. Practice guidelines for medical nutrition therapy provided by dietitians for persons with non–insulin-dependent diabetes mellitus. J Am Diet Assoc 1995;95:999.

Perri MG, et al. Improving the long-term management of obesity. Theory, research and clinical guidelines. New York: Wiley, 1992.

Samovar LA, Mills J. Oral communication: message and response. 8th ed. Dubuque, IA: Wm C. Brown, 1992.

Trudeau E, Dube L. Moderators and determinants of satisfaction with diet counseling for patients consuming a therapeutic diet. J Am Diet Assoc 1995;95:34.

Additional References

The following references provide detailed guidance for interviewing and counseling processes.

Raab C, Tillotson JL. Heart to heart: A manual on nutrition counseling for the reduction of cardiovascular disease risk factors. U.S. Department of Health and Human Services, Public Health Services, National Institutes of Health.

Snetselaar LG. Nutrition counseling skills. Assessment, treatment and evaluation. 2nd ed. Rockville, MD: Aspen, 1989.

Stewart CJ, Cash WB. Interviewing: principles and practices. 6th ed. Dubuque, IA: Wm. C. Brown, 1994.

APPLICATION: A Case for Nutrition Counseling

A nutrition counselor, in this case a Registered Dietitian (R.D.), assesses available information, conducts a focused interview, and initiates intervention by guiding the client in setting goals and beginning to make changes in eating behaviors. This Application builds from the case study in the Application in Chapter 2 and consists of a summary of a counseling session between Ms. Brown, the client who was initially seen in the hospital for an ankle fracture, and Amy Smith, R.D., a registered dietitian who specializes in nutrition counseling. It is designed to demonstrate the following points:

- The two-way exchange of information in a counseling session
- The counseling relationship between dietitian and client
- The flow of a counseling session and the need for subsequent sessions
- The use of anthropometric, biochemical, clinical, and dietary parameters for assessment and problem identification
- Prioritization of goals for changing eating behaviors
- The use of nutrition status information to motivate changes in food behaviors.

The Counseling Session

The orthopedic surgeon, Dr. Blake, who saw Katherine Brown for a fractured ankle following a skiing accident, has referred her to the outpatient clinic for further evaluation due to her low body weight and what he considered her somewhat malnourished appearance. She is scheduled to have blood drawn for tests at 9 a.m., to see a Dr. Wiseman at 9:15, and to meet with Amy Smith, the dietitian, at 10 a.m.

At 10 a.m., Amy walks out into the waiting room. A thin woman, in her early twenties, is sitting in one corner glancing at a magazine. Amy walks toward her, smiles warmly and says, "Hi, are you Katherine Brown? I'm Amy Smith, a registered dietitian." The woman glances up from her magazine, smiles hesitantly and says, "Yes, I'm Katherine."

When they reach Amy's office, she directs Katherine to a chair, helps her with her crutches, and closes the door. She sits down at her desk and forwards her phone calls to the main office to make sure their conversation is not interrupted. Amy pulls the file she had prepared earlier from her drawer. Amy begins the interview "As I mentioned in the waiting room, my name is Amy Smith and I am a Registered Dietitian. Dr. Blake referred you here today. He mentioned that you broke your ankle skiing. Where were you skiing?"

Amy and Katherine briefly chat about skiing. Amy asks if Katherine had a chance to eat something after her blood was drawn, as it is difficult to discuss food and effectively counsel a hungry client.

Katherine replies, "I grabbed something to eat on my way over. I had a really busy morning and it's hard to find a free morning so I could get in here. I'm in graduate school and it seems I never have enough time or money."

AMY: I can appreciate that, I remember when I was in graduate school, it seemed that every minute was filled. Now, Dr. Blake indicated he was concerned about your weight.

KATHERINE: Well, I have always been on the thin side. I am in great health, you know, never sick or anything . . . that's why I couldn't understand why he wanted me to see another doctor and then see you.

AMY: Dr. Blake mentioned he thought by seeing me now you might be able to stay in good health and prevent future health problems. You saw Dr. Wiseman this morning? Katherine shakes her head, yes. "What did he have to say?"

KATHERINE: After they drew some blood, he checked me out. He said that he wanted to hear what you had to say.

AMY: Dr. Wiseman will share the results of the tests with me and when you and I meet again we can talk more specifically about your nutrition status. Today we will be meeting for about an hour. I would like to start by doing some measurements that will help me estimate your body composition. Then we will spend the rest of our time together talking about what you eat.

A private, comfortable setting will make the client feel more at ease. The counselor makes every effort to limit sources of interference.

Frequently, small talk or non-threatening, non-personal conversation can help the counselor establish rapport with the client.

Self-disclosure, a type of listening response, can help build rapport between client and counselor.

Often, in a counseling session the client's medical chart is not available. The counselor may have to depend on the client to provide information about his or her medical condition or health history.

The counselor can make the client feel more comfortable by briefly explaining the anticipated length of the session and the basics of what will be discussed.

KATHERINE: OK. I feel like I have been poked and prodded all morning as it is.

AMY: I will be taking only your height and weight and three measurements—the circumference of your arm, the width of your elbow, and one fatfold thickness on your arm. The fatfold measurement uses these calipers, and it is just a small squeeze.

Amy proceeds to weigh and measure Katherine and records the following on the nutrition screening form:

- height—66 inches
- weight, wearing light clothing—105 lb
- upper arm circumference—20.02 cm
- elbow breadth—2¾ in
- triceps fatfold—10.5 mm

AMY: Now we can sit and talk about what you usually eat.

KATHERINE: What did those measurements tell you?

AMY: I am doing a nutrition assessment. The measurements by themselves don't tell me everything I need to know. I will use these measurements, your medical history, the laboratory results, and what you usually eat. I know that you are busy, but I hope you can find time so that we can meet again next week to go over the test results in more detail.

KATHERINE: I usually have free time on Wednesday mornings and Thursday afternoons.

AMY: Great, we'll schedule a follow-up appointment before you leave today. But now, I want to spend the rest of the time we have today finding out more about you and what you eat. Why don't you start by telling me about your day yesterday. What time did you get up?

KATHERINE: Let me think. Today is Wednesday, so yesterday was Tuesday. I have to teach a class at 9, so I usually get up about 6:30.

AMY: What was the first thing you had to eat or drink?

KATHERINE: Well, I am not a breakfast person. I usually just have coffee . . . and lots of it.

AMY: What type of coffee do you drink?

KATHERINE: Regular, whatever kind is on sale.

AMY: Do you put anything in your coffee? [Katherine shakes her head no.] How many cups would you say you have?

KATHERINE: My coffee-maker makes 10 cups, and I usually have about half a pot before I leave for school in the morning.

AMY: Did you have anything else to eat or drink yesterday before you left for school?

KATHERINE: No, but when I get to school I usually grab something out of the vending machine after my 9 o'clock class.

AMY: What type of something did you grab yesterday?

KATHERINE: I had a package of those little donuts. I think I ate all five of them.

AMY: Did you have anything to drink with your donuts?

KATHERINE: I usually have either a cup of that horrible vending machine coffee or sometimes I fill my thermos with coffee at home and I will have some of that. Yesterday, I just bought a cup from the machine.

AMY: When was the next time you had something to eat or drink?

KATHERINE: At lunchtime I met some friends at the Student Union. I usually grab something fast, you know like a hamburger and fries or a sandwich or something.

AMY: What did you have to eat yesterday?

KATHERINE: Let me see—yesterday I had a hamburger and fries from the burger stand.

AMY: Do you remember what size it was?

KATHERINE: Well, I usually get the lunch special, which is a regular size hamburger and a small fries and then a regular size diet cola.

AMY: "What was on your hamburger?" Amy allows Katherine to answer and then asks additional questions to find out about the type of drink she had, if she put any ketchup or salt on her fries, and how much of each food item she ate.

KATHERINE: I'd say I ate about half of my fries and all of my sandwich.

AMY: Did you have anything else in the afternoon?

An effective way to initiate a recall is by having a client begin with the start of her day. This helps the client think about her entire day, and she is less likely to omit foods eaten.

The counselor needs to avoid leading questions such as "What did you have for breakfast?". To get a truthful and accurate answer, an open-ended question is much more effective.

The counselor notes food preferences but keeps the client focused on the previous day's intake so she can obtain an accurate 24-hour recall.

It is important to know not only what was ordered or put on the plate but how much was eaten.

KATHERINE: Usually I am so full after lunch that I just drink something. If I have my thermos along, I will finish my coffee. If not, I usually run down to the vending machine and will grab a couple of diet sodas. Let me see, yesterday I just had some coffee.

AMY: When is the next time you have something to eat or drink?

KATHERINE: Yesterday I was on campus late for a lecture so I got home about 6. I just threw together a salad.

AMY: What was in your salad?

KATHERINE: I just use whatever greens I have. I don't really like plain lettuce so I usually add some spinach and some endive.

AMY: How much salad would you say you had last night?

KATHERINE: I always use the same plate—it is about this big. Katherine indicates an 8-inch dinner plate.

AMY: Now look at my measuring cups. . . . How many cups would you say you had?

KATHERINE: I would guess about 2 cups of greens.

AMY: What else did you have with your salad?

KATHERINE: All I had was salad.

AMY: Did you put anything on it . . . croutons, meat, cheese?

KATHERINE: I forgot, I usually chop up an egg on it and also add some cheese.

AMY: How much cheese and what kind?

KATHERINE: I buy whatever is on sale, usually cheddar or Colby, and I put about this much on it. She indicates the ½-cup measure.

AMY: Did you put any dressing on your salad?

KATHERINE: I always buy Aunt Sarah's low-fat, low-calorie dressing and then I just use enough to make the salt and pepper stick.

AMY: Did you have anything else with your salad? Any type of roll or bread?

KATHERINE: I had saltines last night. I think I had about 8 of them.

AMY: Did you put anything on your crackers?

KATHERINE: No, I eat them dry.

AMY: Did you have anything else to eat or drink with your salad?

KATHERINE: I had a diet soda.

AMY: Did you eat or drink anything later in the evening?

KATHERINE: Let me see—I just had a couple of diet sodas. My stomach was kind of upset last night, it was really grumbly. I find that if I drink a lot of water or pop it usually quiets it down.

AMY: Let's see if I wrote this down correctly.

She reviews the 24-hour diet recall she has just obtained.
"Is this a typical day for you?"

KATHERINE: That is how I usually eat. Sometimes I have a ham sandwich for lunch with chips, but that is it. For dinner I almost always just have a salad and crackers or sometimes a roll. My friends accuse me of living on coffee and diet soda.

She laughs.

AMY: Does what you eat on weekends differ from the day you just told me about?

KATHERINE: On the weekends, I sleep in . . . in fact, last weekend I didn't get up until noon.

AMY: What do you have to eat then?

Katherine proceeds to tell her that she usually goes to a friend's apartment and they will cook sausage, eggs, and toast. About one weekend day a month she goes out for breakfast and will have bacon and waffles. If she doesn't eat "breakfast" food she will just have her "usual," a ham sandwich with chips. Her usual dinner is a salad every night of the week.

AMY: Are you familiar with the food guide pyramid?

Amy pulls a brochure of the food guide pyramid from the drawer and places it on her desk facing Katherine.

An assortment of measuring tools and food models help the client accurately estimate portion sizes.

A counselor should be familiar with local brand names and specialty food products.

A counselor should always ask if the reported intake was typical. Food consumption and recalls for weekdays and weekends can vary significantly.

The food pyramid is a very effective counseling tool. A check of the reported intake against it can help the counselor and the client make a quick estimate of the adequacy of the diet. It is also a simple tool that the client can use later to assess her diet.

It is important not to criticize or be judgmental about a reported dietary intake. The counselor must offer positive feedback, in addition to offering suggesting changes.

The nutrition counselor should always address alcohol use, as it can contribute significant kilocalories and may be contraindicated in many medical conditions.

There can be many interactions between medications and nutrients or foods that can influence both nutrition status and dietary intake.

AMY: This is designed to help individuals make good choices of what to eat each day. She begins at the bottom of the pyramid. Why don't we go over what you told me your had to eat yesterday and compare it to the food pyramid.

Together they review the 24-hour recall and place checks on the food pyramid for each food item or food group Katherine reported eating.

AMY: From all of our marks on the food pyramid, it looks like your intake of breads, cereals, rice, and pasta is below the 6 to 11 servings recommended each day. Now let us see, you did eat some donuts midmorning, a sandwich bun at lunchtime, and some crackers in the evening. If we stretch it and count the donuts as bread, that adds up to about 4 servings of breads and cereals.

KATHERINE: Are you saying I need to eat twice as much food as I eat now?

AMY: I do think that your intake is below what it needs to be but I don't think you will need to double it. You are making some good choices now. We just need to work on making more good choices. Do you drink milk?

KATHERINE: No, I just got out of the habit of drinking milk. I do eat cheese every day, though.

AMY: That is good. The dairy group includes milk, yogurt, and cheese. It is recommended that women consume at least 3 servings a day. The cheese on your salad would count as a serving. Another serving might be a glass of milk. Do you think that you could choose milk instead of coffee with your midmorning snack? Or to increase your calcium intake you could choose yogurt as an evening snack. [Katherine nods.] From our checks on the pyramid, it doesn't look like you had any fruit or fruit juice yesterday.

KATHERINE: Oh, I can't afford to buy fruit or fruit juice. It is so expensive.

Amy continues through the groups of the food pyramid comparing Katherine's intake with the recommended number of servings. As they review Katherine's intake Amy discusses typical serving sizes for each food group.

AMY: Well, I think I have a pretty good idea of what you usually eat. Is there anything you regularly eat or drink that we didn't talk about?

KATHERINE: No, I try to keep it simple.

AMY: Do you drink alcoholic beverages?

KATHERINE: No, I just don't like the taste of it . . . and it doesn't like me.

AMY: I would like to ask you a few questions about your health history. Do you take any medication regularly?

KATHERINE: No, only an occasional aspirin.

AMY: Do you take any type of vitamin or mineral supplements?

KATHERINE: No, my one friend takes a handful of pills every day but they are so expensive. I figure I am healthy without them.

AMY: Today your weight was 105 pounds. Do you know what your usual weight is?

KATHERINE: I don't weigh myself all the time. I guess I haven't worried about that much this quarter. I know last quarter, or I guess it was about six months ago, I weighed about 130 pounds.

AMY: If you weighed 130 pounds six months ago, that means you have lost almost 25 pounds in six months. Do you think that is possible?

KATHERINE: Yeah, I guess so. All my friends have been telling me that I look too thin, and a lot of my clothes are pretty baggy.

AMY: Why do you think that you have lost the weight?

KATHERINE: I just don't have the time or money to eat.

AMY: Do you receive any type of financial help at school?

KATHERINE: I work as a graduate assistant, which pays my tuition and my rent, but that's about it. My roommate and I have a small apartment and neither of us can afford anything else.

AMY: How do you get money for groceries?

KATHERINE: I do some tutoring part-time.

Amy beings to summarize the information that she has gathered from the dietary recall.

AMY: Katherine, Dr. Blake asked me to see you today because he was concerned about your weight. I found from measuring your elbow that you have a large frame size. Now, just a quick estimate of what health professionals have found to be a good weight for a woman of your height is about 130 pounds. You said that you used to weigh about 130 pounds and, in fact, you said that you have lost about 25 pounds over the last 6 months.

KATHERINE: I didn't think it was a big deal. I've just been busy and haven't had the time or the money or, for that matter, the interest, in eating.

AMY: I appreciate that you are busy and that you are on a very limited income. However, your recent weight loss and the diet you reported to me suggest you may have some serious health problems, both long- and short-term, if you do not make some changes in your eating habits.

KATHERINE: What do I need to do?

AMY: The biggest problem with your diet is that it is low in energy. You are probably only eating around 1100 to 1400 kilocalories. I will run your reported intake through the computer so I can be more specific at our next meeting. For a woman of your age and height who is active I would estimate that you need about 1700 calories.

KATHERINE: What's the big deal?. . . I have lost a little weight and I don't eat enough.

AMY: The problem is you are compromising your long-term health. From your weight history and the measurements I have done here today, you appear to be depleting your energy and protein stores.

KATHERINE: So?

AMY: So, you are not eating enough each day for your body to maintain itself. Just to meet your energy needs, to walk to class, to move around, your body is having to break down stored fat. As you have less fat, your body begins to break down muscle. The long-term health implications are substantial. Women with depleted fat stores can have irregular periods and ultimately may have difficulty getting pregnant. If you were to become ill, your body might not have the reserves to make itself healthy. Your broken ankle needs adequate energy and nutrient reserves to heal properly. In addition, as a woman, you are at risk for osteoporosis. The bones you are building now need to last a lifetime.

KATHERINE: Wow, I didn't think it was that serious. What can I do to improve my diet?

Amy begins to review the Food Guide Pyramid again and makes suggestions about foods to include. She builds from the diet Katherine has reported and adds to it.

AMY: For example, let us take your dinner. A salad is a good place to start. You are choosing a variety of greens. They are a good choice, which add some nutrients to your diet. However, you need to increase the calories in your evening meal and we still are trying to fill in the blanks in the food pyramid.

Katherine begins to list foods that she would consider eating and Amy makes suggestions as to how to work them into her meals.

AMY: Now let us review. The first priority is to increase the amount of food you eat. We decided your second priority is to begin to include more fruits and vegetables in your diet. Your third priority is to work on getting more calcium and iron in your diet. Amy writes down the agreed-upon goals for Katherine to take home with her. "Now to do this what did we talk about that you can do?"

KATHERINE: Let me see—I am going to try to eat something for breakfast.

AMY: That's a great start. Breakfast doesn't have to be anything fancy or even traditional breakfast foods. A peanut butter or ham sandwich with a glass of milk, cheese or yogurt, and a piece of fruit would be fine.

Amy and Katherine continue through each meal and go over very specific suggestions. Katherine begins to make a list of ideas and foods she wants to try when she gets home.

KATHERINE: Now you want me to eat three meals and an evening snack each day? [Amy nods her head yes.] It just seems like so much food . . . plus I can barely afford to feed myself now.

The problems elicited in a counseling session need to be prioritized in order to formulate solutions.

A counselor needs to provide information to a client to help her understand the need for a diet change and the implications of her current eating habits.

It is often more effective to focus on including food sources for the nutrients rather than engaging in a lengthy discussion of individual nutrients.

AMY: I think if you do a little planning, became a little more familiar with the grocery store and begin to spend your grocery money on food rather than diet cola and coffee, you would be surprised. Give it a try for a week and if it really is a struggle, we'll explore some other resources available in the community to help.

KATHERINE: I see now that I do need to change my eating habits. It just seems like so much to do.

AMY: It may seem overwhelming at first but just take it one meal at a time. Even small changes that you can make, like eating something for breakfast or drinking milk or fruit juices instead of coffee, will help. I would like you to meet with me again in a week. By then the laboratory results will be back and we can talk about them. I will have run your diet through the computer and we can talk more about that too. Between now and then I want you to record what you eat and drink for one day. That way we can discuss the changes you have made.

Amy gets a commitment from Katherine to work on what they have discussed and they schedule an appointment for the next week. Amy gives Katherine a copy of the food guide pyramid and a sample meal pattern she has written out, including many of the foods they had talked about. She also gives Katherine her card, which includes her telephone number, in case Katherine has any questions before her next appointment.

After Katherine leaves, Amy completes her notes to include in Katherine's clinic medical record. She outlines her assessment of the diet recall that Katherine gave her. She also lists the goals that they have set for Katherine to work on before the next session. Amy includes her concerns about Katherine's attitudes toward food and her concern about Katherine having adequate money for groceries. Her assessment of Katherine's diet and treatment goals will be outlined in a letter to the referring physician.

The Next Week

Amy begins the counseling session by weighing Katherine. Her weight is 106 pounds. In Katherine's chart are a copy of the laboratory results and the computer printout diet analyses. Katherine has brought a food record for the previous day.

Amy begins the counseling session. "How did the week go for you Katherine?"

KATHERINE: In some ways it was easier and in some ways a lot harder than I thought.

AMY: What do you mean?

KATHERINE: I discovered that I had just gotten out of the habit of eating and, when I started to eat, eating the amounts of food you suggested wasn't hard. I also found that food wasn't as expensive as I thought. Orange juice is cheap compared to coffee these days! I did find that it took a lot of time to cook and shop and eat though.

AMY: It will get easier with time. The food record that you brought in looks great! You were able to eat 3 meals and it looks like you are including something from each food group that we talked about.

KATHERINE: Actually I remembered that I like fruit. I did have a problem drinking milk, though. I think I would rather eat cheese and yogurt.

AMY: Those are good alternatives. We'll talk about them. I do have the information from your lab tests and the computer printout of your diet.

KATHERINE: What did they show?

AMY: As I mentioned last week, I was most concerned about your caloric intake. According to the computer analysis, your caloric level was at 1108 kilocalories. I calculated that you need, just to maintain your weight, about 1700 kilocalories. You actually need somewhat more than that to restore your weight.

Amy continues to review the computer printout comparing Katherine's intake to recommended levels.

AMY: The computerized analysis represents just one day. Your goal is to meet all your energy and nutrient needs over time. According to the lab, your hemoglobin and hematocrit levels were low. In an otherwise healthy person, low levels of these indicate an iron deficiency. Your diet, as you reported it, was also low in iron. Meats, especially red meat, and fortified and enriched breads and cereals are good sources of iron. You eat an egg each day, which is a pretty good source of iron. Since you really don't like red meat, you may want to use more fortified grains.

KATHERINE: What else did my lab results show?

AMY: The laboratory data, the measurements I took last week, and your dietary intake suggest your energy and protein stores are low. This indicates that you have not been eating enough protein or energy to meet your short-term needs.

KATHERINE: Wow, I didn't know I was in such bad shape.

AMY: The biggest concern is the 25 pounds you have lost recently. Your current weight is about 75% of what is considered the reference weight for a woman of your height.

KATHERINE: Well, as I said last week, what do I need to do?

AMY: Last week we talked in detail about what you need to do, and this past week you have done a good job of starting to change you eating habits.

Amy continues to review the goals they had established the previous week comparing the food recall from the previous week with the food record Katherine brought with her. They discuss using yogurt and cheese instead of milk. Amy and Katherine work together to develop strategies to make the changes easier for Katherine.

Amy concludes the counseling session. "I am very pleased with the progress you have made this past week. We have set some specific goals for you to work on over the next four weeks. I truly feel that if you keep working on what you eat, you are on your way to a healthier you. I will see you again in four weeks, but please don't hesitate to call me if you have any questions or problems between now and then."

After Katherine leaves, Amy writes a brief note in Katherine's medical chart to document the counseling session and her recommendations. She indicates the revised goals and plans to meet again in two weeks. Amy also prepares a memo to the referring physician outlining her assessment and mutually agreed treatment goals.

PART II

GROWTH AND DEVELOPMENT

CHAPTER 4

NUTRITION DURING INFANCY

Growth and Development
Assessment of Nutrition Status
Energy and Nutrient Needs

Feeding Infants
Nutrition-Related Concerns During Infancy
Concepts to Remember

Erin is a bright, active 1-year-old and today is her birthday. She is celebrating by playing on her new swing set. With help she can climb to the top of the slide and sail to the bottom. She can sit on one of the swings, but someone has to push her. When the time comes, she will use both a spoon and her hands to eat cake and ice cream with enthusiasm. Last week at her medical check-up she weighed 9.1 kg (20 lb) and was 75.1 cm long (29.5 in). On the day she was born, 12 months ago, Erin measured 3.1 kg (6 lb, 8 oz) in weight and 50 cm (19.7 in) in length. By the time she was 5 months of age, she was 6.4 kg (14 lb) and 64 cm (25 in). Erin has changed dramatically in other ways as well. She started out almost totally dependent—she began with mostly visual exploration of her environment and nonspecific oral expression of her needs to maintaining eye contact and cooing to saying "da da" and "ma ma" to using of several words to communicate. She has progressed from holding her head up to rolling over, sitting up, crawling, standing, and walking short distances.

Erin is a typical example of the progressive growth and developmental changes that occur during the first year of life. These changes depend on many factors, including nutrition.

GROWTH AND DEVELOPMENT

■ What are the gains in length, weight, and head circumference that can be expected for normal, term infants during the first year of life?

■ How would you describe the velocity of growth during this period?

■ How is growth measured and monitored?

■ Describe the physical, neurocognitive, and psychosocial developmental changes that occur from birth to 1 year of age.

At no time are extrauterine growth and development as rapid as during infancy. Although slow by comparison to the rate of **fetal** growth, gains during infancy are rapid in relation to those in the years that follow.

Physical Growth

Differences in patterns of growth among individual infants are a function of genetic, hormonal, nutritional, and environmental influences. The mean birth weight of North American infants is between 3.0 and 3.4 kg (7 and 7.5 lb), and average birth length is approximately 50 cm (20 in) (Lowery, 1986). At birth, the average head circumference

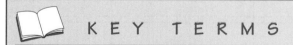

KEY TERMS

fetal: pertaining to the *in utero* growth period of 2 to 9 months

is 33 to 35 cm (13 to 15 in), about one-half its adult size. Overall, the full-term newborn male is slightly longer and heavier and has a larger head circumference than the newborn female. There are substantial increases in these parameters during early life (Fig. 4–1). Although individual growth rates are rapid and highly variable during the first year, the infant generally triples her birth weight and gains about 50% in length and approximately 30% in head circumference.

Healthcare professionals are accustomed to plotting body measurements for infants on gender-specific growth charts for weight and length (Figs. 4–2 and 4–3) and weight-for-length and head circumference (Figs. 4–4, 4–5).

Growth charts from the National Center for Health Statistics (NCHS, 1976) have been devised to represent infants and young children (aged 0 to 36 months) in the United States. They are based on data collected from 867 infants in the Fels Longitudinal Study from Yellow Springs, Ohio. These reference data for weight and recumbent length at various ages are used to compare the size of a particular infant to the reference population and

identify infants with low or high weight or length for age (see Figs. 4–2 and 4–3). Weight for length (plotted on Fig. 4–4 or 4–5) can be an indirect indicator of body fat accumulation, regardless of age. Growth of the skull parallels, to some extent, brain growth during the first 3 years of life (see Figs. 4–4 and 4–5), and head circumference may reflect normality of brain development. **Microcephaly** usually suggests impaired development of the brain.

These growth charts do not consider genetic influences on infant size or individual growth rates, and they may not be representative of infants from non-white populations. However, these charts are useful for tracking an individual infant's growth over time.

Interpretation of Growth Charts

The charts, or grids, shown in Figures 4–2 through 4–5 are divided at the 5th, 10th, 25th, 50th, 75th, 90th, and 95th percentiles. These percentiles represent the distribution of weight, length, and head circumference of the infants in the reference population. The percentile of an infant's weight, height, or head circumference is the point at which the age of the infant on the axis and the measurement along the abscissa intersect. To assess growth accurately, measurements must be accurate (see section on nutrition assessment). When plotted on the growth charts, Erin's birth weight of 3.1 kg (6 lb, 8 oz) and length of 50 cm (19.7 in) are at the 25th percentile and 50th percentile, respectively (see Fig. 4–2). Erin's head circumference, 34.5 cm (13.6 in), is at the 50th percentile (see Fig. 4–4).

Serial length, weight, and head circumference data are used to follow the growth of an individual infant, detect growth abnormalities, monitor nutrition status, and evaluate the effects of nutrition intervention. Erin's height, at the 50th percentile, indicates that 50% of the infants in the reference population were longer than Erin at birth. Her weight, at the 25th percentile, indicates that 75% of the reference infants were heavier. Percentile rankings for head circumference and weight for length are interpreted in the same fashion. Figure 4–6 shows the plotting of serial measurements of weight and length for Erin's growth during infancy.

Successive measurements, plotted on growth charts, can be used to determine whether an infant is maintaining, reducing, or increasing her rate of growth compared to percentile channels or rankings. Such measurements give some indication of growth compared to the reference population by movement across the percentile ranking. For example, an infant who, at 3 months, had a weight at the 15th percentile and at 6 months has a weight at the 75th percentile has gained weight more rapidly than might be expected. Although such a gain may be perfectly normal for that infant, it should trigger the attention of the healthcare professional to carefully assess factors contributing to such an unusual weight gain.

Breast-fed and formula-fed infants gain weight at ap-

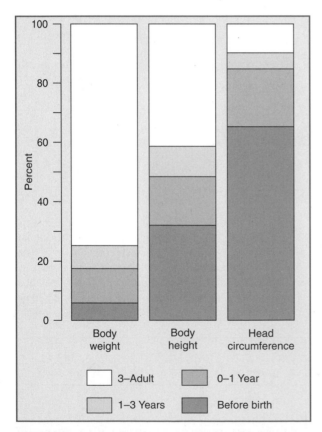

FIGURE 4–1. Growth in body parameters during development. (From Valquist B. The young child: normal. In Jeliffe EF [ed]. Human nutrition—A comprehensive treatise. Vol. 2: Nutrition and growth. New York: Plenum Press, 1979.)

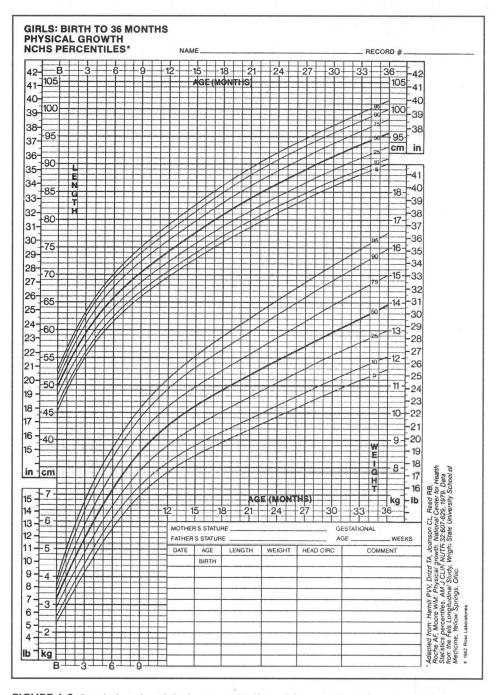

FIGURE 4–2. Growth charts for girls birth to 36 months. National Center for Health Statistics (NCHS) percentiles for length and weight for age. (Used with permission of Ross Products Division, Abbott Laboratories, Columbus, OH 43216 from NCHS Growth Charts. © 1982 Ross Products Division, Abbott Laboratories.)

proximately the same rate during early infancy, but after 4 to 6 months breast-fed infants gain more slowly (Butte et al, 1991). It has been suggested that the NCHS standards may not be appropriate for breast-fed infants because the great majority of the infants in the Fels reference population were bottle-fed or had relatively short periods of breast-feeding. A recent study that compared growth pat-

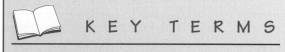

K E Y   T E R M S

microcephaly: head circumference 2 or more standard deviations below the mean for age

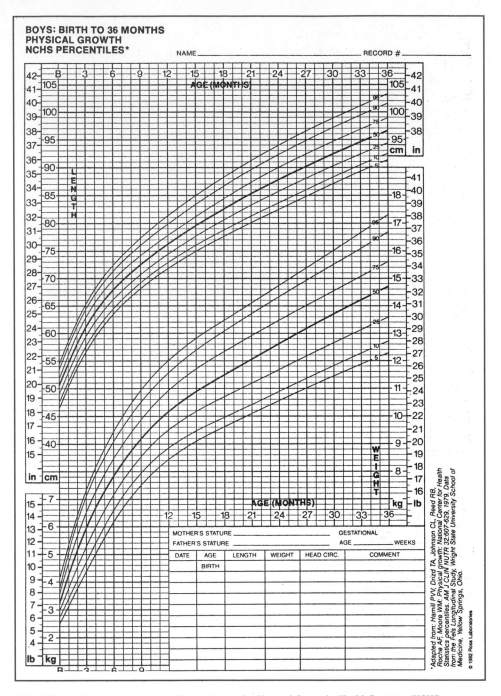

FIGURE 4–3. Growth charts for boys birth to 36 months. National Center for Health Statistics (NCHS) percentiles for length and weight for age. (Used with permission of Ross Products Division, Abbott Laboratories, Columbus, OH 43216 from NCHS Growth Charts. © 1982 Ross Products Division, Abbott Laboratories.)

terns of 226 breast-fed infants from several longitudinal studies to World Health Organization (WHO) and Centers for Disease Control and Prevention reference data found that breast-fed infants grow more rapidly in the first 2 months and less rapidly from 3 to 12 months than the reference standards (Dewey et al, 1995). Breast-fed infants were lighter and shorter than reference data, but mean head circumference was well above the WHO/CDC median for the first year of life.

Velocity of Growth

An infant's length increases by approximately 2.5 cm (1 in) per month in the first 6 months. Gains then decrease to

1.2 cm (0.5 in) per month in the second 6 months. During the first 6 months, the average baby gains close to 1 kg (2.2 lb) per month, or nearly 30 g (1 oz) per day. Over the next 6 months the average increase is about 0.5 kg (1 lb) per month. Head circumference increases about 12 cm (4.7 in) from birth to age 1 year.

Although the NCHS charts allow assessment of changes in size of a specific infant relative to the reference population, such comparisons do not address the magnitude of the gains in length or weight in a specific time frame. Occasionally the growth rate (growth increment divided by time between measurements) can provide a more accurate assessment of growth. Appendix 4 shows the 50th percentile of monthly increments in recumbent length and weight from birth to 12 months for the reference population from the Fels Longitudinal Study (Roche et al, 1989). These tables may be helpful in determining whether an infant's increases are occurring at an appro-

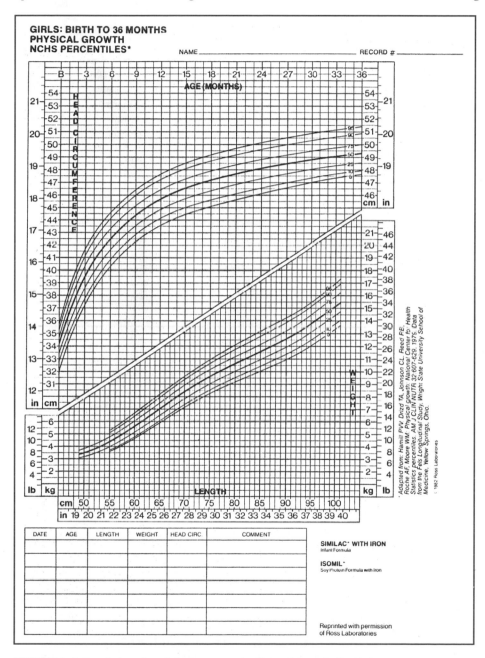

FIGURE 4–4. Growth charts for girls birth to 36 months. National Center for Health Statistics (NCHS) percentiles for head circumference and weight for length. (Used with permission of Ross Products Division, Abbott Laboratories, Columbus, OH 43216 from NCHS Growth Charts. © 1982 Ross Products Division, Abbott Laboratories.)

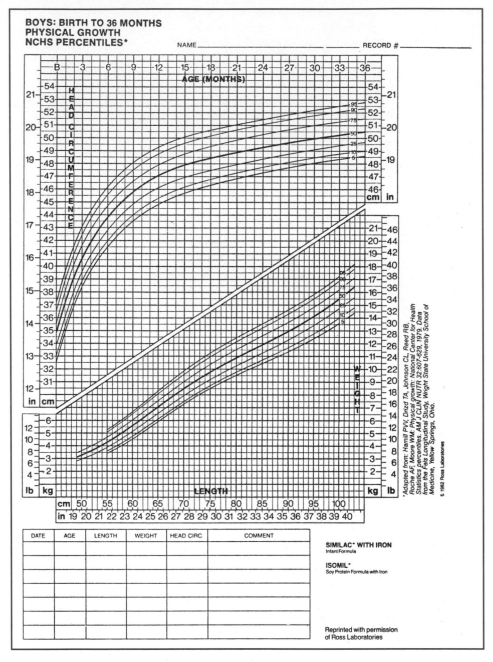

FIGURE 4–5. Growth charts for boys birth to 36 months. National Center for Health Statistics (NCHS) percentiles for head circumference and weight for length. (Used with permission of Ross Products Division, Abbott Laboratories, Columbus, OH 43216 from NCHS Growth Charts. © 1982 Ross Products Division, Abbott Laboratories.)

priate rate and in documenting increased growth in response to nutrition intervention in an undernourished infant.

Recently Lampl and colleagues (1992) confirmed what mothers have known for years—that infants grow in spurts. These researchers measured infants up to 21 months of age and found that increases in length occurred in short-lived growth spurts of 0.5 to 2.5 cm (0.2 to 1.0 in) separated by periods of no apparent linear growth. Caution

must be used, therefore, in interpretating measurements of growth and growth velocity over short periods of time.

Development

As the brief description of Erin illustrated, dramatic developmental changes occur during the first year of life. Some developmental changes and the ages at which they occur are shown in Figure 4–7. Development is complex and encompasses neurodevelopment, cognitive and psychosocial development, and physical development. It is characterized by a progressive and irreversible sequence of events. Table 4–1 illustrates some of the characteristic developmental milestones of the first year of life. Because there is wide variation in the rate at which a normal infant progresses through these developmental stages, the ages at which each stage begins are only approximate. Those given in the table represent the point at which 50% of infants have reached that stage.

Physical Development

Body proportions of the newborn infant are sharply different from those of older infants, children, and adults. The head is relatively larger, and the face is rounder. The chest tends to be rounded rather than flattened, the abdomen is more prominent, and the extremities are proportionally shorter.

Infancy is a period of substantial change in body composition. During the first few days of life a loss of fluid that averages about 6% of body weight occurs. With adequate dietary intake, birth weight is usually regained by day 10. The percentage of body weight that is fat increases from approximately 12% to 14% at birth to about 25% between 6 and 9 months, and then decreases to around 23% by 1 year of age. Protein, approximately 12% of body weight at birth, increases to about 15% by the end of the first year. As a percentage of body weight, fat-free body mass (lean body mass + bone mass) decreases throughout infancy. This is the result of the drop of water content from about 75% at birth to about 60% at 4 months of age and by a rise in body fat content.

In addition to the decline in the percentage of body weight that is water, there is a change in water distribution. At birth, less than one-half of body water is intracellular fluid (ICF), but that increases to about two-thirds as extracellular (ECF) fluid declines. Mineral content, about 3.2% of body weight, is mostly osseous (composed of bone), and gradually increases to about 4.8% at age 18 years.

The human brain is at its peak growth phase at birth and during infancy. By the end of the first year the brain has

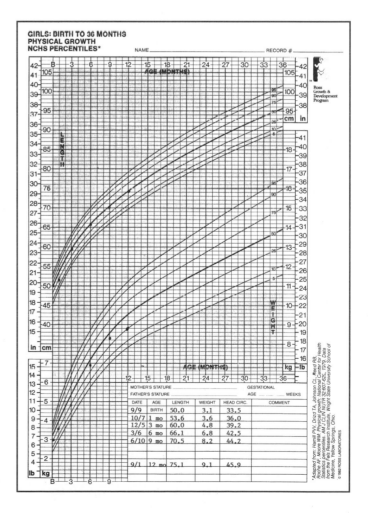

FIGURE 4–6. Example of growth charts for weight and length for Erin.

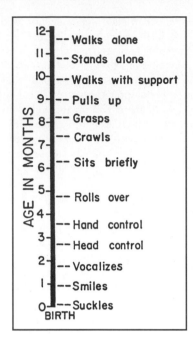

FIGURE 4–7. Behavioral development during the first year of life. (From Guyton AC, Hall JE. Textbook of medical physiology, 9th ed. Philadelphia: WB Saunders, 1996.)

reached two-thirds of adult size. During infancy the first deciduous teeth erupt between 5 and 9 months of age. By 1 year of age, most infants have 4 to 8 teeth.

Neurodevelopment

From the moment of birth, the term infant (38 to 42 weeks) is able to fixate on objects visually and to follow the movements of these objects. When infants are exposed to figures, they give preferential attention to those which resemble the human face. By 2 months of age a supine infant is able to follow an object as it is moved and attempt to make contact with an offered object.

At birth the newborn can turn his head from side to side. By 4 weeks the head is raised momentarily, and at 2 months of age that movement can be sustained. At 5 months, the head can be held erect and steady. This is followed shortly by the ability to roll over. At about the same time, the infant can sit in an upright posture with support. By approximately 6 months of age an infant is able to change the orientation of the entire body to reach out toward a desired object.

Between 6 and 9 months the grasp becomes clearly elaborated into movements involving the thumb and forefinger, and by 9 months the thumb and forefinger can pick up a pellet with a pincer motion. In later infancy, an infant's behavior becomes increasingly imitative. The 9-month-old can wave bye-bye or bring his hands together imitatively; at 12 months he may enter into very simple games with a toy such as a ball.

Cognitive Development

Cognition begins with perception or comprehension of a question or problem, use of memory to determine if the problem resembles a past experience, and generation of ideas to bring about a possible solution. The final process is evaluation as the individual measures the accuracy of his or her conclusions.

In the young infant there is little behavioral evidence of cognitive function, but there is evidence that some perceptual (visual) choices are made when he or she is confronted with different patterns or objects. Later in infancy, selective attention is given to familiar objects, and anticipatory behavior is apparent as demonstrated by the infant quieting at the mother's approach. Another early indication of cognitive development may be curiosity and the exploration of surroundings and objects in the environment.

Cognitive development during the first 2 years of life is characterized by the appearance of repetitive activity that eventually becomes planned, indicating thinking before acting. Two major abilities that develop during this period are **object permanence** and **object recognition**. Later cognitive development is reflected in the infant's efforts to manipulate the environment and imitate people.

Language

An infant is able to make repetitive vowel sounds by 6.5 months and can produce repetitive consonant sounds such as "ba ba" and "ma ma" by 8 months, although he or she does not necessarily associate these sounds with specific objects. By age 8 to 9 months, infants will be attentive to the sounds of their own names, and they may knowingly use a few words by the age of 1 year.

Psychosocial Development

Visual, voice, and physical contact can elicit responses in the neonate. Bonding and attachment consist of those emotional ties and commitments that characterize the relationship between infants and significant persons in their environments to whom they turn for protection, nurturing, and love.

As early as 2 to 6 weeks of age infants can show that they are more comfortable with familiar persons than with strangers. In the early weeks, patterns or rhythms of feeding and sleeping evolve, along with the ability of the infant to control her own state through self-stimulation, such as by finger-sucking or thumb-sucking. The interaction between the mother and the infant in the first weeks of life is initiated by the infant and becomes part of a growing and complex system of signals between her and her mother (or other caregiver). Through these communicative exchanges emotional attachments are formed. In fact, the consistency and promptness of the response of the caregivers to the infant's behavior are more crucial to development than attempts on the part of caregiver's to anticipate the needs of the infant.

TABLE 4-1 Developmental Achievements During Infancy			

4 WEEKS

Motor		
Gross		Poor control of head, neck, and trunk
Fine		Hands fisted
		Hands clench on contact
Adaptive		Regards object in line of vision only
		Follows to midline
		Drops toy immediately
Language		Vague indirect regard (receptive)
		Makes cooing sounds (expressive)
Personal–social		Stares indefinitely at surroundings
		Regards observer's face and diminishes activity

16 WEEKS

Motor		
Gross		Symmetric postures predominate
		Head steady in sitting
		Head lifted 90°; when on stomach, can support weight with straight elbows
Fine		Hands engage
		Reaches, grasps objects, brings to mouth
Adaptive		Eyes follow slowly moving object
		Waves arms on sight of toy
		Regards toy in hand and takes to mouth
		Regard goes from hand to object when sitting
Language		Laughs aloud
		Excites and breathes heavily
Personal–social		Responds to social overture with spontaneous smile or body movements
		Hand play with mutual fingering
		Pulls garment over face
		Anticipates food on sight

28 WEEKS

Motor		
Gross		Sits briefly leaning forward on hands
		Supports large fraction of weight in standing; rolls from back to front
		Bounces actively in supported standing
Fine		Has radial palmar grasp of toy
		Rakes at small pellet with whole hand
Adaptive		Rakes small object toward self
		Bangs and shakes rattle
		Transfers objects from one hand to other
Language		Uses sounds and gestures to communicate
		Talks to toys
Personal–social		Takes feet to mouth
		Reaches for and pats mirror image

40 WEEKS

Motor		
Gross		Sits steadily indefinitely
		Crawls, pulls self up to stand
Fine		Plucks pellet easily with thumb and index finger
Adaptive		Matches 2 objects in hands
		Index finger approach
		Spontaneously rings bell
Language		Says "Mama" and "Dada" with meaning
		Uses one other "word"
Personal-social		Waves "bye-bye" and does pat-a-cakes (or other nursery trick)
		Feeds self cracker and holds own bottle

52 WEEKS

Motor		
Gross		Walks with 1 hand held
		Stands momentarily alone
Fine		Uses thumb and finger to hold small objects
Adaptive		Tries to build tower of 2 cubes
		Releases cube in cup (after demonstration)
Language		Two words besides mama and dada
		Gives toy on request or gesture
Personal–social		Offers toy to image in mirror
		Cooperates in dressing

From Hughes JG and Griffith JF. Synopsis of pediatrics, 6th ed. St. Louis: C. V. Mosby, 1984.

All of these developmental changes are significant in the nurturing of the infant throughout the first year of life.

ASSESSMENT OF NUTRITION STATUS

■ What are the methods of assessment most commonly used for infants and why?

 K E Y   T E R M S

cognition: the means by which an individual accumulates organized knowledge of the world and the use of that knowledge to solve problems and modify behavior

object permanence: knowledge that objects continue to exist although not being perceived

object recognition: use of information acquired to identify an object

■ Describe anthropometric measurement of infants and how it is used in nutrition assessment.

■ Why is accuracy of particular importance in measuring infants?

■ What are the difficulties and advantages of determining dietary intakes of infants?

The basic techniques of nutritional assessment described in Chapter 2 apply to infants. During this period of rapid growth, emphasis is usually placed on growth and hematologic status, but clinical and dietary data are important for a complete assessment.

Anthropometry

Growth changes are relatively large during the first year of life, and monitoring the progression of growth via anthropometry is a primary tool of assessment. Recumbent length, weight, and head circumference are measured on every newborn and are repeated on successive visits to the clinic or physician's office. The keys to successfully monitoring an infant's growth are accuracy and reliability of each measurement (see Chapter 2). When an infant is evaluated in a healthcare setting, the most common reason for an unexpected deviation in measurement is an error in technique. Hence, measurements should be repeated, then recorded and plotted on growth charts immediately to reduce the chance of error. Growth measurements are plotted on standardized charts (such as the NCHS charts in Figs. 4–2 through 4–5) to allow comparison of an individual infant's values with statistical norms.

RECUMBENT LENGTH Recumbent length is measured with the infant in a supine position on a table equipped with a fixed headboard and a movable footboard that are perpendicular to the table surface. A measuring tape is secured along one or both sides of the table. Measurement of recumbent length in infants usually requires two individuals (Fig. 4–8). To get an accurate measurement, the infant is placed so that the crown of the head touches the headboard and the center line of the body is lined up with the center line of the measuring table. The shoulders and buttocks should be flat against the tabletop. One measurer standing behind the end of the table positions the head, ensuring that the baby does not change position, and checks that the body is aligned with the long axis of the table. The legs are extended at the hips and knees to lie flat against the table top. The arms rest against the sides of the trunk. The second measurer places one hand on the knees to ensure that the legs remain flat on the table and, applying firm pressure, moves the footboard against the soles of the feet. The length is recorded to the nearest 0.1 cm or ⅛ inch.

A very young or fussy infant may require gentle restraint to ensure adequate positioning. The more the positioning

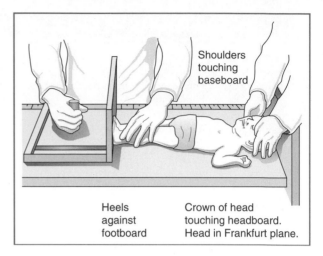

FIGURE 4–8. Measurement of recumbent length.

of an infant deviates from the guidelines, the lower is the reliability of the measurement.

WEIGHT Infants can be weighed using a pan scale with a beam and moveable weights or an electronic scale (Fig. 4–9). The pan of the scale must be large enough to support an older infant or child up to about age 2 years. The scale must be leveled; if the infant is to be weighed with a blanket or diaper, the scale must be calibrated to zero with the blanket or diaper before the infant is weighed. The infant is placed on the scale so that the weight is distributed evenly on the pan. Weight is recorded to the nearest 0.1 kg or 0.25 lb while the infant

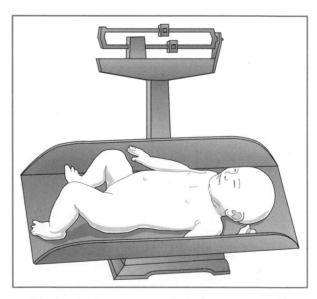

FIGURE 4–9. Infants can be weighed using a pan scale with beam and moveable weights.

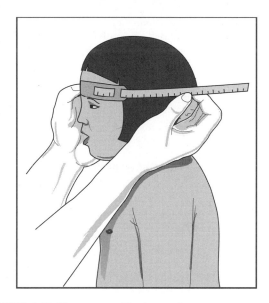

FIGURE 4–10. Measurement of head circumference.

is lying quietly. As with length, weight is recorded in tabular form and plotted on the growth chart. If an infant is restless or crying, it may be better to postpone the measurement and try again later when the infant is calmer.

CIRCUMFERENCES In children younger than 36 months, head circumference is closely related to brain size

and linear growth. Head circumference is measured with a flexible, nonstretch tape about 0.6 inches wide. The infant is seated on the lap of the mother or caretaker, and the measurer positions the tape so that the zero end is on the front of the head. The tape is placed around the head with the ends overlapping so that the zero mark on the tape is underneath the value to be recorded (Fig. 4–10). The tape is placed just above the eyebrows in the front and in the back so that the maximum circumference is measured. The tape must be in the same plane on both sides of the head. The tape is pulled firmly to compress hair, and the measurement to the nearest 0.1 cm is recorded.

The length, weight, and head circumference should be recorded on the form and plotted on growth charts before the infant leaves the office or clinic. If a major discrepancy appears, the measurer can check the accuracy of the plotting and, if necessary, repeat the measurement in question.

FATFOLDS Estimation of body fatness using the fatfold measurement assumes that all components of the body maintain a relatively constant proportion, which is not true of early growth (see the section on body composition).

Fatfolds are not part of routine nutritional screening but can be used to clarify nutrition status when weight for stature is below the 10th percentile or above the 90th percentile. Triceps fatfold measurements have been completed on a population of infants 7 to 13 months of age; percentiles appear in Table 4–2.

Age (months)	n	Mean	SD	5th	10th	25th	50th	75th	90th	95th
							Percentile			
MALES										
7	45	9.2	3.1	—	5.9	7.1	7.5	8.0	11.0	—
8	80	8.8	2.2	5.0	5.9	7.2	8.4	9.2	11.1	11.8
9	95	8.8	2.1	5.2	5.8	7.2	8.6	9.6	11.1	12.1
10	124	9.3	2.3	5.4	6.2	7.4	8.6	9.7	10.8	12.6
11	103	9.3	3.1	5.6	6.8	7.6	8.8	10.3	13.3	15.0
12	68	10.0	3.5	5.6	7.0	7.6	9.3	10.3	13.1	15.9
13	30	9.5	2.5	—	—	—	9.5	—	—	—
FEMALES										
7	46	8.2	2.5	—	3.0	5.2	7.5	9.0	11.0	—
8	88	8.6	2.7	3.0	3.5	5.5	7.5	9.3	10.8	12.0
9	109	8.4	2.5	3.7	4.2	5.6	7.5	9.2	10.8	12.0
10	120	8.7	2.3	3.9	4.6	5.8	7.7	9.5	11.1	13.3
11	95	9.4	3.5	4.4	5.0	6.0	8.3	9.7	11.1	13.8
12	70	9.2	2.7	5.2	5.4	6.4	8.9	10.2	11.1	12.3
13	27	9.5	1.9	—	—	—	9.2	—	—	—

TABLE 4–2 Triceps Skinfold Percentile Values for Infants 7 to 13 Months of Age

From Ryan AS, Martinez GA. Physical growth of infants 7 to 13 months of age: results from a national survey. Am J Phys Anthropo 1987;73:449. © 1987. Reprinted by permission of Wiley-Liss, Inc. a subsidiary of John Wiley & Sons, Inc.

Biochemical Assessment

Blood and urine tests are not used extensively in the assessment of nutrition status of infants. If marginal nutrition status is suspected, biochemical assessment may be initiated using age-specific standards. In an outpatient or clinic setting, an estimate of iron status may be made using a small amount of blood obtained from a finger-stick to determine the hematocrit or hemoglobin level.

The Centers for Disease Control and Prevention recommends that infants and children aged 6 months to 5 years of age be screened for excess blood lead levels. Because infants or children most susceptible for lead toxicity are often those who are also at risk for iron deficiency, both measurements should be made (see Chapter 6 for discussion of lead poisoning).

Dietary Assessment

BREAST-FED INFANTS It is assumed that the breast-fed infant who has ample opportunity to nurse, has an adequate weight gain, and seems satisfied is receiving a sufficient quantity of milk to meet nutritional needs. Other indicators are at least one stool per day and 6 to 8 wet diapers each day. If there is some question regarding the adequacy of the infant's milk intake, it may be necessary to question the mother in detail regarding the frequency and length of nursing periods.

FORMULA-FED INFANTS It is fairly simple to determine an infant's total formula consumption by measuring the amount in the bottle at the beginning of the feeding and subtracting the amount that remains in the bottle after the infant finishes nursing.

SUPPLEMENTARY FOODS Because someone is responsible for feeding the infant, that individual need only record the amount of a food offered (or the proportions in mixed foods such as cereal and milk) and the amount that remains at the end of feeding. After the quantities of breast milk, formula, and supplementary foods consumed have been determined, the infant's intake of energy and nutrients can be calculated from food composition data.

ENERGY AND NUTRIENT NEEDS

■ Compare and contrast the energy and nutrient needs of a term infant to those of an adult.

■ Why do recommendations for energy and protein intakes per kilogram of body weight decrease after 6 months of age?

■ For which nutrients do term infants have body stores at birth?

The rapid growth and major changes in body composition of infancy create high qualitative and quantitative demands for energy and nutrients. In fact, an infant's requirements for many nutrients, per kilogram of body weight, are two or more times those of an adult. Obviously, any inadequacy in intake will have measurable and, potentially long-term, effects on the infant's health and well-being.

Few research studies have investigated the nutrient requirements of infants. Therefore, the Recommended Dietary Allowances (RDA) for the first 6 months of life (Table 4–3) are derived primarily from the average amount of breast milk consumed (assumed to be 750 mL per day) by healthy term infants of well-nourished mothers. Recommended levels for infants 6 to 12 months of age are based on the consumption of 600 mL of breast milk or

TABLE 4–3 Recommended Dietary Allowances for Infants

	Age (years)	
	0.0–0.5	0.5–1.0
Energy	650	850
Protein (g)	13	14
FAT-SOLUBLE VITAMINS		
Vitamin A (μg RE)*	375	375
Vitamin D (μg)†	7.5	10
Vitamin E (mg α-TE)††	3	4
Vitamin K (μg)	5	10
WATER-SOLUBLE VITAMINS		
Vitamin C (mg)	30	35
Thiamin (mg)	0.3	0.4
Riboflavin (mg)	0.4	0.5
Niacin (mg NE)§	5	6
Vitamin B_6 (mg)	0.3	0.6
Folate (μg)	25	35
Vitamin B_{12} (μg)	0.3	0.5
MINERALS		
Calcium (mg)	400	600
Phosphorus (mg)	300	500
Magnesium (mg)	40	60
Iron (mg)	6	10
Zinc (mg)	5	5
Iodine (μg)	40	50
Selenium (μg)	10	15

* Retinol equivalents. 1 retinol equivalent = 1 μg or 6 μg β-carotene.

† As cholecalciferol. 10 μg cholecalciferol = 400 IU of vitamin D.

†† α-Tocopherol equivalents. 1 mg d-α = 1 α-TE.

§ 1 NE (niacin equivalent) is equal to 1 mg of niacin or 60 mg of dietary tryptophan.

Reprinted with permission from Recommended Dietary Allowances, 10th ed. Copyright 1989 by the National Academy of Sciences. Courtesy of the National Academy Press, Washington, D.C.

formula supplemented by increasing amounts of solid foods (National Research Council, 1989).

Energy

The components of energy requirements of the healthy term infant are basal metabolic rate, the thermic effect of food, physical activity, maintenance, growth, and energy losses in urine and feces (Fig. 4–11). The RDA for energy during infancy represents the sum of these expenditures.

The basal metabolic rate that constitutes the largest portion of the energy expenditure has been estimated as 48 to 55 kcal/kg/day (21–25 kcal/lb) and remains relatively constant during infancy. Energy to maintain body temperature in the early extrauterine period, which decreases with time, is a significant component of this expenditure. Growth, the second largest energy cost in early infancy, is the sum of the energy content of the tissue laid down and the energy cost of synthesizing it. The total cost of growth approximates 4 to 6 kcal/g of tissue gained. The proportion of energy expended for growth decreases with time, especially after 6 months. The energy cost of physical activity is low in the neonate, but increases as infancy progresses, offsetting the decreased expenditure of growth. The thermic effect of food is estimated at 5% to 10% of the energy intake, or approximately 4 to 5 kcal/kg/day. Energy lost in excretory products (urine and feces) is relatively small, but is greater than that of adults.

Although energy needs per kilogram of body weight decline during the first year of life, total energy intakes increase. The daily caloric recommendations for a female infant whose weight is at the 50th percentile on the NCHS chart would begin at less than 400 kcal/day shortly after birth and increase to almost 1000 kilocalories over a period of 12 months (Table 4–4).

TABLE 4–4 Projected Daily Energy and Protein Intakes for a Female Infant

Age (mo)	Weight (kg)	Energy (kcal/day)	Protein (g)
Newborn	3.2	350	7
3	5.4	580	12
6	7.2	700	14
9	8.6	840	17
12	9.6	940	19

Protein

Providing sufficient protein for the growing infant involves not only supplying an adequate quantity of protein, but also providing protein of high biologic value and an adequate amount of energy.

PROTEIN QUANTITY Protein requirements have been estimated in 2 ways—factorial estimates and intake levels of healthy breast-fed infants. A factorial estimate is the sum of protein required for growth and for replacement of inevitable losses of nitrogen in urine and feces (1 g nitrogen = 6.25 g protein). Factorial estimations yield a protein requirement of 1.98 g/kg per day during the first month of life, which decreases to 1.18 g/kg per day by 4 to 5 months of age, then continues at that level to age 1 year (Fomon, 1991). Average protein intakes of breast-fed infants in developed countries are 2.04 g/kg per day in the first 3 months and 1.73 g/kg per day in the next 3 months (World Health Organization, 1985). The two estimates are quite similar when a margin of safety is added to factorial estimates. The RDAs for protein (0–6 months, 2.2 g/kg; 6–12 months, 2.0 g/kg) are based on the assumption that the protein consumed will be of the same quality as human milk. For the first 4 months, when such a protein provides 6.5% to 8% of total energy, protein intake will meet the requirements if the energy needs are met. If the protein is of lesser quality, the amounts required will be greater. After 4 to 6 months of age, it may be necessary to add other foods to the breast milk or formula diet of the infant to meet protein needs. The approximate amounts of protein recommended for a female infant whose weight is at the 50th percentile on the NCHS charts are shown in Table 4–4.

Protein intakes in excess of the body's need for maintenance and growth will not enhance growth or health. In fact, excess amino acids require deamination in the liver so that the nonprotein portion can be used for energy. The liver must then convert the nitrogen portion to urea to be excreted by the kidney. Because the infant's ability to concentrate urine is limited, additional excretory products, such as urea from the catabolism of excess protein, require

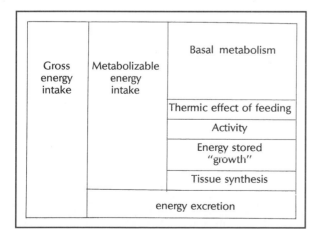

FIGURE 4–11. Components of energy expenditure. (From Butte NF. Energy requirement during infancy. In: Tsang RC, Nichols BL [eds]. Nutrition during infancy. Philadelphia: Hanley & Belfus, 1988.)

TABLE 4–5 Estimated Amino Acid Requirements for Infants 3–4 Months of Age

Amino Acid	mg/kg/day
Histidine	28
Isoleucine	70
Leucine	161
Lysine	103
Methionine + cystine	58
Phenylalanine + tyrosine	125
Threonine	87
Tryptophan	17
Valine	93

a larger volume of water and unnecessarily increase the workload of the kidney.

PROTEIN QUALITY Not all proteins are of equal biologic value or quality. Infants require nine essential amino acids in varying amounts (Table 4–5). Three additional amino acids, cystine, taurine, and tyrosine, have been referred to as conditionally essential or semi-essential because they may be required by young infants under certain circumstances. For example, tyrosine is produced in the body via enzymatic breakdown of phenylalanine. In some very young infants, the enzyme for this conversion may not be fully developed and, therefore, a dietary source becomes necessary. The quality of a protein depends on the amount of essential amino acids it contains in proportion to requirements. The composition of human milk is considered the reference pattern for human infants and, therefore, serve as a guide for the formulation of human milk substitutes and supplementary feeding.

ADEQUATE ENERGY INTAKE Utilization of dietary amino acids for protein synthesis requires an adequate supply of energy. If kilocalories are inadequate, protein is used for energy and protein status suffers. Optimal growth cannot be maintained and, in severe cases, gains in length and weight slow or even cease.

Lipids

More than half of the kilocalories in human milk come from fat. Dietary fat is a concentrated source of energy, a carrier of fat-soluble vitamins, and a source of essential fatty acids. Essential fatty acids provide the substrates for arachidonic acid, docosahexaenoic acid, and their metabolites, which are found in high concentrations in the

phospholipids of all cells, especially membranes of the brain and neural cells. Compared to cow's milk, human milk is higher in polyunsaturated fatty acids, both omega-3 and omega-6 fatty acids, providing 6% of total kcal. The presumed daily requirement of linoleic acid is 2.7% of total calories (American Academy of Pediatrics, 1993a). For a neonate consuming 350 kcal a day, the EFA recommendation would be approximately 1 g per day, increasing to 2 g for the older infant who consumes 600 kcal.

Carbohydrate

Carbohydrate is a major contributor to energy intake and should be prominent in the diet of an infant. Lactose is the carbohydrate source in human milk and many cow's-milk formulas. As infants begin to consume other foods, the percentage of calories obtained from carbohydrate increases as the proportion obtained from fat decreases.

Vitamins

Fat-Soluble Vitamins

The breast milk of a well-nourished mother contains 40 to 70 μg/dL of retinol and a smaller amount of carotenoids (mainly beta carotene) that can be converted to retinol. A daily intake of 750 mL of milk provides the RDA of 375 μg.

Human milk from a vitamin D–sufficient mother provides approximately 2 μg of vitamin D per 750 mL. Vitamin D–deficient rickets has been reported in exclusively breast-fed infants of women with poor vitamin D status and women consuming vegan diets who did not receive vitamin D supplements (Dagnelie et al, 1990). The RDA for vitamin D for infants is 7.5 μg for infants aged 0 to 6 months, and 10 μg for infants 6 to 12 months old. The American Academy of Pediatrics (1993a) recommends vitamin D supplements for breast-fed infants and for formula products developed for infants.

Vitamin E (tocopherol) is required to protect a variety of body cells and compounds from oxidation. The RDA for vitamin E for infants up to the age of 6 months is 3 mg/day, which reflects the tocopherol concentration of human milk. The level increases to 4 mg/day for infants aged 6 to 12 months.

The vitamin K status of the neonate is of concern for several reasons. First, the newborn has low plasma **prothrombin**. Second, human milk contains low levels of vitamin K (2 μg/L), and third, the intestinal microorganisms that synthesize vitamin K in adults are absent at birth and do not become fully active until later in infancy. Therefore, exclusively breast-fed infants are at risk for development of fatal intracranial hemorrhage due to vitamin K deficiency. To prevent this problem, a prophylactic intramuscular injection of 0.5 to 1 mg vitamin K is recommended for all newborns (American Academy of Pediatrics, 1993b).

Water-Soluble Vitamins

VITAMIN C   Vitamin C has several roles in human nutrition, the most carefully documented being the role in the synthesis and maintenance of collagen. The RDA for vitamin C during early infancy (30 mg) is based on the content of human milk plus an adequate margin of safety.

THIAMIN, RIBOFLAVIN, NIACIN, AND VITA-MIN B$_6$ Thiamin, riboflavin, and niacin are essential coenzymes in energy metabolism. The RDAs for these vitamins are based on the average content of breast milk. Vitamin B$_6$ functions as a coenzyme in the metabolism of amino acids, nucleic acids, and lipids. The RDAs of 0.3 and 0.6 mg/day are levels provided in the milk of a mother who has adequate vitamin B$_6$ intake.

FOLATE AND VITAMIN B$_{12}$ As coenzymes, folate and vitamin B$_{12}$ are essential for the synthesis of many body compounds. The newborn infant has small body stores of folate, which are rapidly depleted to meet the requirements for growth. An allowance for folate of 25 μg/day may be met adequately by human milk or cow milk. However, goat's milk contains only 10 μg of folate per liter, and an infant fed goat milk requires a supplement to prevent megaloblastic anemia. Mothers with adequate serum vitamin B$_{12}$ levels appear to supply sufficient vitamin B$_{12}$ to their infants. However, a deficiency associated with irritability, anorexia, **failure to thrive,** and a long-term poor intellectual outcome has been reported in exclusively breast-fed infants of mothers who consumed a diet devoid of animal products and without vitamin B$_{12}$ supplements (Graham et al, 1992).

Major Minerals

Calcium, Phosphorus, and Magnesium

Bone mineralization depends on several nutrients, including protein, vitamin D, calcium, phosphorus, and magnesium. Breast-fed infants retain approximately two-thirds of the 240 mg of calcium in 750 mL of human milk, but retention from cow's milk and commercial infant formulas is less than 50%. Recommended levels of calcium for formula-fed infants are 400 mg per day for the first 6 months and 600 mg for the second 6 months of life. RDAs for phosphorus are based on a calcium-to-phosphorus ratio of 1.3 to 1 during the first 6 months and 1.2 to 1 for the second 6 months. The recommended intakes of 40 and 60 mg/day for magnesium are based on the average magnesium intake of breast-fed infants plus an allowance for variability in growth.

Trace Minerals

Determining specific requirements for trace elements can be difficult because the effects of dietary inadequacies may be subtle and difficult to detect and because bioavailability can be influenced by many factors. In infancy, this is compounded by the movement of an infant from a single food source to a diet supplemented by a variety of supplementary foods, which may change the bioavailability of nutrients in milk.

IRON   A term infant is born with an iron reserve of about 75 mg, which is sufficient to meet iron needs for the first 4 to 6 months of life. Without an additional source, iron stores become depleted at about that time. For infants who are not breast fed, the American Academy of Pediatrics (1993) recommends the use of iron-fortified formulas from birth to the end of the first year of life. Iron deficiency and the concomitant developmental delays and abnormal behaviors can be prevented in infants through the use of iron-fortified formulas (Moffatt et al, 1994) or iron-fortified cereals after 4 months of age (Walter et al, 1993).

ZINC   Zinc is an essential nutrient that functions in growth, reproduction, tissue repair, and cellular immunity. Zinc recommendations of 5 mg/day for breast-fed infants are met from mobilization of liver stores and the approximately 2 mg of zinc obtained each day in breast milk. Formula-fed infants have greater needs due to lesser bioavailability of zinc from formula. Although high amounts of dietary iron have been shown to reduce zinc absorption, the iron in fortified formulas does not appear to have a significant negative impact on zinc status (National Research Council, 1989).

FLUORIDE   The benefits of fluoride in early infancy are somewhat controversial because of the dearth of evidence that fluoride supplements in the first 6 months alter the prevalence of dental caries in the secondary dentition. Unerupted teeth are being mineralized in later infancy, however; consequently supplemental fluoride would be expected to have a beneficial effect during this period. The American Academy of Pediatrics (1995) does not rec-

K E Y   T E R M S

prothrombin: a protein for blood coagulation synthesized in the liver
failure to thrive: deceleration of growth or growth failure due to inadequate food intake or impaired utilization. It may be due to psychosocial or physical factors.

comend fluoride supplementation from birth and doses for 6 months to 3 years (0.25 mg/day) are recommended only when water fluoride content is less than 0.3 ppm.

Fluid and Electrolytes

Water

Infants have proportionally greater water requirements than adults due to their larger surface area per unit of body weight, their higher percentage of both body water and extracellular fluid, and their greater urine volume resulting from a lesser capacity of their kidneys to concentrate the **solute load**. Urea from protein metabolism, sodium, potassium, chloride, and phosphorus is a major contributor to the renal solute load. A daily fluid intake of 1.5 mL/kcal of energy expenditure is adequate to meet the needs of infants. This figure corresponds to the water-to-energy ratio in human milk and commonly used infant formulas. Supplemental water generally is not indicated for healthy infants who are not yet receiving solid foods, except possibly during hot weather for formula-fed infants. When solid foods are introduced, additional water may be required due to the greater renal solute load, and water should be offered to the infant each day.

Infants aged less than 6 months who are vomiting or have diarrhea are at risk for **hyponatremia** particularly if they are fed fluids lacking sufficient sodium. Products containing water and electrolytes for rehydration are available in supermarkets. Hyponatremic seizures have been reported in infants fed excessive amounts of solute-free water (Centers for Disease Control and Prevention, 1994). In addition to seizures, manifestations include altered mental status, hypothermia, and edema. Most commonly hyponatremia has been caused by giving excess tap water or overdiluting formula. In many instances this problem is due inadequate resources to purchase infant formula or a lack of knowledge about the potential dangers of feeding infants solute-free water. Sometimes bottled water products marketed as supplements for infants have been mistaken by parents and other caregivers as an affordable and appropriate feeding supplement or substitute for formula, resulting in hyponatremia.

Sodium, Potassium, and Chloride

Estimated minimum requirements for sodium, potassium, and chloride are listed in Appendix A. Sodium, the major cation in extracellular fluid, is an important regulator of fluid volume. Chloride, the major inorganic anion in extracellular fluid, is essential for maintaining fluid and electrolyte balance. The major cation in intracellular fluid, potassium, is a necessary constituent of each body cell. As lean body mass increases, the need for potassium rises. Both human milk and commercial infant formula contain sufficient sodium, potassium, and chloride.

FEEDING INFANTS

■ What is the feeding relationship and why is it important to the health and well-being of the infant?

■ What are the advantages and possible contraindications of breast-feeding?

■ What adaptations or changes have been made in cow's milk to make it suitable for infant feeding?

■ Should regular cow milk be withheld from an infant until I year of age? Why or why not?

■ Describe the basis for determining when and how supplementary foods should be given to an infant.

■ Do nutrient supplements have a role in infancy? Why?

Normal growth and development depend on the consumption of appropriate amounts and types of food. Breast milk or commercial infant formulas are usually the sole source of energy and nutrients during the first few months of life. Between 4 and 6 months of age, supplementary foods are added to the diet, and there is a gradual progression in the variety, quantity, and consistency of foods until soft table foods can be consumed at about 1 year of age. Recommendations for the introduction of solid foods depend on the individual infant's nutritional needs, physiologic maturation, and developmental and behavioral readiness for feeding (Hendricks and Badruddin, 1992).

The Feeding Relationship

From the earliest moments of life, the infant is dependent on establishment of a social relationship for his nutritional needs and, thus, the maintenance of life and physiologic well being. This relationship (Fig. 4–12) not only provides energy and nutrients but also supports an infant's development. Satter (1990) has characterized three stages of the feeding relationship between the infant and parents—homeostasis, attachment, and individualization. Homeostasis occurs in early infancy as extrauterine biologic functions stabilize and the infant increasingly interacts with the environment. The parents or primary caretakers facilitate development of the feeding relationship by responding promptly to hunger cues (such as crying or fussing), calming the infant, and responding to his or her schedule and feeding capability.

Attachment evolves from birth to about 4 months as the infant achieves **affective** interactions with the parent. The caregiver maintains eye contact, smiles, speaks, and encourages the infant. The infant responds and takes the initiative in indicating readiness for the nipple, and nursing. In fact, an infant may pause during nursing to socialize and then return to feeding. He may indicate satiety by falling asleep, smiling, drawing away from the nipple, and refusing reinsertion of the nipple.

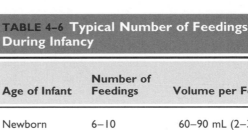

FIGURE 4–12. Infant feeding is both a nutritional and a social experience.

TABLE 4–6 Typical Number of Feedings During Infancy

Age of Infant	Number of Feedings	Volume per Feeding
Newborn	6–10	60–90 mL (2–3 oz)
1 mo	6–8	90–120 mL (3–4 oz)
2–3 mo	5–6	150–180 mL (5–6 oz)
3–6 mo	4–5	180–210 mL (4–7 oz)
7–12 mo	3–4	210–240 mL (7–8 oz)

In the latter half of the first year and beyond, development is characterized by separation and individualization. Based on an increasingly complex sense of self, the infant struggles for autonomy and control. The ability to ingest an appropriate amount of food depends on a positive feeding interaction between the infant and his parents. Parents provide firm and caring support and direction in the development of eating habits and mastery of the feeding situation. The style and quality of caregiver–infant interactions have a strong influence on subsequent feeding behavior. Failure to establish this relationship results in inadequate intake, a major contributor to growth failure. Toward the end of the first year, parents and the infant develop a schedule and pattern in feeding as the intimate feeding relationship evolves into involvement in family meals.

Breast Milk

The physiology of lactation and the process of breast-feeding are discussed in Chapter 10. Breast-feeding is the universally recommended mode of feeding for early infancy. In spite of such recommendations, the prevalence of breast-feeding has changed little, in either the number of mothers initiating lactation or in the duration of breast-feeding.

Health advantages associated with feeding breast milk include a nutritive composition uniquely suited to the human infant, bioavailability of nutrients, and the presence of growth factors, enzymes, hormones, and a number of immune factors. Breast-feeding is associated with reduced incidence and severity of certain infectious gastrointestinal and respiratory diseases, which may be the result of development of a breast milk–induced intestinal mucosal barrier against the penetration of harmful substances (Sheard and Walker, 1988).

Because the capacity of the stomach at birth is only about 7 mL, the amount of breast milk an infant can consume initially is limited. Gastric capacity increases rapidly, about tenfold in the first 2 weeks, when the infant is able to consume 2 to 3 ounces per feeding. An outline of a typical amount and number of feedings of breast milk or formula is found in Table 4–6. Over time the feedings are characterized by greater volume and decreased frequency as solid foods begin to replace some of the energy and nutrients formerly obtained from milk.

Biochemistry of Human Milk

The nutrient content of human milk is variable. There are differences from one mother to another, across the stages of lactation, and even within individual feedings. Specific components in the milk may compensate for limited production of certain compounds by immature systems of the newborn. These include digestive enzymes, immunoglobulins, taurine, and specific long-chain fatty acids (Hamosh, 1992).

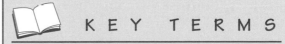

K E Y   T E R M S

solute load: amount of substances that must be dissolved in liquid—in this case, in urine
hyponatremia: low blood levels of sodium
affective: relating to or influencing feelings or emotions

Colostrum

The initial fluid released by the mammary gland, colostrum, is a thick yellow transparent fluid that is higher in protein and lower in fat than mature milk. The abundance of immune factors in colostrum also protects the infant against viral and bacterial infections while his immune system is still developing. After 3 to 6 days, colostrum evolves into transitional milk, and by the seventh to fourteenth day, the change to mature milk has been completed, although protein levels remain high for the first month. Colostrum facilitates the passage of **meco-**

TABLE 4–7 Nutrient Content of Colostrum, Immature (Transitional) and Mature Human Milk, and Cow Milk per Deciliter of Milk

Nutrient	Human Milk			Mature Cow Milk
	Colostrum (1–5 days)	Transitional (Immature; 6–10 days)	Mature	
Energy (kcal)	67	72	74	70
Fat (g)	2.9	3.6	4.5	3.7
Lactose (g)	5.3	6.6	7.2	4.8
Protein (g)	2.7	1.6	0.9	3.3
Casein (g)	1.2	0.7	0.3	2.8
Lactalbumin (g)		0.8	0.3	0.4
Calcium (mg)	31	34	30	125
Phosphorus (mg)	14	17	15	96
Zinc (mg)	0.5	0.4	0.16	0.37
Iron (mg)	0.09	0.04	0.03	0.04
Vitamins				
A (IU)	296	283	240	303
Carotene (IU)	186	63	45	63
D (IU)			5	4
E (mg)	0.8	1.32	0.2	0.06
C (mg)	4.4	5.4	4.3	0.9
K (μg)			2.3	
Folacin (μg)	0.05	0.02	0.52	0.23
Niacin (mg)	0.075	0.15	0.20	0.085
Pantothenic acid (mg)	0.183	0.288	0.18	0.30
Pyridoxine (mg)			0.02	0.048
Riboflavin (mg)	0.029	0.033	0.035	0.16
Thiamin (mg)	0.015	0.006	0.014	0.042
Carnitine (mg)	1.1	1.6	1	2.1
Sodium (mg)	5	19	17	76
Potassium (mg)	74	63	53	152
Chloride (mg)	58	30	37	108
Magnesium (mg)	4.2	3.5	4	13
Iodine (μg)	6	—	6	11
Manganese (μg)	trace	trace	0.3	2.5
Selenium (μg)	—	—	2	4

Adapted from Behrman RE, et al. (eds). Nelson textbook of pediatrics, 14th ed. Philadelphia: WB Saunders, 1996.

TABLE 4–8 Multiple Functions of the Major Nutrients of Human Milk

Nutrient	Amount	Function
PROTEIN	mg/dL	
sIgA	50–100	Immune protection
IgM	2	Immune protection
IgG	1	Immune protection
Lactoferrin	100–300	Antiinfective, iron carrier
Lysozyme	5–25	Antiinfective
Lipase	10	Fat digestion
Lactalbumin	200–300	Calcium carrier
Casein	200–300	Carrier of calcium, phosphate, iron, zinc, and copper
CARBOHYDRATE	g/dL	
Lactose	5.5–6.0	Energy source
Poly-saccharide	1.0–1.5	Prevent bacterial attachment to intestine
FAT	g/dL	
Triglyceride	3.0–4.5	
Long chain polyunsaturated fatty acids		Brain and retinal function
Fatty acids (C12:0, C18:1, C18:2)		Antiviral, antiprotozoan, antibacterial

From Hamosh M. Human milk composition and function in the infant. Semin Ped Gastroenter Nutr 1992;3:4. Reprinted with permission of Decker Periodicals, Inc.

nium, the infant's first stool, and contains the lactobacillus bifidus factor, which facilitates the development of the protective bifidus bacteria in the gut of the young infant. These bacteria limit the growth of **enteropathogenic** organisms and promote the intestinal health of the breastfed infant.

Mature Milk

The nutrient composition of human milk is listed in Table 4–7. Compared to cow milk, mature human milk has a slightly bluish, watery appearance. Its nutritional qualities are especially suited to the needs of the human infant.

Milk from adequately nourished mothers provides approximately 70 kcal per 100 mL of milk, digestible protein, fat, lactose, and adequate levels of vitamins and minerals. Except for fatty acids and vitamins, human milk appears to be relatively independent of the nutritional status of the mother. Maternal undernutrition is more likely to reduce the volume of milk produced than the quantity of a specific component. As illustrated in Table 4–8, the nutrients in milk have more than one function. Recent research indicates that hormones and other bioactive compounds of human milk may aid in development, maturation, and functioning of the physiologic systems of the newborn (Ellis and Picciano, 1992).

Protein

The protein in human milk declines from about 2% in colostrum to 1.3% during the first month of lactation and then to about 0.9 to 1.1% (0.9–1.1 g/100 mL) in mature milk. In human milk whey proteins are dominant; α-lactalbumin makes up the largest single amount of protein in breast milk. Other major whey proteins are lactoferrin and the **immunoglobulin** secretory IgA. Caseins occur only in milk and form large curds when exposed to acid in the stomach. Compared to cow milk, human milk has a low casein content (40% vs 80%) and forms small curds, which are easily digested.

Human milk contains all nine amino acids known to be essential for the human infant in proportion to require-

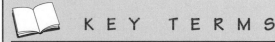

KEY TERMS

meconium: dark green mucilaginous material in the intestine of the newborn

enteropathogenic: *entero*, intestine; *pathogenic*, organism that can be harmful

immunoglobulin: serum globulins that have antibody activity

ments. In fact, the **amino acid pattern** in human milk is used as the reference pattern for formulation of infant formula products (National Research Council, 1989). Compared to cow's milk, human milk is higher in some amino acids that the young infant may not synthesize efficiently, such as cystine, tyrosine, and taurine. The enzymes required for the conversion of methionine to cysteine and phenylalanine to tyrosine develop late in the fetal growth period and may not be at full activity in the neonate, especially the preterm infant. Taurine is present in several body tissues, including fetal brain tissue and bile acids. Because the level is relatively high in human milk, it has been speculated that taurine is of significance in infant nutrition (Sturman, 1988).

Protective Factors

Human milk contains many factors that assist in protecting the infant from infections and viruses (Table 4–9). Many of these factors are relatively resistant to protein digestion and denaturation by the low pH in the stomach. Lactoferrin is an iron-binding protein in milk that reduces the amount of iron available to iron-requiring bacteria in the gastrointestinal tract. The bifidus factor, which promotes "friendly" bacteria, is unique to human colostrum and milk. The suckling infant can be protected by immunoglobulins present in human milk, including IgA, IgG, and IgM. IgA is produced in the mammary gland, but synthesis is probably triggered by **lymphoblasts,** which originate at maternal sites of pathogen exposure, usually the small intestine or respiratory tract.

Secretory IgA (sIgA) is the predominant immunoglobulin in human milk, and specific IgA antibodies protect the infant's gastrointestinal and respiratory tracts from bacteria, viruses, parasites, and fungi, as well as potentially allergenic macromolecules such as food proteins. Other host resistance factors include lysozyme, an anti-infective enzyme, and specific prostaglandins that protect the integrity of the epithelial cells that line the gastrointestinal tract. Lymphocytes in human milk produce the antiviral substance interferon. **Macrophages** in colostrum and mature milk produce **complement,** lactoferrin, lysozyme, and other immune factors.

Lipids

The lipid content of human milk is the major source of energy for the breast-fed infant, providing approximately 50% of the kilocalories in breast milk. The fore milk, that taken from the breast first, is relatively low in fat. Over a nursing period of 10 to 20 minutes there is a gradual increase in the fat content until the last milk (hind milk) has a fat content two to three times that of the fore milk. It is important for a nursing session to be of sufficient length for the infant to consume the high-fat hind milk for satiety and adequate energy for growth. The lipid in human milk is mostly triglyceride but does include phospholipids, cholesterol, and other fats. Human milk contains more essential fatty acids and cholesterol than cow's milk. Higher cholesterol levels may be important to the synthesis of the myelin (a fatlike substance) sheath around certain nerve fibers and may provide stimulus for development of enzymes for cholesterol degradation early in life. In addition to linoleic and linolenic acids, human milk contains the omega-3 fatty acids eicosapentanoic acid and docosahexaenoic acid.

The fatty acid composition of human milk reflects the dietary intake of the mother. If a mother is in negative energy balance and increases mobilization of stored fat for milk synthesis, her milk will reflect the fatty acid composition of depot fat. Human milk contains several lipases, which may be the result of leakage from the mammary tissues. At least one, bile salt–stimulated lipase, is believed to contribute to fat digestion and may partially account for the greater digestibility of fat observed in breast-fed infants. The lipase in human milk may account for the fat breakdown that occurs in expressed breast milk that is refrigerated or frozen for later use.

TABLE 4–9 Protective Factors in Human Milk	
Factor	**Function**
Anti-staphylococcus factor	Inhibits growth of staphylococcal organisms
Bifidus factor	Stimulates growth of bifidobacteria, which antagonizes the survival of enteropathogens
Immunoglobulins: secretory IgA, IgM, IgE, EgD, and IgG	Act against bacterial invasion of the mucosa and/or colonization of the gut.
Interferon	Inhibits intracellular viral replication
Lactoferrin	Iron-binding protein—decreases iron availability for bacterial multiplication
Lactoperoridase	Kills streptococci and enteric bacteria
Lymphocytes	Synthesize secretory IgA
Lysozome	Enzyme that destroys bacteria by breakdown of cell wall
Macrophages	Synthesize lactoferrin, lysozyme; phagocytosis
Vitamin B_{12}–binding protein	Decreases availability of vitamin B_{12} for bacterial growth

Carbohydrate

The carbohydrate in human milk is lactose, which has a positive effect on calcium absorption. If an infant lacks the enzyme required to digest lactose, breast-feeding may be contraindicated or complicated by the need to provide some form of lactase activity.

VITAMINS AND MINERALS In general, breast milk from healthy mothers contains all the infant needs for normal growth. The concentration of major minerals does not appear to be influenced by the mother's diet. The level of fluoride in breast milk is low and varies little, regardless of the level in the water supply. The content of most nutrients will be maintained in breast milk at the expense of maternal reserves. To a greater extent, the vitamin content of human milk is dependent on maternal intake and stores. With poor tissue saturation and chronically low intakes, vitamin levels in human milk, especially of vitamin B_6, B_{12}, A, and D, can be reduced.

Infant Formula

Guidelines to Commercial Formulas

Commercially prepared infant formulas provide an acceptable alternative to breast-feeding. The major goal in preparing human milk substitutes is to formulate an acceptable product that is as nutritionally similar to human milk as possible. The nutrient content of breast milk and several major infant formula products is given in Appendix 5. Guidelines for the minimum amounts of nutrients in commercial infant formulas developed by The Committee on Nutrition of the American Academy of Pediatrics (1993) are found in Appendix 6. The Infant Formula Act of 1980 (Public Law 94-359) gives the Food and Drug Administration the authority to regulate the composition, labeling, and quality assurance of commercial infant formulas sold in the United States. The Act requires that all infant formulas distributed in the United States fall within the limits established by the American Academy of Pediatrics. Infant formulas may be purchased in ready-to-feed bottles (require only the addition of a nipple) or in concentrated liquid and powder preparations diluted with water (boiled or distilled) (Fig. 4–13). These formulas are mixtures of proteins, carbohydrates, emulsified fats, vitamins, and minerals. Most standard infant formulas, like breast milk, have a caloric density of 20 kilocalories per ounce (70 kcal/100 mL).

Protein

The protein levels of most infant formulas range from 1.5 to 2.0 g/100 mL, which is sufficient to promote satisfactory growth in infants if their caloric intake is adequate. The most common source is milk protein or casein or whey proteins. Heat treatment of formulas made with cow's milk produces a smaller, softer curd than pasteurized cow's milk. Recently, infant formulas that contain a whey:casein ratio of 60:40 have been marketed. These proteins have the advantage of forming a smaller curd in the stomach, making them more digestible, and have an amino acid pattern similar to that of breast milk.

Other protein sources for infants intolerant to milk include soy protein and protein hydrolysates (protein partially digested by enzymatic hydrolysis). The hydrolysates are physically or chemically altered proteins, which makes them more digestible and less likely to induce an allergic response. The biologic value of soy protein is somewhat less than that of casein; therefore, these formulas contain slightly greater concentrations of protein. Infants fed soy-based formulas have satisfactory growth and development. The bioavailability of minerals is lower with soy formula than milk-based formulas due to the presence of phytic acid in soy. Increasing the ascorbic acid content or reducing the phytate content improves iron utilization.

Carbohydrate

Lactose, the carbohydrate source in most milk-based formula products, is present in those formulas in amounts similar to that of human milk (4–7 g/100 mL). Several formula products contain corn syrup, sucrose, and modified tapioca starch as their carbohydrate source. The lactose-free characteristic of these formulas make them suitable for feeding infants with gastrointestinal problems that may result from primary or secondary lactase deficiency.

Lipids

In general, formulas contain 45% to 50% of kcal as fat, and the fatty acid profile is designed to be similar to that of human milk. To accomplish this, butter fat is replaced by a

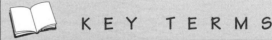

KEY TERMS

amino acid pattern: the amount of individual amino acids present in relation to requirements
lymphoblast: a developing lymphocyte
macrophage: a large cell that engulfs bacteria and other foreign substances
complement: a complex series of enzymatic proteins occurring in normal serum that interact to combine with an antigen–antibody complex, producing lysis when the antigen is an intact cell. Complement includes 11 discrete proteins or 9 functioning components.

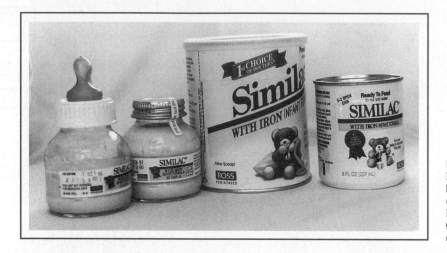

FIGURE 4–13. Infant formula products. Infant formula products include ready-to-eat, bottles, concentrated liquids, and powders. (Used with permission of Ross Products Division, Abbott Laboratories, Columbus, OH 43216. © 1996 Ross Productions Division, Abbott Laboratories.)

variety of vegetable oils, such as palm, soy, corn, coconut, and safflower. These oils, except coconut, are higher in polyunsaturated fatty acids and contain little or no cholesterol. They readily supply linoleic acid, and some formula products also have omega-3 fatty acids added.

Vitamins

The vitamin content of most commercial infant formula products is similar to, or higher than, that of breast milk and, thus, is adequate to meet the requirements of normal healthy infants when they consume approximately 750 mL (26 oz) of formula each day.

Minerals

A calcium-to-phosphorous ratio of 1:1 to 2:1 is suggested for optimal calcium absorption during early infancy. There are both minimum and maximum levels for sodium, potassium, and chloride in formulas. Such levels are sufficient to meet growth needs of the infant while not creating excesses to be excreted by the immature kidney. All formulas contain at least l mg/L of iron, but the American Academy of Pediatrics (1993a) recommends that all formula-fed infants receive iron-fortified formulas that contain 10 to 12 mg/L to prevent iron deficiency. In spite of early concerns about poor tolerance of supplemental iron, there is no evidence that these formulas cause more gastrointestinal problems, such as colic, constipation, diarrhea, or vomiting, than unfortified formulas or that the higher level of iron significantly impairs absorption of other trace minerals (Committee on Nutrition, 1989; Haschke et al, 1993).

Supplementary Food

During the first few months of life, breast milk or iron-fortified infant formula alone provides optimal nutrition for the rapidly growing young infant. As physical and developmental capabilities mature, weaning is begun. Weaning is a developmental process in which semisolid foods are introduced and the composition and consistency of the diet are progressively advanced. Ideally, by 12 months of age the infant is eating a variety of foods from a mixed diet, but breast milk, or formula is the main source of energy and nutrients. Patterns of introduction of supplementary foods should be based on the individual infant's nutritional needs, physiologic maturation, and the development of feeding skills.

Nutritional Needs

By the time the infant is between 4 and 6 months old breast milk or infant formula can no longer meet nutritional needs to support growth. Supplementary foods are introduced initially to provide energy, protein, iron, vitamin C, and, eventually, other nutrients. By the end of the first year of life, solid foods make up one-third to one-half of the infant's dietary intake.

Physiologic Maturation

At birth the kidney performs all its normal functions, but has limited ability to concentrate urine. The functional level of the kidney increases rapidly, so that by 4 months of age the increased solute load of solid foods can be handled, if the foods are introduced gradually. However, additional water should be offered to infants once they begin to receive solid foods.

Adequate enzyme activity and intestinal surface area are essential for efficient digestion and absorption of nutrients in solid foods. In the case of carbohydrate, disaccharidases to digest sugars are readily available at birth in term infants, but salivary and pancreatic amylase levels to hydrolyze starch are low and rise only as infancy progresses. Thus, the young infant has a limited ability to digest starch.

RESEARCH UPDATE
Cow Milk in the Infant Diet

``**M**ilk is for babies,'' or so the old adage goes. But is it? In 1992 the American Academy of Pediatrics recommended that whole cow milk should not replace infant formulas or breast milk in the first 12 months of life (Committee on Nutrition, 1992). Consumption of regular pasteurized cow milk (skin milk or 1% or 2% fat milk) or evaporated milk is associated with several outcomes that make it desirable to withhold cow milk until the second year of life.

Iron Deficiency

Consumption of cow milk during infancy may contribute to iron deficiency. Cow milk contains a low amount of iron which is not very well absorbed. In one study it was observed that infants fed cow milk between 6 and 12 months were at greater risk of iron deficiency than infants who received iron-fortified formulas or iron-fortified cereal (Tunnessen and Oski, 1987). In addition, Ziegler and his coworkers (1990) found that feeding cow milk to normal infants between 6 and 12 months of age resulted in losses of **occult** blood from the gastrointestinal tract, which could contribute to iron deficiency.

Increased Renal Solute Load

Compared to breast- or formula-fed infants, infants fed whole cow milk have higher intakes of protein, calcium, phosphorus, sodium, potassium, and chloride (Ernst et al, 1990). The excess amounts of nitrogenous compounds and minerals must be excreted by the kidneys. Comparisons of dietary intakes of infants consuming cow milk with those receiving formula revealed a renal solute load two to three times greater for those infants consuming cow milk (Martinez et al, 1985). This higher renal solute load requires a larger fluid intake to provide sufficient water for urinary excretion. If fluid needs are not met, the risk of dehydration increases, especially under conditions of fluid loss such as exposure to high environmental temperatures, vomiting, or diarrhea.

Cow Milk Allergy

The most common food allergy in children, which affects 0.4% to 7.5% of infants, is to cow milk protein (Committee on Nutrition, 1992). It is believed that the immature gastrointestinal tract of the infant has increased permeability. Consequently, ingestion of cow milk may result in transfer of intact proteins or peptides, resulting in an allergic response to cow milk. Although more research is needed to define the role of cow milk protein in allergic reactions, delaying introduction of cow milk may result in less sensitivity and, therefore, fewer allergic responses.

Nutrient Content

Infants fed whole cow milk are more likely to have low intakes of iron, linoleic acid, and vitamins E and C compared to formula-fed infants. Milks of reduced fat content—2% or 1% or skim milk—are even more undesirable than whole cow milk during the first year of life because not only do they provide insufficient energy to support growth, they make an even larger contribution to renal solute load and the risk of dehydration. Based on these concerns, recent recommendations are to exclude all forms of regular cow milk from the diet until the infant is 1 year of age (Committee on Nutrition, 1992).

The newborn also has low levels of bile acids and pancreatic lipase and colipase activity to digest and absorb triglycerides. Levels increase significantly during the first months of life, and by 6 months of age, infants can absorb approximately 95% of dietary fat.

Successful adaptation of the infant to the extrauterine environment includes the development of a mucosal barrier against the penetration of harmful substances. At birth many of the intestinal defenses are passive or incompletely developed. Feeding breast milk not only limits the infant's exposure to pathogens and foreign proteins but also provides the stimulus for development of active mechanisms that promote development of a mucosal barrier and eventual readiness for solid foods (Sheard and Walker, 1988).

KEY TERMS

occult: "hidden" blood present in the feces but not readily observable

TABLE 4–10 Developmental Sequence Guide for Nutrition and Feeding During Infancy

Approximate Age	Motor Development	Oral Motor Skills Related to Eating	Self-Help/Social	Food and Appetite
Birth–1 month	Startle (Moro) reflex; minimal head control; hands fisted	Suck and swallow reflex; gag reflex; incomplete lip closure; lip movement in sucking; tongue thrust may be elicited	Looks at people	Breast milk or infant formula
2 months	Head bobs in supported sitting	Weaker suck and swallow reflex	Smiles at people; opens mouth waiting for feeding	
3 months	Head stable; back rounded in sitting; holds toy placed in hands		Anticipates feeding	
4 months	Rolls over to back; head stable and tolerates propped sitting 10–15 min; brings toys to mouth	Tongue thrust present if spoon feeding attempted	Recognizes bottle	
5 months	Back straight in supported sitting; props self on forearms when in prone position; voluntary grasp	Tongue thrust reduced with spoon (may still be seen when cup drinking)	Mouth opens for spoon; brings hands to bottle; knows strangers	Strained, pureed, or blenderized food from spoon
6 months	Pushes up on extended arms in prone position; rolls both ways; briefly sits alone; reach and grasp	Good control with lips and tongue; beginning chewing motion (gumming food); drooling during mouthing	Holds, sucks, and bites cookie	Mashed food without lumps—plain crackers or cookies that are softened by saliva
7 months	Bears weight on legs when held; sits one minute alone; holds one object in each hand	Gag reflex is weaker; makes vowel sounds; attempts to use tongue to move lumps of food	Tries to finger-feed soft food	Mashed but lumpy food by spoon; easily chewed finger foods (large pieces)
8–9 months	Pulls to stand; transfers objects	Cup drinking with improvement in lip control; munching	Recognizes familiar names; fearful of strangers; babbles	Formula or breast milk recommended until end of first year, supplemented with other foods
10–12 months	Cruises, creeps; pincer grasp	Tooth eruption continues; chewing matures; little loss of liquid when cup drinking	Follows simple requests; gestures; plays pat-a-cake; begins to use a spoon	Continued addition of new food with easy-to-chew textures

Developed by Nutrition-Feeding Clinic Faculty, The Nisonger Center University Affiliated Program for Mental Retardation and Developmental Disabilities, The Ohio State University, 1980, Rev. 1995. Work supported in part by U.S. Department of Health and Human Services, Administration on Developmental Disabilities Grant #90DD032902 and Maternal and Child Health Bureau Grant #MCJ399155-04.

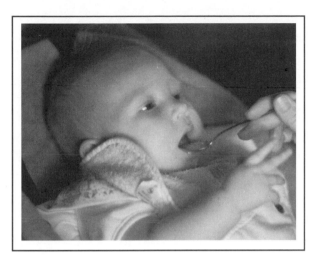

FIGURE 4–14. Adding supplemental foods to the milk diet of the infant depends on developmental readiness.

Infant Feeding Skills

An infant's feeding skills define his or her developmental readiness to progress from nursing to a variety of new foods, textures, and feeding modes. Feeding depends on development of oral, hand-to-mouth, fine motor, body positioning, and communications skills. Table 4–10 outlines typical physical development and corresponding feeding behavior during the first year. As can be seen, by 5 months of age the tongue-extrusion reflex has disappeared, and the infant will accept semi-solid foods placed on the tongue and move them to the back of the mouth for swallowing. Between 5 and 7 months the infant will open her mouth when presented with a spoonful of food and take it from the spoon (Fig. 4–14). By 7 months, the tongue becomes more flexible and the infant can swallow foods with small lumps. The ability to sit without support allows the infant greater ability to manipulate food and to interact during feeding. By 10 months the infant makes definite chewing movements and can take small bites of soft foods. As a pincer grasp develops, the infant begins attempts with self-feeding. By 1 year of age, most infants will accept a variety of foods from all the food groups, can finger feed many foods, and can drink from a cup using two hands.

Introducing the Infant to Solid Foods

The introduction of solid foods to the infant's diet (sometimes called *beikost*) should begin with one single-ingredient food. That food should be given for 3 to 5 days before another is added. Slow introduction gives the infant time to become adjusted to new tastes and permits parents to identify any negative reaction (allergy or intolerance) to a specific food. Repeated dietary exposure to the same food increases acceptance and behavior response to a new food

(Sullivan and Birch, 1994). Table 4–11 outlines foods and amounts appropriate for most babies during the first year. Because iron reserves become depleted at 4 to 6 months, iron-fortified infant cereals mixed with formula or breast milk are added first. The first cereal is usually iron-fortified rice cereal because it is the least **allergenic** cereal. Other cereals are introduced gradually, with wheat and mixed cereals added last. Single strained fruits, vegetables, meats, and egg yolks are other early food choices. Combination foods such as strained cereal with fruit, vegetables with meat, and meat-based dinners may be introduced after single-ingredient foods are well tolerated. Fresh, bottled, or frozen fruit juices are a good source of vitamin C and should be offered once the infant is able to drink from a cup.

The first teeth begin to erupt at about 5 to 6 months. The infant should be given foods that develop the ability to chew. Finger foods should be offered as the infant develops hand and motor skills. Appropriate foods should be selected for ease of handling and chewing without increasing the potential for choking and aspiration (Table 4–12).

Over time a pattern of intake begins to evolve, and gradually the infant's consumption of major nutrient sources centers around family meals, with snacks supporting the overall diet. Diet choices should emphasize foods in the food guide pyramid. Strained and junior desserts and fruit-flavored drinks provide calories and few nutrients; therefore, their use should be limited. Egg whites should be avoided during the first 12 months to minimize the possibility of an allergic reaction.

Some foods are inappropriate for infants even toward the end of the first year. Babies and even young children have difficulty swallowing foods such as popcorn, whole grapes, corn kernels, hot dogs, nuts, raisins, seeds, and potato chips. Honey should never be fed to infants because of the risk of **botulism**.

Supplements

Most healthy infants do not require nutrient supplements. The addition of supplemental foods at 4 to 6 months decreases the risk of nutrient deficiencies by di-

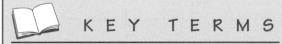

KEY TERMS

allergenic: having the potential to cause a negative reaction in the body due to formation of an antibody in response to a foreign substance (antigen)

botulism: an often fatal illness caused by the ingestion of food containing a toxin produced by *Clostridium botulinum* spores, which grow in improperly canned foods and honey

TABLE 4-11 Suggested Ages for Introduction of Solid Foods

Age	Appropriate Foods	Approximate Amount
0–4 months	Breast milk or iron-fortified formula*	23–29 ounces formula (6–8 feedings a day)
4–6 months†	Breast milk or iron-fortified formula*	26–32 ounces (4–6 feedings a day)
	Iron-fortified infant cereal	1–2 baby spoons 1–2 times a day
	Strained fruits and vegetables	1–2 baby spoons 1–2 times a day
7–9 months††	Breast milk or iron-fortified formula*	24–32 ounces (3–5 feedings a day)
		2–3 tablespoons 2 times a day
	Iron-fortified infant cereal	3–4 ounces a day
	Fruit juice (high in vitamin C)	2–3 tablespoons 2 times a day
	Strained vegetables	2–3 tablespoons 2 times a day
	Strained fruits	1–2 tablespoons 2 times a day
	Strained meats	1–2 tablespoons a day
	Breads, whole-grain or enriched	½–1 serving
10–12 months	Breast milk or iron-fortified formula*	24–32 ounces (3–4 feedings a day)
	Iron-fortified infant cereal	2–4 tablespoons 2 times a day
	Fruit juice (high in vitamin C) in a cup	3–4 ounces a day
	Chopped vegetables (table food)	3–4 tablespoons 2 times a day
	Chopped fruits (table food)	3–4 tablespoons 2 times a day
	Chopped meats (table food)	2–3 tablespoons 2 times a day
	Bread and bread products	½–1 serving a day

* The American Academy of Pediatrics recommends iron fortified formulas for all formula fed infants.
† Infants consuming solid foods should be offered water daily.
†† After 6 months of age, recommendations may be met by using combination foods.

Adapted from Konstant LC et al. Healthy mothers/healthy babies. Volunteer Instructor Guide. Columbia, MO: The Curators of the University of Missouri, 1985.

TABLE 4-12 Some Appropriate Foods for Infant Self-Feeding

Fruits	Soft, fresh or canned, unsweetened, such as bananas, peeled apples, apricots, peaches, or pears
Vegetables	Tender pieces of cooked vegetables such as carrots, potatoes, green beans, summer squash, yellow squash, sweet potatoes
Dairy	Cubes or slices of milk cheese, cottage cheese
Meat, Poultry, Fish	Small, tender pieces of cooked chicken, turkey, or white flaky fish without bones; ground meat such as meat balls, pieces of hamburger patty, or meatloaf
Bread/Cereals	Toast, plain unsalted crackers, teething biscuits, individual cereal pieces
Other	Plain wafer cookies

versifying dietary sources. Nevertheless, about one-third to one-half of infants in the 6- to 12-month age group are given nutrient supplements (Curtis, 1990).

Nutrient supplements may be appropriate in some circumstances. Because the concentration of vitamin D in human milk is low and inconsistent, breast-fed infants may need supplemental vitamin D if the mother and infant have limited exposure to sunlight. Fluoride is considered essential in human nutrition to confer maximal resistance to dental caries. Fluoride supplements are recommended for infants over 6 months if the water supply contains fluoride at a concentration less than 0.3 ppm (American Academy of Pediatrics, 1995).

Full-term exclusively breast-fed infants usually maintain adequate iron status during the first 6 months of life due to mobilization of fetal iron stores and the high absorbability of the iron in human milk. After that time, infants should receive additional iron. If breast-feeding continues, iron-fortified cereals should be added to prevent iron deficiency. Exclusively breast-fed infants of mothers who include no animal products in their diets may require a supplement of vitamin B_{12}. If the infant is weaned to a soy-based commercial infant formula, that formula will contain vitamin B_{12}.

NUTRITION-RELATED CONCERNS DURING INFANCY

■ What is nonorganic failure to thrive and what are its causes?

■ Iron deficiency is a public health problem in North America, but the incidence among infants and young children has been declining. Why?

■ What is baby bottle tooth decay and how can it be prevented?

■ Why is it important to decrease the potential for food allergies during infancy?

■ Why are there concerns about chronic diseases during infancy, and how should they be addressed?

Undernutrition

Failure to Thrive

Failure to thrive (FTT) is a deceleration of growth or growth failure. In the United States, FTT affects up to 10% of children seen in outpatient clinics and accounts for 1% to 5% of all pediatric hospitalizations (Accardo, 1982). The major characteristic of FTT is decreased growth rate. Body weight is affected more than linear growth, especially in infants. Approximately 7% of FTT infants may experience severe **wasting**. **Stunting** is less frequent, depending on the timing, duration, and severity of the nutritional inadequacy.

An infant who has a specific disease or disorder that leads to FFT, such as central nervous system damage, malabsorption, infections or heart disease, is said to have an organic cause (OFFT). However, most cases of FFT appear to be due to factors that are primarily external to the infant. This, called nonorganic failure to thrive (NFTT), is characterized by a syndrome of a low rate of gain in weight and/or length, social and developmental delays, abnormal behavior, and distorted caretaker–infant interactions.

The inadequate food intake and poor growth and development of NFTT often occur in an environment of poverty, dysfunctional relationships, inadequate education, and a dearth of developmentally enriching experiences. NFTT can be related to inadequate knowledge of nutrition and the feeding process as well as erroneous beliefs about infant needs. A disturbance in maternal–infant attachment or in separation/individualization by the infant may lead to food refusal (Chatoor and Eagan, 1983). Counseling of parents and caretakers of NFTT infants may require interaction among social worker, physician, nurse, and dietitian to correct the disordered feeding relationship and to improve nutrition.

Failure to thrive in breast-fed infants may have a nutritional basis due to an inadequate supply of maternal milk. Motil and co-workers (1994) reported a case of a mother whose restricted fat intake appeared to result in "reduced lactation performance" and a decreased growth rate in her infant (Fig. 4–15). A recent report described eight cases of NFTT associated with infants' excessive consumption of fruit juice, which displaced more calorie- and nutrient-dense foods and also caused malabsorption due to the large amounts of fructose and sorbitol consumed (Smith and Lifshitz, 1994).

Iron Deficiency

Iron deficiency affects at least 20% to 25% of the world's babies. In the United States, iron deficiency is most common in infants and children between 6 months and 3 years of age. The prevalence of anemia among low-income children in public health programs is 21% for 1- to 2-year-olds and 10% for those between 3 and 4 years of age. The Healthy People 2000 Objective target is to re-

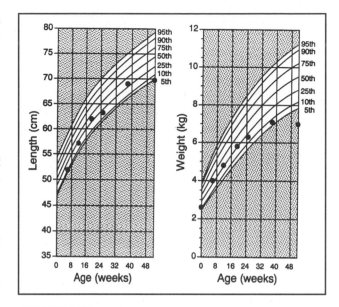

FIGURE 4–15. Length and weight measurements in a breast-fed infant with failure to thrive. (From Motil KJ, et al. Case report: Failure to thrive in a breast-fed infant is associated with maternal dietary protein and energy restriction. J Am Coll. Nutr 1994;13:203.)

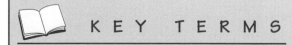

wasting: a greater deficit in weight relative to length
stunting: deficit in length

duce the incidence of iron deficiency among these children by 50%. The incidence of iron deficiency in children has declined somewhat. Contributing factors include increased use of iron-fortified formulas and iron-fortified cereals, which has been enhanced by participation in the Women, Infants and Children (WIC) supplemental food program (Pediatric Nutrition Surveillance System, 1992). The WIC Program is discussed in the Application at the end of Chapter 9.

Iron deficiency during infancy is associated with anorexia, irritability, and lack of interest in surroundings, and can eventually impair growth and development. Infants with iron deficiency perform more poorly on tests of mental and motor development than age-matched, iron-sufficient counterparts. Iron deficiency among infants is of substantial concern because behavior and learning deficits may persist even if iron deficiency is corrected. A 5-year follow-up of children who had had iron deficiency anemia during infancy found that they had lower scores on tests of mental and motor functioning at school entrance than children who were not iron deficient as infants, even though the children had excellent hematologic status and growth at 5 years of age (Lozoff et al, 1991).

Baby Bottle Tooth Decay

Baby bottle tooth decay (BBTD), formerly called the nursing bottle caries syndrome, is a form of rampant tooth decay that affects upper front teeth (incisors) and often the cheek surface of primary upper first molars (Fig. 4–16). Occurring before the age of 2 years, BBTD has its origins in infant feeding practices, specifically with prolonged, inappropriate bottle feeding—i.e., the infant being allowed to fall asleep with a nursing bottle in his or her mouth.

The major dietary factor contributing to BBTD is fre-quent and prolonged exposure of teeth to liquids containing sugars, such as fruit juice and sweetened drinks, as well as milk and formula. Reduced flow of saliva during sleep permits extended exposure of the teeth to a solution that is fermented by plaque-forming microorganisms in the mouth. Acid produced in this fermentation can damage the enamel layer of the newly erupted teeth and lead to dental decay.

BBTD is totally preventable. Contact of the teeth with baby bottle contents can be reduced by not using the bottle as a pacifier and not allowing the infant to fall asleep with a bottle in his or her mouth. A second part of prevention is reducing sugar content of beverages in the nursing bottle. Juices and liquids other than milk or formula should be offered in a cup. Prevention of BBTD is important because once decay occurs, treatment involves extensive and expensive restoration of teeth or extraction of teeth. The Healthy People 2000 Number target is to increase the percentage of parents and caregivers who use feeding practices to prevent BBTD from 55% to 75%.

Allergic Reactions to Food

Food allergies and intolerances are discussed in Chapter 6. They are mentioned here because infant feeding practices involve introduction of food proteins, some of which may induce a food allergy in susceptible infants. Food allergy or hypersensitivity is an immune system–mediated response to dietary **antigens**. Antigenic constituents of cow milk protein, soy protein, or other solid foods may result in negative reactions such as hay fever, asthma, wheezing, vomiting, and dermatitis.

The process by which dietary antigens trigger an immune-mediated reaction is complex and incompletely understood. Factors that influence the immune response include genetic predisposition, the amount of antigen

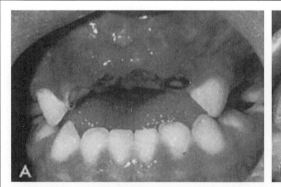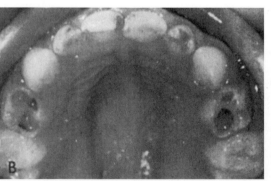

FIGURE 4–16. Baby bottle tooth decay. (From Johnsen D, Nowjack-Raymer R. Baby bottle tooth decay [BBTD]: issues, assessment, and an opportunity for the nutritionist. Copyright The American Dietetic Association. Reprinted by permission from Journal of the American Dietetic Association, 89:1113, 1989.)

introduced, infant's age at the time of exposure to the antigen, maternal immunity, and development of the intestinal mucosal barrier. Determining that adverse reactions are, in fact, immune-mediated responses is often difficult, as is identifying infants at risk for the development of immune-mediated reactions to dietary antigens. Current indicators of risk are increased IgE (one of five classes of immunoglobulins or antibodies) concentrations in cord blood and a parental history of allergy.

Food allergies, particularly to cow milk protein, can occur in some infants. Avoidance of food antigens may have a protective effect in the development of an allergy. Human milk and formulas based on hydrolysates of casein and whey protein are recommended for infants considered at risk for cow's milk protein allergy. Delaying the introduction of solid foods until at least 6 months of age is recommended for these infants. Even greater care must be given in offering new foods gradually and in small portions. Several days should elapse between the introduction of each new food to allow time to recognize whether symptoms of sensitivity appear.

Several investigators have explored manipulation of the maternal diet to prevent the development of food hypersensitivities in infants. Early studies suggested that elimination of highly allergenic foods from the mother's diet during pregnancy and lactation (Chandra et al, 1986) had a protective role for the prevention of allergic responses in the infant. More recently, researchers have failed to show that elimination diets during pregnancy provide any preventive effect (Faith-Magnusson and Kjellman, 1992), and it appears that favorable effects previously reported are due to dietary restrictions during lactation (Sigurs et al, 1992; Arshad et al, 1992). However, not all infants appear to be protected by maternal dietary changes, and the most effective way to reduce allergic responses may be by delaying introduction of cow milk and other potential antigens.

Development of Chronic Diseases

A relationship between specific infant feeding practices and the development of chronic diseases such as obesity, cardiovascular disease, or diabetes mellitus in later life has been much discussed but remains to be established.

Obesity

Breast-fed infants gain weight more slowly than formula-fed infants after the first few months of life. As a result, it has been suggested that breast-feeding may prevent obesity, although there is currently no definitive evidence in support of this theory. There is also little evidence to support a link between excessive weight gain and formula feeding or the early introduction of solid foods.

The lack of a consistent effect of infant feeding practices

on later development of obesity may be related to the many factors that contribute to obesity, particularly heredity and other energy expenditure. For example, Roberts and her coworkers (1988) found that rapid weight gain during infancy and overweight at the age of 1 year were related to reduced energy expenditure and maternal overweight rather than to infant dietary patterns. Body weight during infancy has little relationship to childhood or adult obesity. A recent study investigated feeding practices of more than 300 infants and their relationship to two measures of adiposity—body mass index and the sum of fatfold thicknesses—at 4 years of age (Zive et al, 1992). These researchers found no associations between any of the infant feeding variables, duration of breast-feeding, or introduction to solids and the measures of adiposity.

Cardiovascular Disease

The American Academy of Pediatrics (Committee on Nutrition, 1992) and the National Cholesterol Education Program Expert Panel on Blood Cholesterol Levels in Children and Adolescents (1991) generally agree that diets for infants and children under 2 years of age should not be restricted in kilocalories, fat, or cholesterol. A positive approach involves feeding infants a variety of nutritious foods in response to their appetites.

Unfortunately, some parents restrict their infants' dietary intakes because of concern for subsequent risk of obesity or other health problems. In some instances, such restrictions have been so extreme that the infant or child developed failure to thrive because the diet provided insufficient energy and micronutrients to support normal growth (Pugliese et al, 1987).

Increased blood cholesterol levels are well-documented risk factors for coronary vascular disease. Evidence that the atherosclerotic process begins in childhood has led to concern about a potential role of early dietary habits in the development of coronary artery disease. Human milk is rich in cholesterol, fat, and saturated fatty acids. Infants who are exclusively breast-fed have blood cholesterol levels that are somewhat higher than those of formula-fed infants. A recent study that used stable isotope determination to measure cholesterol synthesis in infants found that an infant who was fed human milk containing approximately 14 mg cholesterol per dL had the lowest level of cholesterol synthesis, compared to infants fed formulas

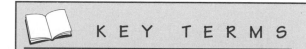

antigen: a foreign protein substance which, in the body, results in formation of an immune response such as antibodies

that contained little or no cholesterol as a result of the replacement of butterfat with vegetable oil or soy formulas with no sources of cholesterol (Cruz et al, 1994).

Serum lipid levels will reflect the fat content of the infant's diet (Fuchs et al, 1994), however, and blood cholesterol levels of children and young adults are not all that different, whether they were formula- or breast-fed as infants (Hamosh, 1988). Although there may be some relationship between early feeding and blood cholesterol levels in later life and the potential of coronary heart disease, there is little evidence to support making changes in the infant's diet (Hardy and Kleinman, 1994).

CONCEPTS TO REMEMBER

▶ Infancy is a period of high nutritional need to support rapid growth and development.

▶ An infant will double his birth weight by 5 months and triple it by 1 year of age. Stature increases approximately 50% during the first 12 months of life.

▶ Per kilogram of body weight, the energy and protein needs of infants are more than twice those of adults.

▶ Because growth is rapid during infancy, nutritional status can be monitored by increases in weight, length, and head circumference.

▶ Due to rapid growth, an infant is more vulnerable to nutritional inadequacies than other age groups.

▶ Breast-feeding is recommended for infants because of the nutritional and immunologic properties of human milk.

▶ Successful infant feeding depends on establishing a social relationship between the infant and mother or primary caregiver.

▶ During the first 4 to 6 months of life, nutritional needs of infants can be met by breast milk or suitable infant formula. To meet nutritional needs after 4 to 6 months, the breast milk or formula diet of the infant is augmented by supplementary foods, starting with iron-fortified infant cereals and gradually progressing to vegetables, fruits, and meats.

▶ Successful introduction of supplementary foods depends on the infant's nutritional needs, physiologic maturation, and developmental readiness.

References

Accardo PJ. Failure to thrive in infancy and early childhood: a multidisciplinary team approach. Baltimore: University Park Press, 1982.

American Academy of Pediatrics. Pediatric Nutrition Handbook. Elk Grove Village, IL: American Academy of Pediatrics, 1993a.

American Academy of Pediatrics. Vitamin K Ad Hoc Task Force. Controversies concerning vitamin K and the newborn. Pediatrics 1993b;91: 1001.

American Academy of Pediatrics. Committee on Nutrition. Fluoride supplementation for children: interim policy recommendations. Pediatrics 1995;95:777.

Arshad SH, et al. Effect of allergen avoidance on development of allergic disorders in infancy. Lancet 1992;339:1493.

Butte NF, et al. Energy requirements of breast-fed infants. J Am Coll Nutr 1991;10:190.

Centers for Disease Control and Prevention. Hyponatremic seizures among infants fed with commercial bottled drinking water. MMWR 1994;43:641.

Chandra RK, et al. Influence of maternal antigen avoidance during pregnancy and lactation on incidence of atopic eczema in infants. Clin Allergy 1986;16:563.

Chatoor I, Egan J. Nonorganic failure to thrive and dwarfism due to food refusal: A separation disorder. J Am Acad Child Psychiatry 1983;22:294.

Committee on Nutrition, American Academy of Pediatrics. Iron-Fortified infant formulas. Pediatrics 1989;84:1114.

Committee on Nutrition. American Academy of Pediatrics. Statement on cholesterol. Pediatrics 1992;90:469.

Committee on Nutrition. American Academy of Pediatrics. The use of whole cow's milk in infancy. Pediatrics 1992;89:1105.

Cruz MI, et al. Effects of infant nutrition on cholesterol synthesis rates. Pediatr Res 1994;35:135.

Curtis DM. Infant nutrient supplementation. J Pediatr 1990;117:S110.

Dagnelie PC, et al. High prevalence of rickets in infants on macrobiotic diets. Am J Clin Nutr 1990;51:202.

Dewey KG, et al. Growth of breast-fed infants deviates from current reference data: a pooled analysis of U.S., Canadian and European data sets. Pediatrics 1995;96:495.

Ellis LA, Picciano MF. Milk-borne hormones: regulators of development in neonates. Nutrition Today, Sept/Oct, 1992.

Ernst JA, et al. Food and nutrient intake of 6- to 12-month-old infants fed formula or cow milk: A summary of four national surveys. J Pediatr 1990;117:S86.

Faith-Magnusson K, Kjellman N-I M. Allergy prevention by maternal elimination diet during late pregnancy—A 5-year follow-up of a randomized study. J Allergy Clin Immunol 1992;89:709.

Fomon SJ. Requirements and recommended dietary intakes of protein during infancy. Pediatrics 1991;30:391.

Fuchs GJ, et al. Effect of dietary fat on cardiovascular risk factors in infancy. Pediatrics 1994;93:756.

Graham SM, et al. Long-term neurologic consequences of nutritional vitamin B_{12} deficiency in infants. J Pediatr 1992;121:710.

Hamosh M. Human milk composition and function in the infant. Seminars in Pediatric Gastroenterology and Nutrition 1992;3:4.

Hardy SC, Kleinman RE. Fat and cholesterol in the diet of infants and young children: implications for growth, development and long-term health. J Pediatr 1994;125:S69.

Haschke F, et al. Iron nutrition and growth of breast- and formula-fed infants during the first 9 months of life. J Pediatr Gastroenterol Nutr 1993;16:151.

Hendricks KM, Badruddin SH. Weaning recommendations: The scientific basis. Nutr Rev 1992;50:125.

Lampl M, et al. Saltation and stasis: a model of human growth. Science 1992;258:801.

Lowery GH. Growth and development of children. 8th ed. Chicago: Year Book Medical Publishers, 1986.

Lozoff B, et al. Long-term developmental outcome of infants with iron deficiency. N Engl J Med 1991;325:687.

Martinez GA, et al. Nutrient intakes of American infants and children fed cow's milk or infant formula. Am J Dis Child 1985;139:1010.

Moffatt ME, et al. Prevention of iron deficiency and psychomotor decline in high-risk infants through use of iron-fortified infant formula: a randomized clinical trial. J Pediatr 1994;125:527.

Motil KJ, et al. Case report: Failure to thrive in a breast-fed infant is associated with maternal dietary protein and energy restriction. J Am Coll Nutr 1994;13:203.

National Center for Health Statistics. NCHS growth charts, 1976. Monthly Vital Statistics Report, vol 25, no 3, suppl (HRA) 76:1120. Rockville, MD; Health Resources Administration, 1976.

National Cholesterol Education Program. Report of the Expert Panel on Blood Cholesterol Levels in Children and Adolescents. National Institutes of Health Publication N4LB1. Rockville, MD: U.S. Department of Health, Education and Welfare, 1991.

National Research Council. Recommended dietary allowances. 10th ed. Washington, DC: National Academy Press, 1989.

Pediatric Nutrition Surveillance System—United States, 1980–1991. MMWR 1992;41:557.

Pugliese MT, et al. Parental health beliefs as a cause of nonorganic failure to thrive. Pediatrics 1987;80:175.

Roberts SB, et al. Energy expenditure and intake in infants born to lean and overweight mothers. N Engl J Med 1988;318:461.

Roche AF, et al. Weight and recumbent length from 1 to 12 months of age: reference data for 1-month increments. Am J Clin Nutr 1989;49:599.

Satter E. The feeding relationship: Problems and interventions. Pediatrics 1990;117:S181.

Sheard NF, Walker WA. The role of breast milk in development of the gastrointestinal tract. Nutr Rev 1988;46:1.

Sigurs N, et al. Maternal avoidance of eggs, cow's milk and fish during lactation: Effect on allergic manifestations, skin-prick tests and specific IgE antibodies in children at age 4 years. Pediatrics 1992;89:735.

Smith M, Lifshitz F. Excess fruit juice consumption as a contributing factor in nonorganic failure to thrive. Pediatrics 1994;93:438.

Sturman JA. Taurine in development. J Nutr 1988;118:1169.

Sullivan SA, Birch LL. Infant dietary experience and acceptance of solid foods. Pediatrics 1994;93:271.

Tunnessen WW, Oski FA. Consequences of starting whole cow milk at 6 months of age. J Pediatr 1987;111:813.

Walter R, et al. Effectiveness of iron-fortified infant cereal in prevention of iron deficiency. Pediatrics 1993;91:876.

World Health Organization (WHO). Energy and protein requirements: Report of a joint FAO/WHO/UNU expert consultation. Technical Report Series 725. Geneva: World Health Organization, 1985.

Ziegler, EE, et al. Cow milk feeding in infancy: Further observations on blood loss from the gastrointestinal tract. J Pediatr 1990;116:11.

Zive MM, et al. Infant-feeding practices and adiposity in 4-year-old Anglo- and Mexican-Americans. Am J Clin Nutr 1992;55:1104.

Additional Resources

Cohen RJ, et al. Determinants of growth from birth to 12 months among breast-fed Honduran infants in relation to age of introduction of complementary foods. Pediatrics 1995;96:504.

Fairweather-Tait F. Bioavailability of iron in different weaning foods and the enhancing effect of a fruit drink containing ascorbic acid. Pediatr Res 1995;37:389.

Gaull GE, et al. Pediatric dietary lipid guidelines. A policy analysis. J Am Coll Nutr 1995;14:411.

Lanting CI, et al. Neurological differences between 9-year-old children fed breast-milk or formula-milk as babies. Lancet 1994;344:1319.

Lapinieimu H, et al. Prospective randomised trial in 1062 infants of diet low in saturated fat and cholesterol. Lancet 1995;345:471.

Lozoff B. Iron deficiency and infant development. J Pediatr 1994;125:577.

APPLICATION: Foods for Infants: The Supermarket

Nutrition Facts		
Serving Size 1/4 cup (15 g)		
Serving Per Container About 30		

Amount Per Serving		
Calories 60		

Total Fat		1 g
Sodium		0 mg
Potassium		50 mg
Total Carbohydrate		10 mg
Fiber		1 g
Sugars		0 g
Protein		2 g

	Infants	Children
% Daily Value	0-1	1-4
Protein	7%	6%
Vitamin A	0%	0%
Vitamin C	0%	0%
Calcium	15%	10%
Iron	45%	60%
Vitamin E	15%	8%
Thiamin	45%	30%
Riboflavin	45%	30%
Niacin	25%	20%
Phosphorus	15%	10%

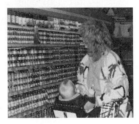

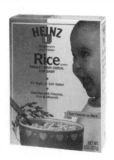

In the early months of life, the infant usually receives a diet consisting of human milk or a commercial formula product with a macro- and micronutrient composition that resembles human milk. Under the Infant Formula Act, the Food and Drug Administration regulates the composition, labeling, and quality assurance of commercial infant formula. To protect the highly vulnerable infant, these products are among the most highly regulated and controlled of all commercially available foods (Fomon, 1987). The introduction of supplementary foods is recommended at 4 to 6 months of age.

In 1942, baby foods were classified as foods for special dietary use under the Federal Food, Drug and Cosmetic Act (Filer, 1993). Under current labeling regulations, labels on foods designated for infants will use the Nutrition Facts format but the information provided is different. A sample food label appears in the margin. Serving sizes are based on average amounts that infants under 2 years of age would consume at one time. Because the current recommendation is that the fat content of an infant's diet should not be restricted, the label lists total calories and total fat, carbohydrate, sodium, and protein per serving but not the distribution of calories from fat, saturated fat, or cholesterol content. The food label for infants (birth to 1 year) and children (under 4 years) lists percentages of the Daily Value for protein, vitamins, and minerals, but does not include daily values for fat, cholesterol, sodium, potassium, carbohydrate, and fiber because they have not been established for children under 4 years of age. Label information is designed to assist the parent or caregiver in making decisions about which foods to purchase to ensure a safe and nutritious diet for the infant.

The milk or formula diet is gradually expanded to include single-ingredient foods, beginning with cereal, then moving on to fruits, vegetables, juice and meats. Eventually the diet will include combination foods and selections from all food groups. An enormous variety of foods for infants is available in the market today. In fact, a stroll down the aisle of any supermarket where baby foods are displayed reveals a confusing array of choices. Variety, balance, and moderation are as applicable to planning the infant's diet as they are to planning for older individuals. Careful selection from available infant foods can provide nutritious, economical diets. Milk is the mainstay of the diet at this time, and other foods are truly supplementary.

Most of the commercial infant food products available in the market today are designed to parallel current feeding recommendations. Textures range from strained to chunky. To assist consumers, foods designed for the first year of life are divided into stages 1, 2, or 3. The designation is displayed on the label to guide the parent in selection of an appropriate level of foods.

Infants generally are ready for stage 1 foods when they have doubled their birth weight, have good control of head movements, can sit with support, and can swallow a spoonful of pureed food easily. Foods in Stage 1, often referred to as "first foods," are single-ingredient foods. The first foods introduced are infant cereals, which are enriched with iron, thiamin, riboflavin, niacin, calcium, and phosphorus. Dry infant cereals do not need cooking. They are mixed with breast milk or formula to a semi-liquid consistency and fed from a spoon. As the baby learns to swallow, the cereal can be made thicker.

Some mothers introduce cereals before 4 months by making a thinner mixture and putting it in the nursing bottle (Solen et al, 1992). This practice is undesirable, however, because it is not necessary to meet the nutrient needs of most young infants and because it increases the potential for choking and for development of food allergies. Ready-prepared cereal in jars is available, but it is more costly than dry baby cereal and requires refrigeration after opening. Once cereals have been accepted and tolerated by the infant, other "first foods," single fruits and vegetables, are offered. These are usually packaged in 2.5-ounce jars.

Fruit juices enriched with vitamin C are usually offered as the infant adjusts to stage 1 foods. Juices for infants are available from single fruits and combinations of fruits and are categorized as stage 1, 2, or 3. Fruit juices should be unsweetened and should be offered from a cup. Four-ounce bottles are sold as singles or in six-packs. Larger bottles ranging in size from 25 to 32 ounces are also available.

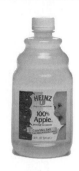

Introduction of stage 2 foods is appropriate when the infant has tried a variety of single-ingredient foods, sits well without support, eats easily from a spoon, and has begun to drink from a cup. The selection of foods designated as stage 2 is much larger. "Second" foods are to be offered to infants from about 6 months of age, after the infant has adapted to "first foods" in the diet. While these foods are still pureed or strained, they have a thicker consistency than "first foods" and, except for meats, are marketed in larger jars (usually 4 ounces). Stage 2 foods include single-item fruits and vegetables as well as combination foods such as mixtures of fruits, vegetables, and mixed dinners. Mixed dinners are available in a variety of food combinations, from turkey with vegetables to beef and macaroni. Strained meats for this stage are in 2.5-oz jars. Puddings and desserts are also available and may be appropriate to include in the diet occasionally. It should be remembered that throughout the first year of life, milk still constitutes a major portion of the diet.

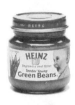

Stage 3 foods are suitable for infants from about 9 months of age who sit alone easily, can handle finely chopped foods, can drink from a cup, and have begun some self-feeding. Foods at this stage include all the foods offered in stage 2 but in greater variety and, in some cases, in larger jars (6 ounces). The mixtures are more complex in consistency and require more chewing than stage 2 foods. Formerly such foods may have been called "junior" foods. Stage 3 food may not be used for many older infants because the infant will move instead to mashed and finely chopped table foods. Table foods are suitable at this age if the consistency is such that the infant can gum and swallow them with ease and seasoning is moderate.

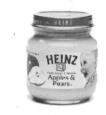

Additional food items, some more advanced than Stage 3, are marketed under various names and may be convenient substitutes for table foods in late infancy and the early toddler period. The consistency of these products is appropriate for use of a spoon, and the pieces are sized for easy chewing and swallowing. They may be in 6-ounce jars, and many come in 6-ounce containers with plastic replaceable lids. They are lower in salt, spices, and seasonings than similar adult foods. Once opened, these products need to be refrigerated promptly to control bacterial growth and should be discarded within 2 days if not used. Additional foods marketed for older infants include desserts, crackers, and finger foods.

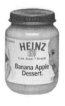

Labels on infant food products must list all ingredients in the product. Virtually all infant foods are prepared without added sodium or monosodium glutamate, most are prepared without flavor or color enhancers, and many are prepared without added sugar. If any of these food additives are present, they must be listed on the label as illustrated in the margin. Ingredients are listed on the product label in the order of greatest presence in the food. Therefore, if water is the first ingredient listed on the label, as in the banana pudding, water is present in the greatest amount. The mixed dinner, often considered a protein source, has three ingredients, including water, that are present in greater quantity than beef, the protein source. This information on the label can assist parents in selecting foods of high nutrient value. It should be remembered, however, that similar foods can be prepared from the family's foods at lesser cost.

ingredients on label of **banana pudding:** water, bananas, high fructose corn syrup (nutritional sweetener), egg yolks, food starch-modified (from corn), modified tapioca starch, citric acid, vitamin C (ascorbic acid)

Commercial infant foods are a convenient, time-efficient, although somewhat costly, means to provide supplementary foods in the diet of the infant. If choices are made wisely, they can make a nutrient-dense contribution to the diet. Table A4–1 gives an example of such a menu for Erin at 8 months of age. The Nutrition Facts and the list of ingredients on the food label provide information to assist in selection of appropriate foods.

ingredients on label of **macaroni, tomato, beef dinner:**

water, tomato puree, carrots, beef, rice flour, enriched macaroni, dehydrated romano cheese made from cow's milk, soy protein concentrate, onion powder, dehydrated sweet pepper, soy bean oil and extracts of celery and oregano

Home Preparation of Baby Foods

Home-prepared infant foods are an important alternative to commercially prepared foods. Using some of the regular family food can be convenient and economical as well as allowing greater flexibility in altering food consistency. However, families that lack

TABLE A4–1 Typical Intake for an 8-Month-Old Infant

Morning	3 tbsp mixed cereal with formula ½ jar of bananas (2 oz) Formula or breast milk
Midmorning	4-oz jar of peaches
Lunch	4 oz of chicken noodle dinner 2 oz sweet potatoes Formula or breast milk
Midafternoon	4 oz pear juice 3 crackers
Dinner	2.5 oz of turkey 4 oz of mixed vegetables 4 oz of applesauce Formula or breast milk
Before bed	Formula or breast milk

variety in their diets should be encouraged to supplement home-prepared foods with commercial foods to achieve a balanced diet. Home preparation of infant foods is not appropriate in homes that lack adequate facilities for refrigeration and freezing or those that have poor sanitation. Home-grown foods should not be prepared for infants if there is any question regarding the lead concentration of the soil in residential areas. Arrangements to test the lead content of soil can be made through the local health department.

Foods to be fed to infants can be prepared by steaming, roasting or broiling, microwave cooking, or boiling. Equipment for preparation can be as simple as a strainer and a blender or a baby food mill that can be used to achieve the desired consistency. If the family's foods are prepared with salt, spices, sugar, or fat, the infant's food should be prepared separately or the baby's portion removed from the family's food before seasonings are added.

Foods that are pureed, ground, or creamed can provide a medium for bacterial growth. Thus, home-prepared infant foods need to be used promptly or stored immediately in the refrigerator or freezer. The practice of freezing infant-size portions in ice cube trays allows thawing of serving sizes when needed. Infant foods should be stored in the refrigerator no more than 2 days. Warming the food to a temperature for feeding creates an ideal environment for bacterial growth. Therefore, only the amount the infant will consume at one meal should be warmed, and this should be done just before serving. Any of that serving that is unused should be discarded.

Home preparation of infant foods can be time-consuming but offers an economical way to provide nutritious meals that can be adapted to the developmental level and preferences of the infant. Care needs to be taken to prepare foods only under sanitary conditions and to provide a variety of foods for a balanced diet.

REFERENCES

Filer LJ. Safe foods for infants—the regulation of milk, infant formula and other infant foods. J Nutr 1993;123:285.

Fomon SJ. Reflections on infant feeding in the 1970s and 1980s. Am J Clin Nutr 1987;46:171.

Solen BJ, et al. Infant feeding practices of low-income mothers. J Pediatr Health Care 1992;6:54.

CHAPTER 5

THE HIGH-RISK INFANT

Nutrition Risk Factors
Assessment of Nutrition Status
Nutrient Needs of High-Risk Infants
Feeding the High-Risk Infant
Growth and Developmental Outcome

Medical/Surgical Conditions Complicating
the Nutritional Management
of High-Risk Infants
Special Concerns
Concepts to Remember

Tiffany is 3 months old and weighs 1880 g (4 lb, 2 oz). She was born at 27 weeks gestation and weighed 680 g (1 lb, 8 oz) at birth. Today she will be discharged home from the neonatal intensive care unit at the regional medical center where she has been hospitalized since birth. Her parents have dressed her in a lacy, flowered doll dress and she smiles when the nurses wish her well as she leaves to go home. Her parents choke back tears as they express deep gratitude to the nursery staff. They have spent the three toughest months of their lives making almost daily trips to the hospital.

When Tiffany was born an extremely preterm infant, the odds were against her. But she was a "fighter" who kicked her little legs and twice grasped and removed the ventilator tubing that kept her alive. She remained on the ventilator for the first month of her life. During this time she was fed purified nutrients (parenteral nutrition) infused into one of her larger veins. Tiffany was also started on small quantities of her mother's milk, which her mom had pumped from her breasts. Eventually Tiffany was weaned from the intravenous nutrition and was fed fortified mother's milk by a tube threaded through her mouth and into her stomach.

Tiffany became strong enough to breathe on her own and then began the process of learning to eat on her own. She alternated nipple feeding and tube feeding until she had the maturity and endurance to stay awake and take all of her feedings by nipple. Her mom was also able to breast-feed her.

On her 3-month "birthday," Tiffany could maintain her temperature (while wrapped in a blanket) in a normal room environment. She was also able to breathe on her own and fully nipple or breast-feed (without tube feedings). Her proud parents, nurses, doctors, and other healthcare team members were excited to see her "graduate" from the neonatal intensive care unit and go home.

Contributed by Melody Thompson

■ Define the preterm, low-birthweight infant and describe the factors that place this infant at high nutritional risk.

Infants born before 38 weeks gestation are considered to be **preterm or premature. Low-birthweight (LBW)** infants weigh 2500 grams or less at birth (AAP/ACOG, 1992). Being preterm and/or LBW is associated with an increase in morbidity and mortality when compared with a full-term, normal-weight baby. Thus, preterm and LBW infants are considered to be "high-risk" infants. Advances in the technology of infant intensive care have allowed smaller and smaller babies to survive (Roth et al, 1995). Thus, birth weight categories have been further subdivided to define **very-low-birthweight (VLBW)** infants as those weighing 1500 g or less, and **extremely-low-birthweight (ELBW)** infants as those weighing 1000 g or less (Hay, 1991). Lower birth weight and younger gestational age are associated with higher medical and nutritional risk.

Infants who are preterm are often LBW, but these conditions do not necessarily occur together. Some babies are LBW because they did not grow properly in utero. These babies are small for gestational age (SGA) or have suffered intrauterine growth retardation (IUGR). For example, a 40-weeks gestation baby weighing 2300 g is the product of a mother who smoked 2 packs of cigarettes a day. (Maternal cigarette smoking can have a negative effect on fetal growth.) This infant may behave like a mature infant but have problems related to LBW. On the other hand, preterm babies can be of normal birth weight. For example, a 36-weeks gestation baby weighing 3500 g is the product of a diabetic mother. This baby is considered large for gestational age (LGA) and may have problems related to prematurity but not to birth weight.

In the United States, the incidence of LBW is 7.1% and VLBW is 1.3% of live births (U.S. Department of Health and Human Services, 1994). Preterm and/or LBW infants may require prolonged hospitalization before they are big, strong, and mature enough to be taken care of at home.

NUTRITION RISK FACTORS

High-risk infants are hospitalized to treat their medical or surgical problems. They also need time for nutritional rehabilitation and growth. Several factors put these babies at high nutritional risk.

Limited Nutrient Reserves

The majority of nutrient transfer and fetal weight gain occurs during the third trimester of pregnancy. At this time, the fetus can gain 30 g daily. This transplacental transfer

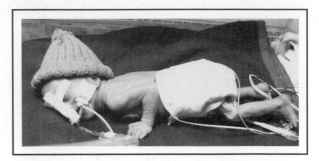

FIGURE 5–1. A 1000-g baby. Note the absence of subcutaneous fat stores.

of nutrients is abruptly interrupted by preterm birth. A striking visual example of this is the absence of subcutaneous fat stores in a tiny preterm baby (Fig. 5–1). Fat is important for thermoregulation, organ support and insulation, and storage of fat-soluble vitamins and essential fatty acids, and, most importantly, as an energy source. Thus, tiny babies are vulnerable to problems caused by inadequate fat stores. They need to be kept in incubators that help to regulate their body temperatures. They need adequate supplies of fat-soluble vitamins and essential fatty acids. And they need exogenous energy sources to help preserve and build their small fat reserves.

Another good example of limited nutrient stores involves calcium. During the third trimester, the placenta is pushing calcium into the fetus against a concentration gradient. Two-thirds of bone mineralization occurs at this time. Thus, a baby born early in the third trimester has undermineralized bones that may be susceptible to fractures unless an adequate mineral intake is insured.

Increased Nutrient Needs

The increase in nutrient needs of high-risk infants relates to inadequate nutrient stores and rapid growth rates. For example, during the third trimester, the fetus receives 130 milligrams per kilogram per day (mg/kg/d) of calcium through the placenta. In order to duplicate this calcium retention rate, a preterm infant must ingest 200 mg/kg/d of calcium, which has an absorption rate of 65% (Koo and Tsang, 1991). In contrast, a full-term, normal-weight infant whose bones are adequately mineralized needs only 60 mg/kg/d of calcium. Adults need only 10 to 20 mg/kg/d of calcium. Providing this high calcium intake to high-risk infants poses clinical challenges to the medical team. Often, these infants receive intravenous (IV) nutrition. Because there are limits to the solubility of minerals in IV solutions, infants are rarely able to receive the minerals they need by this route. When these infants are enterally fed, high-mineral formulas or supplements must be chosen.

Immature Alimentary Tract

Immaturities in the preterm infant's alimentary tract make it difficult to feed this baby by the enteral route. The infant's sucking and/or swallowing are immature and uncoordinated until 32 to 34 weeks gestational age (Lebenthal, 1995). The gastric capacity may limit the amount of formula that is tolerated. For example, a 1500-g infant has a stomach capacity of only 3 milliliters (mL) at birth. By the end of the first week, this infant's gastric capacity is 30 mL, or 2 tablespoons (Groh-Wargo, 1994).

The motor function of the preterm infant's intestinal tract is underdeveloped. Peristaltic waves and segmentation do not propel the food bolus as effectively as they do in mature infants. There may also be enzyme and cofactor immaturities, which may limit digestion and absorption of nutrients. For example, preterm infants have limited amounts of pancreatic lipase and half of the bile acid pool that term infants have (Lebenthal and Leung, 1988). This is thought to limit their ability to handle a normal intake of long-chain triglycerides (LCT). Thus, they are often fed diets containing medium-chain triglycerides (MCT) (Hamosh et al, 1989).

Metabolic Immaturities

Adaptation to extrauterine life requires that high-risk infants regulate their own fluid, electrolyte, and glucose levels. Immature organs may limit their ability to do this effectively. The SGA infant, for example, may have hypoglycemia (low blood sugar) due to inadequate glycogen stores. On the other hand, the LGA infant also may have hypoglycemia, due to the abrupt interruption in glucose supply with birth resulting in relatively high insulin and low glucose levels. Both of these infants require an immediate source of glucose to correct low serum levels and prevent neurologic problems associated with prolonged or profound hypoglycemia (Kliegman, 1993).

Medical Complications/Stresses

Some high-risk infants are born with or develop complications that have an effect on their nutritional status or nutrient needs. Some infants, for instance, are born with their intestines protruding through a defect in the abdominal wall. This condition is called gastroschisis. These edematous and malrotated intestines often function poorly and are too large to fit immediately into the infant's small abdominal cavity. The intestines are suspended in a plastic sheath until the swelling goes down and they fit comfortably in the abdomen. Meanwhile, the infant must be fed completely by the intravenous route. Need for protein may be elevated due to surgical stress and excess losses (Valentine, 1994).

ASSESSMENT OF NUTRITION STATUS

■ What are the elements of nutrition assessment, and how does each element apply to the high-risk infant?

Nutrition assessment of high-risk infants involves the same elements as nutrition assessment of other populations, i.e., anthropometric, biochemical, clinical, and nutrient intake data. Additionally, assessment of the infant's gestational age and size is important.

Determination of Gestational Age and Size for Age

Because the clinical problems of infants differ according to their gestational age and size for age, accurate estimation of gestational age is important. Several methods are used to determine gestational age. If the mother knows the date of her last menstrual period, this can be used to calculate the infant's gestational age. Because this method relies on the mother's memory, it may be subject to error.

Alternatively, gestational age can be estimated by fetal measurements performed during ultrasound examinations early in the pregnancy. Measurements of the fetal head diameter and/or length are compared to established standards to assess the gestational age more accurately.

When the infant is born, physical and neuromuscular examinations are used to assess his or her maturity. For example, muscle flexion is associated with maturity. The more flexed the posture of the baby, the more mature he or she is. Flaccid, extended posture is associated with extreme immaturity. Infants are scored on at least 12 physical and neuromuscular parameters. The summation of the scores correlates with a particular gestational age (Ballard et al, 1979). This examination has recently been standardized for even very immature infants and is considered a reliable estimate of gestational age (Ballard et al, 1991).

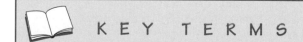

K E Y   T E R M S

preterm/premature: <38 weeks gestation
low-birthweight: ≤2500 grams at birth
very-low-birthweight: ≤1500 grams at birth
extremely-low-birthweight: ≤1000 grams at birth

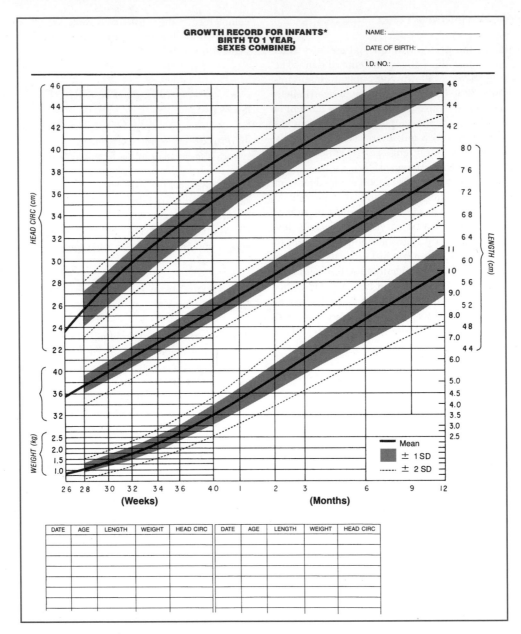

FIGURE 5–2. Intrauterine growth chart used to assess size for gestational age and plot successive growth measurements. (From Babson SG, Benda GJ. Growth graphs for the clinical assessment of infants of varying gestational ages. J Pediatr 1976; 89:814)

In order to assess size for gestational age, the infant's weight, length, and head circumference measurements are plotted on an intrauterine growth chart (Fig. 5–2). If birth weight is less than two standard deviations from the mean, the infant is classified as small for gestational age (SGA). If the birth weight is greater than two standard deviations from the mean, the infant is classified as large for gestational age (LGA).

Anthropometric Assessment

Assessment of weight, length, and head circumference for high-risk infants involves the same techniques used for term infants (see Chapter 4). A few differences may be noted, however. For small babies requiring intensive care, the scale should be accurate to the nearest 5 g. Medical apparatus (e.g., ventilator tubing, IV tubing) must be supported while the baby is removed from the bed and placed on the scale for weighing. Some babies are too unstable to be moved from the bed to the scale. Bed scales are available that allow the babies to remain on scales in their beds for prolonged periods.

Small, plastic length boards are available to measure the lengths of tiny babies. As for larger infants, two people are required to hold the infant's head and feet for accurate measurement. Measurement of head circumference is accomplished as for term infants (see Chapter 4).

High-risk infants are weighed at least once daily. Weight correlates with fluid status and growth. Initially, small babies, like term babies, lose weight with diuresis of extracellular fluid. When fluid status stabilizes and they are provided with adequate calories, they gain weight with tissue growth. Normal weight gain is considered to be 10 to 20 g/kg/d (Shaffer et al, 1987). Weight is one of the most important measurements in the neonatal intensive care unit (NICU). Fluid, calorie, and many other nutrient needs are expressed in terms of the infant's weight.

Length and head circumference are usually measured weekly in the NICU. Expected growth in length is 0.8 to 1.1 cm per week for babies from 28 to 40 weeks gestation. Normal head circumference growth from 28 to 40 weeks gestation is 0.5 to 0.8 cm per week (Crouch, 1994). If abnormal head growth is suspected, the head circumference is measured more frequently.

To assess the infant's progress, anthropometric measurements are plotted regularly on intrauterine growth charts (see Fig. 5–2). It is important to plot the measurements at the correct gestational age. An infant born at 28 weeks gestation who is 2 weeks old chronologically, has a "corrected age" of 30 weeks gestation. When the infant is 12 weeks, or 3 months, old, her corrected age will be "fullterm." Once the infant's corrected age reaches term, it is acceptable to use standard National Center for Health Statistics (NCHS) growth charts to plot the infant's subsequent progress (see Chapter 4).

Skinfold or fatfold measurements are not routinely performed in high-risk infants. The friable skin of tiny babies makes this measurement potentially invasive because skin puncture can occur. Variations in fluid status also make this measurement unreliable. The upper mid-arm circumference and the mid-arm circumference to head circumference ratio reflect muscle and fat stores and the relationship of these stores to brain growth, respectively (Sasanow et al, 1986). Although not routinely taken, these measurements may be used for individual babies.

Biochemical (Laboratory) Assessment

The infant's initial laboratory measurements, if performed shortly after birth, reflect the mother's biochemi-

cal status. Over the first several days of life, blood gases, blood count, and electrolyte measurements are performed in the laboratory to assess the high-risk infant's adaptation to the extrauterine environment. If the infant remains on IV nutrition, laboratory measurements are made several times weekly to monitor the safety and effectiveness of this therapy. Once the infant is stable and few changes are being made in the IV solutions, weekly biochemical assessments are made. Infants who are enterally fed have less frequent biochemical assessments.

An infant's blood volume is approximately 90 mL/kg of body weight (Moyer-Mileur, 1994). Thus, an infant weighing 700 g will thus have a total blood volume of approximately 63 mL. Laboratory testing is minimized, therefore, to preserve the infant's blood volume. When tests are performed, the laboratory uses microtechniques whenever possible. Microtechniques require very small amounts of blood. Often, NICU nurses keep track of how much blood the infant has had withdrawn for various tests. When a certain percentage of blood volume has been removed, a blood transfusion may be given. Blood transfusions are avoided unless absolutely necessary, because donor blood can contain viruses that are then passed to the baby. Blood screening procedures are used to minimize this possibility. Nonetheless, laboratory tests are ordered prudently in the NICU.

The infant's urine is tested by a NICU nurse for pH, specific gravity, blood, and various metabolites. The infant's wet diaper is used for these spot-checks. Urine collections over a number of hours are difficult to perform and are seldom used in the NICU. Urine bags do not adhere well to immature skin, which is damaged in their removal, leaving abraded skin that is susceptible to infection. Thus, tests requiring urine collections, such as creatinine-height index, are not performed for high-risk infants.

Clinical Assessment

Clinical assessment of the high-risk infant involves observing the baby's general condition. Clinical assessment can be supportive of laboratory and anthropometric data in determining the baby's state of hydration, for example. A baby who is **dehydrated** can have sunken eyes and fontanelle, poor skin turgor, decreased urine output, and increased urine specific gravity, as well as elevated laboratory values (hemoconcentration) and weight loss. A baby

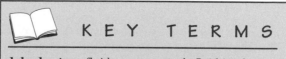

KEY TERMS

dehydration: fluid output exceeds fluid intake

who is **overhydrated** can have dependent edema; puffy hands, feet, and eyes; as well as depressed laboratory values (hemodilution) and excessive weight gain. Clinical signs, observed in concert with other assessment parameters, can be used as a guide for adjusting the infant's therapy.

Feeding tolerance frequently is assessed clinically. The NICU nurse measures the infant's abdominal girth, checks the contents of the infant's stomach, records vomiting or emesis if it occurs, and records the characteristics of the infant's stools. These clinical observations are used to determine if the infant's feedings need to be halted or can be safely advanced.

Intake Assessment

Nutrient intake assessment can be qualitative and quantitative. **Qualitative assessment** involves evaluation of nutrient sources in relation to an infant's needs. Infant formulas contain a variety of nutrient sources. Lactose, the carbohydrate in mammalian milk, is common in many formulas, for example. Because an infant who has galactosemia cannot properly metabolize lactose or galactose, a lactose-free formula is indicated.

Quantitative assessment involves calculating the quantities of nutrients that the infant receives and comparing the results to recommended intakes. The infant's 24-hour intake is often used to perform calculations. Total intakes of fluid, calories, and protein are calculated. For parenterally fed infants, intakes of IV carbohydrate (glucose) and fat are calculated as well. With either enteral or parenteral nutrition, other nutrients may be calculated in addition, depending on the infant's particular problems. Computer programs are available to assist in calculating multiple nutrient intakes for infants who require intensive care (Thompson, 1994).

NUTRIENT NEEDS OF HIGH-RISK INFANTS

■ Why are the needs for fluid, energy, and protein greater for the high-risk infant than they are for the term, healthy infant?

What constitutes optimal nutrient intake and growth in the high-risk infant is unknown and is the subject of some controversy. In 1993 the American Academy of Pediatrics reaffirmed its contention that the goal of nutritional care for preterm infants is to resume growth at an intrauterine rate. Actual growth rates of LBW infants often fall short of this goal. Metabolic and excretory limitations of high-risk infants can preclude resuming intrauterine nutrient accretion and growth. Whether intrauterine-type growth is optimal or better than the slower growth customarily seen remains to be proved (Hay, 1991).

TABLE 5–1 Approximate Fluid Requirements for LBW Infants		
Birth Weight (g)	**Transition (mL/kg/day)**	**Maintenance (mL/kg/day)**
<1000	100	120–160
1000–2000	80	100–140
>2000	60	80–120

From Shaffer SG, Weismann DN. Fluid requirements in the preterm infant. Clin Perinatol 1992;19:239. Used with permission.

In the NICU, nutrient intakes and needs are often expressed as the amount of nutrient per kilogram body weight per day rather than the absolute quantity of the nutrient per day. This expression is necessary because the size of the infants in an NICU varies. A 500-g baby and a 4000-g baby may both require intensive care. The large baby weighs eight times more than the small baby and needs much larger quantities of nutrients. Each baby may grow on 100 kcal/kg/d. For the 500-g baby this is 50 kcal/d, whereas for the 4000-g baby, this is 400 kcal/d. Thus nutrient intakes and needs are often expressed *per kilogram* per day.

Fluid and Electrolytes

Fluid needs are quite variable for high risk neonates. Fluids are lost through urine, stool, respiratory tract, and skin. Small babies lose much fluid (called **insensible water loss**) through their immature skin and respiratory tracts. They may, therefore, need a lot more fluid per kilogram of body weight than a larger baby needs. Fluid needs in the first several days of life (transition) are lower than in the maintenance phase (Table 5–1). A high-risk infant's immature kidneys do not conserve electrolytes as well as those of a mature baby do, so his electrolyte needs are often higher than those of a term baby.

Energy

The high-risk infant needs energy to perform body functions and to grow. Categories of energy expenditure include basal metabolic rate (resting caloric expenditure), activity, cold stress, specific dynamic action (SDA), stool losses, and growth (Table 5–2). The average caloric need for the enterally fed high-risk infant is 120 kcal/kg/d. Because the parenterally fed infant does not use as many calories for activity, cold stress, SDA, or stool losses, the parenterally fed baby may need only 80 to 90 kcal/kg/d (Groh-Wargo, 1987). As in other age groups, calorie needs differ among individuals and must be assessed for each patient in relation to that child's growth and medical problems.

Protein

The high-risk infant needs protein to build and repair body tissues. Smaller babies need to accrete more nitrogen-containing tissue and thus have higher protein needs per kilogram than larger babies do. Infants who weigh less than 2000 g may need 3.5 g protein/kg/d or more (American Academy of Pediatrics Committee on Nutrition, 1993). Parenterally fed preterm infants need 2.5 to 3 g protein/kg/d in the form of crystalline amino acids (Heird et al, 1991). If inadequate energy is supplied, protein will be broken down and used as an energy source. Thus, enough calories must be provided as carbohydrate and fat to "spare" the protein (Jones et al, 1995).

Minerals and Vitamins

Because of their low nutrient stores and high needs for growth, high risk infants often have micronutrient needs that exceed those of term, normal-weight babies. Small infants have particularly high needs for the minerals (calcium and phosphorus) that provide structure for skeletal mass. Their stores of iron, trace elements, and vitamins are depleted more quickly than are the stores of a mature baby. Sources of these nutrients must be ensured (Zlotkin et al, 1995). Parenteral needs for these nutrients may differ from enteral requirements. Intestinal absorption rates are considered in developing recommended enteral intakes (Table 5–3).

TABLE 5–3 Guidelines for Selected Daily Nutrient Intakes of Enterally-Fed Preterm Infants

Nutrient	Recommended Intake
Protein	3–4 g/kg
Calcium	150–230 mg/kg
Phosphorus	100–140 mg/kg
Iron	2–4 mg/kg
Sodium	2–3 mEq/kg
Vitamin A	700–1500 IU/kg
Vitamin D	400–600 IU/d
Thiamine	180–240 μg/kg
Riboflavin	250–360 μg/kg
Vitamin C	18–24 mg/kg

Adapted from Groh-Wargo S. Recommended enteral nutrient intakes. In: Groh-Wargo S, Thompson M, Cox JH, eds. Nutritional care for high risk newborns. Chicago: Precept, 1994:155.

FEEDING THE HIGH-RISK INFANT

■ Describe the impact of physiological development on the choice of feeding method for the high-risk infant.

■ What are the unique features of fortified preterm human milk and preterm formulas?

Physiologic Development

The fetus demonstrates sucking in utero at 24 weeks (Groh-Wargo, 1994). The preterm infant, however, cannot effectively coordinate sucking, swallowing, and breathing until approximately 32 to 34 weeks gestational age. Before that time, the infant needs to receive tube feedings because the risk of aspiration with nipple feedings is too great. Preterm infants are given pacifiers during tube feed-

TABLE 5–2 Estimated Caloric Requirement in a Typical Growing Premature Infant

	kcal/kg/day
Resting caloric expenditure	50
Intermittent activity	15
Occasional cold stress	10
Specific dynamic action	8
Fecal loss of calories	12
Growth allowance	25
Total	120

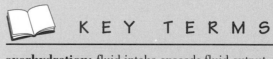

KEY TERMS

overhydration: fluid intake exceeds fluid output
qualitative assessment: evaluation of nutrient sources
quantitative assessment: calculation of nutrient intake quantities and comparison to recommendations
insensible water loss: water lost through immature skin and respiratory tract

ings to give them practice sucking and to promote the association of sucking with satiety. This is called **nonnutritive sucking** (Kimble, 1992). Infants who engage in nonnutritive sucking interventions are able to bottle feed and are discharged from the hospital sooner than infants who do not have this sucking practice (Schwartz et al, 1987). Nutritive sucking (taking formula from a nipple) often starts with one feeding daily. Preterm infants are capable of giving subtle cues to caregivers about their readiness to feed by mouth. Experienced NICU nurses recognize and respond to these cues. Eager sucking and swallowing that allows effective formula intake in a reasonable time period indicates that the infant is ready for more nipple feedings daily. Poor sucking, poor state control (falling asleep during feeding), or poor autonomic control (loss of control in respiration, color, and/or heart rate) may mean that the infant is not ready to progress on an oral feeding regimen. This infant receives tube feedings to replace or supplement oral feedings as needed (VandenBerg, 1990).

Mode of Feeding

Parenteral

The medical conditions of high-risk infants often preclude enteral feeding immediately after birth. An IV of glucose in water is started, therefore, to maintain fluid balance and to spare body tissues from being broken down for energy. When the baby has shown adequate urine output, usually within 24 hours, electrolytes are added to the glucose water IV solution. At this time or the next day, all other IV nutrients are added to the solution. This is called parenteral nutrition (PN). These nutrients are in forms (e.g., sterile, "predigested") and quantities needed for infants. Prepackaged IV vitamins, minerals, and trace elements that meet the unique needs of high-risk infants are available. Pediatric crystalline amino acid solutions (the IV protein source) are available that contain the proper proportions of amino acids to meet high-risk infants' needs while reducing the risk of metabolic complications (Heird, 1995). Intravenous fat emulsions may be infused separately or added to the solution to provide a source of essential fatty acids and calories. These nutrients are combined under sterile conditions in the hospital pharmacy to provide a complete IV nutrient mixture for each infant. In many cases, standard solutions that supply the same proportions of nutrients to all infants can be used. For infants with special needs, individual combinations of nutrients must be prepared. Investigators continue to define the unique parenteral nutrient needs of the LBW infant (Lipsky and Spear, 1995; Lacey et al, 1996).

Enteral

As mentioned earlier, high-risk infants receive enteral feedings by nipple or by tube. Traditionally, enteral feedings were withheld from high-risk infants for the first several weeks of life because their gastrointestinal tracts were thought to be too immature to handle feedings. Recent evidence shows that small-volume feedings are trophic to the infant's gastrointestinal tract. If the infant is medically stable, these **priming feedings** (also called **gut stimulation** or **hypocaloric feedings**) are started at 10 to 20 mL/kg/d and are not advanced for the first week or two. Priming feedings are associated with improved feeding tolerance, improved hormonal surges, and earlier intestinal maturation (Berseth, 1995; Meetze et al, 1992; Lucas et al, 1986). Early feeding also has beneficial effects on indirect hyperbilirubinemia, cholestatic jaundice, and osteopenia of prematurity (Dunn et al, 1988). It is important to advance feedings very slowly to avoid overwhelming the infant's digestive and absorptive capabilities, because this can lead to intestinal disease (McKeown et al, 1992). The preferred feedings for high-risk infants are human milk and preterm formula.

HUMAN MILK The benefits of human milk for the high-risk infant include superior digestibility and the presence of host resistance factors not available in current formulas. Additionally, nutrient composition of the milk of mothers who deliver preterm is different from the milk of mothers who deliver at term (Gross et al, 1980; Lemons et al, 1982; Sann et al, 1981). Preterm mothers' milk (PTM) is better suited to the preterm infant's needs than is term mothers' milk (TM). PTM contains higher amounts of protein and electrolytes than does TM, which is a bonus for high-risk infants, who need more of these nutrients. PTM does not, however, contain enough calcium and phosphorus to mineralize the bones of VLBW infants (Atkinson et al, 1980, 1983). These babies can develop osteopenia of prematurity and even fractured bones unless their mothers' milk is fortified with minerals (Steichen et al, 1987). Commercially available **human milk fortifiers** are added to PTM to enrich the mineral content and also to provide extra calories and vitamins (Thompson and McClead, 1987). High-risk infants who are fed fortified PTM demonstrate improved bone mineralization and growth (Raschko et al, 1989; Schanler, 1995). Although fortifiers are usually discontinued when the baby is discharged from the hospital, there is evidence that tiny babies may benefit from continued fortification at home (Abrams et al, 1989; Hall et al, 1989).

Although some NICUs accept donor milk, most prefer milk only from the infants' own mothers. Like donor blood, donor milk may contain viruses that can cause illness in the infant receiving the milk. Providing milk for her baby is a unique contribution that a mother can make to the care of her high-risk infant.

PRETERM FORMULAS Formulas designed specifically for preterm infants are more suited to their nutritional needs than are standard term infant formulas (Greer et al, 1982; Shenai et al, 1980). Preterm formula (PTF) differs from term formula in nutrient sources and nutrient quantity (Brady et al, 1982). The protein in PTF (whey-predominant cow's milk protein) is easier for the infant to digest and contains amino acids that preterm infants need. PTF contains two sources of carbohydrate (lactose and glucose polymers) and two sources of fat (LCT and MCT). Because high-risk infants have immature intestinal tracts and may not be able to handle a full load of any one carbohydrate or fat, two of each are used. Each uses different enzymes and absorptive mechanisms, with a resulting increase in overall nutrient retention (Shulman et al, 1995). Ongoing studies have implications for future modifications of preterm formulas (Koletzko et al, 1995; Farquharson et al, 1995).

Because high-risk infants have limited nutrient stores and high needs, and can often tolerate only limited formula volume, PTF is highly fortified with nutrients. The protein, mineral, and vitamin content of PTF is higher than that of standard formula (Table 5–4). In practice, PTF is generally used for infants weighing less than 2000 g at birth. When the baby is well enough to go home, the formula is often changed to a term infant formula because PTF is expensive and difficult to find outside of the hospital. There is concern, however, that term formula cannot meet the ongoing nutrient needs of high-risk infants. Additionally, some babies in follow-up have shown subclinical nutrient deficiencies, suggesting the continued need

for nutrient-dense formulas following hospital discharge (Ziegler, 1985). Special preterm discharge formulas have promoted improved growth in high-risk infants at home during the first year of life (Lucas et al, 1992; Friel et al, 1993). One such formula, Similac NeoCare (Ross Products Division, Abbott Laboratories, Columbus, OH) is currently available in the United States.

OTHER FORMULAS Standard term infant formulas and protein hydrolysate formulas are not suited to the high-risk infant's needs. If these formulas must be used for prolonged periods, they require nutrient fortification. The use of soy-based formulas has been associated with osteopenia of prematurity, because the minerals in soy formula are not as well absorbed as are the minerals in cow's milk-based formulas (Shenai et al, 1981). Even when it is supplemented with minerals, the use of soy formula in VLBW infants is associated with slower growth and lower serum protein status than that achieved with PTF (Hall et al, 1984). Soy formulas are not recommended for high-risk infants, therefore (American Academy of Pediatrics Committee on Nutrition, 1993).

LACTATION MANAGEMENT The high-risk infant may be unable to breast-feed for a prolonged period of time. The mother who wishes to eventually nurse her baby will need to pump the milk from her breasts to establish and maintain a milk supply. Breast milk production follows the law of supply and demand. If the milk is removed from the breasts regularly, the body will produce more. Electric breast pumps, which effectively remove milk and assist in maintaining a milk supply over a prolonged period, are available. Other methods of breast pumping (e.g., hand expression, manual pumps) are not as effective for long-term pumping (see page 621) (Lawrence, 1994).

Expressed milk is placed in sterile containers, labeled, and stored in a refrigerator or freezer. This milk can be fortified in the NICU and fed (by tube or bottle) to the high-risk infant. Eventually, the baby will be able to nurse directly from the breast. Because pumped human milk is not sterile and is a good growth medium for microorganisms, the milk may be cultured before it is fed to the baby (Lawrence, 1994). The milk can be contaminated by

Nutrient	Standard Infant Formula*	Preterm Infant Formula[†]
Protein	1.5 g	1.8–2.0 g
Calcium	47–51 mg	111–122 mg
Phosphorus	32–39 mg	56–61 mg
Iron	1.2 mg	1.2 mg
Sodium	0.8 mEq	1.1–1.3 mEq
Vitamin A	203–209 IU	460–840 IU
Vitamin D	41–42 IU	100–180 IU
Thiamin	53–68 μg	135–170 μg
Riboflavin	101–105 μg	200–420 μg
Vitamin C	5.5–6.1 mg	24–25 mg

TABLE 5–4 Selected Nutrient Comparison in 100 mL of Formula

* Ranges of nutrients contained in Similac with Iron 20, Ross Products Division, Abbott Laboratories, Columbus, OH and Enfamil with Iron 20, Mead Johnson Nutritionals, Evansville, IN.

[†] Ranges of nutrients contained in Similac Special Care with Iron 20, Ross Products Division, Abbott Laboratories, Columbus, OH and Enfamil Premature Formula with Iron 20, Mead Johnson Nutritionals, Evansville, IN.

K E Y   T E R M S

nonnutritive sucking: sucking on a pacifier
priming feedings: small volume feedings that are trophic to the GI tract and help in its maturation
human milk fortifiers: nutrients added to boost the nutritional value of human milk for high-risk infants

soiled pumping equipment or poor handwashing techniques. It is thus important to have policies and procedures for handling, storing, culturing, and feeding human milk in a NICU.

GROWTH AND DEVELOPMENTAL OUTCOME

■ What factors affect the high-risk infant's growth rate and developmental outcome?

Several factors affect the high-risk infant's growth rate: birth weight, gestational age, nutrient intake, medical problems, home environment, and genetic potential. LBW infants are, by definition, smaller than average term neonates at birth. **Catch-up growth** may occur during the first 1 to 3 years of life in infants without residual illness (Ernst et al, 1990; Casey et al, 1990 and 1991). Catch-up growth in head circumference usually precedes that in weight and length (Manser, 1984). Preterm infants who are appropriately grown for their gestational age are more likely to eventually catch up to their full-term peers than are SGA infants (Sung et al, 1993).

Recent investigations have explored the relationship of early diet (i.e., in the first month of life) to neurodevelopmental outcome (Lucas, 1987). Low-birthweight infants fed preterm formula in the first month of life scored significantly higher in developmental tests at 18 months of age than did those fed term formula in the first month (Lucas et al, 1990). Male infants and SGA infants showed particularly striking advantages in mental and motor development if they had received preterm formula. Moderate developmental impairment was considerably more common in the group fed term formula. Infants fed preterm formula also showed a slight advantage in social maturity quotient.

Follow-up studies in 7- to 8-year-old former LBW infants demonstrate a significant improvement in intelligence quotient (IQ) in infants who received their mother's milk compared to those who received no maternal milk (Lucas et al, 1992). The infants received the milk by tube, which eliminates the possibility that the act of breast-feeding itself conferred this advantage. There was a dose-response relationship between the proportion of mother's milk in the diet and subsequent IQ. These results persisted after adjusting for differences in maternal education and social class. Receiving mature donor human milk (as opposed to term formula) may also promote superior neurodevelopmental outcome in preterm infants (Lucas et al, 1994).

These initial outcome studies underscore the importance of early nutrition for LBW infants. Whether the positive influences of preterm formula and mother's milk are related to specific nutrients, nutrient ratios, or other components is unknown. Additional outcome studies are needed.

MEDICAL/SURGICAL CONDITIONS COMPLICATING THE NUTRITIONAL MANAGEMENT OF HIGH-RISK INFANTS

Hyperbilirubinemia

Hyperbilirubinemia (or jaundice) is a condition defined by high amounts of the pigment bilirubin in the blood. Bilirubin is produced from the breakdown of heme-containing proteins, particularly red cell hemoglobin. Hyperbilirubinemia is common in immature infants because their livers are not as capable of breaking down the bilirubin pigment as are the livers of term babies. Hyperbilirubinemia occurs more frequently in breast-fed than in formula-fed infants, for unknown reasons.

If too much bilirubin builds up in the bloodstream, it can cross the blood-brain barrier and cause mental retardation. Fortunately, bilirubin can be changed to a water-soluble isomer by certain wavelengths of light. The infant receives phototherapy, and bilirubin is then excreted in the baby's stool or urine.

Nutrition plays only a small, complementary role in treating hyperbilirubinemia. Feedings may be started or advanced to enhance intestinal movement and excretion of bilirubin. Breast-fed infants should be fed more often, because feeding frequency is inversely related to serum bilirubin concentrations in these infants (DeCarvalho et al, 1982). If jaundice persists, interruption of nursing (i.e., feeding formula or alternating formula and breast-feeding) for 24 to 48 hours usually resolves hyperbilirubinemia related to breast-feeding (Newman and Maisels, 1992; American Academy of Pediatrics, 1994). Providing water supplements to breast-fed infants has no impact on serum bilirubin levels (DeCarvalho et al, 1981; American Academy of Pediatrics, 1994).

Respiratory/Cardiac/Renal Problems

High-risk infants can have medical problems that involve their respiratory, cardiac, or renal systems. Often, they may be sensitive to high fluid intakes, which make their conditions worse, leading to respiratory distress, congestive heart failure, or acute renal failure, respectively. These babies need alterations in their fluid and electrolyte intakes. They may need higher-calorie formula because they have fluid restrictions and are often too sick or tired to eat well (Wahlig and Georgieff, 1995; Pereira et al, 1994; Karlowicz and Adelman, 1992).

Gastrointestinal Problems

Infants who have gastrointestinal problems may need to "rest" their intestines until they heal. Thus, they receive parenteral nutrition during this time. When the intestines have healed, enteral feedings are gradually reintroduced (Kern et al, 1990; Kanto et al, 1994).

Bone Problems

Osteopenia of prematurity can occur in infants with undermineralized bones, inadequate mineral intake, or excessive mineral losses. Treatment involves providing high intakes of calcium and phosphorus to mineralize the bones (Koo and Tsang, 1991). Adequate intake of vitamin D helps in calcium absorption and bone remodeling (Specker et al, 1988).

SPECIAL CONCERNS

■ Describe the impact of maternal substance abuse or HIV on the infant.

Effects of Maternal Substance Abuse

Maternal substance abuse encompasses the use of alcohol, cigarettes, and/or illicit drugs during pregnancy. The effects on the fetus vary with the frequency and dose of the substance received and the stage(s) of pregnancy in which the substance is used. Fetal effects can be caused directly by the substance itself or indirectly by maternal self-neglect. Because drug abuse, alcohol abuse, and cigarette smoking frequently coincide, it is difficult to isolate the effects of one substance from the other in studies of pregnant substance-abusing women (Jacobson et al, 1994).

Alcohol

Alcohol and its primary metabolite, acetaldehyde, are directly toxic to the developing fetus and are capable of producing abnormalities. Infants of mothers who drink heavily during pregnancy may be afflicted with fetal alcohol syndrome (FAS). FAS includes physical and developmental abnormalities specific to infants with this condition. The infant is SGA and has microcephaly, postnatal growth deficiency, developmental delay, and distorted facial features. Adequate nutrition does not reverse the infant's growth delay (Lee and Leichter, 1982). Children who are exposed to alcohol during the entire pregnancy demonstrate worse performance on developmental testing than do those exposed to alcohol during the first trimester only (Autti-Ramo et al, 1992). Thus it behooves a mother to curtail alcohol consumption as soon as possible during pregnancy. Binge drinking during the first trimester, however, may be as dangerous to the fetus as steady exposure throughout gestation (Clarren et al, 1992).

When compared to his or her peers, the school-aged child with FAS has a lower IQ and may have learning disabilities. Because no one knows how much alcohol during pregnancy is "too much," alcohol use during pregnancy is not recommended.

Smoking

Cigarette smoking by pregnant women has been associated with an increased risk of spontaneous abortion, stillbirth, prematurity, and intrauterine growth retardation. The degree of growth retardation is directly related to the number of cigarettes smoked. This growth failure may be irreversible in the postnatal period (Friesen and Fox, 1986). The exact mechanism of the adverse effect of cigarette smoking on pregnancy is unknown. Smoking in the same room as the infant also increases the risk for sudden infant death (Klonoff-Cohen et al, 1995).

Illicit Drugs

Illicit drug use during pregnancy can have profound negative effects on the fetus. Infants who are exposed to drugs in utero are often growth-retarded and may be drug-addicted at birth (Kliegman et al, 1994). The symptoms of neonatal withdrawal syndrome are primarily neurologic: jitteriness, restlessness, tremulousness, irritability, and hypertonicity. Alimentary tract symptoms include poor sucking and swallowing, vomiting, and diarrhea. Providing calorie/nutrient supplements, small, frequent feedings, and tube feedings when needed may help to attenuate problems with nutrition and growth (Torrence and Horns, 1989; Rice-Asaro et al, 1990).

Drug-exposed infants may have delayed postnatal growth, especially in head circumference. Small head size correlates with suboptimal developmental outcome (Chasnoff et al, 1992; Singer et al, 1994).

Human Immunodeficiency Virus

Human immunodeficiency virus (HIV) is the virus that causes acquired immunodeficiency syndrome (AIDS). The most common cause of pediatric HIV infection is perinatal transmission from an infected mother (Frenkel and Gaur, 1994). Another rare cause is transmission of HIV in

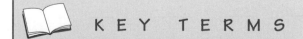

KEY TERMS

catch-up growth: growth at a faster-than-expected rate following a period of attenuated growth

---

RESEARCH UPDATE
Team Approach to Neonatal Nutrition Management

Because management of the nutritional care of high-risk infants occurs in the hospital, a team of professionals is involved. Key members of the team are physicians (MDs), nurses (RNs), and dietitians/nutritionists (RDs). The MD is responsible for writing orders that prescribe the nutrition care that the infant receives. The RN implements the feeding orders (i.e., administers IV nutrition and enteral feedings) and notes the infant's reac-

tions to feedings. The RD develops individual nutrition care plans and provides consultation to MDs and RNs on infant nutrient needs, product composition, and growth expectations (Thompson, 1994). The nutrition team can also include a clinical pharmacist, developmental therapist, and lactation specialist. These health care professionals work together to provide optimal nutrition to high-risk infants (Thompson et al, 1994; Institute of Medicine, 1992).

---

human breast milk (Black, 1996). Maternal-infant transmission of HIV can be reduced with medication (zidovidine); antenatal HIV testing and counseling is encouraged, therefore (Peckham and Gibb, 1995).

The diagnosis of HIV infection in newborns is difficult because of the transplacental transport of maternal antibody to HIV. Because maternal antibody may persist for up to 15 months, the Centers for Disease Control and Prevention recommends serologic diagnosis of HIV infection only after the infant reaches 15 months of age. Serologic testing before that time can be misleading. Approximately 70% of newborns who are seropositive at birth are seronegative and free of symptoms by 18 to 24 months of age (Blanche et al, 1989).

Children with HIV infection who become symptomatic (develop AIDS) succumb to the disease more quickly than do adults (Pizzo, 1990). Symptoms of HIV infection in the pediatric population include generalized lymphadenopathy (swollen glands), hepatomegaly (enlarged liver), splenomegaly (enlarged spleen), failure to thrive (poor growth), diarrhea, and fever. Multiple nutritional deficiencies, particularly protein-calorie malnutrition, may develop. Malabsorptive disorders contribute to nutritional problems (Miller et al, 1991). Nutrition intervention may include protein-calorie supplementation and vitamin/mineral assessment and supplementation as needed. Tube feedings may be necessary if oral intake is insufficient; parenteral nutrition is indicated if the gastrointestinal tract is nonfunctional (Nicholas et al, 1991).

SUMMARY

The high-risk infant is usually preterm and/or low-birth-weight. This infant is at high nutritional risk due to limited nutrient reserves, increased nutrient needs, immature alimentary tract, metabolic immaturities, and medical com-

plications or stresses. Assessing the infant's nutrition status includes determination of gestational age and size for age, as well as anthropometric, biochemical, clinical, and intake assessments. Nutrient needs are usually higher for these infants than they are for term, normal-weight infants. Parenteral nutrition may be emphasized until physiologic maturity allows advancement to full enteral feedings. Pediatric parenteral products, preterm formulas, and fortified mother's milk are appropriate nutrient sources for high-risk infants. Infants who are AGA may catch up in growth to their term, normal-weight peers; SGA infants are less likely to catch up. Medical/surgical conditions complicate the nutritional management of high-risk infants. Maternal substance abuse (alcohol, cigarettes, illicit drugs) has a negative impact on growth, development, and nutritional status of infants. Management of the high-risk infant's nutritional care is the responsibility of a team of health professionals.

CONCEPTS TO REMEMBER

▶ The high-risk infant is usually preterm, low-birth-weight, or both.

▶ Nutritional risk factors include limited nutrient reserves, high nutrient needs, physiologic and metabolic immaturities, and medical complications.

▶ Nutrient needs are usually higher for these infants than they are for term, normal-weight infants.

▶ Pediatric parenteral products, preterm formulas, and fortified mother's milk are appropriate nutrient sources for high-risk infants.

▶ Growth in weight, length, and head circumference is the best measure of nutritional outcome.

◗ Maternal substance abuse has a negative impact on the growth, development, and nutritional status of infants.

References

Abrams SA, Schanler RJ, Tsang RC, Garza C. Bone mineralization in former very low birth weight infants fed either human milk or commercial formula: one-year follow-up observation. J Pediatr 1989;114:1041.

American Academy of Pediatrics/American College of Obstetricians and Gynecologists. Guidelines for perinatal care, 3rd ed. Elk Grove, IL: American Academy of Pediatrics, 1992.

American Academy of Pediatrics Committee on Genetics. Issues in newborn screening. Pediatrics 1992;89:345.

American Academy of Pediatrics Committee on Nutrition. Alternate formulas: soy formulas. In Pediatric nutrition handbook. 3rd ed. Elk Grove Village, IL: American Academy of Pediatrics, 1993:17.

American Academy of Pediatrics Committee on Nutrition. Nutritional needs of preterm infants. In Pediatric nutrition handbook. 3rd ed. Elk Grove Village, IL: American Academy of Pediatrics, 1993:64.

American Academy of Pediatrics Committee on Nutrition. Nutritional needs of low-birth-weight infants. Pediatrics 1985;75:976.

American Academy of Pediatrics Provisional Committee for Quality Improvement and Subcommittee on Hyperbilirubinemia. Practice parameter: management of hyperbilirubinemia in the healthy term newborn. Pediatrics 1994;94:558.

Atkinson SA, Radde IC, Anderson GH. Macromineral balances in premature infants fed their own mothers' milk or formula. J Pediatr 1983; 102:99.

Atkinson SA, Radde IC, Chance GW, Bryan MH, Anderson GH. Macromineral content of milk obtained during early lactation from mothers of premature infants. Early Hum Dev 1980;4:5.

Autti-Ramo I, Korkman M, Hilakivi-Clarke L, Lehtonen M, Halmesmaki E, Granstrom ML. Mental development of 2-year-old children exposed to alcohol in utero. J Pediatr 1992;120:740.

Ballard JL, Khoury JC, Wedig K, Wang L, Eilers-Walsman BL, Lipp R. New Ballard score, expanded to include extremely premature infants. J Pediatr 1991;119:417.

Ballard JL, Novak KK, Driver M. A simplified score for assessment of fetal maturation of newly born infants. J Pediatr 1979;95:769.

Berry HK. Special and therapeutic formulas for inborn errors of metabolism. In: Tsang RC, Nichols BL, eds. Nutrition during infancy. Philadelphia: Hanley & Belfus, 1988:340.

Berseth CL. Minimal enteral feedings. Clin Perinatol 1995;22:195.

Black RF. Transmission of HIV-1 in the breast-feeding process. J Amer Diet Assoc 1996;96:267.

Blanche S, Rouzioux C, Moscato M-LG, Veber F, Mayaux M-J, Jacomet C, et al. A prospective study of infants born to women seropositive for human immunodeficiency virus type 1. N Engl J Med 1989;320:1643.

Brady MS, Rickard KA, Ernst JA, Schreiner RL, Lemons JA. Formulas and human milk for premature infants: a review and update. J Amer Diet Assoc 1982;81:547.

Burton BK. Inborn errors of metabolism: the clinical diagnosis in early infancy. Pediatrics 1987;79:359.

Casey PH, Kraemer HC, Bernbaum J, Tysen JE, Sells JC, Yogman MW, et al. Growth patterns of low birth weight preterm infants: a longitudinal analysis of a large, varied sample. J Pediatr 1990;117:298.

Casey PH, Kraemer HC, Bernbaum J, Yogman MW, Sells JC. Growth status and growth rates of a varied sample of low birth weight preterm infants: a longitudinal cohort from birth to three years of age. J Pediatr 1991;119:599.

Chasnoff IJ, Griffith DR, Freier C, Murray J. Cocaine/polydrug use in pregnancy: two-year follow-up. Pediatrics 1992;89:284.

Clarren SK, Astley SJ, Gunderson VM, Spellman D. Cognitive and behavioral deficits in nonhuman primates associated with very early embryonic binge exposures to ethanol. J Pediatr 1992;121:789.

Crouch J. Anthropometric assessment. In: Groh-Wargo S, Thompson M, Cox JH, eds. Nutritional care for high risk newborns. Chicago: Precept 1994:11.

DeCarvalho M, Hall M, Harvey D. Effects of water supplementation on physiological jaundice in breast-fed babies. Arch Dis Child 1981;56: 568.

DeCarvalho M, Klaus MH, Merkatz RB. Frequency of breast-feeding and serum bilirubin concentration. Am J Dis Child 1982;136:737.

Dunn L, Hulman S, Weiner J, Kliegman R. Beneficial effects of early hypocaloric enteral feeding on neonatal gastrointestinal function: Preliminary report of a randomized trial. J Pediatr 1988;112:622.

Ernst JA, Bull MJ, Rickard KA, Brady MS, Lemons JA. Growth outcome and feeding practices of the very low birth weight infant (less than 1500 grams) within the first year of life. J Pediatr 1990;117:S156.

Farquharson J, Jamieson EC, Abbasi KA, Patrick WJA, Logan RW, Cockburn F. Effect of diet on the fatty acid composition of the major phospholipids of infant cerebral cortex. Arch Dis Child 1995;72:198.

Frenkel LD, Gaur S. Perinatal HIV infection and AIDS. Clin Perinatol 1994;21:95.

Friel JK, Andrews WL, Matthew JD, McKim E, French S, Long DR. Improved growth of very low birthweight infants. Nutr Res 1993;13:611.

Friesen C, Fox HA. Effects of smoking during pregnancy. Kans Med 1986;87:7.

Greer FR, Steichen JJ, Tsang RC. Effects of increased calcium, phosphorus, and vitamin D intake on bone mineralization in very low-birth-weight infants fed formulas with Polycose and medium-chain triglycerides. J Pediatr 1982;100:951.

Groh-Wargo S. Gastrointestinal development. In: Groh-Wargo S, Thompson M, Cox JH, eds. Nutritional care for high risk newborns. Chicago: Precept 1994:139.

Groh-Wargo S. Prematurity/low birth weight. In: Lang CE. Nutritional support in critical care. Rockville, MD: Aspen, 1987:287.

Gross SJ, David RJ, Bauman L, Tomarelli RM. Nutritional composition of milk produced by mothers delivering preterm. J Pediatr 1980;96:641.

Hall RT, Callenbach JC, Sheehan MB, Hall FK, Thibeault DW, Kurth CG, et al. Comparison of calcium- and phosphorus-supplemented soy isolate formula with whey-predominant premature formula in very low birth weight infants. J Pediatr 1984;3:575.

Hall RT, Wheeler RE, Montalto MB, Benson JD. Hypophosphatemia in breast-fed low-birth-weight infants following initial hospital discharge. Am J Dis Child 1989;143:1191.

Hamosh M, Bitman J, Liao TH, Mehta NR, Buczek RJ, Wood DL, et al. Gastric lypolysis and fat absorption in preterm infants: effect of medium-chain triglyceride or long-chain triglyceride-containing formulas. Pediatrics 1989;83:86.

Hay WW Jr. Nutritional needs of the extremely low-birth-weight infant. Semin Perinatol 1991;15:482.

Heird WC. Amino acid and energy needs of pediatric patients receiving parenteral nutrition. Pediatr Clin North Am 1995;42:765.

Institute of Medicine. Committee on Nutritional Status during Pregnancy and Lactation. Nutrition services in perinatal care. 2nd ed. Washington, DC: National Academy Press, 1992.

Jacobson JL, Jacobson SW, Sokol RJ, Martier SS, Ager JW, Shankaran S. Effects of alcohol use, smoking, and illicit drug use on fetal growth in black infants. J Pediatr 1994;124:757.

Jones MO, Pierro A, Garlick PJ, McNurlan MA, Donnell SC, Lloyd DA. Protein metabolism kinetics in neonates: effect of intravenous carbohydrate and fat. J Pediatr Surg 1995;30:458.

Kanto WP, Hunter JE, Stoll BJ. Recognition and medical management of necrotizing enterocolitis. Clin Perinatol 1994;21:335.

Karlowicz MG, Adelman RD. Acute renal failure in the neonate. Clin Perinatol 1992;19:139.

Kern IB, Leece A, Bohane T. Congenital short gut, malrotation, and dysmotility of the small bowel. J Pediatr Gastroenterol Nutr 1990;11: 411.

Kimble C. Nonnutritive sucking: adaptation and health for the neonate. Neonatal Network 1992;11:29.

Kliegman RM, Madura D, Kiwi R, Eisenberg I, Yarnashita T. Relation of maternal cocaine use to the risk of prematurity and low birth weight. J Pediatr 1994;124:751.

Kliegman RM. Problems in metabolic adaptation: glucose, calcium, and magnesium. In: Klaus MH, Fanaroff AA, eds. Care of the high risk neonate. 4th ed. Philadelphia: WB Saunders, 1993:289.

Klonoff-Cohen HS, Edelstein SL, Lefkowitz ES, Srinivasan IP, Kaegi D, Chang JC, et al. The effect of passive smoking and tobacco exposure through breast milk on sudden infant death syndrome. JAMA 1995;273: 795.

Koletzko B, Edenhofer S, Lipowsky G, Reinhardt D. Effects of a low birthweight infant formula containing human milk levels of docosahexaenoic and arachidonic acids. J Pediatr Gastroenterol Nutr 1995;21: 200.

Koo WWK, Tsang RC. Mineral requirements of low-birth-weight infants. J Amer Coll Nutr 1991;10:474.

Lacey JM, Crouch JB, Benfell K, Ringer SA, Wilmore CK, Maguire D, et al. The effects of glutamine-supplemented parenteral nutrition in premature infants. J Parent Ent Nutr 1996;20:74.

Lawrence R. Breastfeeding: A guide for the medical profession. 4th ed. St Louis: Mosby–Year Book, 1994:607, 621.

Lebenthal E. Gastrointestinal maturation and motility patterns as indicators for feeding the premature infant. Pediatrics 1995;95:207.

Lebenthal E, Leung YK. Alternative pathways of digestion and absorption in the newborn. In: Lebenthal E, ed. Textbook of gastroenterology and nutrition in infancy. New York: Raven, 1989:3.

Lebenthal E, Leung YK. Feeding the premature and compromised infant: gastrointestinal considerations. Pediatr Clin North Am 1988; 35:215.

Lee M, Leichter J. Alcohol and the fetus. In: Jelliffe EF, Jelliffe DB, eds. Adverse effects of foods. New York: Plenum, 1982:245.

Lemons JA, Moye L, Hall D, Simmons M. Differences in the composition of preterm and term human milk during early lactation. Pediatr Res 1982;16:113.

Lipsky CL, Spear ML. Recent advances in parenteral nutrition. Clin Prenatal 1995;22:141.

Lucas A. Does diet in preterm infants influence clinical outcome? Biol Neonate 1987;52:141.

Lucas A, Bishop NJ, King FJ, Cole TJ. Randomised trial of nutrition for preterm infants after discharge. Arch Dis Child 1992;67:324.

Lucas A, Bloom SR, Aynsley-Green A. Gut hormones and "minimal enteral feeding." Acta Paediatr Scand 1986;75:719.

Lucas A, Morley R, Cole TJ, Gore SM, Lucas PJ, Crowle P, et al. Early diet in preterm babies and developmental status at 18 months. Lancet 1990;335:1477.

Lucas A, Morley R, Cole TJ, Lister G, Leeson-Payne C. Breast milk and subsequent intelligence quotient in children born preterm. Lancet 1992;339:261.

Lucas A, Morley R, Cole TJ, Gore SM. A randomised multicentre study of human milk versus formula and later development in preterm infants. Arch Dis Child 1994;70:F141.

Manser JJ. Growth in the high-risk infant. Clin Perinatol 1984;11:19.

McCabe ERB, McCabe L. Issues in the dietary management of phenylketonuria: breast-feeding and trace-metal nutriture. Ann NY Acad Sci 1986;477:215.

McKeown RE, Marsh TD, Amarnath U, Garrison CZ, Addy CL, Thompson SJ, et al. Role of delayed feeding and of feeding increments in necrotizing enterocolitis. J Pediatr 1992;121:764.

Meetze WH, Valentine C, McGuigan JE, Conlon M, Sacks N, Neu J. Gastrointestinal priming prior to full enteral nutrition in very low birth weight infants. J Pediatr Gastroenterol Nutr 1992;15:163.

Miller TL, Orav EJ, Martin SR, Cooper ER, McIntosh K, Winter HS. Malnutrition and carbohydrate malabsorption in children with vertically transmitted human immunodeficiency virus 1 infection. Gastroenterology 1991;100:1296.

Moyer-Mileur L. Laboratory assessment. In: Groh-Wargo S, Thompson M, Cox JH, eds. Nutritional care for high risk newborns. Chicago: Precept, 1994:34.

Newman TB, Maisels MJ. Evaluation and treatment of jaundice in the term newborn: a kinder, gentler approach. Pediatrics 1992;89:809.

Nicholas SW, Leung J, Fennoy I. Guidelines for nutritional support of HIV-infected children. J Pediatr 1991;119:S59.

Peckham C, Gibb D. Mother-to-child transmission of the human immunodeficiency virus. N Engl J Med 1995;333:298.

Pereira GR, Baumgart S, Bennett MJ, Stallings VA, Georgieff MK, Hamosh M, et al. Use of high-fat formula for premature infants with bronchopulmonary dysplasia: metabolic, pulmonary, and nutritional studies. J Pediatr 1994;124:605.

Pizzo PA. Pediatric AIDS: Problems within problems. J Infect Dis 1990;161:316.

Platt LD, Koch R, Azen C, Hanley WB, Levy HL, Matalon R, et al. Maternal phenylketonuria collaborative study, obstetric aspects and outcome: the first 6 years. Am J Obstet Gynecol 1992;166:1150.

Raschko PK, Hiller JL, Benda GI, Buist NR, Wilcox K, Reynolds JW. Nutritional balance studies of VLBW infants fed their mothers' milk fortified with a liquid human milk fortifier. J Pediatr Gastroenterol Nutr 1989;9:212.

Rice-Asaro M, Wasek N, Franklin P, Dixon SD. Nutritional concerns for children born to drug abusing women. Nutrition Focus 1990;5:1.

Roth J, Resnick MB, Ariet M, Carter RL, Eitzman DV, Curran JS, et al. Changes in survival patterns of very low-birth-weight infants from 1980 to 1993. Arch Pediatr Adolesc Med 1995;149:1311.

Sann L, Bienvenu F, Lahet C, Bienvenu J, Bethenod M. Comparison of the composition of breast milk from mothers of term and preterm infants. Acta Paediatr Scand 1981;70:115.

Sasanow SR, Georgieff MK, Pereira GR. Mid-arm circumference and mid-arm/head circumference ratios: standard curves for anthropometric assessment of neonatal nutritional status. J Pediatr 1986;109:311.

Schanler RJ. Suitability of human milk for the low-birthweight infant. Clin Perinatol 1995;22:207.

Schmidt H, Mahle M, Michel U. Continuation vs discontinuation of low-phenylalanine diet in PKU adolescents. Eur J Pediatr 1987; 146(Suppl 1):A17.

Schwartz R, Moody L, Yarandi H, Anderson GC. A meta-analysis of critical outcome variables in nonnutritive sucking in preterm infants. Nurs Res 1987;36:292.

Seashore MR, Friedman E, Novelly RA, Bapat V. Loss of intellectual function in children with phenylketonuria after relaxation of dietary phenylalanine restriction. Pediatrics 1985;75:226.

Shaffer SG, Quimiro Cl, Anderson JV, Hall RT. Postnatal weight changes in low birth weight infants. Pediatrics 1987;79:702.

Shenai JP, Reynolds JW, Babson SG. Nutritional balance studies in very-low-birth-weight infants: enhanced nutrient retention rates by an experimental formula. Pediatrics 1980;66:233.

Shenai JP, Jhaveri BM, Reynolds JW, Huston RK, Babson SG. Nutritional balance studies in very low-birth-weight infants: role of soy formula. Pediatrics 1981;67:631.

Shulman RJ, Feste A, Ou C. Absorption of lactose, glucose polymers, or combination in premature infants. J Pediatr 1995;127:626.

Singer LT, Yamashita TS, Hawkins S, Cairns D, Baley J, Kliegman R. Increased incidence of intraventricular hemorrhage and developmental delay in cocaine-exposed, very low birth weight infants. J Pediatr 1994; 124:765.

Specker BL, Greer F, Tsang RC. Vitamin D. In: Tsang RC, Nichols BL, eds. Nutrition during infancy. Philadelphia: Hanley & Belfus, 1988:264.

Steichen JJ, Krug-Wispe SK, Tsang RC. Breastfeeding the low birth weight preterm infant. Clin Perinatol 1987;14:131.

Sung I, Vohr B, Oh W. Growth and neurodevelopmental outcome of very low birth weight infants with intrauterine growth retardation: Comparison with control subjects matched by birth weight and gestational age. J Pediatr 1993;123:618.

Thompson M, McClead RE. Human milk fortifiers. J Pediatr Perinat Nutr 1987;1:65.

Thompson M. Computer use in neonatal nutrition information management. In: Groh-Wargo S, Thompson M, Cox JH, eds. Nutritional care for high risk newborns. Chicago: Precept, 1994:41.

Thompson M. Perspectives on the neonatal nutritionist's role. In: Groh-Wargo S, Thompson M, Cox JH, eds. Nutritional care for high risk newborns. Chicago: Precept, 1994:391.

Thompson M, Price P, Stahle DA. Nutrition services in neonatal intensive care: A national survey. J Amer Diet Assoc 1994;94:440.

Torrence CR, Horns KMH. Appraisal and caregiving for the drug addicted infant. Neonatal Network 1989;8:49.

US Department of Health and Human Services. Public Health Service. Healthy People 2000, Review 1993. National Health Promotion and Disease Prevention Objectives. DHHS Publication No (PHS)94-1232-1. Washington, DC: US Government Printing Office, 1994.

Valentine C. Congenital anomalies of the alimentary tract. In: Groh-

Wargo S, Thompson M, Cox JH, eds. Nutrition care for high risk newborns. Chicago: Precept, 1994:299.

VandenBerg KA. Nippling management of the sick neonate in the NICU: the disorganized feeder. Neonatal Network 1990;9:9.

Wahlig TM, Georgieff MK. The effects of illness on neonatal metabolism and nutritional management. Clin Perinatol 1995;22:77.

Ward JC. Inborn errors of metabolism of acute onset in infancy. Pediatr Rev 1990;11:205.

Ziegler EE. Infants of low birth weight: special needs and problems. Amer J Clin Nutr 1985;41:440.

Zlotkin SH, Atkinson S, Lockitch G. Trace elements in nutrition for premature infants. Clin Perinatol 1995;22:223

APPLICATION: Inborn Errors of Metabolism

An inborn error of metabolism (IEM) is a genetic disorder that involves the blocking of specific metabolic pathways due to missing or defective enzymes. IEMs can be considered the biochemical counterparts of structural malformations. If an enzyme is missing or defective, it cannot carry out its catalytic function of enhancing biochemical reactions in the body. The substrate requiring the enzyme builds up in the bloodstream and may be excreted in the urine; or it may be converted to another intermediary metabolite. This abnormal accumulation of substrate can result in mental retardation, coma, or even death. Because substrate or intermediary metabolites may take several days or weeks to build up to toxic levels in the infant's bloodstream, the IEM may not be detected immediately. Presenting signs for many IEMs include some or all of the following: vomiting, diarrhea, poor growth, lethargy, seizures, respiratory distress, hypoglycemia, and metabolic acidosis (Ward, 1990; Burton, 1987). Because early diagnosis and early treatment improve the outcome, most states require that all newborns be screened for the most common inborn errors of metabolism within the first few days after birth (American Academy of Pediatrics Committee on Genetics, 1992).

Nutrition management of patients with IEMs involves eliminating or restricting the intake of the harmful nutrient. Often the nutrient cannot be removed from the diet completely because it is essential. The intake of the offending nutrient must be adequate to promote growth, therefore, but not enough to be toxic. Nutrients beyond the metabolic block must be provided as well as all other nutrients needed for adequate growth and development. This involves careful calculations and diet planning by the health professional as well as adequate understanding and implementation by the infant's caregiver. Periodic laboratory tests detect whether the intake of the nutrient has been properly restricted or needs to be liberalized.

Special formulas have been developed for treating IEMs in infancy and childhood. These products eliminate the offending nutrient altogether or provide it in restricted amounts. They also provide varying amounts of vitamins, minerals, and energy-providing nutrients. It may be necessary to add measured quantities of a standard infant formula to provide an adequate amount of the targeted nutrient. As the infant grows, the diet is expanded to include foods free from the targeted nutrient, or controlled quantities of foods containing the targeted nutrient are allowed. For most IEMs, dietary treatment is a lifelong process. The disorder can be controlled by diet but is never eliminated.

Phenylketonuria

Phenylketonuria (PKU) involves a defect in the enzyme phenylalanine hydroxylase, which catalyzes the conversion of phenylalanine to tyrosine. Phenylalanine and its metabolites accumulate in the bloodstream and are excreted in the urine—thus the name phenylketonuria. Because phenylalanine is an essential amino acid, it must be supplied in the diet. Too little inhibits growth and normal development; too much in infants with PKU can lead to deterioration of intellect, and, if untreated, severe mental retardation develops.

Phenylalanine → phenylalanine hydroxylase → tyrosine

The requirement for phenylalanine varies from baby to baby and within the same child throughout life. Published recommendations for infants with PKU are consulted (Table A5–1) and adjusted according to the baby's blood phenylalanine level. For optimal therapeutic effects, serum phenylalanine level should be maintained between 3 and 8 mg/dL (Berry, 1988).

A special low-phenylalanine or phenylalanine-free formula is substituted for standard infant formula, which is added in small quantities to meet phenylalanine requirements. Breast-feeding can be continued in a limited fashion based on the baby's phenylalanine levels (McCabe and McCabe, 1986). The balance of the baby's nutrient needs are met by a phenylalanine-free formula. Foods added to the diet later in infancy should be low in phenylalanine. Relaxation of the phenylalanine restriction later in childhood has been associated with decreased mental functioning (Schmidt et al, 1987; Seashore et al,

TABLE A5–1 Recommended Daily Intakes of Nutrients for Infants with Phenylketonuria

Age	Phenylalanine (mg/kg)	Protein (g/kg)	Calories/kg
0–3 mo	50–60	2.2–2.5	110–120
4–6 mo	40–50	2.0–2.5	110–120
7–12 mo	30–40	2.0–2.5	110

Adapted from Berry HK. Special and therapeutic formulas for inborn errors of metabolism. In: Tsang RC, Nichols BL, eds. Nutrition during infancy. Philadelphia: Hanley & Belfus, 1988:346.

1985). Additionally, pregnant women who have PKU have a higher incidence of congenital anomalies in their offspring if they do not follow a phenylalanine-restricted diet during pregnancy (Platt et al, 1992). Thus, patients with PKU may benefit from lifetime restriction of phenylalanine.

References

American Academy of Pediatrics Committee on Genetics. Issues in newborn screening. Pediatrics 1992;89:345.

Berry HK. Special and therapeutic formulas for inborn errors of metabolism. In: Tsang RC, Nichols BL, eds. Nutrition during infancy. Philadelphia: Hanley & Belfus, 1988:340.

Burton BK. Inborn errors of metabolism: the clinical diagnosis in early infancy. Pediatrics 1987; 79:359.

McCabe ERB, McCabe L. Issues in the dietary management of phenylketonuria: breast-feeding and trace-metal nutriture. Ann NY Acad Sci 1986;477:215.

Platt LD, Koch R, Azen C, Hanley WB, Levy HL, Matalon R, et al. Maternal phenylketonuria collaborative study, obstetric aspects and outcome: the first 6 years. Am J Obstet Gynecol 1992;166:1150.

Schmidt H, Mahle M, Michel U. Continuation vs discontinuation of low-phenylalanine diet in PKU adolescents. Eur J Pediatr 1987;146(Suppl 1):A17.

Seashore MR, Friedman E, Novelly RA, Bapat V. Loss of intellectual function in children with phenylketonuria after relaxation of dietary phenylalanine restriction. Pediatrics 1985;75:226.

Ward JC. Inborn errors of metabolism of acute onset in infancy. Pediatr Rev 1990;11:205.

CHAPTER 6

NUTRITION DURING GROWTH: PRESCHOOL AND SCHOOL YEARS

Ramon is 6 years old today. He is excited because it is also his first day at school and he gets to stay all day. He's been to the Head Start Program and half-day kindergarten before, but this is school! He came on the bus with his sister, Juanita, this morning. His grandmother packed his favorite lunch—a peanut butter and jelly sandwich, an apple, and three chocolate chip cookies. He was so nervous this morning that he could hardly eat his breakfast. Now he's really hungry.

At lunch time the cafeteria is so busy and noisy that Ramon hardly has time for lunch. Everything happens so fast. He hurries through lunch so he can go outside to the playground with the other children. He didn't even take time to eat his apple. He won't tell Nina he threw it away. But he drank the milk he got in the cafeteria. Some of the kids in his class made fun of the blue and white bag in which he brought his lunch. The teacher said he would be eligible for the lunch program, so tomorrow he will probably have hot lunch, which would be better.

Ramon is so proud to have a sister in the fifth grade at his school, and he is lucky because she can show him around. She is out on the playground with the other older kids playing basketball. Just now she doesn't have much time for Ramon, but he understands that she has her own friends and doesn't want a little brother hanging around. Juanita is as good a basketball player as any of the boys in her class. She's taller than most of them too. In fact she grew 2 inches this summer. At home Juanita is really picky about what she will eat, but she always eats the hot lunch at school, as do most of the kids in her class. Besides, she is hungry by lunch time. But Juanita says that when she goes to middle school next year she won't eat the school lunch because, according to her older friends in the neighborhood, nobody does.

Ramon and Juanita are each at a transition point of childhood. Ramon's home- and family-bound preschool years are behind him, and he is eagerly moving into the early school years. He will be increasingly influenced by what his peers at school think and do. As Juanita approaches the end of her childhood years, there are still few gender differences in body size or performance, but her recent growth signals that that is about to change as she begins puberty. Already her social patterns are assuming major peer orientation.

GROWTH AND DEVELOPMENT

Childhood, the period between infancy and adolescence, encompasses great diversity in size, age, growth rates, and

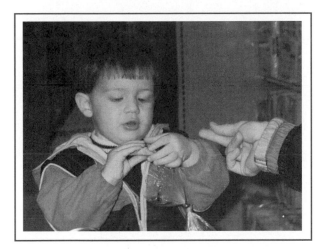

FIGURE 6–1. Toddlerhood is a transition between infancy and childhood.

developmental skills. The timing and pattern of growth and development are influenced by heredity, hormones, and environment, including nutrition. Growth patterns are highly individual, erratic at times, with spurts in height and weight followed by periods of little or no growth. In healthy children these patterns usually correspond to similar changes in appetite and food intake.

An adequate intake of energy and nutrients is essential to maintain health and support growth. In addition, childhood is a critical period for development of the attitudes and behaviors that can influence lifestyle and health habits through adolescence into adulthood. During this time, there are rapid changes in physiologic, psychological, and social growth and development, which may place some children at nutritional risk.

In this chapter, childhood growth is divided into two periods. The preschool period includes the year between 1 and 2, often designated as late infancy or toddlerhood (Fig. 6–1), and ages 2 to 6 years. Compared to infancy, the preschool years are characterized by a decreased rate of growth, and a child's interest in eating may diminish during this period. The ages of 6 to 10 years in girls and 6 to 12 years in boys are often referred to as the "latent growth period," a period during which growth is slow and steady, preceding the prepubertal growth spurt.

Growth and Body Composition

■ What gains in stature and weight can be expected for normal preschool and school-age children?

■ How does the velocity of growth differ between the preschool and school-age periods?

■ How is growth monitored?

■ What changes occur in body appearance and composition during the preschool and school-age periods?

As in infancy, the growth of a child is measured in terms of gains in stature and weight and, in the first 3 years, head circumference. During childhood there is a general deceleration in the rapid incremental height and weight gains that were characteristic of infancy. The 50th percentile values for stature and weight from the National Center for Health Statistics growth charts are given in Table 6–1. Annual increments are about 2.5 kg (5–6 lb) and 12 cm (5 in) during the second and third year of life and approximately 6 to 8 cm (2.5–3.5 in) and 2 kg (4.5 lb) from 3 to 5 years of age.

During the early school years the velocity of growth slows but remains relatively steady until the preadolescent growth spurt at about 10 years of age in girls and 12 in boys. Increments in height are generally 6 cm (2 in) per year, and increments in weight are 3 to 3.5 kg (7 lb) per year (see Table 6–1). Limb length increases more than trunk length, resulting in a change in body proportions (Fig. 6–2). The upper to lower body segment ratio is about 1.3 at 3 years, 1.1 at 6 years, and 1.0 at 10 years of age.

Growth of the brain decelerates after infancy, and head circumference, a rough indicator of brain growth, is usually monitored only until 36 months of age (see Figs. 4–4 and 4–5 in Chapter 4). Whereas head circumference increases approximately 12 cm (4.5 in) during infancy, the gain is only 2 cm (0.75 in) in the second year. After the

TABLE 6–1 Stature and Weight of Children (50th Percentile on NCHS Growth Charts)

Age (y)	Stature (cm)		Weight (kg)	
	Male	Female	Male	Female
1	76.1	74.3	10.2	9.5
2	86.8	86.8	12.3	11.8
3	94.9	94.1	14.6	14.1
4	102.9	101.6	16.7	15.9
5	109.9	108.4	18.7	17.7
6	116.1	114.6	20.7	19.5
7	121.7	120.6	22.9	21.8
8	127.0	126.4	25.3	24.8
9	134.8	132.2	28.1	28.4
10	137.5	138.3	31.4	32.6
11	143.3	144.8	35.3	36.9
12	149.7	151.5	39.8	41.5

From Hamill PVV, et al. Physical growth: National Center for Health Statistics percentiles. Am J Clin Nutr 1979;32:607. © Am J Clin Nutr. American Society for Clinical Nutrition

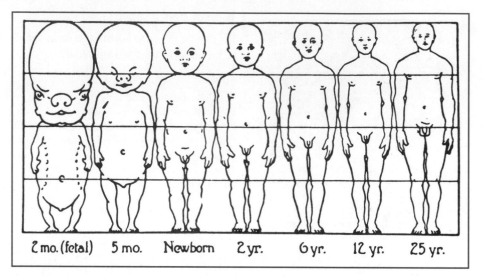

FIGURE 6–2. Body proportions change with growth and development. (From Robbins. Growth. New Haven: Yale University Press, 1928.)

third birthday, increases in head circumference are limited. In fact, only 2 to 3 cm are gained between 3 and 12 years of age. By age 12, the brain has reached virtually adult size, although neuronal development continues.

Major body compartments are water, protein, fat, and minerals. By the time the child is 2 to 3 years of age, the proportion of body weight that is water is 60% to 65%, similar to that of an adult. Because of the growth of new cells, the extracellular fluid compartment decreases to about 20% to 25%, while intracellular fluid increases to about 35% to 40% of body weight. Rapid shifts of fluid between intracellular and extracellular compartments are less likely, making the child less vulnerable to dehydration than the infant. Throughout the childhood years the percentage of weight as fat remains relatively constant, while fat-free body mass (skeletal muscle, bone, and soft tissue protein) increases. By 10 years of age, lean body mass has reached approximately 17% in boys and 15% in girls. Mineral content, less than 3.5% in infancy, increases gradually throughout childhood to reach 4.8% of body weight by the end of puberty.

Development

■ Describe the typical physical, neurologic, cognitive, language, and psychosocial developmental changes of the preschool and school-age periods.

The Preschool Years (Ages 1 to 6)

The preschool years, ages 1 to 6 years, are a period of rapid social, intellectual, and emotional growth. As overall physical growth is decelerating, motor skills are being fine-tuned. A summary of developmental achievements associated with ages 1 through 6 years appears in Table 6–2. These changes influence the development of eating skills and the child's successful participation in the feeding process.

PHYSICAL DEVELOPMENT Although there are only limited increases in head size after 2 years of age, there are significant changes in facial configuration during the preschool period. The length of the skull increases, and the face tends to grow proportionately more than the cranial cavity. The jaw widens to accommodate development of permanent teeth.

As the second year progresses some of the subcutaneous "baby" fat is lost, and the plump infant slowly evolves into a lean and muscular child. During the third, fourth, and fifth years, most children are lean in comparison with their earlier body configuration. The protuberant (projecting) abdomen characteristic of the second and third years of life generally disappears by the fourth year.

NEURODEVELOPMENT Toddlers and children in this age group derive pleasure from the exercise of new skills. During the second year the child moves from an awkward upright stance and wobbly walk to a high degree of locomotor control. At 18 months he or she is able to run stiffly, and by 24 months, he or she runs easily. Motor skills become more sophisticated. By the end of the fourth year the child can ascend and descend stairs, and a year later he or she can hop and skip.

Fine motor skills also progress rapidly during the preschool years. At 12 months a toddler is able to pick up and release a pellet or piece of food, and by 18 months he or she is able to put it into and dump it out from a small bottle. An 18-month-old can spontaneously scribble; a

TABLE 6–2 **Developmental Achievements During the Preschool Years**

15 MONTHS

Motor

Gross	Toddles independently
	Crawls upstairs
Fine	Puts pellet into bottle
Adaptive	Builds tower of two cubes
	Puts six cubes in and out of cup
Language	Jargon
	Four to six words, including names
	Pats pictures in book
Personal-social	Says "thank you" or equivalent
	Points or vocalizes wants
	Hugs parents
	Throws objects in play or refusal

18 MONTHS

Motor

Gross	Walks, seldom falling; runs stiffly
	Sits in small chair and climbs into adult chair
	Hurls ball in standing position
Fine	Turns two or three pages of book at once
Adaptive	Builds tower of three or four cubes
	Imitates scribbling with a crayon
	Dumps pellet from bottle
Language	Ten words, names pictures
	Identifies one or more body parts
	Carries out one or two directions
Personal-social	Pulls toy on string
	Carries and hugs doll
	Feeds self in part, with spilling
	Seeks help when in trouble

2 YEARS

Motor

Gross	Runs well, no falling
	Walks up and down stairs, one step at a time
	Climbs, jumps
Fine	Turns pages of book singly
Adaptive	Builds tower of six or seven cubes
	Aligns cubes for train
	Circular scribbling
Language	Three-word sentences; vocabulary of 50–75 words
	Carries out four directions with toy ("on the table," "on the chair," "to mother," "to me")
Personal-social	Verbalizes toilet needs consistently
	Helps undress
	Handles spoon well
	Listens to stories

3 YEARS

Motor

Gross	Alternates feet going upstairs
	Stands momentarily on one foot
	Rides tricycle
Fine	Holds crayon with fingers
Adaptive	Builds tower of nine or ten cubes
	Names own drawing
	Copies circle and imitates cross

3 YEARS (cont.)

Language	Counts three objects
	Gives action in picture book
	Knows full name and gender
	Obeys two prepositional commands ("on," "under," "over")
Personal-social	Feeds self well
	Puts on shoes and unbuttons buttons
	Knows a few rhymes or songs
	Plays simple games
	Plays "parallel" with other children

4 YEARS

Motor	Walks downstairs alternating feet
	Hops on one foot
	Throws ball overhand
Adaptive	Draws man with two to four parts besides head
	Copies cross and square
	Counts three objects with correct pointing
	Imitates construction of five-cube bridge
Language	Names one or more colors correctly
	Obeys five prepositional commands ("on," "under," "in back," "in front," "beside")
Personal-social	Tells a story, washes and dries face and hands; brushes teeth
	Distinguishes front from back of clothes
	Plays with several children

5 YEARS

Motor	Skips, alternating feet
	Stands on one foot for several seconds
Adaptive	Builds two steps with cubes
	Draws unmistakable man with body, head, etc.
	Draws triangle
	Prints a few letters
	Counts ten pennies correctly
Language	Knows four colors
	Five-word sentences
	Descriptive comment on pictures
	Follows three directions
Personal-social	Dresses and undresses without assistance
	Asks meaning of words
	Domestic role-playing

6 YEARS

Motor	Advanced throwing
	Stands on each foot alternately, eyes closed
Adaptive	Knows right from left
	Draws man with neck, hands, and clothes
	Adds and subtracts within 5
	Copies diamond
Language	Composes a complex five- or six-word sentence
	Comprehends "if," "because," "why"
Personal-social	Ties shoelaces
	Differentiates morning and afternoon
	Knows right from left
	Increased interaction with peers

From Hughes JG and Griffith JF. Synopsis of pediatrics, 6th ed. St. Louis: C.V. Mosby, 1984.

3-year-old can imitate crudely the drawing of a cross; a 5-year-old can copy figures in correct proportions. These skills are reflected in the progression from using hands to eat finger foods to effective use of a spoon and fork.

COGNITIVE DEVELOPMENT Healthy preschool children are often described as alert and curious as they actively explore their environment. From ages 1 to 6 years, the imitative and conceptual behavior of infancy continues to evolve. During the second year the child develops a sense of self. She demonstrates memory, anticipation, and original thinking and becomes capable of taking initiative and making choices in behavior. The preschool child becomes increasingly concerned with the expectations of adults.

The preschool child learns to use speech for communication with increasing precision. The child who has a vocabulary of 10 words at 18 months of age has progressed to putting three words together by the second birthday. The 3-year-old can use short sentences and sustain a brief conversation. Longer conversations occur in the 4th year, and by age 5 language is used in most social functions.

PSYCHOSOCIAL DEVELOPMENT During the second year imitative behavior extends from parents to siblings and playmates. Play is generally solitary, with occasional contests with other children over possession of objects or toys. Frustration or anger with societal expectations may result in temper tantrums and other outbursts.

As children progress through the preschool period they become increasingly aware that they will become larger children and eventually adults and begin to emulate role models. Often they enter play activities with other children and eventually act out imaginative roles. Late in this period, peer groups begin to influence the child's preferences and behavior.

Early School Years

PHYSICAL DEVELOPMENT Although there is great variation in body fat among individual children at any stage of growth, body fat remains a relatively constant percentage of body weight during the school years (Fig. 6–3). Because of shifts in accumulation and location of body fat, most children develop a slimmer appearance as childhood progresses. With the increase in skeletal muscle, the child becomes stronger. Development of skeletal muscles means an increase in intracellular water, because skeletal muscles have a high water content.

Throughout life, bone is continually remodeled or rearranged in response to the stress of body weight and exercise. This is especially true of **trabecular bone**. Bone is in a dynamic state of formation and resorption. The outer shell, cortical bone, grows by adding new tissue on the outer surface and resorbing from the inner surface. In the growing years, bone formation exceeds resorption and

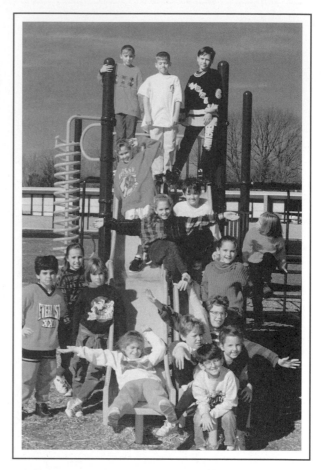

FIGURE 6–3. School-age children are of varying sizes and grow at different rates.

there are gradual increases of mineral mass. As growth occurs, the **bone shaft** lengthens until the **epiphyses** close after puberty (Fig. 6–4).

NEURODEVELOPMENT The school years are a time of vigorous physical activity. The spine becomes straighter, but the child's body is flexible. The motor skills developed in earlier years, such as running and climbing, become increasingly directed toward physical activities and games that require specialized motor and muscular skills.

COGNITIVE DEVELOPMENT During the early school years the child develops an increasing ability to monitor his or her own mental processes. Intuitive thinking advances to the concrete operational level. Concepts of conservation of volume and mass are achieved. In art, the notion of perspective evolves. Speech becomes reasoning and expressive.

PSYCHOSOCIAL DEVELOPMENT The early school years are complex as children grow physically and

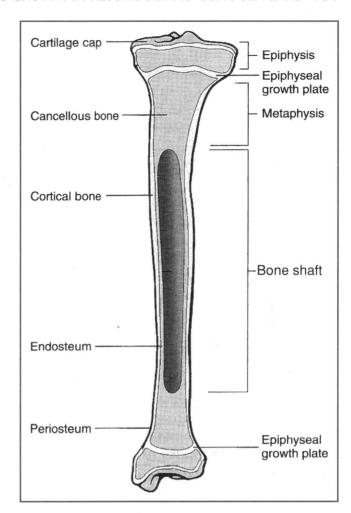

FIGURE 6–4. The long bone has a central part (shaft) and two terminal parts (epiphysis). The shaft of the bone consists of cancellous bone on the outside and trabecular bone on the inside. The epiphyseal growth plate allows bone lengthening. When the epiphyses close, linear growth ceases. (From Applegate EJ. The anatomy and physiology learning system: Textbook. Philadelphia: WB Saunders, 1995: 393.)

emotionally. They develop a sense of responsibility and of realistic accomplishment. By ages 5 and 6 years, school has assumed a central role in their lives. As they become increasingly independent, friends and acquaintances become a significant influence in forming standards of behavior. The habits and patterns that children develop during these years are strong influences on later dietary patterns, health, and well-being.

ASSESSMENT OF NUTRITION STATUS

■ What tools are most frequently used to assess the nutrition status of children?

■ How are growth charts used in nutrition assessment and in defining under- and overweight?

■ What are the limitations of the methods of determining children's dietary intakes?

Nutrition assessment of children includes anthropometric, biochemical, clinical, and dietary measures.

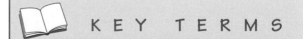

K E Y   T E R M S

trabecular bone: the spongy bone in the ends of the long bones, the iliac crest, scapula and vertebrae
bone shaft: the long slender portion of bone between the wider ends
epiphysis: the end of the long bone. During growth the epiphyses are separated from the main portion of the bone by cartilage. This space closes as maximum height is attained.

The most commonly used techniques are those that assess growth changes. Techniques for measurement of height and weight were described in Chapter 2. Children younger than 2 years of age may have stature measured in the recumbent position, as described in Chapter 4, until they are able to stand independently to be measured.

Anthropometry

Measurements of stature and weight can be recorded on growth charts from the National Center for Health Statistics (NCHS) for birth to 36 months (see Figs. 4–2 and 4–3 in Chapter 4) or those for children aged 2 to 18 years (Figs. 6–5 and 6–6). (Interpretation of growth charts is

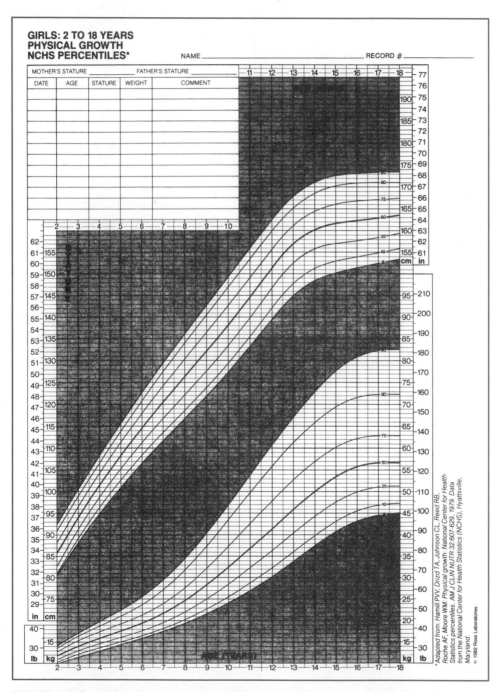

FIGURE 6–5. Growth charts for girls 2 to 18 years: NCHS percentiles for stature and weight for age. (Used with permission of Ross Products Division, Abbott Laboratories, Columbus, OH 43216 from NCHS Growth Charts. © 1982 Ross Products Division, Abbott Laboratories.)

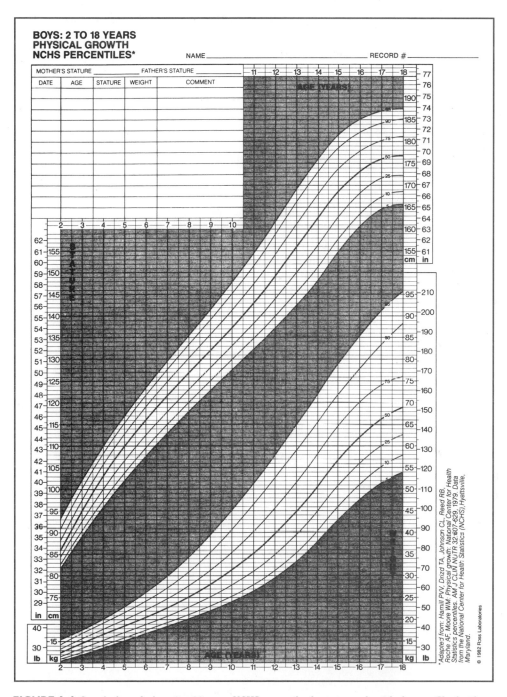

FIGURE 6–6. Growth charts for boys 2 to 18 years: NCHS percentiles for stature and weight for age. (Used with permission of Ross Products Division, Abbott Laboratories, Columbus, OH 43216 from NCHS Growth Charts. © 1982 Ross Products Division, Abbott Laboratories.)

discussed in Chapter 4.) As in infancy, the most commonly used nutrition assessment technique for children is documentation of increases in stature and weight.

For this purpose, height and weight are recorded periodically and plotted over time on growth charts. A growth pattern usually emerges, with successive measurements falling around the same percentile on the growth chart.

Growth rates will vary among children, however, and within an individual child's growth pattern. Rapid growth and slowing of growth usually reflect the spurts and latent periods that are typical of normal growth. However, if such periods are prolonged, a more thorough evaluation of nutrition status is merited.

Inadequate dietary intake can influence the velocity of

growth, at first by decreases in the rate of weight gain and eventually in a diminishing of gains in height. Declining weight gain is a sensitive indicator of short-term inadequate nutrition status; diminished increases in height indicate long-term inadequate nutrition status. It is essential for any child who loses weight to receive immediate evaluation to determine the cause, because weight loss is an indicator of severely inadequate dietary intake or a health problem. Growth charts for prepubescent girls and boys on which weight for stature is plotted can be found in Appendices 7A and 7B. These charts can be useful in identifying a risk of obesity or severe undernutrition unrelated to age, especially for children at either extreme of height.

FATFOLD MEASUREMENTS   Fatfold measurements can be useful for assessment of body fat. Triceps and subscapular fatfold thicknesses are the measurements most commonly used to assess energy reserves. Percentile values from NHANES data for triceps fatfolds (skinfolds) for various groups appear in Appendices 3A and 3B. Fatfolds are not employed for routine nutrition screening in children, but they can be useful in clarifying the nutrition status of children for whom weight for height falls above the 90th or below the 10th percentile.

Biochemical

Laboratory measurements used for assessment of nutrition status are discussed in Chapter 2. These same tests are appropriate for children but may require age-specific standards.

Clinical

Although much of the assessment of nutrition status is based on growth parameters, advanced stages of undernutrition are manifested in physical and, in a more subtle fashion, behavioral signs. Table 6–3 lists some common physical signs of well-nourished and undernourished children. Such clinical changes appear more rapidly in undernourished children than in adults because of the higher nutritional demands of growth. Interpretation of any clinical sign of undernutrition must be made with caution.

Dietary

Dietary intakes of children can be estimated using dietary records, 24-hour recalls, and food frequency questionnaires. Obtaining accurate dietary information for young children requires cooperation of the parent or primary caregiver. In addition, if the youngster is in daycare, preschool, or school, complete intake information requires input from teachers or other individuals who care for the

TABLE 6–3 Physical Signs of Well-Nourished and Undernourished Children

Well-Nourished	Undernourished
HAIR	
Shiny, firmly in the scalp	Dull, brittle, dry, loose and falls out easily
EYES	
Bright, clear, membranes pink	Pale membranes, spots, redness, slow adjustment to dim light
FACE	
Good complexion	Off-color; scaly, flaky, cracked skin; lack of fat under the skin
GLANDS	
No lumps	Swollen at front of neck, cheeks
SKIN	
Smooth, firm, good color	Dry, rough, "sandpaper" feel, spotty, or sores
LIPS	
Smooth, good color	Red, swollen, cracks at corners of mouth
TONGUE	
Red, rough, bumpy	Sore, smooth, purplish, swollen
TEETH AND GUMS	
No pain or cavities, gums firm, teeth bright	Missing teeth, bad color, decay; gums bleed easily, swollen, spongy
NAILS	
Firm, pink	Spoon-shaped, brittle, ridged
MUSCLES AND BONES	
Good muscle tone, posture; long bones straight	"Wasted" appearance of muscles; swollen bumps on skull or ends of bones; small bumps on ribs; bowed legs or knock-knees; pain
INTERNAL SYSTEM	
Heart rate, rhythm, and blood pressure normal; normal GI function; reflexes, psychological development normal	Heart rate, rhythm, or blood pressure abnormal; liver, spleen enlarged; GI dysfunction; mental irritability, confusion; burning, tingling of hands, feet; loss of balance, coordination

Adapted from Christakis A. Nutritional assessment in health programs. Am J Public Health 1973;63(Suppl):19. Reprinted with permission of the American Public Health Association, Inc.

child. Young children may be able to report what they ate at school or at the babysitter's but are seldom able to give accurate estimates of amounts consumed. For very young children it is important to assess feeding skill development and psychosocial factors that influence nutrient intake as well as actual foods consumed. Similar problems may impair accuracy of intake data during the early school years.

As children reach fourth or fifth grade they may be able to report their food intake with some accuracy (Domel et al, 1994) but have difficulty quantifying portion size, particularly in estimating how much they actually ate (Lytle et al, 1993). In addition, this age group is very responsive to nutrition and health education. Recent exposure to such information may bias their responses on dietary records or to questionnaires. An accurate evaluation of food intake may require the use of more than one method.

ENERGY AND NUTRIENT NEEDS OF CHILDREN

■ Compare recommended levels of energy and nutrients for children to those for infants and adults.

■ What is the most accurate basis for determining energy and protein recommendations for children?

■ How do recommended levels for energy, protein, vitamins, and minerals change across childhood?

■ How does iron deficiency influence cognitive function?

■ How does nutrition contribute to tooth development and oral health?

■ How much dietary fiber is appropriate for children?

Children's nutritional needs are determined by the individual child's size and rate of growth. Because children come in many sizes, and because growth rates change from day to day, nutritional needs and dietary intakes vary widely. The Recommended Dietary Allowances (RDAs) for children from 1 to 10 years that appear in Table 6–4 make no distinction between boys and girls. Much of the information used to determine these recommendations was extrapolated from data from studies of adults. As for all of the RDAs except energy, a margin of safety or sufficiency over requirements is included, which means that recommended levels exceed the physiologic requirements for most children. It should be remembered that the RDAs are meant to be applied to groups, not to individual children. Recommended allowances for individuals over 10 years of age are discussed in Chapter 7.

Energy

The diversity of energy needs of healthy children is related to differences in the energy expended for growth, basal metabolism, physical activity, and the thermic effect of food. The energy allowances are based on age groups of 1 to 3 years, 4 to 6 years, and 7 to 10 years. A reference weight and height is established for each age group.

Because the size of children varies, and because growth occurs in spurts, age alone is not an adequate criterion for energy needs. Kilocalories per kilogram (kcal/kg) of body weight is an appropriate reference for children between the 15th and 85th percentiles on the NCHS growth charts, but kcal/kg would be misleading for underweight and overweight children. Kilocalories per centimeter (kcal/cm), as shown in Table 6–5, would yield a more appropriate estimate of energy needs for an individual child. For example, on the RDA chart, the energy recommendation for a child 4 to 6 years old is 1800 kcal. If a 5-year-old is 112 cm (44.1 in) tall, it is an appropriate level. However, a 5-year-old who has short parents and is 100 cm (39.4 in) tall would require only 1600 kcal, whereas a tall child of 125 cm (49.2 in) might need 2000 kcal each day. Such energy recommendations are only guidelines, and the child's appetite is a better indicator of day-to-day needs.

Protein

Adequate protein is essential to support optimal growth in children. For dietary protein to be utilized effectively, sufficient energy must be consumed to make amino acids available for protein synthesis. Recommendations for protein intake range from 0.18 to 0.21 g/cm of height for ages 1 to 10 years (see Table 6–5). The values established for protein assume the diet contains a mixture of animal and vegetable protein and that energy intake is adequate to support growth.

Data from the USDA Food Consumption Survey (1985) indicate that American children consume approximately 16% of their kilocalories from protein, a level that exceeds the RDA. Children who have low food intakes and must use protein for energy may be at risk for malnutrition.

Vitamins and Minerals

Minerals and vitamins are essential to adequate nutrition. Although studies of food consumption of children in the United States indicate that intakes of some nutrients are likely to be low, clinical signs of vitamin or mineral deficiencies are rare. Intakes below recommended levels are found most frequently for calcium, iron, ascorbic acid, vitamin A, folate, and Vitamin B_6 (USDA, 1985). Children at particular risk for inadequate diets are those from low-income families and other groups with limited food and health resources, particularly homeless families.

VITAMINS Vitamins function in numerous metabolic processes. Vitamin needs are often dependent on en-

TABLE 6-4 Recommended Dietary Allowances for Young Children

	Age (years)		
	1–3 (13 kg/90 cm)	4–6 (20 kg/112 cm)	7–10 (28 kg/132 cm)
Energy (kcal)	1300	1800	2000
Protein (g)	16	24	28
FAT-SOLUBLE VITAMINS			
Vitamin A (μg RE)*	400	500	700
Vitamin D (μg)†	10	10	10
Vitamin E (mg-TE)‡	6	7	7
Vitamin K (μg)	15	20	30
WATER-SOLUBLE VITAMINS			
Vitamin C (mg)	40	45	45
Thiamin (mg)	0.7	0.9	1.0
Riboflavin (mg)	0.8	1.1	1.2
Niacin (mg NE)§	9	12	13
Vitamin B_6 (mg)	1.0	1.1	1.4
Folate (μg)	50	75	100
Vitamin B_{12} (μg)	0.7	1.0	1.4
MINERALS			
Calcium (mg)	800	800	800
Phosphorus (mg)	800	800	800
Magnesium (mg)	80	120	170
Iron (mg)	10	10	10
Zinc (mg)	10	10	10
Iodine (μg)	70	90	120
Selenium (μg)	20	20	30

* RE, retinol equivalents. 1 retinol equivalent = 1 μg or 6 μg β-carotene.
† As cholecalciferol. 10 μg cholecalciferol = 400 IU of vitamin D.
‡ δ-Tocopherol equivalents. 1 mg d-δ = 1 δ-TE.
§ 1 NE (niacin equivalent) = 1 mg of niacin or 60 mg of dietary tryptophan.
Reprinted with permission from Recommended Daily Allowances, 10th ed., Copyright 1989 by the National Academy of Sciences. Courtesy of the National Academy Press, Washington, DC.

ergy intake or the levels of other nutrients. Most of the RDAs for children have been extrapolated from studies on infants and adults.

CALCIUM   Children require calcium not only to maintain existing bone but also to support growth of new bone. Approximately 100 mg of calcium are retained as bone each day, and this amount doubles and triples during peak periods of adolescent growth (Matkovik et al, 1990). The RDA for calcium is only a guide because of the large variability in calcium requirements. Calcium needs of individual children are influenced by the velocity of growth, the efficiency of calcium absorption, and the availability of other nutrients, including phosphorus, vitamin D, and protein.

An adequate intake of calcium throughout childhood, adolescence and early adulthood is needed to attain peak bone mass (Johnston et al, 1992), which is believed to di-

minish the risk of bone loss later in life (Matkovik et al, 1990).

Bone mineral density in children may be enhanced by calcium intakes greater than the current RDA. A recent study compared bone mineral density of 22 pairs of prepubertal identical twins. One twin of each pair consumed 1600 mg of calcium a day and the other 900 mg per day. After 3 years, the twin who had the higher calcium intake had a greater bone density. A similar increase in total body and spine bone was observed in 12-year-old girls who increased their calcium intake by 30% for 18 months (Lloyd et al, 1993).

Because dairy products are the major sources of calcium, children with limited amounts of these foods in their diets are at risk for calcium deficiency. Attention also must be given to vitamin D intake because it has a major role in calcium absorption and metabolism. For children with limited exposure to sunshine, meeting the RDA of 10 μg

TABLE 6-5 RDA for Energy and Protein per Centimeter of Height				
Age (y)	Weight (kg)	Height (cm)	kcal/cm	Protein/cm
1-3	13	90	14	0.18
4-6	20	112	16	0.21
7-10	28	132	15	0.21

from a dietary source becomes critical. Dietary sources of vitamin D are limited and variable. In the United States, vitamin D–fortified milk is the primary food source. Other dairy products are seldom fortified with vitamin D, so a child who consumes two to four servings of cheese and yogurt gets sufficient calcium but consumes little vitamin D. If such a child has infrequent exposure to sunlight, vitamin D levels may be inadequate to facilitate optimum utilization of dietary calcium.

IRON Iron is needed to maintain hemoglobin concentration and to support growth. Dietary requirements depend on the rate of growth, iron stores, and the efficiency of the absorption of iron from food sources. Iron requirements increase during rapid growth and, therefore, the RDA may just meet the child's needs on some days but exceed them on others. The dietary intake needed by a 10-year-old child to establish adequate body stores of iron are as great as those of an adult male. The recommended levels are based on the assumption that 10% to 15% of dietary iron is absorbed. Absorption of nonheme iron can be enhanced by consumption of foods containing vitamin C.

Chronic iron deficiency in childhood may have adverse effects on growth and development. The prevalence of iron deficiency is higher in African-Americans than in white children and is substantially higher in children from families with incomes below the poverty level. An important objective of the Healthy People 2000 initiative is to reduce the incidence of iron deficiency to less than 3% among American children aged 1 through 4 years and to 4% for children aged 3 through 4 years. The potential for iron deficiency to influence cognitive function is discussed later in this chapter.

Fluoride and Oral Health

■ Describe the role of nutrition in tooth development and prevention of dental disease.

Oral health is essential to the consumption of an adequate diet, and nutrition is essential to the maintenance of oral health. Inadequate nutrients for tooth formation can result in structurally weak teeth that are susceptible to injury and decay, which interferes with mastication of food.

Even in developmentally sound teeth, poor dietary habits can contribute to tooth decay, and periodontal disease can result in poor dentition and tooth loss.

TOOTH STRUCTURE Teeth are specialized structures of mineralized tissue that encase a highly vascular dental pulp and its ample supply of nerves (Fig. 6–7). Dental enamel forms a hard, protective coating over the tooth. This coating consists mostly of calcium, carbonate, calcium phosphate, and other ions in a **hydroxyapatite**-like structure. The second layer, dentin, has no vascular components but, compared to enamel, is more readily permeable to fluids from blood via dentinal tubules. Overlying the dentin and the root of the tooth below the gums and alveolar bone is cementum, a bone-like connective tissue that assists in tooth support. The support structures of the periodontium include the gingiva and the periodontal ligament or membrane that joins the root cementum to the alveolar bone.

Primary teeth usually erupt between the ages of 6 and 24 months. The hard tissue of permanent dentition begins to form as early as birth, but completion of root formation, the last stage of development, does not occur until the mid-teens. Permanent teeth erupt between age 6 years and the early teens. During the pre-eruptive period, formation of healthy tooth structure is fostered by adequate dietary protein, calcium, phosphorus, magnesium, and vitamins C and D. Saliva is supersaturated with calcium and phosphorus, the major minerals found in the hydroxyapatite of the dental enamel and dentin. The dental enamel is bathed with saliva, promoting continuous exchange of calcium and phosphorus, typically in equilibrium.

DENTAL CARIES Initiation of dental caries involves interactions among the susceptible tooth, **cariogenic** bacteria in **plaque**, and a substrate, preferably fermentable carbohydrate. Fermentable carbohydrates (mono- and disaccharides and some cooked or processed starches) are all metabolized by the bacteria in plaque. The byproduct of that metabolism is organic acids. When the pH falls to about 5.7, the organic acids diffuse through the tooth surface, reaching susceptible surfaces where

K E Y   T E R M S

hydroxyapatite: crystalline structure of bones and teeth, composed of calcium phosphate and calcium carbonate in a collagen matrix, gives strength and rigidity to bone
cariogenic: promoting tooth decay
plaque: a mass adhering to the enamel surface of a tooth, composed of a mixture of bacteria, cells, and fermentable carbohydrate

RESEARCH UPDATE
Iron Deficiency and Cognitive Function

Iron deficiency is the most common nutrient deficiency in the United States and the world. It has been estimated that 15% to 20% of the United States population under 18 years old is iron deficient. In spite of differences in ways of measuring cognitive function, there are consistent observations that **iron deficiency anemia** (IDA) is associated with poor performance on infant developmental scales, IQ and learning tasks in preschool children, and educational achievement among school-age children. Although it has been observed that children with iron deficiency are less attentive and have greater difficulty learning than iron-replete children, the mechanism by which low levels of iron affect learning and behavior is unclear. It has been suggested that iron deficiency causes a decline in hemoglobin concentration, resulting in reduced oxygen availability to the brain or decreased levels of iron-dependent neurotransmitter receptors in the brain (Pollitt, 1993). In two double-blind randomized clinical trials in which iron was administered for 4 months to infants with IDA, there was consistent improvement in developmental scores (Aukett et al, 1986) and the psychomotor development index (Idjradinata and Pollitt, 1993). Changes in developmental scores in infants who received a placebo were negligible. Duration of IDA also may be a factor in cognitive development. In Costa Rica, 5-year-old children with histories of chronic and moderately severe IDA during infancy scored lower in a wide range of tests of cognition and fine and gross motor proficiency than children who had not been iron deficient (Lozoff et al, 1991).

Infants and Toddlers (0–24 Months)

Infants with IDA are often unhappy, tense, fearful, or withdrawn. They are less responsive and less goal directed and generally obtain poorer scores on developmental scales than iron-replete infants (Idjradinata and Pollitt, 1993). Following iron therapy, however, the atypical affective state changes and the infants' responsiveness to their social environment becomes equivalent to that of iron-replete infants (Oski and Honig, 1978). Although there are statistically significant differences between developmental scores of infants with replete iron stores and infants with IDA, it does not necessarily indicate that infants with iron deficiency anemia are developmentally delayed. The mean developmental scores of infants with moderate IDA have been within the range of performance expected in healthy, average infants in the United States.

Preschool and School-Age Children

Preschool children with IDA perform more poorly on tests of intelligence and cognitive processes than iron-replete children (Soewondo et al, 1989), regardless of income level. For instance, a child with IDA takes more trials to learn how to discriminate between very similar visual stimuli than those who are iron replete.

IDA among school children (older than 6 years) has been associated with poor performance on tests of cognitive processes such as short-term memory and attention (Pollitt et al, 1989; Soemantri, 1989). However, the magnitude of the differences between subjects with IDA and subjects who are iron replete is small.

In general, among preschool and school-age children with IDA, iron interventions that lasted for 2 months or more resulted in major improvements in performance on one or more tests of cognitive processes (e.g., attention, visual perception organization, short-term recall). In contrast, the changes in test performance observed among IDA subjects who received placebo were inconsequential (Soewondo et al, 1989; Soemantri, 1989).

---

they dissolve calcium and phosphate. As mineral loss continues, the enamel breaks down, producing visible tooth destruction.

The ability of a food to be cariogenic is related to its ability to produce acid. Foods should be selected on the basis of their nutritional contribution to the diet but, because ingestion of carbohydrates presents an acid challenge to the teeth, it is desirable to limit the frequency of food consumption and encourage brushing following meals and snacks (American Dietetic Association, 1996).

The fluoride ion, when present at the tooth surface, acts to inhibit enamel demineralization and encourages calcium and phosphorus to leave saliva and remineralize the tooth as well as inhibit formation of dental plaque. For

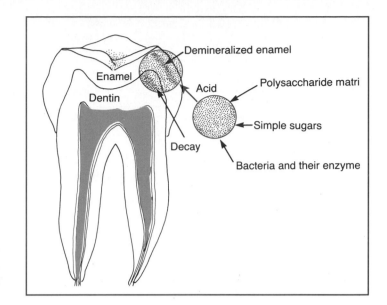

FIGURE 6–7. Parts of a tooth and its supporting structure. (From Mahan K, Arlin MT. Krause's food, nutrition, and diet therapy. 8th ed. Philadelphia: WB Saunders, 1992.)

children, the optimal intake of fluoride is 0.5 mg/kg body weight (Committee on Nutrition, 1993), a level provided when water is fluoridated at a level of 1 ppm. For children who live in areas where the water supply is not fluoridated, supplementation is recommended (Committee on Nutrition, 1993).

In addition to fluoride, a program to avoid accumulation of plaque and prevent dental caries and periodontal disease includes brushing, regular use of dental floss and regular professional care beginning by 2 years of age.

Fiber Consumption of dietary fiber in childhood is associated with important health benefits, particularly the promotion of normal laxation (Williams et al, 1995). It may also help reduce future risk of cardiovascular disease, some cancers, and adult-onset diabetes. In 1995, the Conference on Dietary Fiber in Childhood concluded that current dietary fiber intakes of children in the United States are suboptimal (Saldanha, 1995) and recommended increasing dietary fiber in childhood by increasing consumption of fruits, vegetables, and cereals and other grain products. According to these recommendations, children older than 2 years should increase their fiber to an amount equal to or greater than their age plus 5 g. Thus, fiber intake would increase from 8 g/day at age 3 years to 25 g/day by age 20. Examples of how these recommendations might be met at ages 2, 6, and 12 appear in Table 6–6.

High-fiber diets are not recommended for children younger than 1 year of age, and caution should be exercised in the use of high-fiber foods for older children. Foods high in fiber usually have low caloric density and, if consumed in large quantities, the total diet may not provide adequate calories for growth. A high fiber intake may impair the absorption of certain essential minerals, such as calcium, iron, zinc, copper, magnesium, and phosphorus (Committee on Nutrition, 1993).

FACTORS INFLUENCING FOOD INTAKE

■ Describe factors that influence dietary intakes of preschool and school-age children. How do they differ by age group?

Poverty

Poverty is a significant risk factor threatening the health of children. Nationwide, one out of every five children lives in a family whose income is below the poverty level. Despite the availability of food and nutrition programs (discussed in Application 6), economically disadvantaged children have a greater prevalence of short stature (Yip et al, 1993) and an increased risk of nutrient deficiencies, especially among subgroups (Drake, 1991) and homeless children (Taylor and Koblinsky, 1993).

The 1990–92 Consumer Expenditure Survey reveals that poor households with children spend 32% of their income on food, compared to 16% for non-poor families. However, the annual expenditure for food of poor households was approximately $2,500 less, even when poor households included more people (Lino, 1996).

Data from the Food Consumption Surveys in the United States and Canada (USDA, 1986; USDA, 1993; Evers and Hooper, 1995) indicate that average kilocalorie intake

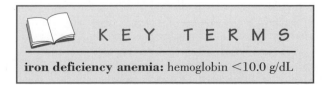

KEY TERMS

iron deficiency anemia: hemoglobin <10.0 g/dL

TABLE 6–6 Examples of Foods to Meet Fiber Recommendations for Children at Ages 2, 6, and 12 Years

2 Years		6 Years		12 Years	
Food	Fiber (g)	Food	Fiber (g)	Food	Fiber (g)
I slice whole wheat bread	2	I c Cheerios	3	Frosted Miniwheats	6
½ c cornflakes	I	I raw carrot	3	10 dried apricots	3
I banana	2	2 tbsp peanut butter	2	I oz almonds	3
½ c applesauce	2	I medium apple	3	2 c popped popcorn	2
Total	7		11		17

levels for children are less than those recommended but that mean nutrient intakes exceed the recommended levels for many nutrients. Mean levels of intakes in large surveys can mask large swings in intake, however. Although more than 80% of children in these surveys met target levels for nutrients, obviously, many did not.

In one survey, questions were asked about household food insecurity. Children were asked if enough food and enough of the kinds of food they wanted were available. As responses moved from more food secure to less food secure, the mean level of energy intake for children fell and levels of fat and saturated fat increased (Kennedy and Goldberg, 1995).

Family

The infant's rapid growth is reflected in her insistent demands for food. As infancy ends and toddlerhood begins, the slowed rate of growth is accompanied by a dramatic decrease in appetite. During early childhood, growth is steady but sporadic. Because a child's appetite ordinarily reflects his or her rate of growth, food intake is often inconsistent. Parents may become concerned that their young child is not eating enough. Such concern can lead to unnecessary anxiety over the child's eating habits and even create a battlefield between the parent and child in the kitchen and at the dinner table. In reality, studies of daily intakes of children have found that, although there was a high degree of variability from meal to meal, overall energy and nutrient intakes were relatively constant (Birch et al, 1991, Shea et al, 1992).

Dietary habits are formed early in life and often establish patterns that are carried into adulthood. Dietary patterns are shaped by the availabile choices and depend on food availability as well as cultural, environmental, and societal factors. Feeding young children depends on providing a variety of nutritious foods to meet nutritional needs and a social and emotional environment conducive to the enjoyment of food and the development of positive eating behaviors. In the preschool years, parents usually determine what foods are available to children and how they are presented. Not unexpectedly, there is a significant correlation between parents' and children's food preferences and attitudes toward food (Borah-Giddens and Falciglia, 1993). Parents are responsible for providing young children with foods that are nutritionally and developmentally appropriate at regular mealtimes and snacks. Although parents provide food to the child, it is the child who determines how much he will eat or even if he will eat. Allowing a child to make that decision, within limits, creates a structure that promotes positive eating behaviors (Birch et al, 1991).

Social and economic changes during recent decades have affected the family significantly. There are more single-parent families, most of which are headed by women. In addition, more mothers are employed outside the home, which may influence food patterns due to less time available for food shopping and preparation, and more meals eaten away from home. An analysis of the nutrient contents of the diets of children 2 to 5 years of age in the Nationwide Food Consumption Survey, however, found that maternal employment alone did not diminish the quality of the child's diet (Johnson et al, 1992). A recent survey conducted by the Food Marketing Institute and *Better Homes and Gardens* magazine found that having dinner together is a strong commitment of American families. Forty-three percent of families with young children indicated they ate dinner together 7 days a week, and another 28% said they ate together 4 to 6 times weekly (Food Marketing Institute, 1995).

Peers

As children move into daycare, preschool, or school, food choices are influenced increasingly by people outside the home. In the daycare or preschool setting, meal and snack times may provide an opportunity to expand a child's exposure to and acceptance of new foods. As the child becomes increasingly concerned with peer acceptance, eating becomes more of a social activity away from home.

Media and Advertising

Television reaches many children before they are capable of verbal communication. It has been estimated that children and adolescents in the United States watch 22 to 25 hours of television each week (Huston et al, 1992). Preschool children usually are not able to discriminate between regular programming and commercial messages and often watch commercials more closely than older children. Because commercial messages are based on emotional or psychological appeal and often promote products of low nutrient density, they may not support development of positive eating habits. Approximately 60% of all advertising shown during children's programming is for food products (Sylvester et al, 1995), most commonly for sweetened breakfast cereals, snack foods, candy, cookies or other desserts, and fast food restaurants.

There has been much discussion of the potential contribution of television viewing to the development of obesity in childhood. It may be that excess television viewing promotes increased snacking and inactivity, a lifestyle that is consistent with the development of obesity (DuRant et al, 1994). Insofar as it precludes other activities that require greater energy expenditure, extensive television viewing may promote inactivity. It has been observed that leaner children watch less television and are more physically active, and it is likely that television viewing is a manifestation of an individual who chooses to be less active.

Nutrition Knowledge and Education

The education level and nutrition knowledge of parents are important factors in determining foods available to their children. Young children are knowledgeable about nutrition. They can name the five food groups, and are able to understand the general relationship of food to exercise, body fat, and health (Murphy et al, 1995). Children who are allowed control over their food intake are significantly more aware of the role of foods in energy balance and are more likely to make healthful food choices (Anliker et al, 1992). Although the use of pressure or rewards may result temporarily in a child eating a certain food or meal, the long-term effects of such behavior may have a negative impact on food habits (Birch et al, 1984).

RECOMMENDATIONS FOR FOOD INTAKE

■ What are the developmental events that mark progress in self-feeding?

■ Describe the recommended amounts from each of the food groups for children aged 1 to 12 years.

■ Why is it important to promote positive food habits in young children?

■ What factors must be considered in planning vegetarian diets for children? What are the risks?

Feeding the Preschool Child

Early in the preschool years, the child is developing self-feeding skills using large motor skills, a process that involves frequent spills and the use of fingers and hands. These somewhat messy behaviors are a normal part of the development and maturation of young children (Table 6–7). The shift from large motor to fine motor skills provides a greater precision in eating and marks a time when preschoolers can participate in food preparation. The preschool years are important in the development of positive attitudes toward food and learning to make food choices. This process is promoted by an eating environment that is pleasant, both physically and emotionally. It includes a positive atmosphere with companionship and gentle guidance in fostering food-related behaviors.

A guide for types of foods and portion sizes appropriate for children aged 1 to 6 years appears in Table 6–8. Children require smaller portions than adults but will eat more often. In general, an appropriate portion size is a tablespoon of each type of food for every year of the child's age. More can be provided according to the child's appetite.

Because a young child has a smaller capacity and variations in appetite, she needs snacks as well as regularly scheduled meals. Snacks should be planned to provide nutrient-dense foods and timed so that they contribute to total nutrient intake but do not interfere with meals. Overall, preschool children prefer unmixed dishes with mild flavors at moderate temperatures that can be handled easily with utensils or hands.

Children aged 3 years and younger are at greatest risk for choking on food and require supervision while eating. The foods that most often cause choking are hot dogs, hard pieces of fruit or vegetables, peanut butter, popcorn, and nuts (Harris, 1984). Almost any other food can also cause problems with choking if the mouth is too full or if the child is running while eating.

Parents are often concerned when a toddler shows decreased interest in eating and refuses some favorite foods. Appetites may become erratic and unpredictable. Rejection of meats and vegetables is common. Children may refuse milk or may want to drink it to the exclusion of other foods. Often the preschool period is characterized by food jags during which the child may eat only a few foods or may want the same food meal after meal. Most jags (e.g., peanut butter and jelly sandwiches) last only a few days or weeks. When they are treated casually, they become passing food behaviors that are soon forgotten. However, placing greater importance on them may increase rather than

TABLE 6–7 Developmental Sequence Guide for Nutrition and Feeding During Childhood

Age (Approximate)	Motor Development	Oral Motor Skills Related to Eating	Self-Help/Social	Food and Appetite
12–24 mos	Walking; climbing; mature pincer grasp	Chewing using rotary motion; refined cup drinking	Enjoys eating; uses words; refined spoon feeding skills; eats with family	Bite-size foods; good appetite; avoid foods associated with easy choking
24–36 mos	Runs; jumps; three-jaw chuck (finger) grasp; uses fork	Straw drinking; independent cup drinking	Phrases and sentences; negativism emerges; toilet training in progress	Growth slows with decrease in appetite; avoid foods associated with easy choking
3–4 y	Hops; rides tricycle; static tripod (3-finger) grasp		Asserts independence; conversational body language; pours liquids	Picky eater; avoid foods associated with easy choking
5–6 y	Rides bicycle; refinement of grasp to adult pattern; ability to use one upper extremity for one task, other for a different task		Beginning to use knife and fork for cutting; acceptable table manners; peers becoming more important	Appetite more regular as rate of growth stabilizes; supervise eating of foods associated with easy choking

Developed by Nutrition-Feeding Clinic Faculty, The Nisonger Center University Affiliated Program for Mental Retardation and Developmental Disabilities, The Ohio State University, 1980. Revised 1995. Work supported in part by U.S. Department of Health and Human Services, Administration on Developmental Disabilities Grant #90DD032902 and Maternal and Child Health Bureau Grant #MCJ399155-04.

decrease such behavior, which may influence long-term food habits. Table 6–9 addresses solutions to some common feeding concerns in young children.

Feeding the School-Age Child

The period from 7 to 12 years of age is one of slow but steady growth. As appetite increases, so does food intake. Most food-related behavior problems of the preschool years have been resolved. Older children develop more autonomy with eating and take the initiative in making changes, usually accepting a wider variety of foods. They make their own eating decisions, but parents still exert an influence in terms of family food habits, attitudes, and expectations.

Because children spend much of their day in school, they do not eat as often as preschoolers. Individuals who work with children recognize the "barter and swap" environment of eating at school. The acceptance of a school lunch meal or a lunch packed at home is decided less by the foods themselves than by the preferences of peers. After-school snacks are almost universal. In the elementary school years, children increasingly assume responsibility for their own meals and snacks. Because of working parents and demanding schedules, many children are responsible for getting themselves off to school, packing their own lunches, and finding snacks. Participation in organized sports and other after-school activities may reduce the frequency of family meals. In addition, children in the early school years may be forced to assume responsibility for family shopping and preparation of the evening meal. As a result, children are targets of sophisticated advertising for a wide variety of food products.

Vegetarian Diets for Children

As the number of adults adopting vegetarian life styles increases, it is expected that more children will become vegetarians (Committee on Nutrition, 1993). The diets that sustain health in adult vegetarians are not necessarily appropriate for periods of rapid growth, however. The form of vegetarianism that is practiced determines the nutritional adequacy of the child's diet. The vegan diet, which excludes all animal products, may pose a risk for deficiencies of protein, calcium, iron, zinc, riboflavin, vitamins B_6 and B_{12}, and vitamin D (Dwyer, 1993).

Decreased growth of children following vegan-like diets compared to omnivore children has been reported, but the differences are small (Dwyer, 1993; Tayter and Stanek, 1989). Meal planning, especially for young children, may be complicated by limited food choices and the restriction of the number of meals and snacks. Because of the high fiber content and low caloric density of a vegetarian diet and the smaller stomach capacity of children, a child may be unable to consume a sufficient volume of food to meet his or her needs (Sanders and Reddy, 1994). Caloric density can be improved by emphasizing cereals, nut butters, and legumes. Diets that include dairy products are lower in fiber and provide several of the nutrients often lacking in strict vegan diets.

Vegetarian diets that include a variety of foods can be planned to provide all the nutritional requirements for growth (Sabate et al, 1991; O'Connell et al, 1989). As for all children, however, special attention must be paid to ensure adequate intake of energy, protein, vitamins B_{12} and D, calcium, zinc, and iron.

Dietary Intakes of Children

Adequate energy and nutrient intakes are easily achieved from dietary sources. Data from nationally representative surveys of the United States population found that energy intakes are stable or declining slightly but are consistent with recommended levels (Kennedy and Goldberg, 1995). In the USDA Continuing Food Consumption Survey, children from 0 to 5 years and 6 to 11 years of age consumed between 82% and 92% of the RDA for energy. For a majority of children intakes exceeded 75% of the RDA for all nutrients except for calcium, iron, and zinc.

Use of nutrient supplements is a common practice in the United States. Up to 60% of children use vitamin and mineral supplements regularly or occasionally (USDA, 1993), but supplement use declines with age (Bowering and Clancy, 1986). Parents of young children may assume that giving a supplement compensates for poor or marginal dietary intakes, but this is not necessarily true. For example, a child who consumes no dairy products may have a diet

TABLE 6–8 Food Guide for Preschool Children

Type of Food	Suggested Portion for:					Servings/Day
	1 y	2 y	3 y	4 y	5 y	
MILK, CHEESE, YOGURT						Total intake of 16–24 oz
Milk, yogurt	4 oz	5 oz	6 oz	6 oz	6 oz	
Cheese	½ oz	½ oz	¾ oz	¾ oz	1 oz	
PROTEIN FOODS						3–4
Meats, fish, poultry	½ oz	1 oz	1 oz	1 oz	1 oz	
Egg	1	1	1	1	1	
Cooked legumes	1 tbsp	2 tbsp	3 tbsp	4 tbsp	4 tbsp	
FRUITS						4–5
Fresh*	½ piece	½ piece				
Canned	1–2 tbsp	2–3 tbsp	3–4 tbsp	¼ c	¼–½ c	
Juice	2 oz	2–3 oz	3–4 oz	4 oz	4 oz	
VEGETABLES						4–5
Dark green, leafy or yellow vegetable	1 tbsp	2 tbsp	3 tbsp	4 tbsp	5 tbsp	
Other	1 tbsp	2 tbsp	3 tbsp	4 tbsp	5 tbsp	
Raw*	—	2–3 pieces	2–3 pieces	few pieces	few pieces	
BREADS AND GRAINS						4–5
Whole grain/enriched bread	¼ slice	¼ slice	½ slice	½ slice	½ slice	
Cooked cereal	1 tbsp	2 tbsp	3 tbsp	⅓ c	⅓ c	
Dry cereal	2 tbsp	¼ c	⅓ c	½ c	½ c	
Rice/pasta	2 tbsp	2 tbsp	3 tbsp	⅓ c	⅓ c	

*Should be given to young children only when they can chew well.

Adapted from McWilliams M. Nutrition for the growing years. New York: Wiley, 1986. Reprinted by permission of Prentice Hall, Upper Saddle River, NJ.

TABLE 6-9 Common Feeding Concerns in Young Children

Common Concern	Possible Solutions
Refuses meats	Offer small, bite-size pieces of moist, tender meat or poultry Incorporate into meatloaf, spaghetti sauce, stews, casseroles, burritos, pizza Include legumes, eggs, cheese Offer boneless fish (including canned tuna and salmon)
Drinks too little milk	Offer cheeses and yogurt, including cheese in cooking, e.g., macaroni and cheese, cheese sauce, pizza Use milk to cook hot cereals; offer cream soups, milk-based puddings and custards Allow child to pour milk from a pitcher and use a straw Include powdered milk in cooking and baking, e.g., biscuits, muffins, pancakes, meatloaf, casseroles
Drinks too much milk	Offer water if thirsty between meals Limit milk to one serving with meals or offer at end of meal; offer water for seconds If bottle is still used, wean to cup
Refuses vegetables and fruits	If child refuses vegetables, offer more fruits, and vice versa Prepare vegetables that are tender but not overcooked Steam vegetable strips (or offer raw if appropriate) and allow child to eat with fingers Offer sauces and dips, e.g., cheese sauce for cooked vegetables, dip for raw vegetables, yogurt to dip fruit Include vegetables in soups and casseroles Add fresh or dried fruit to cereals Prepare fruit in a variety of ways, e.g., fresh, cooked, juice, in gelatin, as a salad Continue to offer a variety of fruits and vegetables
Eats too many sweets	Limit purchase and preparation of sweet foods in the home Avoid using as a bribe or reward Incorporate into meals instead of snacks for better dental health Reduce sugar by half in recipes for cookies, muffins, quick breads, etc. Work with staff of daycare, preschools to reduce use of sweets

From Lucas B. Normal nutrition from infancy through adolescence. In: Queen PM, Lang CE (eds). Handbook of pediatric nutrition. Gaithersburg, MD: Aspen, 1993. © 1993, Aspen Publishers, Inc.

low in calcium, which probably would not be provided in a pediatric supplement. A balanced diet rather than supplementation is the best source of nutrition for healthy children (except for fluoride supplementation in areas where the fluoride level of water is below that which is consistent with prevention of dental caries).

Giving a child a single-dose, standard pediatric multivitamin presents no risk of nutrient excess. However, giving large or multiple doses of single nutrients or small groups of nutrients, particularly of vitamins A and D, is inappropriate. An important caution is to keep all vitamin preparations out of the reach of children. The most common cause of pediatric poisoning deaths reported to poison control centers in the United States is the accidental ingestion of iron supplements. Of the 5144 ingestions of iron supplements reported to poison control centers during 1991, 69.9% were in children less than 6 years of age, and 11 cases were fatal (Litovitz et al, 1992).

UNDERNUTRITION

■ What factors contribute to the development of protein energy undernutrition?

■ Describe the effects of undernutrition on growth and development.

■ What is catch-up growth?

■ How does short-term fasting influence cognition?

Severe Undernutrition

With favorable conditions, a child will follow a genetically predetermined growth curve. Growth retardation is the inevitable consequence of inadequate food intake, however. In developing countries, growth retardation is primarily the result of a synergistic relationship between inadequate food intake and infection, whereas in developed countries it is more frequently the result of inadequate absorption, chronic disease, psychological stress, or nonorganic failure to thrive (see Chapter 4). The overall impact on an individual child's growth is determined by the type, timing, and duration of the nutritional deficit.

Successful nutrition rehabilitation depends on correction of the underlying condition and improvement of nutrient and energy intake. Initial dietary management begins with small, frequent feeding, with progressive increases in volume and concentration. The term "catch-up growth" is used to describe the acceleration in growth that occurs when a period of growth retardation ends and favorable conditions are restored. Weight gain may occur at a rate several times faster than that of normal healthy children the same age. The energy cost of weight gain can range from 10 kcal/g of muscle gained to 2 kcal/g of fat (Solomon, 1985).

Undernutrition and Cognition

Severe undernutrition occurs infrequently in North America, but the impact of moderate undernutrition or inadequate food intake is of concern. Recent investigations have explored the subtle behavioral and cognitive consequences of inadequate intake and short-term fasting. Such studies have been hampered by difficulty in measuring cognition and distinguishing the effects of nutrition from those of genetics and other environmental factors.

Measuring Cognition

Most development in the human brain occurs prenatally and during the first 2 years of postnatal life. Cognition in infants has been measured using developmental scales, most commonly the Bayley Scales of Mental and Motor Development (BSMMD). These scales assume that observed behavior is a reflection of intelligence or mental competence. For preschool and school-age children, IQ tests, learning tasks (such as discrimination and oddity learning), and school achievement are used most often to estimate cognitive development.

Short-Term Fasting and Cognition

For decades it has been accepted that good nutrition has a positive effect on a child's ability to learn and that skipping a meal, especially breakfast, can have a negative impact on learning. In the 1950s, a series of studies suggested academic performance was improved when children consumed breakfast, but, due to small sample sizes and poor experimental designs, no definitive benefits could be documented.

In the 1980s, carefully controlled experimental studies in a controlled setting measured problem-solving performance of well-nourished 9- to 11-year-old children after they ate breakfast and after they skipped breakfast (Pollitt et al, 1982; Simeon et al, 1989). When the children ate breakfast they made fewer errors on tasks of picture identification, response to stimulus on a computer display, and arithmetic tests than when they had skipped breakfast.

The acute effects of skipping breakfast involve the short-term physiologic changes associated with a diminished supply of nutrients to the brain. Under normal short-term fasting conditions, homeostatic mechanisms attempt to maintain blood glucose within physiologic ranges to ensure adequate brain function. A prolonged fast requires more adaptation on the part of the body to maintain blood glucose levels. It may be that a decline (even within normal physiologic range) results in metabolic changes that influence cognition.

Over the past several years there has been increasing evidence that a moderate elevation of blood glucose regulates a variety of brain functions, including memory and learning. Brain scans show that cognitive functions increase the rate at which glucose is metabolized, and there is some evidence that moderate increases in blood glucose levels improve cognitive functioning in children (Hall et al, 1989). One proposed mechanism by which raised blood glucose levels may influence cognition is through the synthesis of acetylcholine, a neurotransmitter that has a well-established role in memory functions.

These recent studies led participants in a 1995 International Symposium on Breakfast and Performance and Health to conclude that children who skip breakfast are less efficient in problem solving, have reduced recall of newly acquired information, and have decreased verbal fluency and creativity (Pollitt, 1995). The conferees encouraged development of policies to promote recognition of the importance of breakfast and intervention to ensure that breakfast is available to children.

Eating breakfast also has a long-term impact on an individual's nutrient intake. When breakfast is skipped, the nutrients usually consumed at the breakfast meal are not recovered from intake during the remainder of the day (Nicklas et al, 1993). Nonetheless, examination of data from national surveys indicates a decline in breakfast consumption across all age groups. It is estimated that on any given day as many as half of school-age children skip breakfast, but a school breakfast program is associated with decreased absenteeism and tardiness (Pollitt, 1995).

NUTRITION-RELATED CONCERNS

■ How can nutrition status or diet influence behavior?

■ How do food allergies develop?

■ How are food allergies identified and treated?

■ What are the risks to children of lead exposure? How can the risk be minimized?

■ What is the role of nutrition in avoidance of or recovery from lead toxicity?

Diet and Behavior

Since the mid-1970s, relationships between diet or nutrition and behaviors such as hyperactivity, minimal brain dysfunction, and learning disabilities have been postulated. Evidence for many such associations is anecdotal or subjective in nature, however. In recent years a more systematic, scientific approach has suggested that there are some such relationships, the details of which are yet to be explored.

NEUROTRANSMITTERS Many dietary substances function as **neurotransmitters** or are precursors to neurotransmitters. For example, the amino acids glutamate and aspartate are neurotransmitters. However, ingestion of large quantities of these amino acids has little effect on brain function because they do not readily cross the **blood–brain barrier** (Fernstrom, 1994). Tyrosine and phenylalanine are precursors for norepinephrine and dopamine, which are also neurotransmitters. Administration of large amounts of these precursors can alter levels of the neurotransmitters and potentially alter brain function, but the changes are minimal.

Tryptophan is a precursor to the neurotransmitter serotonin, which is the one that has been studied most extensively. The effect of tryptophan on brain function is contingent upon getting the tryptophan into the brain. Large neutral amino acids, namely tryptophan and the **branched-chain amino acids** (BCAA), compete for the same carrier to cross the blood–brain barrier. When carbohydrate is ingested, insulin is released and blood levels of BCAA decline, creating a relative excess of tryptophan in the blood. Proportionately higher levels of tryptophan in the blood mean that the carrier will transport more tryptophan and less BCAA. The overall effect is an increase in tryptophan in the brain and increased synthesis of brain serotonin, which, in turn, has been postulated to induce sleepiness. If a meal consisting only of protein and fat is eaten, blood tryptophan levels rise, but so do levels of the branched chain amino acids; consequently, there is no increase in the uptake of tryptophan in the brain. Thus, it appears that very high carbohydrate ingestion can increase brain levels of serotonin, but the effect on behavior is speculative.

Attention Deficit Hyperactivity Disorder

Attention deficit hyperactivity disorder (ADHD), a persistent pattern of inattention with or without hyperactivity-impulsivity, is one of the most common childhood developmental disorders. The prevalence of ADHD varies from 1% to 20% of elementary school children (Murphy and Hagerman, 1992). The diagnostic criteria for ADHD are listed in Table 6–10. Children with ADHD experience inattention, impulsivity, and overactivity to a degree that is inappropriate for their age or developmental levels, resulting in major problems in home, school, and peer adjustment. Therapy for ADHD conditions centers on behavior management, medication, and special education.

It has been postulated that dietary factors such as food additives, sugar, and food allergies may be linked to ADHD. In the 1970s, a popular diet for children with behavioral disturbances involved removing foods containing salicylates from their diets. Presentation of this hypothesis to physicians at medical meetings and to the public via a best-selling book quickly enhanced its popularity (Feingold, 1976). Proponents and critics offered widely differing estimates of its value. Eventually the hypothesis was tested in several **double-blind challenge** clinical trials. These studies concluded that the data did not support a relationship between diet and ADHD except in a very small percentage of children (Lipton and Mayo, 1983; Kaplan et al, 1989). However, because the diet altered so many factors in the child's life, it has been difficult to determine whether the positive changes resulted from the dietary regimen or from other lifestyle changes that occurred because of the diet.

Children with ADHD are commonly treated with stimulant medications such as methylphenidate (Ritalin) or dextroamphetamine (Dexedrine), which reduce symptoms of irritability, restlessness, and short attention span by stimulating the brain. Anorexia, which has the potential to reduce food dietary intake and impair growth, is a frequent side effect of these drugs (Farris et al, 1986; Harper et al, 1978). To minimize the anorectic effect of these medications, they should be given with or after meals, and growth should be monitored carefully in children on such drugs.

Sucrose

Sugar (sucrose) has been reported in popular literature and the media to cause behavior problems in children and even delinquency in adolescents. All of the media publicity suggesting an association between sugar and behavior may prime parents to expect the adverse behavior and conclude that their child is "sensitive to sugar." Studies using sugar, aspartame, and saccharin reveal that none of these substances has any effect on behavior, attention, or academic performance (Wolraich et al, 1994). A meta-analysis was performed of studies that used a **within-subject design** to compare sucrose to a placebo in trials for which both parents and researchers were blinded to the substance given. These researchers concluded that sugar does not affect the behavior or cognitive performance of children (Wolraich et al, 1995). However, there are many valid reasons for reducing sugar consumption, such as improving dental health and increasing the nutrient density of the child's diet.

Caffeine

Caffeine is the most widely ingested stimulant in North America. This naturally-occurring legal stimulant is readily available in carbonated beverages, chocolate-containing foods, coffee and tea, and over-the-counter medications. In the Bogalusa Heart Study (Arbeit et al, 1988), at least 77% of children 76 months of age had caffeine in their diet.

The effects of caffeine in preschool children have been essentially unstudied, and observations in school-age children do not indicate any clear negative effects from caffeine in normal children (Leviton, 1992). A double-blind placebo-controlled crossover design on children between 8 and 12 years of age found that caffeine improved performance on some measures of attention and on a test of mental dexterity. There was a concurrent trend toward an increased level of self-reported anxiety. Children reported feeling significantly less sluggish after caffeine than after placebo ingestion (Bernstein et al, 1994).

Food Hypersensitivities

Food hypersensitivities, or allergies, are characterized by abnormal or exaggerated responses to specific food allergens (antigens that trigger a response of the immune system). Most potential food antigens are prevented from entering the body by mechanisms in the gastrointestinal tract, but very small amounts of antigenic molecules may be absorbed and transported throughout the body. If these antigens reach **immune competent** cells, the antibody **IgE** is produced, resulting in **sensitization**, so that subsequent exposure to the specific antigen induces an allergic response. The most common food allergies are to eggs, cow's milk, nuts, wheat, soy products, whitefish, and shellfish. IgE-mediated allergic reactions (hypersensitivities) to foods are manifested by a variety of symptoms. Most allergic reactions to food are immediate (within 2 hours) and may cause symptoms of the gastrointestinal tract, with cramping, bloating, vomiting, and diarrhea. In other cases, the antigen spreads through the bloodstream and lymphatic system, causing symptoms to appear in 2 to 24 hours. These may include itchy skin and hives (eczema and uticaria), cough and wheeze (asthma), runny nose (rhinorrhea), itchy eyes (conjunctivitis), and in rare cases anaphylaxis.

Adverse reactions to food are often **food intolerances** rather than actual allergies, but the symptoms are similar. Dietary proteins, sugars, lipids, toxins, and food additives are among the most common causes of reactions due to food intolerance (Anderson, 1986).

Incidence

Allergic reactions to food are found in all age groups, but they occur most frequently in the first few years of life. Between 4% and 6% of infants have food allergies (Sampson, 1992). Fortunately, most children outgrow or develop a tolerance for allergens after about 3 years of age (Bock, 1987). If the food allergen can be identified and excluded from the diet for 1 to 2 years, adults and older children may also lose their sensitivity to that specific allergen (Sampson and Scanlon, 1989; Pastorello et al, 1989).

Diagnosis

It is difficult to identify specific allergens. Manifestations of an allergic response are influenced by the child's age, the integrity of the bowel mucosa, the state of the food

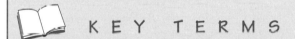

KEY TERMS

neurotransmitters: substances released from neurons on excitation that travel to target cells either to excite or inhibit

blood–brain barrier: a membrane structure that allows selective transport of nutrients into the brain via a carrier system

branched-chain amino acids (BCAA): valine, leucine, isoleucine

double blind: a research design in which neither the researcher nor the subjects know who is receiving the control diet or the experimental diet until the study is completed

challenge: the withholding of a substance suspected to cause a reaction until there are no symptoms and then giving that substance to ascertain whether it will cause a reaction

within-subject design: the treatments (in this case sugar and placebo) are administered to each subject so that they serve as their own control for comparison of treatments

immune competent: able to produce an immune response to antigens

IgE: a specific antibody triggered by a food antigen

sensitization: initial exposure of an individual to a specific antigen, resulting in an immune response

food intolerance: reaction to food or chemical substances in food that is not mediated via IgE

TABLE 6–10 Diagnostic Criteria for Attention Deficit Hyperactivity Disorder

SYMPTOMS

Either six (or more) of the symptoms of inattention (Group 1) or hyperactivity–impulsivity (Group 2) have persisted for at least 6 months to a degree that is maladaptive and inconsistent with developmental level:

GROUP 1

Inattention

Often fails to give close attention to details or makes careless mistakes in schoolwork, work, or other activities

Often has difficulty sustaining attention in tasks or play activities

Often does not seem to listen when spoken to directly

Often does not follow through on instructions and fails to finish schoolwork, chores, or duties in the workplace (not due to oppositional behavior or failure to understand instructions)

Often has difficulty organizing tasks and activities

Often avoids, dislikes, or is reluctant to engage in tasks that require sustained mental effort (e.g., schoolwork or homework)

Often loses things necessary for tasks or activities (e.g., toys, school assignments, pencils, books, or tools)

Often is easily distracted by extraneous stimuli

Often is forgetful in daily activities

GROUP 2

Hyperactivity

Often fidgets with hands or feet or squirms in seat

Often leaves seat in classroom or in other situations in which remaining seated is expected

Often runs out or climbs excessively in situations in which it is inappropriate (in adolescents or adults, may be limited to subjective feelings of restlessness)

Often has difficulty playing or engaging in leisure activities quietly

Is often "on the go" or often acts as if "driven by a motor"

Often talks incessantly

Impulsivity

Often blurts out answers before questions have been completed

Often has difficulty awaiting turn

Often interrupts or intrudes on others (e.g., butts into conversations or games)

OTHER CRITERIA

Hyperactivity

Some hyperactive–impulsive or inattentive symptoms that caused impairment were present before age 7 years.

Some impairment from the symptoms is present in two or more settings (e.g., at school [or work] and at home).

There must be clear evidence of clinically significant impairment in social, academic, or occupational functioning.

The symptoms are not better accounted for by another developmental or mental disorder.

Reprinted with permission from the Diagnostic and Statistical Manual of Mental Disorders, Fourth Edition. Copyright 1994 American Psychiatric Association.

(cooked foods are usually less allergenic than raw foods), and the presence of other foods or substances that may influence the response or cause a reaction of their own.

Diagnosis involves identification of the suspected food, demonstration that ingestion of that food causes an adverse reaction, and confirmation that ingestion of the food is associated with an immune response, i.e., increased levels of IgE. Skin testing by subcutaneous administration of an extract of the suspected food antigen can elicit an IgE-mediated response (a positive test) as indicated by a **wheal** and **flare** reaction. Blood tests can demonstrate the presence of a specific IgE response to a food allergen. However, both types of tests for food allergies give false positive results 60% to 65% of the time (Sampson, 1992).

The double-blind placebo-controlled food challenge (DBPCFC) is considered the gold standard for diagnosis of food allergies (Bock et al, 1988). It involves giving increasing amounts of an extract of the suspected food until symptoms are provoked or until a total of 10 g of the food has been given. If there is a reaction (recurrence of symptoms), the offending food is eliminated from the diet for 6 to 12 weeks. If symptoms are then reduced or eliminated, it is assumed that the food was the source of the allergic reaction. In some instances a challenge with the food itself is used to confirm the diagnosis.

Treatment

Successful treatment of a food allergy involves elimination of the offending allergen. Some individuals may need to avoid the offending foods completely, but others can control symptoms by limiting the amounts consumed. The tolerable level depends on exposure to other allergens, health status, and the level of stress the individual is experiencing. If more than a few foods must be eliminated from the diet, careful attention has to be given to food selection to ensure an adequate diet. Medications are available that help to control allergic symptoms, but they do not affect the allergy itself.

Lead: The Silent Health Threat to Children

Lead toxicity, or plumbism, is the number one environmental health threat to infants and children. It is insidious, because minute amounts can impair a child's growth and cause irreversible damage to the nervous system, resulting in lowered IQ and learning disabilities. Unfortunately, for many children, the physical symptoms may be absent or vague until lead accumulation in the body reaches very high levels. The Centers for Disease Control (CDC) estimates that at least 17% of children under the age of 6 years have blood lead levels in the toxic range of 10 mg/dL (CDC, 1991).

Sources of Lead

Sources of lead contamination are ubiquitous. Lead is found in thousands of products, such as batteries, gasoline, newspaper ink, shotgun ammunition, pesticides, water pipes, lead solder on copper pipes (lead solder was banned in 1986), housewares, and leaded crystal. Pollution created by incineration, factory emission, and automobile exhaust releases lead into the air and onto the soil. Although lead-containing paints were banned in the United States in 1978, their legacy persists. Lead toxicity is frequent among young children who have **pica**, specifically those who eat chips of lead-containing paint from walls, woodwork, furniture, or toys. The greatest risk, however, is exposure to lead-containing dust particles in older homes in which walls are still coated with leaded paint. Levels are especially high when lead paint is being sanded and scraped.

All foods contain some lead due to air and soil pollution. Lead solder is used to seal the seams in less than 4% of American-produced food cans. However, for those in which lead is used, lead can be leached from the solder into the food, particularly by acidic foods such as fruits, fruit juices, and tomatoes. Therefore, such foods should not be stored in the can after it has been opened. Lead-containing paints and glazing compounds used on ceramics and pottery can leach into foods prepared or stored in them. Lead paint and glazes have been banned in the United States, so the main risk is from old dishes or imported ceramics and china.

The Effects of Lead

Blood lead levels at which symptoms occur are shown in Figure 6–8. Symptoms of plumbism are uncommon unless lead levels are very high. However, many **epidemiologic** studies have documented that low-level lead exposure in children, even in the absence of symptoms, is associated with lower IQ, impairment in learning and visual motor skills, increased behavior abnormalities, and learning disabilities (Bellinger et al, 1990).

Young children are at greatest risk for plumbism because they engage in more hand-to-mouth activities, they

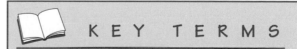

KEY TERMS

wheal: a localized area of edema on the body surface, often accompanied by severe itching and redness
flare: an area of redness on the skin around the point of application of an irritant such as a food allergen
pica: consumption of nonfood substances
epidemiologic: factors that influence the frequency and distribution of diseases in humans

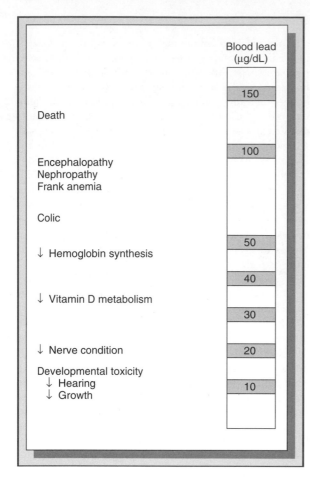

Blood lead
(µg/dL)

	150
Death	
	100
Encephalopathy	
Nephropathy	
Frank anemia	
Colic	
	50
↓ Hemoglobin synthesis	
	40
↓ Vitamin D metabolism	
	30
↓ Nerve condition	20
Developmental toxicity	
↓ Hearing	10
↓ Growth	

FIGURE 6–8. Observed effect levels of inorganic lead in children. (From Agency for Toxic Substances and Disease Registry [ASTDR]. Case studies in environmental medicine: lead toxicity. Atlanta: 1990.)

absorb lead more efficiently than adults (50% vs 10%), and they have relatively rapid growth between 6 months and 3 to 4 years of age, particularly in the brain and central nervous system, which is susceptible to lead-induced neurologic damage. **Glial** replication and differentiation and **cerebellar** growth are most rapid during the first 18 months of life, and **myelination** continues into the third or fourth year. Excess body lead can interfere with this development. Infants whose mothers were exposed to high levels of lead during pregnancy experience cognitive and growth defects in infancy and are particularly vulnerable when exposure continues postnatally (Dietrich et al, 1993). If postnatal lead levels remain below 10 µg/dL, however, prenatally exposed children tend to catch up to normal growth and development patterns by 2 years of age (Shukla et al, 1991).

Long-term studies reveal that children with early lead exposure are six times more likely than others to have learning disabilities and seven times more likely to drop out of high school (Needleman et al, 1992). Thus, blood lead levels in late infancy and early childhood may compromise a child's long-term performance.

Role of Diet

The body handles lead by making use of existing transport systems for metal nutrients. Consequently, some nutrients may influence the handling of lead. Exposure to excess lead results in high blood lead levels even in the presence of an adequate diet. However, lead toxicity is more common in infants and children who are at nutritional risk, e.g., urban, poor, and nonwhite children. Lead uptake is greatly enhanced in the fasting state. Deficiencies of calcium, phosphate, iron, or zinc may make children more susceptible to lead intoxication.

Studies of animals and human infants have shown inverse relationships between the absorption and distribution of dietary calcium and levels of lead in the blood (Mushak and Crocetti, 1996). Furthermore, data from the NHANES survey indicate that children with elevated blood levels of lead have low dietary intakes of calcium (Mahaffey et al, 1986). Such preliminary data suggest that increasing calcium intake might have value in secondary prevention of plumbism by minimizing lead absorption (Koo et al, 1991). Recent research studies indicate that phosphate as well as or in conjunction with calcium reduces lead toxicity (Mushak and Crocetti, 1996).

Iron deficiency anemia and high blood levels of lead are likely to occur in the same child. At first it was assumed that lead caused microcyte anemia by impairing iron utilization, but it is now recognized that iron deficiency and excess lead both impair hemoglobin synthesis. Iron deficiency may enhance lead intoxication because decreased iron in the intestine can allow absorption of a larger portion of ingested lead (Yip et al, 1981). Therefore, children with elevated blood lead levels should be screened for iron deficiency and treated appropriately. Preliminary animal studies indicate that adequate amounts of zinc, the amino acid methionine, and copper may decrease intestinal absorption of lead and thus have a protective effect (Flora et al, 1991).

Acceptable Blood Levels

In 1991, the Centers for Disease Control defined lead toxicity at 10 micrograms per deciliter (µg/dL). This standard is based on evidence of permanent damage to the nervous, **hematopoietic**, and renal systems from lead levels higher than 10 µg/dL. Under this definition 54% of African-American inner-city and 6% of white suburban children are at risk for neurotoxic impairment.

Treatment/Prevention

Prevention is the most important treatment for lead toxicity. Suggestions for decreasing intake of excess lead ap-

TABLE 6–11 Ways to Decrease Excess Exposure to Lead in Foods and Beverages

Run cold tap 30–60 seconds before using for drinking or cooking whenever faucet hasn't been used for several hours.

Use cold water (boiling concentrates lead).

Investigate water supply and, if necessary, have water analyzed for lead content.

Do not use leaded crystal on a daily basis. Do not store liquids in it.

Check cans of imported foods for lead solder. If type of solder cannot be determined, limit consumption.

Avoid using old or imported ceramic products for food or beverages.

Never store acidic foods in open cans.

Wash vegetables; discard outer leaves.

Consume adequate amounts of calcium, iron, and zinc.

Do not use inside-out colored bread packaging to store or transport food.

Make sure children's hands are clean before they eat.

pear in Table 6–11. Screening for blood lead levels is a cornerstone of prevention. The Centers for Disease Control (1991) recommends that all children from 6 to 36 months of age have a blood test for lead. More frequent screening is recommended for youngsters in environments with increased exposure to lead, such as those who live in old houses, near a smeltery or processing plant, or in areas of heavy traffic.

The most important factor in the management of the child with lead poisoning is to control the level of exposure to lead (Ruff, 1993). Blood lead levels greater than 25 μg/dL may be treated with **chelating** agents, which act to filter lead out of the blood and increase its excretion in the urine. However, for any treatment to be effective, exposure to lead must be reduced concurrently.

PROMOTING OPTIMAL NUTRITION FOR CHILDREN

What are appropriate dietary recommendations for children to promote long-term health? Atherosclerosis is a life-long disease process that begins with fatty streak formation in childhood and adolescence and progresses to fibrous plaques leading to coronary heart disease (CHD) in adulthood (National Cholesterol Education Program, 1992). Many of the risk factors associated with coronary heart disease, such as diets high in total and saturated fat, obesity, hypertension, and lack of exercise, may originate early in life. Substantial evidence implicates elevated blood cholesterol levels in childhood in the eventual development of coronary artery disease (Lauer et al, 1988).

It has been suggested that the cardiovascular disease process can be slowed or prevented by modifying risk-related behaviors early in life. The National Cholesterol Education Panel (NCEP) has issued recommendations for a population-wide reduction in the average levels of blood cholesterol through changes in eating patterns of children 2 years and older. These recommendations, the same as those recommended as Step One for adults, include a distribution of energy sources as approximately 55% carbohydrate, 15% protein, and 30% fat, with almost equal amounts from polyunsaturated, monounsaturated, and saturated fatty acids, and a dietary cholesterol less than 300 mg/day.

It is important to emphasize that the primary role of diet is to provide sufficient kilocalories and nutrients to support normal growth and development and that caution must be exercised when decreasing the fat intake of children (Sigman-Grant et al, 1993). Severe restriction of children's fat intake with the intention of reducing the risk of heart disease will have a negative impact on growth (Lifschitz and Moses, 1989). Although dietary fat can be restricted safely to approximately 30% of kilocalories, care in planning is necessary to ensure an adequate energy and nutrient intake. This means including all food groups and making low-fat choices within each group, such as low-fat milk and fish, lean meats and poultry, and a wide variety of foods in moderation.

A sedentary lifestyle is also linked to development of CHD and other chronic diseases. Regular physical activity results in substantial health benefits for adults and children. In addition, the energy expended allows larger amounts of food to be consumed with a decreased risk of obesity.

According to the survey "Food, Physical Activity and Fun: What Kids Think" conducted by the Gallup Organization (1995), most American children have positive attitudes about food, nutrition, and physical activity. The children surveyed agreed that a balanced diet and regular physical activity are important for health. They also indi-

KEY TERMS

glial: specialized cells and their processes that form the supporting structure of the brain and spinal cord
cerebellar: pertaining to the hindbrain; concerned with coordination of movements
myelination: production of fat-like substance forming a sheath around certain nerve fibers
hematopoietic: red blood cell–forming
chelating: capable of binding lead and therefore depleting the soft and hard skeletal tissues of lead, thus reducing its toxicity

cated that they were aware of the importance of eating a variety of foods and a willingness to try new foods. While recognizing that physical activity is good for health, most children reported they were physically active because it was fun and they enjoyed it.

The best preparation for a long, healthy life is a healthy lifestyle that includes a balanced, varied diet and enjoyable physical activity. Efforts to improve the nutrition and health of children must target families, schools, and others who work with children to encourage them to involve and motivate children to appreciate that physical activity is fun and that healthful eating tastes good (Borra et al, 1995; Luepker et al, 1996).

CONCEPTS TO REMEMBER

▶ Overall, childhood is a period of slow, steady growth, the rate of which is determined by genetic and environmental factors.

▶ In the short term, growth is characterized by spurts and latent periods.

▶ Children's energy and nutrient needs are determined by body size, body composition, rate of growth, and level of activity.

▶ Physical activity enables children to expend more calories and, therefore, to have more flexibility in energy and food intake.

▶ Because of day-to-day variation in the rate of growth, energy and, nutrient needs and, therefore, dietary intakes of children will vary.

▶ Undernutrition during childhood can slow the rate of growth and impair physical and cognitive development.

▶ During childhood, appetite reflects growth and nutrition needs.

▶ It is the responsibility of parents to offer developmentally and nutritionally appropriate foods and to provide an environment conducive to development of positive attitudes toward and acceptance of food that will influence long-term food habits.

▶ As children grow older, food preferences are increasingly influenced by peers and other factors outside the home.

▶ Nutrition concerns of childhood center on ensuring a nutritionally adequate diet to support growth and to minimize the risk of chronic disease.

▶ An important area of nutrition research is exploring the role nutrition may play in behavior and cognitive development.

▶ Special nutrition and diet-related concerns include dental health, food allergies, and exposure to lead.

References

American Dietetic Association. Position of The American Dietetic Association: Oral health and nutrition. J Am Diet Assoc 1996;96:184.

Anderson JA. The establishment of common language. J Allergy Clin Immunol 1986;78:140.

Anliker JA, et al. Mothers' reports of their three-year-old children's control over foods and involvement in food-related activities. J Nutr Educ 1992;24:285.

Arbeit ML, et al. Caffeine intakes of children from a biracial population: the Bogalusa Heart Study. J Am Diet Assoc 1988;88:466.

Aukett MA, et al. Treatment with iron increases weight gain and psychomotor development. Arch Dis Child 1986;61:849.

Bellinger D, et al. Low-level lead exposure and children's cognitive function in the preschool years. Pediatrics 1991;87:219.

Bernstein CA, et al. Caffeine effects on learning, performance, and anxiety in normal school-age children. J am Acad Child Adolesc Psych 1994;33:407.

Birch LL, et al. Eating as a "means" activity in contingency: effect on young children's food preference. Child Dev 1984;55:431.

Birch LL, et al. The variability of young children's energy intake. N Engl J Med 1991;324:232.

Bock SA. Prospective appraisal of complaints of adverse reactions to foods in children during the first 3 years of life. Pediatrics 1987;79:683.

Bock SA, et al. Double-blind placebo-controlled food challenge as an office procedure: a manual. J Allergy Clin Immunol 1988;82:986.

Borah-Giddens J, Falciglia GA. A meta-analysis of the relationship in food preference between parents and children. J Nutr Educ 1993;25:102.

Borra ST, et al. Food, physical activity and fun: inspiring America's kids to more healthful lifestyles. J Am Diet Assoc 1995;95:816.

Bowering J, Clancy KL. Nutritional status of children and teenagers in relation to vitamin and mineral use. J Am Diet Assoc 1986;86:1033.

Centers for Disease Control. Preventing lead poisoning in young children. Atlanta: U.S. Department of Health and Human Services, October 1991.

Committee on Nutrition. In: Bruness LA (ed). American Academy of Pediatrics Pediatric Nutrition Handbook. 3rd ed. Elk Grove Village, IL:1993.

Dietrich KN, et al. The developmental consequences of how to moderate prenatal and postnatal lead exposure: intellectual attainment in the Cincinnati Lead Study Cohort following school entry. Neurotoxicol Teratol 1993;15:37.

Domel SB, et al. Accuracy of fourth- and fifth-grade students' food records compared with school-lunch observations. Am J Clin Nutr 1994;59:S218.

Drake MA. Anthropometry, biochemical iron indexes, and energy and nutrient intake of preschool children: comparison of intake at daycare centers and at home. J Am Diet Assoc 1991;91:1587.

DuRant RH et al. The relationship among television watching, physical activity, and body composition of young children. Pediatrics 1994;4:449.

Dwyer JT. Vegetarianism in children. In: Queen PM, Lang CE (ed). Handbook of pediatric nutrition. Gaithersburg, MD: Aspen, 1993.

Evers SE, Hooper MD. Dietary intake and anthropometric status of 7- to 9-year-old children in economically disadvantaged communities in Ontario. J Am Coll Nutr 1995;14:595.

Farris RP, et al. Macronutrient intakes of 10-year-old children, 1973 to 1982. J Am Diet Assoc 1986;86:765.

Feingold BF. Why your child is hyperactive. New York: Random House, 1975.

Fernstrom JD. Dietary amino acids and brain function. J Am Diet Assoc 1994;94:71.

Flora, SJ et al. Interaction of zinc, methionine or their combination with lead at gastrointestinal or post-absorptive level in rats. Pharmacol Toxicol 1991;68:3.

Food Marketing Institute and Better Homes and Gardens Magazine. Meal Watch. Summer 1995.

Gallup Organization. Food, physical activity and fun: what kids think. Chicago, IL and Washington, DC: American Dietetic Association and International Food Information Council in cooperation with the President's Council on Physical Fitness and Sports, 1995.

Hall JL, et al. Glucose enhancement of performance on memory tests in young and aged humans. Neuropsychologia 1989;27:1129.

Harper PH, et al. Nutrient intakes of children on the hyperkinesis diet. J Am Diet Assoc 1978;73:515.

Harris CS, et al. Childhood asphyxiation by food: a national analysis and overlook. JAMA 1984;251:2231.

Huston AC, et al. Big world, small screen: the role of television in American society. Lincoln, NE: University of Nebraska, 1992.

Idjradinata P, Pollitt E. Reversal of developmental delays among iron deficient anemic infants treated with iron. Lancet 1993;341:1.

Johnson RK, et al. Maternal employment and the quality of young children's diets: empirical evidence based on the 1987–1988 nationwide food consumption survey. Pediatrics 1992;90:245.

Johnston CC, et al. Calcium supplementation and increases in bone mineral density in children. N Engl J Med 1992;327:82.

Kaplan BJ, et al. Dietary replacement in preschool-aged hyperactive boys. Pediatrics 1989;83:7.

Kennedy E, Goldberg J. What are American children eating? Implications for public policy. Nutr Rev 1995;53:111.

Koo WWK, et al. Serum vitamin D metabolites and bone mineralization in young children with chronic low to moderate lead exposure. Pediatrics 1991;87:680.

Lauer RM, et al. Factors affecting the relationship between childhood and adult cholesterol levels: The Muscatine Study. Pediatrics 1988;82:309.

Leviton AL. Behavioral correlates of caffeine consumption by children. Clin Pediatr 1992;26:742.

Liftschitz F, Moses N. Growth failure: a complication of dietary treatment of hypercholesterolemia. Am J Dis Child 1989;43:537.

Lino M. Income and spending of poor households with children. Fam Econ Nutr Rev 1996;9:2.

Lipton MA, Mayo JP. Diet and hyperkinesis—an update. J Am Diet Assoc 1983;83:132.

Litovitz TL, et al. 1991 annual report of the American Association of Poison Control Centers. National Data Collection System. Am J Emerg Med 1992;10:452.

Lloyd T, et al. Calcium supplementation and bone mineral density in adolescent girls. JAMA 1993;270:841.

Lozoff B, et al. Long-term developmental outcome of infants with iron deficiency. N Engl J Med 1991;325:687.

Luepker RV, et al. Outcomes of a field trial to improve children's dietary patterns and physical activity. JAMA 1996;275:768.

Lytle LA, et al. Validation of 24-hour recalls assisted by food records in third-grade children. J Am Diet Assoc 1993;93:1431.

Mahaffey KR, et al. Blood lead levels and dietary calcium intake in 1- to 11-year-old children: The Second National Health and Nutrition Examination Survey, 1976 to 1980. Pediatrics 1986;78:257.

Matkovic V, Fontana D, Tominac C. Factors that influence peak bone mass formation: a study of calcium balance and the inheritance of bone mass in adolescent females. Am J Clin Nutr 1990; 52:878.

Murphy AM, Hagerman RJ. Attention deficit hyperactivity disorder in children: diagnosis, treatment, and follow-up. J Pediatric Health 1992;6:2.

Murphy AS, et al. Kindergarten students' food preferences are not consistent with their knowledge of the Dietary Guidelines. J Am Diet Assoc 1995;95:219.

Mushak P, Crocetti AF. Lead and nutrition: biologic interactions of lead with nutrients. Nutrition Today 1996;31:12.

National Cholesterol Education Program (NCEP) Expert Panel on Blood Cholesterol Levels in Children and Adults. National Cholesterol Education Program (NCEP): Highlights of the Report of the Expert Panel on Blood Cholesterol Levels in Children and Adults. Pediatrics 1992;89:495.

Needleman H, et al. The long-term effects of exposure to low doses of lead in childhood: An 11-year follow-up report. N Engl J Med 1990;322:83.

Nicklas TA, et al. Dietary studies of children: The Bogalusa Heart Study experience. J Am Diet Assoc 1995;95:1127.

Nicklas TA, et al. Breakfast consumption affects adequacy of total daily intake in children. J Am Diet Assoc 1993;9:886.

O'Connell J, et al. Growth of vegetarian children: The Farm study. Pediatrics 1984;84:475.

Oski FA, Honig AS. The effects of therapy on the developmental scores of iron-deficient infants. J Pediatr 1978;92:21.

Pastorello EA, et al. Role of the elimination diet in adults with food allergy. J Allergy Clin Immunol 1989;84:475.

Pollitt E. Iron deficiency and cognitive function. Ann Rev Nutr 1993;13:521.

Pollitt E. Does breakfast make a difference in school? J Am Diet Assoc 1995;95:1134.

Pollitt E, et al. Iron deficiency and educational achievement in Thailand. Am J Clin Nutr 1989;50(Suppl):687.

Pollitt E, et al. Fasting and cognitive function. J Pediatr Res 1982;17:169.

Ruff HA. Declining blood lead levels and cognitive changes of moderately lead-poisoned children. JAMA 1993;269:1641.

Sabate J, et al. Attained height of lacto-ovo vegetarian children and adolescents. Eur J Clin Nutr 1991;45:51.

Saldanha LG. Fiber in the diet of US children: results of national surveys. Pediatr 1995;96:S995.

Sampson HA, Metcalfe DD. Food allergies. JAMA 1992;268:2840.

Sampson HA, Scanlon SN. National history of food sensitivity in children with atopic dermatitis. J Pediatr 1989;115:23.

Sanders TA, Reddy S. Vegetarian diets and children. Am J Clin Nutr 1994;59:1176S.

Shea S, et al. Variability and self-regulation of energy intake in young children in their everyday environment. Pediatrics 1992;90:542.

Shukla R, et al. Lead exposure and growth in the early preschool child: a follow-up report from the Cincinnati Lead Study. Pediatrics 1991;88:886.

Sigman-Grant M, et al. Dietary approaches for reducing fat intake of preschool-age children. Pediatrics 1993;91:955.

Simeon T, et al. Effects of missing breakfast on the cognitive functions of school children with differing nutritional studies. Am J Clin Nutr 1989;49:646.

Soemantri S. Preliminary findings on iron supplementation and learning achievement of rural Indonesian children. Am J Clin Nutr 1989;50(Suppl):698.

Soewondo S, et al. Effects of iron deficiency on attentional learning processes in preschool children: Bandung, Indonesia. Am J Clin Nutr 1989;50(Suppl):667.

Solomon NW. Rehabilitating the severely malnourished child. J Am Diet Assoc 1985;85:28.

Sylvester GP, et al. Children's television and nutrition: friends or foes? Nutrition Today 1995;30:6.

Taylor ML, Koblinsky SA. Dietary intake and growth status of young homeless children. J Am Diet Assoc 1993;93:464.

Tayter M, Stanek KL. Anthropometric and dietary assessment of omnivore and lacto-ovo-vegetarian children. J Am Diet Assoc 1989;89:1661.

USDA Human Nutrition Information Services. Nationwide Food Consumption Survey. Continuing survey of food intakes by individuals: women 19–50 years and their children 1–5 years, 4 days. Washington, DC: CSFII Report 86–3, 1986.

USDA Human Nutrition Information Services. Food and nutrient intakes by individuals in the United States, 1 day, 1989. Nationwide Food Consumption Survey 1987–88. Washington, DC: NFCS Report 87–1-1, 1993.

Williams CL, et al. A new recommendation for dietary fiber in childhood. Pediatr 1995;96:S985.

Wolraich M, et al. Effects of diets high in sucrose or aspartame on the behavior and cognitive performance of children. N Engl J Med 1994;330:301.

Wolraich ML, et al. The effect of sugar on behavior or cognition in children: a meta-analysis. JAMA 1995;274:1617.

Yip R, et al. Iron status of children with elevated blood-lead concentrations. J Pediatr 1981;98:922.

Yip R, et al. Trends and patterns in height and weight status of low income children. Crit Rev Food Sci Nutr 1993;33:409.

APPLICATION: Meals at School

School Lunch Program

Ramon and Juanita, at the beginning of this chapter, were eligible for free lunch at their school. There had also been a meal program at Ramon's Head Start program the year before. Ramon and Juanita are just two of the approximately 25 million American students who participate each day in the National School Lunch Program (NSLP), which is administered by the United States Department of Agriculture (USDA). Almost all public schools and 83% of private schools participate in school lunch programs (Burghardt et al, 1995). Meal pattern requirements have been established for food groups and portion sizes so that the "type A" lunch provides approximately one-third or more of the RDA for children and students at various ages (Table A6–1). The Special Milk Program supplements the NSLP and provides a subsidy for milk served in a school.

The NSLP, established in 1946 by the School Lunch Act, is supported by cash reimbursements and provision of supplemental food commodities to participating schools. Each state is required to match every dollar of federal money with $3 from sources within the state. In addition to meeting nutritional standards, participating schools are required to operate on a nonprofit basis, serve meals at a regular meal hour, and provide lunches free or at reduced cost to those unable to pay. Eligibility for free and reduced price meals is determined by household size and income (Burghardt and Daveny, 1995). In 1991,

Free meals: family incomes are 130% or less of the poverty guidelines

Reduced price meals: family incomes are between 130% and 180% of the poverty guidelines

TABLE A6–1 School Lunch Pattern

Components		Minimum Quantities Per Lunch				Recommended Quantities for Group V: 12 y and Older; Grades 7–12*
		Group I: Age 1–2 y; Preschool	Group II: Age 3–4 y; Preschool	Group III: Age 5–8 y; Grades K–3	Group IV: Age 9 y and Older; Grades 4–12	
Milk	Whole and unflavored lowfat must be offered (flavored or skim milk may also be offered)	¾ c	¾ c	½ pint	½ pint	½ pint
Meat or meat alternate (quantity of the edible portion as served)	Lean meat, poultry, or fish	1 oz	1½ oz	1½ oz	2 oz	3 oz
	Cheese	1 oz	1½ oz	1½ oz	2 oz	3 oz
	Large egg	½	¾	¾	1	1½
	Cooked dry beans or peas	¼ c	⅜ c	⅜	½ c	¾ c
	Peanut butter or an equivalent quantity of any combination of any of above	2 tbsp	3 tbsp	3 tbsp	4 tbsp	6 tbsp
Vegetable or fruit	2 or more servings of vegetable or fruit or both	½ c	½ c	½ c	¾ c	¾ c
Bread or bread alternate	Must be enriched or whole-grain. 1 serving = 1 slice of bread; or ½ cup of cooked rice, macaroni, noodles, other pasta or cereal; 1 biscuit, roll or muffin	1 (5/wk)	1+ (8/wk)	1+ (8/wk)	1+ (8/wk)	2 (10/wk)

*The *minimum* portion sizes for these children are the portion sizes for group IV.

From Food and Nutrition Service, US Department of Agriculture. Meal pattern requirements and offer versus serve manual, FNS-265. Washington, DC: 1990.

over one-half of the children participating in the school lunch program received free or reduced price lunches.

The school lunch program has been criticized for excessive plate waste; high levels of fat, sugar, and salt in the food served; and competition from vending machines. In at least one study it was observed that children eating a sack lunch prepared at home or eating from vending machines consumed fewer nutrients than the school lunch meal, however (Ho et al, 1991). As part of the School Nutrition Dietary Assessment Study, analysis of menus from 515 NSLP schools found that less than 5% of the schools offered lunches that provide a 5-day average close to the dietary guidelines for fat (Chapman et al, 1995); the amounts of fat and saturation fat offered exceeded the Dietary Guidelines. The School Meals Initiative for Healthy Children changes standards for school meals, provides a variety of menu planning alternatives, and streamlines program administration. It requires compliance with the 1990 Dietary Guidelines by the 1996–97 school year. It will also measure a school's compliance with the nutrition standards weekly rather than daily (Federal Register 1995).

Schools must offer the five required food items each day. To improve food acceptance, high school students have the option of selecting three (one must be an entree) of the five designated items of the Type A lunch. At the discretion of the school authority, students at senior high level may be permitted to decline one or two required food items. This "offer versus serve" policy is believed to improve student participation, but the effect on nutrient intake has not yet been assessed.

Other changes in the school lunch program include involving students in menu planning and offering popular items, such as pizza, tacos, and hamburgers, more frequently. To encourage development of menus with a lower fat content, many schools have added salad bars and reduced the number of baked desserts.

5 required food *items:*
Milk
Meat or alternate
2 vegetable/fruits
Bread or alternate

School Breakfast Program

The Child Nutrition Act of 1966 provided funds for the School Breakfast Program in the United States. The School Breakfast Program is operated predominantly in schools where children travel long distances to school and where many are from low income families. In 1992, average daily participation in the School Breakfast Program was 4.9 million. Approximately 85% of children participating in the School Breakfast Program receive free or reduced-price breakfasts (Burghardt et al, 1995). The breakfast is planned to provide one-fourth of the RDA, and consists of one serving of fruit or juice, one half-pint of milk, and one serving of cereal (Table A6–2). This program may improve the overall quality of the children's diet.

A recent study of 10-year-old children who ate breakfast versus those who did not found that children who skipped breakfast consumed 200 to 500 fewer kilocalories and less than the RDAs for vitamins A, E, D, B_6, and calcium (Nicklas et al, 1993). Such a deficit may be difficult to make up in the remaining meals and snacks of the day.

A recent survey of children conducted by the Kellogg Foundation found that children learn about food and nutrition from their parents and from school. The Child and Adolescent Trial for Cardiovascular Health (CATCH) is an 8-year (1987–1995) multicenter trial designed to assess the effectiveness of a school-based intervention for promoting healthful behaviors in elementary school children in third through fifth grades in order to reduce their subsequent risk for cardiovascular disease. The specific interventions of the program include classroom curricula and school environmental modifications related to food consumption, physical activity and initiatives to support nonsmoking, and a family program that complements the school curriculum. In particular, it targets the school food service through training sessions, educational materials, and ongoing support visits to effect positive changes in school meals. Four major areas of change were identified and addressed at training sessions and in the development of intervention strategies: menu planning, food purchasing, food preparation, and program promotion.

A report of that intervention found that in school lunches, the percentage of energy intake from fat fell significantly more (from 38% to 31.9%) than in control lunches (38.9%

TABLE A6–2 Food Servings Required for the School Breakfast Program

Food Components	Minimum Quantities		
	Ages 1 and 2 y	Ages 3–5 y	Grades K–12
MILK			
As a beverage, on cereal, or both	½ c	¾ c	½ pint
JUICE/FRUIT/VEGETABLE*			
Fruit and/or vegetable; or full-strength fruit juice or vegetable juice	¼ c	½ c	½ c
BREAD/BREAD ALTERNATES†			
Bread (whole-grain or enriched)	½ slice	½ slice	1 slice
Biscuit, roll, muffin or equal serving of cornbread (whole-grain or enriched meal flour)	½ serving	½ serving	1 serving
Cereal (whole-grain or enriched or fortified)	¼ c or ⅓ oz	⅓ c or ½ oz	¾ cup or 1 oz
MEAT/MEAT ALTERNATES			
Meat, poultry, or fish	½ oz	½ oz	1 oz
Cheese	½ oz	½ oz	1 oz
Egg (large)	½	½	½
Peanut butter or other nut or seed butters	1 tbsp	1 tbsp	2 tbsp
Cooked dry beans and peas	2 tbsp	2 tbsp	4 tbsp
Nuts and/or seeds (as listed in program guidance)‡	½ oz	½ oz	1 oz

* A citrus juice or fruit or a fruit or vegetable juice that is a good source of vitamin C (see Menu Planning Guide for School Food Service, PA-1260) is recommended to be offered daily.

† See Food Buying Guide for Child Nutrition Programs, PA-1331 (1984) for serving sizes for breads and bread alternates.

‡ No more than 1 oz of nuts and/or seeds may be served in any one meal.

From Food and Nutrition Service, US Department of Agriculture, Washington, DC. Meal pattern requirements and offer versus serve manual. FNS-265. 1990.

to 36.2%). The intensity of physical activity in physical education classes during the CATCH intervention increased significantly in intervention schools. Self-reported daily energy intake from fat among students in the intervention schools was significantly reduced, from 32.7% to 30.3%, compared to 32.6% to 32.2% among students in the control schools. Intervention students reported significantly more daily vigorous activity than controls (58.6 minutes versus 46.5 minutes). Blood pressure, body size, and cholesterol measures did not differ significantly between treatment groups. No evidence of deleterious effects of the intervention on growth or development was observed (Luepker et al, 1996).

Throughout the country school lunch menus are changing. Children will be eating lunches that are lower in fat and sodium and have more variety. These changes reflect an historic policy advancement—the School Meals Initiative for Healthy Children.

Team Nutrition is a network of public and private partnerships that span the country linking USDA to all those who touch children's lives. The network brings together organizations in agriculture, the food industry, consumer health and nutrition advocates and educators, the media, and federal and state agencies to reach out and amplify its nutrition education message to help children change their behavior. The new policy of updating school meals' nutrition standards to reflect the Dietary Guidelines for Americans under the School Meals Initiative for Healthy Children is the most significant reform of the school meals program since it began in 1946. A complementary school program fostered by the USDA is the Team Nutrition Schools Program. It showcases healthy changes in school meals and new nutrition education programs. Team Nutrition Schools will model the involvement of Team Nutrition partners and supporters at the local level and actively promote school meals that offer more healthful choices.

REFERENCES

Burghardt JA, et al. The School Nutrition Dietary Assessment Study: summary and discussion. Am J Clin Nutr 1995;61:252S.

Burghardt JA, Devaney BL. Background of the school dietary assessment study. Am J Clin Nutr 1995;61:178S.

Chapman N, et al. Factors affecting the fat content of National School Lunch Program lunches. Am J Clin Nutr 1995;61:199S.

Federal Register 1995; 60N.113.

Ho CS, et al. Evaluation of the nutrient content of school, sack and vending lunch of junior high students. Sch Food Serv Res Rev 1991;15:85.

Luepker RV. Outcomes of a field trial to improve children's dietary patterns and physical activity. The child and adolescent trial for cardiovascular health (CATCH). JAMA 1996;275:768.

Nicklas TA, et al. Secular trends in dietary intake and cardiovascular risk factors of 10-year-old children: The Bogalusa Heart Study (1973–1988). Am J Clin Nutr 1993;57:930.

USDA's Team Nutrition Schools. Food and Consumer Service, United States Department of Agriculture. Alexandria, VA: 1995.

CHAPTER 7

NUTRITION DURING ADOLESCENCE

Growth and Development
Assessment of Nutritional Status
Energy and Nutrient Needs
Factors That Influence Food Habits

Nutrition-Related Concerns of Adolescence
Promoting Positive Food Habits
Concepts to Remember

When David was 12 years old, he was an easy going seventh grader who performed well in school and participated in several outside activities. His life centered around his family, especially his younger brother and sister. In the autumn, when David began eighth grade, he was 140 cm (55 in) tall and weighed 34 kg (75 lb). That year he began to "shoot up," and by Christmas he was an inch and a half taller and the jeans purchased for school in the fall were well above his shoe tops. He seemed to have more friends and was spending much of his time with them.

By the time David was 13 years old, he had grown 14 cm (5 in) and gained 11 kg (24 lb). Increased body hair and sexual development were becoming apparent, but he was concerned because he had "no muscles." He seemed to eat all the time. A usual breakfast consisted of two bowls of cereal, fruit juice, and some kind of toast or pastry, with two large glasses of milk. He ate two or more portions of everything at the dinner meal. For years David had been "brown bagging" his lunch to school, but when high school began, he wanted to eat in the cafeteria or nearby fast food establishments. His first stop upon arriving home after school was at the refrigerator for a snack.

At the end of his freshman year, David was 168 cm (66 in) tall and weighed 55 kg (121 lb). That summer he worked at the local swimming pool and played baseball. It seemed he was never home except to eat and sleep. David's life became even busier when he returned to school. He tried out for and made the basketball team. This meant long hours of practice, and now he really was hungry all the time. He returned to taking his lunch to school because his lunch allowance did not buy enough "to fill him up." He would carry two lunches—one for noon and one for after school. Each included two sandwiches, fruit, and cookies. At noon he would add milk and potato chips from the cafeteria. After school he would have a soft drink from the vending machine. David ate dinner when he got home and then had a large dish of ice cream and a glass of milk before bedtime. Weekends found David either playing ball or just hanging out with friends.

At the time of his physical examination in the fall of his junior year, David was 174 cm (68 in) tall and weighed 62 kg (136 lb). He was disappointed that he had not grown more and started lifting weights to "build himself up." He developed some problems with acne, which made him very self-conscious. A friend suggested a product he had bought at the drug store to "dry up" the "zits," which seemed to help. Even though David was seldom home for family meals, he did consume large quantities of food there. When at home, he spent much of his time in his room with the door closed. He was impatient with the family and rejected many of the foods which had been his favorites.

By the time David entered his senior year, he was 177 cm (70 in) in height and 67 kg (147 lb) in weight. While he was still not pleased with his body weight and shape, he had more muscle than a year ago. He felt lifting weights had helped. His acne was less bothersome than it had been. He still had a huge appetite, especially during basketball season, but he was not quite as ravenous as he had been the last couple of years. His relationships at home seemed more harmonious and he felt his parents were beginning to respect him as an individual.

As David approached the close of his high school years, he was very different from that 12-year-old. He had grown another 2 inches and gained 8 pounds during his senior year, and will continue to grow slowly after he leaves high school. His muscle mass and bone mass will continue to increase as he "fills out." David has a part-time job at a local restaurant. He is saving some of his earnings for a car. He is planning for his future after he leaves high school.

David's story is a rather benign example of the transitions of adolescence. In the United States there are approximately 30 million teenagers, constituting about 17% of the population (Committee on Nutrition, 1993). Adolescence, spanning the ages 10 to 20 years, is the bridge from childhood to adulthood. It is a period of multiple transitions to physical maturity, a coherent sense of self, and emotional independence (Table 7–1). The term *puberty* refers to the rapid somatic growth, changes in body composition, and sexual development that accompany reproductive maturation. Because the time of onset of puberty varies among individuals and because the progression of puberty is uneven, chronologic age is a poor indicator of physiologic maturity. Adolescence is of longer duration than the defined stages of puberty. Except for increases in bone mass, the physical changes of puberty are usually completed around 17 years of age, but the overall transition from adolescence to young adulthood is generally reached between the ages of 17 and 20 years. Understanding the growth and development patterns of adolescence is essential to the determination of nutritional needs and formulation of dietary recommendations for this age group.

GROWTH AND DEVELOPMENT

■ What are the characteristics of the growth and changes in body composition of puberty, and how do males and females differ?

■ What is the significance of the stage of sexual maturation (SMR) in interpreting growth measurements?

■ How do hormonal changes of puberty influence growth and development?

■ Describe the cognitive and psychosocial changes of adolescence.

Except for the first 2 years of life, there is no time when growth and development are as rapid as during the early teens. Puberty begins at different times for girls (8 to 13 years) than for boys (9.5 to 13.5 years) and at widely divergent times among age cohorts of boys and girls. The typical duration of puberty is 3 to 4 years, but it can be much shorter or longer. Developmental stages of pubescence are considered the best guide of growth and maturation. The most frequently used sexual maturity ratings (SMR), developed by Tanner (1962), appear in Table 7–2. The changes described, once initiated, follow a consistent pattern regardless of chronologic age. The stages of SMR, ranging from prepubertal (SMR 1) to adult (SMR 5), are defined by the development of primary and secondary sex characteristics in females (pubic hair and breasts) and males (pubic hair and mature genitalia).

Stage 1, characterized by rapid growth but no discernible physical changes, lasts 0.5 to 2 years in boys and 0.2 to 1.2 years in girls. The middle stage (SMR 3 and 4) begins at 12 to 14 years in girls and 12.5 to 15 years in boys and lasts from less than 1 to more than 2 years. Mean age of the onset of menarche is 12.8 years (SMR 3 or 4), but the normal range is from 10 to 16.5 years. Late puberty (SMR 5) has its onset at 14 to 16 years in girls and 14 to 17 years in boys.

Physiologic or **skeletal age** can be assessed by comparing an x-ray of the wrist and hand to standard radiographs from a reference population (Cameron, 1993). The skeletal age of the individual adolescent is the chronologic age of the standard that his or her x-ray most closely resembles.

Growth

Height

The magnitude of growth during puberty is reflected in gains in height (Fig. 7–1). At the onset of puberty (skeletal age of 10 years in females and 12 years in males), girls

TABLE 7–1 Characteristics of Stages of Adolescent and Pubertal Development

Adolescence: General Characteristics	Puberty: Physical Development Characteristics
EARLY (10–13 y)	**EARLY (onset: males, 10.5–14 y, females, 10–13 y)**
Onset of puberty; concern with developing body; expands social radius beyond family; concentrates on relationship to peers; cognition is usually concrete	Rapid growth; observable sexual maturation begins—small amount of pubic hair, beginning of changes in genitalia
MIDDLE (14–16 y)	**MIDDLE (males 12.5–15 y, females 12–14 y)**
Pubertal development usually complete; peer groups sets many of behavioral standards; family values still persist; conflicts over independence; cognition begins to be abstract	Increased pubic hair; larger penis and scrotum in males; increased breast tissue, onset of menses in females; peak height and weight velocity in males
LATE (17–20 y)	**LATE (males 14–16 y, females 14–17 y)**
Physical maturation complete; body image established; relationships more giving and sharing; more individual than peer group; idealistic, emancipation nearly secured; cognitive development is complete; functional role begins to be defined	Adult-type pubic hair distribution and genitalia

Adapted from Behrman RE et al (eds). Nelson textbook of pediatrics. 14th ed. Philadelphia: WB Saunders, 1992.

and boys have attained 84% of their ultimate height. They will acquire 95% of their ultimate height by a skeletal age of 13 years for girls and 15 years for boys (Roche and Davila, 1972).

Girls will add 23 to 28 cm (9 to 11 in) during pubertal development. Peak height velocity, the point at which the increase in height is at its greatest rate, occurs approximately 1 year after breast development begins and about 1 year before menarche, after which gains range from 4.3 to 10.6 cm (1.7 to 4.2 in), as shown in Figure 7–2. An adolescent female who has reached menarche is in the decel-eration phase of growth. Girls who mature early will be taller sooner and attain their final height at a younger age, but final height is greater in girls who mature later because they have a longer preadolescent growth spurt.

Compared to girls, boys have a longer period of childhood growth before the adolescent spurt and achieve a higher peak height velocity at about 13.9 years (Fig. 7–3). They accumulate an average of 28 cm (11 in) in the pubertal phase, resulting in an average final height that is 13 cm (5.2 in) taller than that of females (Slap, 1986; Tanner, 1985).

With this rapid linear growth and increasing height comes lengthening of long bones and increased skeletal mineral mass. Adolescents gain about 40% of their eventual skeletal mass between SMR 3 and 4 for males and in SMR 2 for girls (Matkovik, 1993). The **epiphyses** are found at the ends of long bones, on the margins of flat bones and at **tubercles**. During skeletal growth, the epiphyses are separated from the main portion of bone by a specialized fibrous connective tissue called **cartilage**. The final stage of skeletal maturation occurs at a median age of 17.3 years in females and 21.2 years in males when, under the influence of the gonadal hormones of puberty, the epiphyses fuse with the main portion of the bones (Roche and Davila, 1972). When this process is complete, growth in stature ceases (Tanner, 1962), but increases in bone mass continue well into the mid-twenties.

Weight

The rate of weight gain during adolescence parallels the increase in stature. In females, peak weight velocity occurs 6 to 9 months prior to peak height velocity (Gong and Spear, 1988). From ages 10 to 17 years, girls gain an average 24 kg (53 lb), approximately 42% of their young adult weight. The onset of menses occurs with attainment of a critical body weight or body fatness (Merzenich et al, 1993). In males, peak height velocity coincides with peak

KEY TERMS

skeletal age: a physiologic age determined from x-ray examination of the number and size of epiphyseal centers, the sharpness of outline of the ends of the bones and distance separating the epiphyseal center and the bone shapes and the degree of fusion between these two elements

epiphyses: the end of the long bone, usually under the shaft and either entirely cartilaginous or separated from the shaft by a cartilaginous disk

tubercles: a nodule or rough, rounded prominence on a bone

cartilage: a specialized fibrous connected tissue

TABLE 7–2 Stages of Sexual Maturation (Sexual Maturity Ratings)

Male	Pubic Hair	Genital Development	Female	Pubic Hair	Genital Development
Stage 1	None	Prepubertal	Stage 1	None	Prepubertal
Stage 2	Small amount at outer edge of pubis; slight darkening	Enlargement of scrotum and testes Scrotum reddened and changed in texture Beginning penile enlargement	Stage 2	Small amount; downy on labia majora	Elevation of breast as small bud Enlargement of areola diameter
Stage 3	Darker, coarser and curled; sparsely covers pubis	Enlargement of penis Growth of testes and scrotum	Stage 3	Increase over junction of pubis; darker and curly	Further enlargement and elevation of breast and areola
Stage 4	Adult type; does not extend to thighs	Increased size of penis Testes and scrotum larger Scrotal skin darker	Stage 4	More abundant; coarse	Increased size of breast; areola and nipple form secondary mound
Stage 5	Adult type; now spread to thighs	Genitalia adult size and shape	Stage 5	Adult type; now spread to thighs	Adult distribution of breast tissue; continuous outline

Adapted from Tanner JM. Growth at adolescence. 2nd ed. Oxford: Blackwell, 1962.

weight velocity. During the same period, ages 10 to 17 years, boys accumulate an average of 32 kg (70 lb), which accounts for 51% of their adult body mass.

Development

Hormonal Changes That Influence Growth and Development

Sexual development is governed by hormones. Androgens are steroid sex hormones that promote development of masculine characteristics; estrogens are feminizing. Both types of hormones are normally secreted by both sexes. The testes secrete large amounts of androgens, principally testosterone, but they also secrete small amounts of estrogens. The ovaries secrete large amounts of estrogens and small amounts of androgens. Androgens are also secreted by the adrenal gland in both sexes. The ovaries also secrete progesterone, which has special functions in preparing the uterus for pregnancy. The role of hormones in the normal menstrual cycle is discussed in Chapter 8.

In males, androgens promote the accumulation of proportionately more muscle mass, less fat, greater linear growth, a heavier skeleton, and greater red blood cell mass than females. In addition to promoting growth and changes in body composition, testosterone stimulates development of the genitalia. For both males and females, elevated levels of androgens produced by the adrenal gland promote growth and are responsible for initiation of the growth of pubic and **axillary** hair. Another effect of androgens is increased size and secretions of the **sebaceous glands**. These effects are the forerunners of acne.

Estrogens and progesterone promote the deposition of proportionately more fat than lean body mass in females. Estrogens secreted in response to the follicle-stimulating hormone (FSH) from the pituitary gland stimulate growth of the ovaries and enlargement of the uterus and also influence breast development.

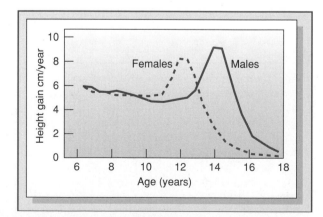

FIGURE 7–1. Maximum height gain (cm/y) for girls and boys from the peripubertal to pubertal period. (From Tanner JM. Growth at adolescence. 2nd ed. Oxford: Blackwell, 1962.)

Physical Development

Puberty is characterized by accelerated muscular, skeletal, endocrine, and emotional development. During pu-

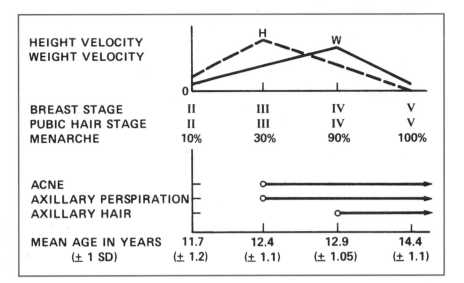

FIGURE 7–2. Sequence of maturational events in females. (From Marshall WA, et al. Variations in pattern of pubertal changes in girls and boys. Arch Dis Child 1969;44:291.)

berty, the size of many of the abdominal organs increases. Skeletal changes other than those related to linear height become apparent. In males, the obvious changes are a development of a more muscular torso and broader shoulders. Increases in shoulder width and leg length are more pronounced in males than in females. For males, the increases in lean body mass (LBM) and testosterone during late puberty are associated with a marked increase in muscular strength. Females experience an increase in the width of the hips, associated with a significantly broadened pelvic girth, as well as increased fat deposition.

Alterations in craniofacial proportions entail mandibular (lower jaw) growth, with a more prominent chin and sharpening of the features. The well-recognized voice changes that occur in boys during puberty are the consequence of growth of the larynx and laryngeal muscles. By early adolescence the cuspids (canines) and first molars of the primary dentition are shed and permanent cuspids, first and second premolars, and molars erupt during this period.

Body Composition

LEAN BODY MASS   Throughout childhood lean body mass (LBM) is approximately the same in both sexes (Fig. 7–4). Males and females accumulate lean body mass during puberty, but males have a more rapid growth spurt of longer duration so that their final LBM exceeds that of females by almost 50% (Bartlett et al, 1991). Shortly after the gain in stature is completed, muscle mass peaks. For females this occurs at SMR 3–4, usually by age 16 to 18 years, and for males at SMR 5, approximately 3 years later. As a percentage of body weight, LBM increases in males from 80% to 90% of total body weight, whereas in females LBM *decreases* from 80% to 75% as females accumulate proportionally greater amounts of body fat. Lean body mass is related to height, and taller individuals have a larger LBM.

BODY FAT   There are great differences between males and females in body fat and lean body mass upon completion of the rapid body changes of puberty (see Fig. 7–4). The percentage of body weight that is fat in girls is about twice that in boys. The mean body fat in boys increases from about 4% to 11% early in puberty (usually SMR 1–2) and remains relatively constant into adulthood. In females, each successive stage of pubertal development is associated with an increase in body fat content, which can range from 15% to 27% of weight. Females characteristically have more subcutaneous adipose tissue in the pelvic, breast, upper back, and arm areas.

BONE MINERAL MASS   From birth through about 16 years of age there is rapid bone growth and **modeling**. Puberty is a critical period for accumulation of bone mass; gains may be 7% to 8% per year (Fig. 7–5) (Matkovik, 1990). **Peak bone mass** is achieved well into the third

KEY TERMS

axillary: upper chest, medial side of the arm, armpit

sebaceous glands: glands located at the base of the hair follicle which secrete sebum, a thick substance composed of fat and epithelial debris from cells

modeling: a continuing process of bone resorption and formation associated with general shaping of bones from adjustment to changes in body weight, stature and proportion

peak bone mass: the maximum amount of bone an individual will accumulate

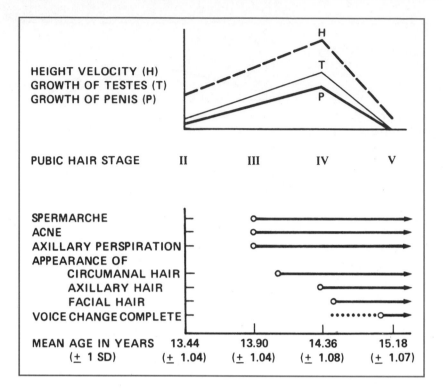

FIGURE 7–3. Sequence of maturational events in males. (From Marshall WA, et al. Variations in pattern of pubertal changes in girls and boys. Arch Dis Child 1969;44:291.)

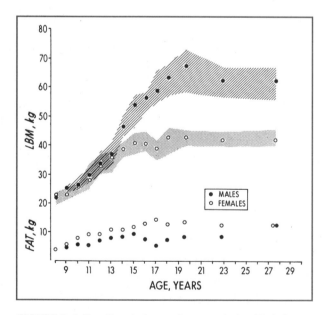

FIGURE 7–4. Plot of lean body mass (upper portion) and body fat (lower portion) for males and females, aged 9 to 29 years. Shaded areas embrace the 25th and 75th percentiles; the dots are at the 50th percentile. (From Forbes GB. Growth of lean body mass in man. Growth 1972;36:325.)

decade of life. After that period, the skeleton is in a constant process of remodeling throughout life, but the accumulation of bone mass declines. Achievement of maximal bone mass at skeletal maturity is considered to be the best protection against age-related bone loss and subsequent fracture in later life.

BODY WATER As a percentage of body weight, total body water decreases gradually across childhood and adolescence. Muscle tissue contains a relatively large amount of cellular water. As LBM increases, the proportion of water in the intracellular compartment increases and the proportion of extracellular water decreases. By approximately 16 years of age, body water is approximately 58% of total body weight, and about 66% of that water is intracellular (Grande and Keys, 1980).

Neurodevelopment

Early adolescence is a period of continuing neurodevelopmental maturation. By 12 years of age most individuals manifest a "mature" response to all items of a standardized neurodevelopmental assessment, including the ability to distinguish left from right and to perform refined finger movements.

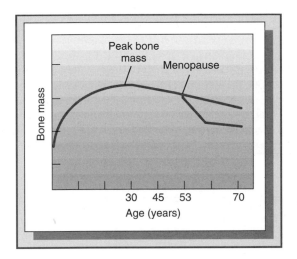

FIGURE 7–5. Bone mass rises in adolescent years and declines with aging.

Cognitive Development

The rapid physical growth and maturation of early adolescence are associated with impulsive behavior. The adolescent has little ability to understand the etiology of that behavior, however. During this period logical thought development begins and the individual learns to organize (see Table 7–1). Middle adolescence is characterized by rapid growth in cognition as the adolescent begins to understand complex abstract concepts and becomes capable of generating hypotheses to be tested before action is initiated. Such understanding allows him or her to consider possible consequences of behavior and to modulate impulsive behavior. The final stage, in late adolescence, is characterized by establishment of personal identity and a functional role in society.

As adolescents become capable of understanding complex abstract concepts, they can consider options and make choices. Adolescence is an important time for development of positive health behaviors and sound nutritional practices because the individual is able to understand the potential consequences of behavior and make choices accordingly.

Psychosocial Development

Cognitive and psychosocial development are intertwined in adolescence. The developmental tasks of early, middle, and late adolescence change as the adolescent progresses toward independence. The psychological changes of adolescence are often described as storm and stress. The adolescent must function in three arenas: family, peer group,

and school, and the criteria for success may be different in each arena. The major psychosocial developmental change of early adolescence is initiating independence from the family. During this time, rebellion may disrupt family homeostasis as an adolescent's need for limits comes in conflict with her need for autonomy.

In early adolescence the individual begins to expand his or her social radius beyond family and concentrate on relationships with peers (Fig. 7–6). Middle adolescence is characterized by conflicts over independence. By late adolescence, emancipation is complete, and the budding young adult develops giving and sharing relationships. Conflict tends to subside after completion of puberty because there is a general shift in family relations as the adolescent begins to assume adult responsibilities. As is discussed later in this chapter, these sometimes turbulent changes affect the dietary intake of the adolescent as focus shifts from family food habits to peer group influence and, eventually, to her own independent patterns.

ASSESSMENT OF NUTRITIONAL STATUS

■ Describe the nutrition assessment techniques used for adolescents.

■ What are the difficulties in interpreting assessment data for adolescents?

Nutrition assessment of adolescents involves anthropometric measurements, biochemical studies, clinical observations, and evaluation of dietary habits. Implementation and interpretation of these techniques are discussed in Chapter 2. The three important features of the adolescent growth spurt that must be considered in nutrition assessment are time of onset, duration, and magnitude.

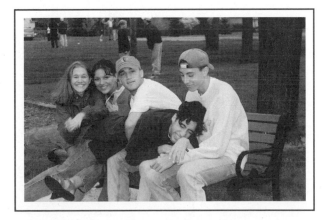

FIGURE 7–6. During adolescence relationships with peers become very important.

Anthropometry

Because adolescence is a period of rapid growth, much of nutrition assessment centers on changes in growth parameters. Monitoring growth or growth velocity is one of the most sensitive means for evaluation of the status of an adolescent, because it reflects genetic makeup as well as adequacy of nutrition and the environment (Underwood, 1991). Measurements of height, weight, and weight for height should be recorded and plotted on growth charts such as the NCHS growth charts for boys and girls up to 18 years (see Figs. 6–3 and 6–4 in Chapter 6). David's gains in stature and weight are plotted in Figure 7–7. These charts are divided at the 5th, 10th, 25th, 50th, 75th, 90th, and 95th percentiles. The area between any two percentiles on the growth chart is referred to as a growth channel. Crossing from one growth channel to another occurs frequently during the rapid growth of puberty. When

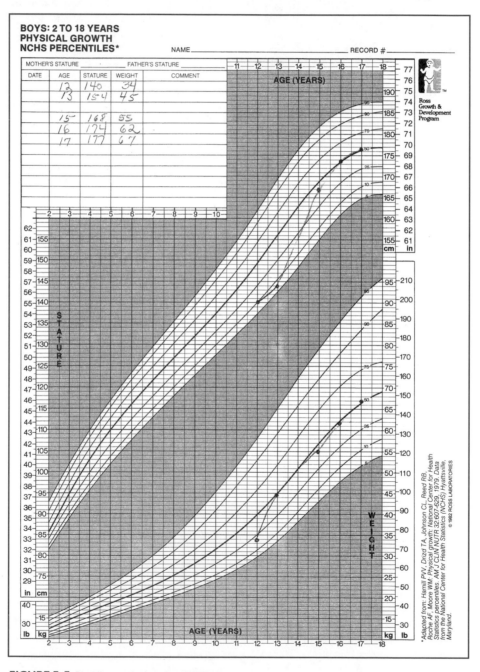

FIGURE 7–7. David's growth plotted on NCHS chart.

two or more channels are crossed, further evaluation of nutrition status may be appropriate to identify factors contributing to changes in growth patterns.

During puberty, girls accumulate substantial body fat, which is sustained into adulthood. Although boys also acquire some fat in early adolescence, overall their body fat stabilizes or even declines. Hence, neither body weight nor height suffices as an accurate indicator of nutrition status. Fatfolds at various body sites, most frequently triceps and subscapular, are used to estimate body fat stores. The adolescent's measurement can be compared with age and gender percentiles from the NHANES data, which appear in Appendices 3A and 3B. The midarm muscle circumference, or midarm muscle area, can be calculated using the midarm circumference and the triceps fatfold (see page 36). Comparison of these indicators to gender- and age-specific percentiles from the NHANES data (Appendices 3C and 3D) provides an estimator of somatic protein status.

Anthropometric assessment of nutrition status during puberty is complicated by the fact that the ratio of lean body mass and fat to height changes during normal growth and development. If the SMR of an adolescent is known, some assumption can be made about the composition of weight changes and the nutritional significance of growth deviations. For example, for a girl at SMR 4, a weight and triceps fatfold at the 85th percentile may indicate she has excess body fat that may continue into adulthood, whereas for a girl of the same chronologic age who is at stage 1, the same values may be viewed as an indication of weight and fat accumulation preceding the pubertal growth spurt.

Biochemical

The biochemical measurements of nutritional status discussed in Chapter 2 are appropriate for assessment of visceral protein and hematologic status in adolescence.

Clinical Evaluation

Clinical evaluation is based on overt symptoms and signs of deficiency states. Table 2–7 in Chapter 2 outlines signs associated with various nutrient deficiencies. Because of their rapid growth, nutrition deficiencies become apparent in adolescents more quickly than in adults. However, even though they show up quickly, they do reflect advanced stages of undernutrition, and accurate interpretation of clinical signs and symptoms requires an experienced clinician.

Dietary Intake

Dietary records, 24-hour dietary recalls, or food frequency questionnaires can be used to obtain dietary intake data from adolescents. A detailed nutrition history can yield information regarding typical dietary intakes. Each of these methods requires time and cooperation of the teenager. Because adolescents are likely to have irregular eating patterns, it may be difficult to get accurate information from some youngsters, and a combination of these tools may be appropriate.

Overall nutrition assessment and identification of potential nutrition risk require integration of data from anthropometric, biochemical and dietary assessments. As discussed in the Application at the end of this chapter, determination of substance use or abuse is an essential component of health and nutrition assessment in this age group.

ENERGY AND NUTRIENT NEEDS

■ What are the needs of adolescents for energy and nutrients?

■ How well nourished are American adolescents?

■ For which nutrients are there special concerns for adolescents?

The section on growth and development makes it clear that the rapid changes of puberty markedly increase nutritional needs. Because little experimental evidence is available to determine exact requirements during this period, the Recommended Dietary Allowances (RDAs) are based on data from animal studies or extrapolated from research with adults or children. As for other age groups, the levels of the RDAs for adolescence are those considered to be sufficient for growth and health (Food and Nutrition Board, 1989).

For practical reasons, the RDAs for adolescents are categorized by chronologic age rather than sexual maturation rating. The RDAs for adolescence are divided by gender and into two age groups: 11 to 14 years and 15 to 18 years (Table 7–3).

Energy

Energy is required for growth, muscular activity, and synthesis of body compounds. The current recommendations for energy are estimated from average energy intakes of adolescents based on average body weights (Food and Nutrition Board, 1989). Because of the wide variability in rates of growth and development as well as levels of physical activity, it is difficult to estimate specific energy requirements for adolescents.

Energy intake is related to growth rate. Studies of the caloric intakes of girls across the pubescent growth period found that the highest intakes occurred during the growth spurt, i.e., the peak height velocity (Daniel, 1982). Therefore, the best index for determining energy needs is thought to be kilocalories per unit (centimeter) height (Table 7–4).

TABLE 7–3 The Recommended Dietary Allowances for Adolescents

	Age 11–14 y		Age 15–18 y	
	Male 45 kg 157 cm	Female 46 kg 157 cm	Male 66 kg 176 cm	Female 55 kg 163 cm
Energy (kcal)	2500	2200	3000	2200
Protein (g)	45	46	59	44
FAT-SOLUBLE VITAMINS				
Vitamin A (μg RE)*	1000	800	1000	800
Vitamin D (μg)†	10	10	10	10
Vitamin E (mg α-TE)‡	10	8	10	8
Vitamin K (μg)	45	45	65	55
WATER-SOLUBLE VITAMINS				
Vitamin C (mg)	50	50	60	60
Thiamin (mg)	1.3	1.1	1.5	1.1
Riboflavin (mg)	1.5	1.3	1.8	1.3
Niacin (mg NE)§	17	15	20	15
Vitamin B_6 (mg)	1.7	1.4	2.0	1.5
Folate (μg)	150	150	200	180
Vitamin B_{12} (μg)	2.0	2.0	2.0	2.0
MINERALS				
Calcium (mg)	1200	1200	1200	1200
Phosphorus (mg)	1200	1200	1200	1200
Magnesium (mg)	270	280	400	300
Iron (mg)	12	15	12	15
Zinc (mg)	15	12	15	12
Iodine (μg)	150	150	150	150
Selenium (μg)	40	45	50	50

* RE, retinol equivalent. 1 retinol equivalent = 1 μg or 6 μg β-carotene.

† As cholecalciferol. 10 μg cholecalciferol = 400 IU of vitamin D.

‡ α-Tocopherol equivalents. 1 mg d-α = 1 α-TE.

§ 1 NE (niacin equivalent) 1 mg of niacin or 60 mg of dietary tryptophan.

In the first Health and Nutrition Examination Survey (U.S. Department of Health, Education and Welfare, 1974) and the National Food Consumption Survey (U.S. Department of Agriculture, 1984) mean energy intakes were below the RDA for females aged 12 to 17 years, older boys, all African-American adolescents, and adolescents from economically deprived families.

Protein

The RDAs for protein are based on data for body composition and calculations of growth rate. As with kilocalories, the protein needs of the adolescent correlate more closely with the growth pattern than with chronologic age, making grams of protein per centimeter of height the most accu-

TABLE 7–4 Recommendations for Energy and Protein Intake Based on Height

Age Group (y)	Males			Females		
	Reference Height (cm)	Energy (kcal/cm)	Protein (g/cm)	Reference Height (cm)	Energy (kcal/cm)	Protein (g/cm)
11–14	157	15.9	0.29	157	14.0	0.29
15–18	176	17.0	0.34	163	13.5	0.27
19–24	164	16.4	0.33	164	13.4	0.28

rate method for estimating protein allowances. The daily protein recommendations for adolescents range from 0.29 to 0.34 g/cm height for males and 0.27 to 0.29 g/cm for females (see Table 7–4).

For most Americans, including adolescents, daily protein intakes exceed the RDA (National Center for Health Statistics, 1979). Adolescents at risk of poor protein nutriture are those who severely restrict total food intake or exclude major food groups providing protein and those in low-income groups.

Carbohydrate and Fat

The Food and Nutrition Board (1989) has not established recommended levels for dietary carbohydrate or fat, but levels sufficient to meet energy needs are necessary to "spare" dietary protein. The same Dietary Guidelines for adults are appropriate for adolescents—more than 55% of kilocalories consumed should be from carbohydrate and less than 30% of total kilocalories from fat.

Minerals and Vitamins

The 1977–78 Nationwide Food Consumption Survey (U.S. Department of Agriculture, 1984), and the National Health and Nutrition Examination Surveys I and II (National Center for Health Statistics, 1979) have identified low dietary intake and deficient or low biochemical measures of some vitamins (folate, riboflavin, B_6, A, and C) and minerals (calcium, iron, and zinc). Female adolescents and those of low socioeconomic status are at particular risk.

Minerals

CALCIUM The skeletal development of infancy and childhood accelerates during puberty, and continues slowly into the third decade of life. The percentage of trabecular bone surface covered with **osteoids** is high during this period and declines in early adulthood, remaining low thereafter. Because of increased bone formation and accelerated muscular and endocrine development, calcium needs are greatest during puberty. A calcium deficiency during skeletal formation and maturation may be associated with a decrease in peak bone mass, which could contribute to increased risk of fracture later in life.

If optimal peak bone mass is to be achieved, the adolescent must be in positive calcium balance. This means that both calcium intake and absorption have to be adequate to compensate for **obligatory losses** and to provide a surplus for skeletal growth. Accumulation of bone mass is optimal when the **threshold calcium balance** is met or exceeded. The RDA for calcium increases to 1200 mg during adolescence. It has been suggested that this level of intake may be insufficient to foster the development of peak bone mass, however, because the threshold calcium values determined during childhood and adolescence appear to be higher than the current RDAs (Matkovik, 1993). (See the Research Update for some views on calcium needs.) Optimal utilization of dietary calcium requires adequate levels of vitamin D, a 1:1 calcium to phosphorus ratio, and adequate levels of other nutrients, including protein, magnesium, and vitamin C.

According to dietary surveys, males, except for African-Americans, have diets that approximate their RDA for calcium (Eck and Hackett-Renner, 1992). In contrast, calcium intakes of adolescent females tend to be 400 to 700 mg below the RDA (Eck and Hackett-Renner, 1992; Barr, 1994). Limited use of calcium-rich dairy products, fewer total meals and snacks consumed each day, and increased consumption of soft drinks are largely responsible for inadequate calcium intakes in adolescents (Barr, 1994; Guenther, 1986). Substituting carbonated beverages for milk may substantially increase phosphorus intake, creating an unfavorable environment for bone formation. In African-Americans, lactose intolerance may be a major contributing factor to low consumption of milk and other dairy products.

The National Health Objectives, Healthy People 2000 have established a goal of increasing calcium intake so that at least 50% of youths age 12 through 24 years consume three or more servings daily of foods rich in calcium. A serving is considered to be one cup of milk or an equivalent that provides approximately 300 mg of calcium. Three servings would supply three-fourths of the RDA.

IRON The increase in iron requirements during puberty is associated with the sharp increase in lean body mass, blood volume, and red cell mass. More iron is needed for synthesis of myoglobin in muscle and hemoglobin in blood.

Dietary intake and absorption must be sufficient to compensate for losses through feces, urine, skin, and menstruation and to provide for tissue growth. The RDAs for iron needed to reach adulthood with a storage level of 30 mg of iron are 12 mg for males and 15 mg for females.

The iron content of the American diet is approximately 6 mg per 1000 kilocalories (Marino and King, 1980). For

KEY TERMS

osteoids: sites of new bone formation

obligatory losses: amount lost through urine, feces and skin in normal metabolic processes

threshold calcium balance: the level of calcium intake below which skeletal accumulation of calcium varies with intake and above which it remains constant

RESEARCH UPDATE
Do Adolescents Need Calcium Supplements?

An important factor in lifelong bone health is the level of bone mass achieved in early life (Food and Nutrition Board, 1989). Genetics and a variety of lifestyle factors can influence whether that peak is attained and maintained. Prominent among those factors are dietary intake, smoking, and physical activity. The role of diet, particularly dietary calcium, is of considerable interest. A **meta-analysis** of studies of the relationship between calcium intake and bone density in adults shows a significant positive correlation between the amount of calcium consumed and bone density, particularly for premenopausal, and, to a lesser extent, for postmenopausal women (Cumming, 1990). An important factor in lifelong bone health, however, is the level of peak bone mass achieved in early life (Heaney, 1996).

Retrospective studies of calcium intake and bone mass in early adulthood have demonstrated that calcium intake in adolescence can have a great impact on bone mineral density (Nieves et al, 1995). Observations of calcium intake and excretion in young girls showed that retention of calcium and, thus, gastrointestinal absorption was significantly greater in early puberty (Weaver et al, 1995; Abrams and Stuff, 1994).

Other studies have addressed calcium requirements with experimental approaches. A unique 3-year **clinical trial** measured bone mass at three sites (spine, radius, and hip) in male and female identical twins 6 to 14 years of age assigned to a placebo or a calcium supplement (Johnston et al, 1992). In the 19 pubertal twin pairs no significant differences in bone measures were observed; however, calcium supplementation enhanced the rate of increase in bone mineral density in the 22 prepubertal twin pairs.

In another study, Lloyd and co-workers (1993) assessed the effect of a placebo or calcium supplement on bone mineral measures in 12-year-old Caucasian girls over an 18-month period. Mean calcium intakes were 1370 and 935 mg per day for supplemented and placebo groups, respectively. Bone mineral density was assessed at baseline and at 6-month intervals up to 18 months with **dual x-ray absorptiometry**. The increases for spine bone mineral density, spine bone mineral content, and total bone mineral density were significantly greater in the supplemental group than the placebo group.

Although the results obtained by Lloyd and co-workers (1993) suggest that calcium intakes in the range of 1300 mg/day allow greater increases in bone mineral measures, the level of calcium intake or the critical time when a high amount is required for achievement of optimal peak mass is still unclear.

The National Institutes of Health (NIH, 1994) Consensus Development Conference on Optimal Calcium Intake suggested a daily dietary intake of calcium between 1200 and 1500 mg for individuals between ages 11 and 24 years (Levenson and Bockman, 1994). Further research is needed before calcium supplements are recommended for adolescents. It is not known whether the early increase in bone mass will be maintained or to what extent a deficit in calcium intake during one phase of growth may be made up later. Until more data are available, it is important to encourage adolescents, especially young adolescents, to consume at least 1200 mg of calcium each day from dietary sources.

---

adolescent females, who typically have caloric intakes well below the RDA, and those involved in vigorous physical activity, inadequate iron intake is a problem.

ZINC Zinc is essential for healthy growth and sexual maturation. Although there have been no controlled studies on the zinc requirements of adolescents, growth retardation and hypogonadism in adolescent males with zinc deficiency have been reported in developing countries. Body zinc levels appear to decline during puberty (Thompson et al, 1986), which may reflect either an increased need for zinc during growth or a redistribution of plasma zinc due to hormonal changes. Recommended levels for adolescents are the same as for adults.

OTHER MINERALS Very little information is available on the requirements for other trace minerals during adolescence. Current recommendations have been extrapolated from adult values.

Vitamins

Data on vitamin requirements for adolescents are even more limited than those for minerals. The RDAs are extrapolated from data for other age groups, with estimates of increments for growth. Due to the increased energy demands of growth, the need for thiamin, riboflavin, and niacin is elevated. There are also heightened demands for vitamin B_6, folate, and vitamin B_{12}, which are required for normal DNA and RNA synthesis and protein metabolism. The recent association of adequate folate intake during embryonic development with prevention of neural tube defects emphasizes the importance of adequate folate in the diets of teenage girls. Folate supplements have been recommended for any female who might become pregnant (Centers for Disease Control, 1991). Vitamin C, an antioxidant, participates in collagen synthesis and a number of other biologic reactions. The RDAs for vitamin C are based on those for adults.

VITAMIN D Vitamin D is necessary for maintaining homeostasis of calcium and phosphorus in mineralization of bone. The RDA for vitamin D is 10 μg per day throughout adolescence. Because peak bone mass is not achieved before the third decade, this level is continued through 24 years of age. The major source of dietary vitamin D is fortified milk, which may be consumed in decreasing amount by adolescents, especially females.

Until further research provides data for more precise nutrition recommendations for adolescents, the consumption of a varied diet remains the best assurance of adequate and safe intake levels of nutrients.

FACTORS THAT INFLUENCE FOOD HABITS

■ Describe the eating habits of teenagers.

■ How does psychological development influence dietary patterns?

■ What social factors influence the food choices and nutrition status of teens?

■ How does knowledge of nutrition science affect dietary intake?

The eating patterns of adolescents are complex, influenced by an array of interwoven factors (Fig. 7–8). These influences on food behavior are environmental (family, peers, idols, and sociocultural factors) and personal (individual physiologic needs, development of self-concept, and food preferences). The food habits of adolescents are important not only in ensuring an adequate diet to support growth and development, but also in developing lifelong patterns for maintenance of health.

Eating Practices of Teenagers

The dietary habits of adolescents are a reflection of those of the population in general. As adolescents make the

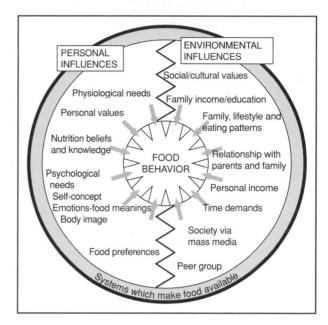

FIGURE 7–8. Illustration of factors that act in concert to influence the food behavior of adolescents.

transition to adulthood, their dietary intakes become less consistent due to busy schedules, the search for self-identity, peer group acceptance, and preoccupation with body weight, shape, appearance, or athletic prowess. For a teenager, eating the recommended number of servings from the groups in the food pyramid has a low priority. Dieting, skipping meals, snacking, eating away from home, consuming fast foods, trying unconventional diets, and attempting to gain or lose weight are characteristic food behaviors among adolescents that relate to their physical, emotional, and social development.

K E Y   T E R M S

meta-analysis: meta-change or transformation; analysis-determine component parts. Generally interpreted as a "scientific overview" of multiple studies in one topic area

retrospective: something in the past, in this instance comparing bone mass based on previous calcium consumption

clinical trial: a controlled study of treatment vs. controls in a patient population

dual x-ray absorptiometry: a technique used to measure bone mineral content in which the individual is scanned with photons from an x-ray source

Eating Away from Home

Teenagers can obtain food from many places. Many earn their own money and can buy food they prefer to eat and discard foods they don't like. Adolescents often eat away from home. Sources of food include schools, fast food establishments, restaurants, vending machines, concessions at sporting events and movies, friends' houses, and ready-to-eat convenience foods and snacks from almost anywhere.

In the past three decades fast foods have become popular with most segments of the American population, but they have special appeal for teenagers. According to the Forecast Magazine Survey (1989), 75% of teens eat at fast food restaurants. Because it is relatively inexpensive, fast food fits into the budget of an adolescent. The menu items are well accepted and can be eaten with a minimum of utensils. In addition, fast food restaurants provide a casual environment where teens feel comfortable.

A major criticism of fast food restaurants is that the menu items tend to be calorically dense, high in fat and sodium, and low in fiber. In addition, they may be low in several vitamins and minerals, including vitamins A and C, calcium, riboflavin, and folate.

Table 7–5 lists the nutrient content of menu items from one fast food restaurant chain. Some of these foods, such as Chicken McNuggets and Big Mac, contain as much as 50% of kilocalories from fat. Fortunately, many restaurants have begun to offer salads and sandwiches with lower fat content. Although they are lower in fat, such

items can still provide more than 30% of their kilocalories as fat. A salad can be low in kilocalories and fat, but adding dressings, croutons, bacon bits, cheese, ham, and eggs can increase the fat content greatly. For example, a chef salad with many of these items provides 47% of its energy from fat (see Table 7–5). Given the prominent place of fast foods in the diet, it is important to encourage teens to make nutritious choices as well as to lobby the food industry to continue to offer more foods that are high in nutrient density and low in fat, sugar, and sodium.

Snacks and Meals

Although their overall patterns of food intake appear to meet nutrient needs, adolescents tend to skip more meals and eat more snacks. For example, only 21% of the adolescents interviewed in the Rand Youth Poll (1990) reported eating three meals a day, and 40% of the adolescents participating in the National Adolescent Student Health Survey (U.S. Department of Health and Human Services, 1991) reported that they ate breakfast on only 2 or fewer days during the previous week.

For many Americans, adolescents in particular, snacks have become the fourth meal, contributing significant amounts of energy and nutrients. (See Table 7–6 for the nutrient content of some popular snack foods. Those low in fat are highlighted.) Over 90% of teenagers eat between meals (U.S. Department of Health and Human Services, 1991). Although 61% of these teens (The Nationwide

TABLE 7–5 Energy, Macronutrient, Cholesterol, and Sodium of Selected Fast Food Items

Item	Serving Size	Energy (kcal)	Protein (g)	Carbohydrate (g)	Fat (g)	% Fat (kcal)	Saturated Fat (g)	Cholesterol (mg)	Sodium (mg)	Fiber (g)
Chicken McNuggets (6-piece)	4 oz	400	20	26	23	52	5	85	870	0
McGrilled Chicken w/ mayonnaise	6.5 oz	340	25	32	13	34	2	55	560	1
Big Mac	7.5 oz	490	24	49	27	50	9	90	890	2
McLean Delux w/Cheese	5 oz	370	24	35	14	34	5	75	890	3
Chef salad	9 oz	170	17	8	9	47	4	110	400	2
Chunky chicken salad	9 oz	150	25	7	4	1	1	80	230	2
Ranch dressing	1 pkg	230	1	10	21	82	3	23	580	0
Chocolate milkshake	16 oz	350	13	62	6	15	4	25	240	0
Orange juice	6 oz	150	0	20	0	0	0	0	20	0
Coke	16 oz	150	0	38	0	—	—	—	—	0
1% lowfat milk	8 oz	100	8	13	2.5	23	1.5	10	115	0

Data from McDonald's Nutrition Information Center, McDonald's Corporation, Oak Brook, IL 60521.

TABLE 7–6 **Nutrient Content of Popular Snack Foods**						
Item	Serving Size	Energy (kcal)	Protein (g)	Carbohydrate (g)	Fat (g)	Sodium (mg)
BREAKFAST DRINKS						
Carnation Instant Breakfast	1 oz	130	7	23	1	136
CAKE						
Angel food	2 oz	142	4	32	0	142
Chocolate cupcake	1 oz	130	2	21	5	120
Yellow cake w/icing	2 oz	268	3	40	11	191
CANDY						
Caramels/chocolate	1 oz	115	1	22	3	74
Chocolate-coated peanuts	1 oz	160	5	11	12	19
Fudge	1 oz	115	1	21	3	54
M&Ms	1.5 oz	220	3	31	10	—
Jellybeans	10			17		1
Hard candy	1 oz	110		28		9
CEREALS						
Cheerios	1 c	88	3	16	1	246
Bran Chex	1 c	156	5	39	1	455
Corn Flakes	1 c	88	2	20		281
Trix	1 c	108	1.5	25		179
Product 19	1 c	126	3	27		378
Lucky Charms	1 c	125	2	26	1	227
COOKIES						
Chocolate chip	1	50	.5	7	2	38
Oatmeal raisin	1	62	.7	9	3	37
Chocolate cookie sandwich	1	50	.5	7	2	63
CRACKERS						
Ritz	10	180		20	10	320
Cheddar snacks	10	70	1.5	11	2.5	140
Graham	4 (1 oz)	120	2	22	3.5	128
Wheat Thins	10	90	1	12	3.5	
Saltines	5	63	1	10	1	185
ICE CREAM						
10% fat	1 c	269	4	32	14	116
2% fat	1 c	223	8	38	5	163
SHERBET						
2% fat	1 c	270	2	59	4	88
YOGURT						
Lowfat	1 c	144	13	16	2	159
Nonfat	1 c	127	13	17	.5	174
POPCORN						
Light butter	6 c	150	0	25	7	310
Plain-air popped	5 c	125	5	25	0	
SOUP						
Cream of mushroom	1 c	203	6	15	14	1076
Vegetarian vegetable	1 c	72	2	12	2	823
Chicken noodle	1 c	75	4	9	2	1107
Tomato	1 c	86	2	16	2	872

TABLE 7–7 Examples of Nutrient-Dense, Low-Fat Snack Foods

1%, 0.5% low-fat or skim milk
Low-fat cheese, low-fat or nonfat yogurt

Fresh or unsweetened fruits
Raw vegetables

Fruit juices or vegetable juices

Pretzels, air-popped popcorn, bagels, baked tortilla chips

Sandwiches; turkey, lean roast beef, lean ham, low-fat cold cuts, low-fat cheese, water-packed tuna with reduced-fat mayonnaise or salad dressing, peanut butter and jelly

Hamburger/sloppy joes made with ground turkey

Chicken tacos, enchiladas, bean burritos made with low-fat cheese

Pizza with vegetables and low-fat cheese

Frozen low-fat or nonfat yogurt, ice milk, sherbet, frozen fruit bars, fruit sorbets, pudding made with skim milk, commercial fat-free pudding

Food Consumption Survey, USDA, 1984) said they snacked on foods high in fat and/or sugar, low in fiber, and of low nutrient density (Bigler-Doughten and Jenkins, 1987), almost 39% reported they selected nutritious snacks such as yogurt, milk, juice, and fruits and vegetables. For these adolescents, snacks provided up to one-third of daily dietary energy as well as significant amounts of calcium, magnesium, and vitamin C.

Snacking can be a liability, an asset, or a necessity, depending on the needs and choices of the adolescent. Many adolescents, especially those who are growing rapidly and are physically active, have high energy needs that require high-calorie snacks. For others with lower energy requirements, snacks can have a negative impact on the diet if they replace needed nutrient-dense foods. When chosen wisely and consumed in moderation, however, snacks can improve the adolescent's overall dietary intake and may, indeed, be essential for an adequate diet. Table 7–7 lists some nutritious snack food alternatives that are low in fat, sugar, and sodium.

Factors That Influence Food Behavior

Successful transition from childhood to adulthood is contingent on the interplay of physical, psychological, and social forces. For example, an adolescent's characteristic repeated attempts to change his physical appearance and body shape to emulate a perceived desirable image is not simply a desire to conform to social and peer expectations but the result of the struggle to integrate the physical changes of puberty into a stable body- and self-image and to establish individuality and autonomy.

Psychological Influences

SELF-CONCEPT Self-concept includes attributes an individual perceives he or she possesses as well as the perception of how others view him or her. Self-esteem, a facet of self-concept, involves perception of one's position in the social structure and how one sees himself or herself as a social object. Self-concept encompasses self-perceived attributes of physical appearance (including body image), personality features, and moral characteristics. Adolescents struggle to varying degrees to establish their own self-concept. Self-concept is one factor that can be a significant influence on eating patterns and, thus, on nutrient intakes (Witte et al, 1991).

EMOTIONAL DEVELOPMENT Eating habits have an emotional basis. Individuals eat not only because they are hungry but also to fulfill myriad social and psychological needs. Eating when "lonely" or "bored" or "treating oneself to special food as a reward" are simple examples of the emotional use of food. More complex manifestations include denial of hunger or overeating associated with stress or anxiety, all of which can interfere with nutritional well-being. Adolescents become prone to these behaviors as they struggle to establish emotional independence.

BODY IMAGE It is normal for adolescents to be self-conscious about or dissatisfied with their changing bodies. A society that emphasizes slimness and the bombardment of advertising that promises thinner thighs and slimmer waists or bigger muscles and a wonderful body create a standard to which teenagers compare themselves, no matter how unrealistic that standard may be. An acute sense of how their bodies differ from the "ideal" may wreak havoc on adolescents' self-esteem. Girls are particularly prone to obsessing about the shape of their bodies, but boys are not immune.

Approximately two-thirds of adolescent girls report they are dissatisfied with their weight, and slightly more than half are dissatisfied with the shape of their bodies (Moore, 1993). These percentages increase as body weight increases. African-American girls are less likely to consider themselves overweight than whites or Hispanics (Serdula et al, 1993). Specific concerns of girls are about perceived excess size of their thighs, hips, waist, and buttocks. Boys are more likely to be satisfied with their body weight, but approximately one-third of males expressed dissatisfaction with their body shape, desiring to appear strong and muscular, particularly in the upper body (Moore, 1993). Adolescents who attempt to lose weight or who struggle to maintain weight are not necessarily overweight by usual standards but perceive themselves as overweight (Emmons, 1994). Such teens tend to have poorer body images and self-esteem than those who are satisfied with their body weight and shape (Allen et al, 1993).

Social Influences

CULTURE   Each individual requires the same nutrients to meet physiologic needs, yet the foods that are consumed to supply these nutrients are as different as the environments in which people live. Culture represents the way in which people have adapted to their environment and reflects national, ethnic, and religious backgrounds as well as geographic, social, and economic environments. A composite of these factors provides the background against which the adolescent eventually forms his or her individual food habits.

Financial Status

The increased nutrition needs of adolescents translate into a demand for a greater quantity of food. This can stress the family budget. Because adolescents eat at home less often, those with limited financial resources may find they are restricted in the amount of food they can afford or the food choices they can make when eating out. For example, a teenager may be able to afford to buy lunch in the school cafeteria but not to join friends at fast food establishments or restaurants.

The School Lunch Program provides free or reduced-cost lunches for youngsters from low-income families (see the application in Chapter 6). It is important that such programs, if they are to be successful, provide not only nutritious meals but also meals that are acceptable to the adolescent. Often, families of children who receive free lunches are eligible to receive additional assistance through the use of food stamps. Dollar amounts allotted for food stamps are based on the USDA's food plans, which estimate the cost of food prepared at home. Although food stamps increase the availability of food to a family, the level of support is insufficient to afford "eating out."

TIME PRESSURES   In the hectic life of the typical teenager, the biggest obstacle to meeting nutrition needs may be making time to eat. A lunch period when both time and food are available is scheduled at school, but there are no guarantees that teens will use that opportunity to eat or, if they do eat, that they will make nutritious choices. After-school activities, sports, and employment create demands that interfere with regular eating patterns. Many teens may not eat until they arrive home hours after school is over. Possible solutions to this problem, such as packing an additional lunch at home to be eaten after school and planning ahead for nutritious snack alternatives, may be limited by time and financial resources.

Many adolescents must assume some responsibility for purchasing and preparing food for themselves, younger siblings, and even the whole family. A survey of American teens revealed that 80% (50% of females and 30% of males) shop at supermarkets or grocery stores each week (American Medical Association, 1991).

FAMILY   Throughout childhood the family is the predominant influence on food habits and lifetime eating patterns. The family mediates a child's food behavior in two essential ways. The first, and most obvious, is the direct influence of the family as the main provider of food. The second, which shapes lifetime eating habits, is the influence exerted through the transmission of food attitudes, preferences, and patterns. Superimposed on this is the emotional component of food as a channel for interpersonal communication of love, approval, or even disapproval. These influences can have a positive or negative impact on food-related behavior.

The family can be an important unit for promoting healthy food habits, and positive family relationships are associated with acceptance of a wide variety of foods. Those teens who eat with their families on a regular basis usually have more nutritious diets than those who eat alone or with friends. During adolescence, the child in each individual struggles to become an adult. This transition becomes evident in eating patterns, as the teen rejects family food traditions or preferences and seeks to assert his or her own autonomy. Difficulties during this transition are exaggerated by disordered family relationships. Adolescents whose parents are authoritarian and structured in relation to food patterns may use food to express rebellion against parental authority. Permissive parents and situations in which there is a breakdown in family relationships give teens little guidance with respect to eating and may consequently foster poor eating habits.

PEERS   There is no doubt that during adolescence the peer group defines what is socially acceptable and determines behavior standards (Fig. 7–8). It is commonly assumed that adolescents are strongly influenced by the eating habits of their peers, but there is little research to support or contradict this assumption (Farthing, 1991). However, adolescents spend a lot of time with friends, and eating is an important part of their recreation and socialization. In a group context, at least, it appears that foods may be selected to meet the approval of the peer group. For example, many young adolescent girls who like and drink milk at home may choose to consume soft drinks when with their friends.

MASS MEDIA   The extent to which adolescent food choices are influenced by the mass media is difficult to document. Today's adolescents have grown up in a time when mass media, via advertising and programming, have promoted the desirability of slim, trim, beautiful bodies and the fun and luxury of "good eating." Prominent among foods promoted for "good eating" are soft drinks, fast foods, and other foods high in calories and fat and low in fiber. Although adolescents are better able than younger children to deal with the apparent contradictions between slimness and high energy foods, a lifetime of television viewing may have made them an almost ingrained value. In addition, the physical, emotional, and social transitions of adolescence make adolescents especially susceptible to certain advertising, such as weight control programs, diet aids, and body-building products.

NUTRITION KNOWLEDGE   Today's teenagers have had extensive exposure to nutrition information. Nutrition is incorporated into the curriculum as early as preschool or first grade, and several studies have reported that adolescents are aware of and knowledgeable about nutrition (Anderson, 1991). However, this knowledge is not necessarily a major determinant of food choices. For example, adolescents participating in the Rand Youth Poll (1990) acknowledged the importance of breakfast, but the National Food Consumption Survey revealed that two-thirds of teens surveyed ate a limited or no breakfast (Bigler-Doughten and Jenkins, 1987). Of more than 11,000 adolescents who responded to the National Adolescent Student Health Survey questionnaire, 34% scored low on knowledge of fat and could not identify foods of high fiber content (Portnoy and Christenson, 1989).

Story and Resnick (1986), in a survey of 900 high school students, found that while the adolescents were well informed about good health and could easily identify undesirable nutrition practices (e.g., skipping meals, unbalanced meals, too much snacking), they often failed to make healthy food choices. These students cited lack of time, lack of discipline, and lack of a sense of urgency as barriers to choosing better diets.

NUTRITION-RELATED CONCERNS OF ADOLESCENCE

■ Beyond achieving a nutritionally adequate diet to support growth, what are the areas of concern related to nutrition for adolescents?

■ How does nutrition relate to control of acne in teenagers?

■ What role does nutrition play in the prevention of chronic disease in adolescence?

Adolescence is a relatively healthy period of life, but because of the dramatic physical and lifestyle changes, the teenager is often worried that something is or will go wrong. Their concerns often relate to appearance, body image, and body weight. The increased physiologic demands of stresses such as pregnancy and athletic performance can place them at nutritional risk. It is important for their diets to provide a sound foundation to meet the demands during adolescence and to foster eating patterns and practices that will sustain them well into a healthy adulthood and even into old age.

Adolescent Pregnancy

In the United States, birth rates have consistently declined for all females of reproductive age except those under 15 years of age, making adolescent pregnancy a major public health concern. Although pregnancy is a normal physiologic state, there are increased maternal, fetal, and neonatal risks for pregnant teens who are still growing. The nutrition status of the pregnant adolescent is influenced by the psychological and social factors discussed in this chapter. In fact, they may actually contribute to increased risk through poor dietary habits and inadequate weight gain. (Adolescent pregnancy is discussed in detail in Chapter 9.)

Acne

Through the generations acne has been a scourge for teenagers. During no other time of life is appearance so important for self-esteem and peer acceptance. The face, the primary locus in determining attractiveness, is also a primary site of pilosebaceous follicles, the source of the blackheads and pimples known as acne vulgaris.

Acne is a disease of the pilosebaceous unit in the skin. This unit is made up of a hair follicle and a sebaceous gland, which are connected to the surface of the skin by a duct though which the hair passes (Fig. 7–9). The sebaceous gland produces sebum, which helps keep the skin and the hair moist. Sebum also carries cells shed by the glands to the surface of the skin, a process called follicular keratinization. Pilosebaceous units are found all over the body, but they are more frequent on the face, upper chest, and back, which explains why acne usually occurs in these places.

Development

Acne develops when the sebaceous glands produce increased amounts of sebum, making the skin more oily. In the anaerobic depths of the sebaceous follicle, sebum provides a substrate for bacteria, resulting in the production of a wide variety of antigenic substances, which induce an immune response such as inflammation. In response, cells stick together to form a thick layer that blocks the duct. As more cells and sebum pile up behind this layer, a compact plug called a comedo is formed.

If the sebum and accumulated cells remain below the skin surface, a "closed" comedo or white head is formed. If the orifice of a closed comedo dilates, the plug enlarges and pops out of the duct. This is called an "open" comedo or blackhead. The discoloration is due to a buildup of melanin, the dark pigment in skin. If the wall of a closed comedo ruptures and releases its contents into the dermis, an inflammatory lesion results.

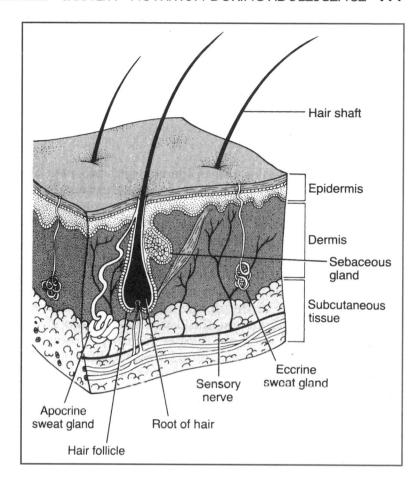

Hair shaft

Epidermis

Dermis

Sebaceous gland

Subcutaneous tissue

Eccrine sweat gland

Sensory nerve

Root of hair

Apocrine sweat gland

Hair follicle

FIGURE 7–9. A pilosebaceous unit. (From Betz CL, et al. Family-centered nursing care of children. 2nd ed. Philadelphia: WB Saunders, 1994.)

Approximately 80% of all teenagers develop some form of acne with the onset of puberty. The exact cause is unknown, but heredity and androgens that stimulate sebaceous glands are contributing factors. Males are usually more severely affected than females. However, attractiveness has a greater impact on the social status of girls and, therefore, acne may be a greater concern for them. In females, acne often worsens during the premenstrual period.

Most adolescents develop what is called "noninflammatory acne," which usually involves the eruption of just a few blackheads or whiteheads every now and then. For some, a more severe form, called "inflammatory acne," causes a constant outbreak covering the face and sometimes the neck, back, chest, and groin. The pus-filled pimples and cysts can cause deep pitting and scarring.

For generations, certain foods such as chocolate, nuts, cola drinks, potato chips, french fries, and other foods have been indicted in causing or exacerbating acne. There is no scientific evidence to support these claims, but some adolescents do notice that certain foods seem to increase outbreaks for them. A nutritious, balanced diet is important for overall health of the adolescent, including the skin, to minimize the effects of acne.

Treatment

Mild acne can be controlled by washing the face once or twice daily. If these measures are not effective, the next line of treatment is over-the-counter preparations that are applied directly to the skin. They may contain benzoyl peroxide, sulfur, resorcinol or salicylic acid, all of which are approved by the Food and Drug Administration (FDA) for treating acne. Acne that does not respond to over-the-counter preparations requires medical consultation. Prescription drugs include both topical and oral antibiotics, such as tetracycline and erythromycin, and a derivative of vitamin A, tretinoin (Retin-A) that comes in cream, gel, or liquid form. Because tretinoin is applied externally, there appears to be no danger of toxicity.

A small percentage of adolescents and young adults develop deep **subcutaneous** severe cystic acne, which can cause scarring. These individuals can be treated with another derivative of vitamin A. **Isotretinoin**, 13-cis-retinoic acid, known as Accutane, is approved for the treatment of severe cystic acne (Committee on Drugs, 1992). Accutane is administered orally, usually over a period of 15 to 20 weeks, until the total cyst count is decreased by 70%. Use of this drug is associated with a reduction in sebaceous gland size and a 75% to 90% decrease in sebum excretion. A course of treatment usually results in significant clearing of acne lesions, and prolonged remission often follows.

However, isotretinoin is a potent human **teratogen** and, if administered during pregnancy, can result in serious congenital anomalies in the offspring (Lammer et al, 1985). Exposure to isotretinoin during embryosis produces defects in the central nervous system (e.g., hydrocephalus, microcephaly, microphthalmia), ears (e.g., microtia, anotia), and cardiovascular system as well as other abnormalities. Even exposed infants who have no external abnormalities show subnormal intelligence and other neuropsychological impairments (Adams, 1990). Therefore, Accutane is prescribed with caution for any female and is contraindicated in situations in which a girl might become pregnant.

Preoccupation with Body Weight

Data on body mass index and triceps fatfold thicknesses obtained from national surveys indicate that between 15% and 25% of American adolescents are obese. The National Health Objectives, Healthy People 2000 includes as one of its goals the reduction of overweight to a prevalence of no more than 15% among adolescents aged 12 through 19 years, to be accomplished through sound dietary practices combined with regular physical activity. In addition, there is evidence that anorexia nervosa, bulimia nervosa, and compulsive eating disorders are also on the rise among adolescents (Neumark-Sztainer, 1995). Eating disorders are discussed in Chapter 13.

This prevalence of eating disturbances is reflected in attitudes and eating behaviors of adolescents. Weight—too much or too little—is an actual or anticipated problem for many teenagers. For example, the Youth Risk Behavior Survey, a national survey of health risk behaviors of more than 11,000 students in grades 9 through 12, found that 44% of female and 15% of male students were trying to lose weight (Serdula et al, 1993). An additional 26% of females and 15% of males reported they were trying to keep from gaining more weight. Preoccupation with body image, weight, or shape is apparent in behaviors, and especially in weight control practices. Students in the Youth Risk Behavior Study reported using a variety of measures to control body weight, including exercise, skipping meals, taking diet pills, and inducing vomiting (Serdula et al, 1993). Chronic dieting is a risk factor for eating disorders (Neumark-Sztainer, 1995).

On the other hand, many adolescents attempt to gain weight or increase muscle mass by using a variety of nutrient or food supplements, following highly restrictive diets, or becoming engaged in rigorous physical training (aerobic or resistance exercise). To appear muscular and athletic, some teenagers may resort to taking **anabolic steroids** to stimulate muscle growth. Although these substances are controlled and require a prescription, 2.2% of high school students reported using steroids without a doctor's prescription (Kann et al, 1995). While steroid pills are readily available on the "black market" to supply athletes, at least one-fourth of high school boys are not aware of the health risks associated with anabolic steroid use (Wang et al, 1994). In the short term, these drugs can cause problems such as fatigue, acne, **hirsutism**, and combative behavior (often referred to as "roid rages"). Long-term use increases the risk of early heart disease, osteoporosis and liver tumors.

Physical Fitness

Despite the fact that more teenagers are participating in athletics, the overall fitness level of the entire adolescent population remains uncertain. Only 50% of adolescents engage in vigorous physical activity on a regular basis (American Medical Association, 1991). There is substantial evidence, however, that increased physical activity results in an improved level of fitness, lower body fat, and a more favorable lipid profile (Sutter et al, 1993). The role of physical activity throughout the life span is discussed in Chapter 14.

Cardiovascular Disease

PREVENTION   The adolescent years are often considered the healthiest. Infectious childhood illnesses are in the past, and it appears that chronic health problems of adulthood, particularly coronary heart disease, are in the distant future. There is substantial evidence, however, that atherosclerosis or precursors of atherosclerosis have their origins in childhood and adolescence, progressing slowly into adulthood (National Heart, Lung and Blood Institute, 1991).

Fatty streaks are the earliest grossly visible lesions of the atherosclerotic process. Autopsy studies following untimely deaths of children, adolescents, and young adults (Strong, 1986) have revealed that fatty streaks appear in the coronary arteries and other blood vessels during early childhood and into the second decade of life. **Fibrous plaques**, the lesions that begin to narrow the arteries, appear in the coronary arteries of some young persons as

TABLE 7–8 National Cholesterol Education Program Step One and Step Two Diet for Children and Adolescents

Nutrient	Recommended Diet	
	Step One Diet	Step Two Diet
Total fat	Average of no more than 30% of total calories	Same as Step One Diet
Saturated fatty acids	<10% of total calories	<7% of total calories
Polyunsaturated fatty acids	≤10% of total calories	Same as Step One Diet
Monounsaturated fatty acids	Remaining dietary fat calories	Same as Step One Diet
Cholesterol	<300 mg/d	<200 mg/d
Carbohydrates	About 55% of total calories	Same as Step One Diet
Protein	About 15% of total calories	Same as Step One Diet
Calories	To promote growth and development	Same as Step One Diet

From National Cholesterol Education Program (NCEP). Report of the Expert Panel on Blood Cholesterol in Children and Adolescents, 1992.

early as the second decade. For youth and adults, blood levels of total cholesterol and LDL cholesterol are related to the development of early atherosclerotic lesions. There is evidence that identifying youngsters at risk of CHD and preventing or reducing the effects of major risk factors (e.g., high blood lipid levels, hypertension, obesity, smoking, physical activity) can have long-term health benefits (National Heart, Lung and Blood Institute, 1991).

Arthereosclerotic lesions are more prevalent in the arteries of adolescents who are obese or hypertensive or who smoke cigarettes (Newman et al, 1991), and loss of body weight is associated with a reduction of blood levels of the **atherogenic** factors (Wabitsch et al, 1994). Dietary intervention to reduce body weight and fat is more effective when exercise is also included (Jacobson et al, 1993; Sutter et al, 1993). In addition, greater reductions in systolic and diastolic blood pressure occur in combined programs (Rocchini et al, 1993).

NATIONAL CHOLESTEROL EDUCATION PROGRAM (NCEP) The Dietary Guidelines from the U.S. Departments of Agriculture and Health and Human Services, discussed in Chapter 1, are recommendations to promote healthy eating to decrease the long-term risk of disease. In addition, the federally sponsored National Cholesterol Education Program (NCEP) has developed a two-phase approach to reduce the risk of CHD in children and adolescents (NCEP, 1992). The first phase provides nutritional guidelines intended for all healthy children

and adolescents over the age of 2 years (see Step One diet, Table 7–8). Analysis of the diets of school-age children and adolescents following these recommendations indicates that they do not compromise the level of vitamins and minerals consumed (McPherson et al, 1990).

The guidelines can be implemented readily with moderation and common sense by selecting low-fat dairy products as well as protein alternatives that are low in total fat and saturated fat, such as poultry, fish, and legumes. In-

K E Y   T E R M S

subcutaneous: immediately beneath the skin
isotretinoin: 13-cis retinoic acid, a drug used to treat severe acne
teratogen: a substance which can cause physical defects in the developing embryo
anabolic steroids: synthetic versions of testosterone which stimulate muscle growth
hirsutism: abnormal or excessive body hair
fatty streaks: lipid accumulation on the intima (inside surface) of the artery
fibrous plaques: fatty streaks with an accumulation of connective tissue and various blood components
atherogenic: promote changes which contribute to the development of artherosclerosis

creasing the intake of fruits, vegetables, and whole-grain products can have the benefits of reducing fat in the diet and increasing fiber content. Introduction of low-fat nutrient-dense snack foods enhances nutritional adequacy (see Table 7–7). The more varied the diet, the more likely it is that the teenager's nutrient needs will be met.

The second approach in the NCEP program is screening by measuring blood lipid levels of children and adolescents at high risk for CHD. These youngsters are identi-

fied as those who have parents or grandparents diagnosed with coronary heart disease or a cardiac event before age 55 or parents with a serum cholesterol of 240 mg/dL or above.

Youngsters who have blood lipid levels that are borderline for LDL cholesterol level (range 110 to 129 mg/dL) should be encouraged to follow the Step One dietary guidelines and have their lipoprotein evaluation repeated in 1 year. Youngsters deemed to have high LDL choles-

TABLE 7–9 Concerns and Possible Solutions in Adolescent Nutrition and Health

Concern	Suggested Solutions
Consuming fast foods	Teach and model healthful ways to eat at fast-food restaurants.
	Assist in preparing similar meals and discussing healthier alternatives.
	Accept that fast foods are going to be eaten on occasion.
	Be familiar with nutrient information on fast-food items.
Snacking on high-fat foods or food of little nutritional value	Make more nutritious snack alternatives available at home.
	Encourage schools to incorporate nutritious foods into vending or snack offerings.
Preparing food when time is limited	Have family member share responsibility for preparing meals.
	Prepare nutritious meals and snacks in serving size portions that can be heated in the microwave.
	Selected nutritious ready-to-eat products when shopping.
	Plan simple meals that require little preparation.
	Plan meals for which preparation can be done in advance.
Controlling body weight	Provide positive role models in food selection; exercise and share activities with the adolescent on a regular basis.
	Make nutritious, low-fat snacks readily available, such as fruit, vegetables, low-fat yogurt, fortified cereals.
	Encourage school and community programs to support adolescents with weight concerns.
	Help adolescents to understand and accept normal body changes.
	Assist adolescents in making food choices from those available at school or in their social environment.
	If there are any indications of serious eating problems, seek professional assistance.
Encouraging physical fitness	Provide a positive role model in physical activity and leisure-time activities.
	Limit sedentary activities, such as television and video games.
	Encourage more physical activity in daily activities.
	Teach or share sports-related skills that can be enjoyed in adulthood.
	Encourage schools, parks, and community to make available programs and facilities to increase physical activity.
	Encourage physical activities at school that attract students and encourage lifetime participation.

Adapted from Targets for Adolescent Health: Adolescent Nutrition and Physical Fitness. Chicago: American Medical Association and The American Dietetic Association, 1991.

terol levels (>130 mg/dL) should be encouraged to follow the same recommendations. If blood lipid levels do not decline in a year, intake guidelines should be reduced to less than 7% of kilocalories from saturated fat and a cholesterol intake of less than 200 mg per day (Step Two Diet).

PROMOTING POSITIVE FOOD HABITS

■ Why is it important to strive to improve the dietary intakes of adolescents?

■ What are the long-term benefits of positive dietary habits in adolescents?

Although many adolescents consume diets that approach nutritional adequacy, the habitual intakes of a significant proportion fall short of nutrient needs and dietary recommendations. Typical dietary patterns of adolescents are not consistent with dietary guidelines. A national survey of dietary intakes of adolescents found that approximately 36% of calories came from fat and 13% from saturated fat (Kimm et al, 1990). Early results from NHANES III indicate that the percentages of energy from saturated fat were highest for those aged 16 to 19 (Morbidity and Mortality Weekly Report, 1994). Because lifestyle habits observed in youth tend to persist over time, promotion of positive health and nutrition habits in adolescence seems to be warranted.

Creative approaches are needed to improve the overall health and nutrition status of adolescents. Effective nutrition education requires community-based support from parents, schools, health care professionals, and agencies to accomplish positive changes in knowledge, attitudes and behaviors. Late adolescence is a period when youngsters can consider possible consequences of their behaviors in making decisions about their dietary practices. The most effective changes occur when adolescents are armed with knowledge about nutrition and are in an environment in which standard or normative behaviors among their peers support sound health practices.

Some suggestions of how parents, teachers, and others who work with adolescents can deal with improving adolescent nutrition and fitness appear in Table 7–9. If changes are to be made, it is important to recognize the special emotional, physical and psychological, and social needs of adolescents and to create programs that are sensitive and responsive to those needs.

CONCEPTS TO REMEMBER

▶ Adolescence, ages 11 to 20 years, is a period of major physical, emotional, cognitive, and social transition.

▶ Puberty is a period of rapid physical growth, sexual maturation, and changes in body composition, which typically lasts 3 to 4 years.

▶ Specific energy and nutrient needs, at their peak during puberty, are related more to the stage of physiologic development than to chronologic age.

▶ Due to the physical, social, and emotional changes of adolescence, eating habits become increasingly variable and can place some adolescents at nutritional risk.

▶ The food habits of adolescents are influenced by a multitude of personal and environmental factors.

▶ Nutrition-related concerns for adolescents include overweight, eating disorders, low levels of physical fitness, poor dietary intake, acne, teenage pregnancy, and the future risk of chronic disease.

References

Abrams SA, Stuff JE. Calcium metabolism in girls: current dietary intakes lead to low rates of calcium absorption and retention during puberty. Am J Clin Nutr 1994;60:793.

Adams J. High incidence of intellectual deficits in 5-year-old children exposed to isotretinoin "in utero." Teratology 1990;41:614.

Allen KM, et al. Relationships between expectancies and adolescent dieting. J Sch Health 1993;63:176.

American Medical Association and The American Dietetic Association. Targets for Adolescent Health. Adolescent nutrition and physical fitness. Chicago, IL: AMA ADA, 1991.

Anderson JB. The status of adolescent nutrition. Nutr Today 1991;26:7.

Barr SI. Association of social and demographic variables with calcium intakes of high school students. J Am Diet Assoc 1994;94:260.

Bartlett HL, et al. Fat-free mass in relation to stature: ratios of fat-free mass to height in children, adults and elderly subjects. Am J Clin Nutr 1991;53:1112.

Bigler-Doughten S, Jenkins RM. Adolescent snacks. Nutrient density and nutritional contribution to total intake. J Am Diet Assoc 1987;87:1678.

Cameron N. Assessment of growth and maturation during adolescence. Horm Res 1993;36(Suppl 3):9.

Centers for Disease Control. Recommendations for the use of folic acid to reduce the number of cases of spina bifida and other neural tube defects. MMWR 1991;41:1.

Committee on Drugs. Retinoid therapy for severe dermatological disorders. American Academy of Pediatrics. Pediatrics 1992;90:119.

Committee on Nutrition, American Academy of Pediatrics. Pediatric Nutrition Handbook. Elk Grove Village, IL, 1993.

Cumming RG. Calcium intake and bone mass: a quantitative review of the evidence. Calcif Tissue Int 1990;47:194.

Daniel WA. Nutritional requirements of adolescents. In: Winick M (ed). Adolescent nutrition. New York: Wiley, 1982.

Eck LH, Hackett-Renner C. Calcium intake in youth: sex, age, and racial differences in NHANES II. Prev Med 1992;21:473.

Emmons L. Predisposing factors differentiating adolescent dieters and nondieters. J Am Diet Assoc 1994;94:725.

Farthing MC. Current eating patterns of adolescents in the United States. Nutr Today 1991;26:35.

Food and Nutrition Board. National Research Council. Recommended Dietary Allowances, 10th ed. Washington, DC: National Academy of Sciences, 1989.

Forecast Magazine and Food Processing Magazine and Food & Beverage Marketing Magazine. 1989 Food and Nutrition Study. A National Survey of Teenagers. Fifth Annual Study. Forecast Magazine, 1989.

Gong EJ, Spear BA. Adolescent growth and development: implication for nutritional needs. J Nutr Educ 1988;20:273.

Grande F, Keys A. Body weight, body composition and calorie status. In: Goodhart RS, Shils ME (eds). Modern nutrition in health and disease. 6th ed. Philadelphia: Lea & Febiger, 1980.

Guenther PM. Beverages in the diets of American teenagers. J Am Diet Assoc 1986;86:493.

Heaney RP. In: Krummel DA, Kris-Etherton PM (eds). Nutrition in women's health. Gaithersburg, MD: Aspen, 1996.

Jacobson MS, et al. Adolescent obesity and cardiovascular risk: a rational approach to management. Ann NY Acad Sci 1993;699:220.

Johnston CC Jr, et al. Calcium supplementation and increases in bone mineral density in children. N Engl J Med 1992;327:82.

Kann L, et al. Youth risk behavior surveillance—United States, 1993. MMWR 1995;44:1.

Kimm SYS, et al. Dietary patterns of U.S. children: Implications for disease prevention. Prev Med 1990;19:432.

Lammer E, et al. Retinoic acid embryopathy. N Engl J Med 1985;313:837.

Levenson DI, Bockman RS. A review of calcium preparations. Nutr Rev 1994;52:221.

Lloyd TL, et al. Calcium supplementation and bone mineral density in adolescent girls. JAMA 1993;270:841.

Marino DD, King JC. Nutritional concerns during adolescence. Pediatr Clin North Am 1980;27:125.

Matkovik V. Calcium intake and peak bone mass. N Engl J Med 1993;327:119.

Matkovic V, et al. Factors which influence peak bone mass formation: a study of calcium balance and the inheritance of bone mass in adolescent females. Am J Clin Nutr 1990;52:88.

McPherson RS, et al. Intake and food sources of dietary fat among school children in the Woodlands, Texas. Pediatrics 1990;86:520.

Merzenich H, et al. Dietary fat and sports activity as determinants for age at menarche. Am J Epidemiol 1993;138:217.

Moore DC. Body image and eating behavior in adolescents. J Am Coll Nutr 1993;12:505.

Preliminary findings from NHANES III. MMWR 1994;43:116.

National Center for Health Statistics. Caloric and selected nutrient values for persons 1–74 years of age. First Health and Examination Survey, 1971–1974. DHEW Pub. No. (PHS) 79–1657. Series 11, No. 209. Hyattsville, MD: US Dept of Health, Education and Welfare, 1979.

National Cholesterol Education Program Expert Panel on Blood Cholesterol Levels in Children and Adolescents. National Cholesterol Education Program (NCEP): Highlights of the Report of the Expert Panel on Blood Cholesterol Levels in Children and Adolescents. Pediatrics 1992;89:495.

National Heart, Lung and Blood Institute. National Cholesterol Education Program: Report of the Expert Panel on Blood Cholesterol Levels in Children and Adolescents. Bethesda, MD: National Heart, Lung and Blood Institute, 1991.

National Institutes of Health, Consensus Development Conference on Optimal Calcium Intake. Bethesda, MD: National Institutes of Health, 1994.

Neumark-Sztainer D. Excessive weight preoccupation. Nutr Today 1995;30:68.

Newman WP, et al. Autopsy studies in U.S. children and adolescents. Relationship of risk factors to atherosclerotic lesions. Ann NY Acad Sci 1991;623:16.

Nieves JW, et al. Teenage and current calcium intake are related to bone mineral density of the hip and forearm in women aged 30–39 years. Am J Epidemiol 1995;141:342.

Portnoy B, Christenson GM. Cancer knowledge and related practices: results from the National Adolescent Student Health Survey. J Sch Health 1989;59:218.

Rand Youth Poll. The marketing characteristics of American teenagers. New York: Rand Youth Poll, 1990.

Rocchini AP. Adolescent obesity and hypertension. Pediatr Clin North Am 1993;40:81.

Roche AF, Davila GH. Late adolescent growth in stature. Pediatrics 1972;50:874.

Serdula MK, et al. Weight control practices of U.S. adolescents and adults. Ann Int Med 1993;119:667.

Slap GB. Normal physiological and psychological growth in the adolescent. J Adolesc Health Care 1986;7:13S.

Story, M Resnick MD. Adolescents' views on food and nutrition. J Nutr Educ 1986;18:188.

Strong J. Coronary atherosclerosis in soldiers: a clue to the natural history of atherosclerosis in the young. JAMA 1986;256:2863.

Sutter E, Hawes MR. Relationship of physical activity, body fat, diet, and blood lipid profile in youths 10–15 yr. Med Sci Sports Exerc 1993;25:748.

Tanner JM. Developmental age and the concept of physiological maturity. In: Growth at adolescence. Oxford; Blackwell, 1962.

Tanner JM, Davies PSW. Clinical longitudinal standards for height and weight velocity for North American children. J Pediatr 1985;107:317.

Thompson PR, et al. Zinc status and sexual development in adolescent girls. J Am Diet Assoc 1986;86:892.

Underwood LE. Normal adolescent growth and development. Nutr Today 1991;26:11.

US Department of Agriculture. Nationwide Food Consumption Survey, Nutrient Intakes: Individuals in 48 states, Year 1977–78. Report No. 1–2. Hyattsville, MD, 1984.

US Department of Health and Human Services, Am Sch Health Assoc, Assoc Adol Health Educ, Soc Public Health Educ, Inc. The National Adolescent Student Health Survey: A Report of the Health of America's Youth. 1989. Oakland, Third Party, 1991.

US Department of Health, Education and Welfare. First health and nutrition examination survey, United States, 1971–1972: Dietary intake and biochemical findings. Health Resources Administration (HRA) 74-219-1. Rockville, MD; National Center for Health Statistics, 1974.

Wabitsch M, et al. Body-fat distribution and changes in the atherogenic risk-factor profile in obese adolescent girls during weight reduction. Am J Clin Nutr 1994;60:54.

Wang MQ, et al. Desire for weight gain and potential risks of adolescent males using anabolic steroids. Percept Motor Skills 1994;78:267.

Weaver CM, et al. Differences in calcium metabolism between adolescent and adult females. Am J Clin Nutr 1995;61:577.

Witte DJ, et al. Relationship of self-concept to nutrient intake and eating patterns in young women. J Am Diet Assoc 1991;91:1068.

Wright LS. Physiological development in adolescence. In: Mahan LK, Rees JM (eds). Nutrition in adolescence. St. Louis: Times Mirror/Mosby, 1984.

APPLICATION: Substance Use During Adolescence

Mark came to high school from the same elementary and middle school as David. They had been friends since they were in the second grade. Mark was also interested in basketball, and he played some on their eighth grade team, but mostly he sat on the bench.

When Mark did not make the basketball team in high school, he and David seemed to drift apart. They still rode the bus to and from school together but didn't seem to have much in common anymore. David noticed that Mark seemed to miss school frequently and, when in school, he often missed the bus to go home. A couple of times when David did something with Mark, he thought Mark smelled like cigarettes and even whiskey, the way Aunt Dorothy did, and he worried a little about his old friend. When he tried to ask Mark about it, Mark became very quiet, almost sullen.

Mark's father traveled a great deal and his mother tried hard to be a "good parent," but she worked long hours and often did not get home until after 8 p.m. She was concerned about Mark. He spent a lot of time away from home but not with his old neighborhood friends. From what she had seen she didn't care much for his new friends. Mark never seemed to do any homework, saying he had finished it at school, and refused to discuss what was going on at school. When she discussed it with Mark's dad, he assured her it was just part of being a teenager.

At the end of the fall term of his sophomore year, two of Mark's teachers requested a conference to discuss his performance. When his mother returned from the conference, she was very angry with Mark, and their discussion of his failures at school turned into a shouting match that ended with Mark stamping out of the house. The next morning they talked more calmly, and Mark promised to work harder and to spend less time out with his friends, but he seemed withdrawn and not very enthusiastic. His mother wanted to help him all she could, but she was so busy. They agreed that she would call him each day after school to make sure he was home and doing his homework.

Things were better for a while. Mark was home more and seemed to have fewer mood swings. His mother thought she smelled liquor on his breath once when he came in late after a school activity, but she didn't say anything. She also found a pack of cigarettes in his jacket pocket, which he insisted his father had given him to hold for him several weeks earlier.

In a short time, Mark became moody and irritable and spent most of his time in his room with the music turned up. He skipped meals and was not interested in food. The snacks his mother always had bought for him stayed on the shelf. He frequently violated curfew, but whenever his mother confronted him about it, he would promise to do better. Mark was socializing with a group of older teenagers. His mother began to notice money missing from her purse or the "kitty" she kept in the kitchen cupboard.

At midterm the school counselor requested an appointment with Mark and his parents about Mark's poor academic performance and truancy. Mark's father came home especially to attend. At the session it was apparent that Mark was having problems. At first he denied any substance use except an occasional beer with friends and a few cigarettes. Eventually he did admit to drinking liquor "most days" and to smoking cigarettes, including marijuana, occasionally. He denied using any other drugs but said some of his friends did.

The school counselor assisted them in locating a local clinic for family counseling. After several sessions they discovered that Mark had been drinking up to a pint of hard liquor almost every day, some taken from home and the rest purchased by older friends. If his mother left for work before the school bus came, he might stay home and drink in his room much of the day. If he took the bus to school he would often leave campus before the day began or at lunch. He and his friends hung out in a nearby vacant house where they could smoke and drink.

Together through family and individual counseling they began to work out a plan to help Mark control his substance abuse and get his life back on track.

Just as adolescence is an important time for the formation of food habits, it is a critical period in vulnerability for other behaviors, including substance use. Alcohol, tobacco, and marijuana are the most widely used substances among teenagers. As illustrated by Mark's case, teens can move rapidly to abuse, often of multiple substances. The initiation of alcohol or tobacco use during adolescence often becomes the beginning of a lifetime pattern of substance use with long-term negative heath consequences. Because the use of alcohol and tobacco usually precedes the use of illicit substances, and because drug use among teenagers has recently been on the increase, the prevention of substance use and abuse is a primary public health concern.

Tobacco

Cigarette smoking is the major preventable cause of premature disease and death in the United States. It has been causally linked to cancer, pulmonary disease, coronary heart disease, and a wide array of serious health consequences (Centers for Disease Control, 1989). Despite three decades of explicit health warnings, the number of adolescents starting to smoke has continued to rise (Cummings et al, 1995; Lee et al, 1993; Winkleby et al, 1993). Currently more than three million adolescents smoke cigarettes and over one million, mostly males, use smokeless tobacco (Centers for Disease Control, 1994). Tobacco use is greater among white students (15.4%) than Hispanic (6.8%) or African-American (3.1%) students (Centers for Disease Control, 1992).

Social factors, particularly friends who smoke, are important in the early initiation of smoking by adolescents (Botvin et al, 1992). Other important determinants are perceived acceptability of smoking and intrapersonal factors such as self-efficacy and self-esteem (Bertrand and Abernathy, 1993). Compared to non-users, students who use tobacco have lower self-image, are less independent and mature, are less involved with school and academic achievement, are of lower socioeconomic status, and have greater susceptibility to advertising and promotional activities.

Active smoking during growth can reduce the rate of lung growth and the maximum level of lung function attained. Compared to nonsmokers, young smokers are more likely to experience shortness of breath, coughing spells, wheezing, and overall diminished physical health. Long-term health consequences of smoking are a function of the duration (years) and the intensity (amount) of use. Nicotine is highly addictive, and initiating smoking at an early age increases the probability of being an adult smoker. Adolescent use of tobacco increases the life years of exposure and possibly the intensity, thereby attenuating the risk of serious health consequences.

A comparison of the nutrient content of diets of smokers and non-smokers suggests that smokers have lower intakes of fiber, vitamins, and minerals. Both cigarette smokers and users of smokeless (chewing) tobacco have lower plasma levels of vitamins C and E (Giraud et al, 1995). The RDA for vitamin C for smokers is 100 mg/day, reflecting an increased need due to reduced plasma concentrations associated with an increased metabolic turnover.

Tobacco is often considered a "gateway drug" because it is generally the first drug used by young people in a sequence that can include alcohol, marijuana, and other illicit drugs. One recent study reported that 85% of adolescents admitted to substance treatment facilities were smokers (Myers and Brown, 1994). There is, in fact, a strong dose-dependent relationship between smoking and the use of alcohol and illicit drugs.

Smokeless (chewing) tobacco use has become popular with both school-age children and adolescents. Use of smokeless tobacco has been reported by more than 10% of high school students, most of whom were male (Centers for Disease Control, 1992). Health consequences of chewing tobacco range from halitosis to periodontal degeneration, soft tissue lesions, and various forms of oral cancer. Smokeless tobacco use is as addictive as cigarette smoking, and users are likely to become cigarette smokers.

Because tobacco use by young people has substantial implications for long-term health, two of the national health promotion and disease prevention objectives for the year 2000 are related to tobacco use in young people.

Health Risks of Cigarette Smoking:
Lung cancer
Other fatal malignancies
Pulmonary disease
Coronary artery disease
Stroke
Peripheral vascular disease

Health Objectives for the Year 2000:
Reduce the initiation of cigarette smoking by children and youth so that no more than 15% become regular cigarette smokers by age 20

Reduce smokeless tobacco use by males aged 12 through 24 to a prevalence of not more than 4%

Alcohol Use and Abuse

Although ethanol provides 7 kcal/g, it is not considered a nutrient. Beverages that contain alcohol provide few if any nutrients, and displacement of food calories by alcohol calories reduces the total nutrient intake, even if caloric intake is the same or increased.

Ethanol is rapidly absorbed from the gastrointestinal tract. About 20% is absorbed through the lining of the stomach; the remainder enters the duodenum and, when absorbed, is carried via the portal vein to the liver. Alcohol dehydrogenase, the enzyme required for the oxidation of ethanol, converts it to acetaldehyde. As shown in the margin, acetaldehyde is metabolized to acetyl coenzyme A (CoA), which enters the tricarboxylic acid cycle to provide energy.

In the liver, alcohol is metabolized preferentially, e.g., before carbohydrate and fat, but the rate of metabolism is limited by the availability of alcohol dehydrogenase. About 1 ounce of ethanol can be oxidized every 2 hours. Some beverage equivalents of 1 ounce of ethanol in drinks are listed in the margin. When ethanol ingestion exceeds the amount that can be metabolized, ethanol enters the general circulation, reaching the brain, where it can influence the function of brain cells.

Small amounts of ethanol induce a sense of euphoria, the effect drinkers seek. The blood level of ethanol after two to three drinks increases to 0.05%, reducing inhibitions, restraint, and judgment. This level can double to 0.10% with 4 to 5 drinks and continue to rise to a level of 0.30, which is associated with stupor. Large amounts of ethanol depress the motor area of the brain, impairing muscle coordination, reflexes, speech, and auditory and visual discrimination. Acute alcohol poisoning can occur if a large amount of alcohol is ingested rapidly, as in drinking contests.

The long-term consequences of alcohol abuse can effect nearly every organ. In the liver, the major site of alcohol metabolism, the influx of large amounts of ethanol over time changes glucose, fat, and protein metabolism. Prolonged abuse results in a "fatty liver" due to decreased fat oxidation, increased fatty acid synthesis, and mobilization of fat from body stores. In the early stages of alcohol abuse, fat accumulation can be reversed by abstinence from alcohol, but with prolonged abuse, liver cells become damaged and replaced by fibrous tissue, leading to cirrhosis.

Alcohol abuse is associated with reduced food intake, leading to malnutrition. In time inadequate intake is compounded by the effects of alcohol on the liver and the gastrointestinal tract. Because of the central role of the liver in metabolism, alcohol-induced changes have far-reaching implications. In addition to these changes, fat and glucose utilization is impaired, and eventually there are defects in protein synthesis and transport and storage of vitamins and minerals. The undernutrition of alcoholism has many causes.

Alcohol consumption in the United States seems to be an accepted practice. Long before a youngster enters high school he or she is likely to have had some experience with alcohol. Drinking that first beer or shot of whiskey often is one of the rebellious adolescent rites of passage. More than 90% of teenagers report drinking alcohol, usually beginning around the age of 11 or 12 years (Centers for Disease Control, 1992). Unfortunately, many youngsters get hooked. In a national survey, 45% of high school senior boys and 28% of girls reported at least one episode of binge drinking or consuming more than five drinks at one time in the month prior to the survey (Johnston et al, 1986). Today, alcohol abuse ranks as the number-one drug problem among young people and is a major cause of morbidity and mortality (American Medical Association, 1986).

Drinking during adolescence has biologic, social, psychological, and economic consequences. Less alcohol is needed in teenagers than in adults to impair reflexes and bring about loss of control. Because of their smaller, lighter bodies, girls are not able to handle ethanol as well as boys. In addition, females have only about half as much alcohol dehydrogenase as males (Frezza et al, 1990).

Family socialization processes are important influences on behavior. Children from families that are too controlling or too lax and unsupportive tend to have more problems during adolescence. Both extremes of family support and control are associated with increased adolescent alcohol use (Foxcroft and Lowe, 1991).

Structure of ethanol:

Oxidation of ethanol:

Ethanol
(alcohol dehydrogenase)
↓
Acetaldehyde
(acetaldehyde dehydrogenase)
↓
Fatty → Acetyl ← Glucose
acids   CoA
↓
Tricarboxylic acid
cycle

Equivalents of a Drink (1 ounce of ethanol) in Alcoholic Beverages:
A drink is equal to:
3 to 4 oz wine (8% to 14% alcohol)
10 oz wine cooler (5% to 6% alcohol)
12 oz beer (4% to 6% alcohol)
1.5 oz distilled liquor (whiskey, scotch, rum, vodka, gin, tequila) (30% to 40% alcohol)

Effects of Blood Alcohol Concentration on Behavior:

Blood Alcohol (%)	Behavior
0.03	Relaxation, euphoria
0.05	Relaxed inhibitions, restraint, and judgment
0.10	Slight staggering; impaired coordination; reduced digital dexterity; delayed reaction time; impaired peripheral vision; exaggerated emotional responses
0.15	Slurred speech; blurred vision; staggered walk; decreased motor response
0.20	Double vision; need for assistance walking; emotional liability; uninhibited behavior
0.30	Stupor; confusion; inability to comprehend
0.40–0.50	Unconsciousness; coma

---

cirrhosis—a condition in which liver cells and function are irreversibly lost

Alcohol abuse by adolescents is often concurrent with use of other drugs. Although little is known about the extent and pattern of polydrug use in adolescents, a recent study of 72 alcohol abusers admitted to an inpatient treatment center found that 96% of males and females also used drugs other than alcohol (Martin et al, 1993).

Marijuana

After smoking and alcohol, marijuana is the substance most frequently used by teenagers. Over 40% of high school seniors report having used marijuana (Farrow et al, 1987), but recent increases in use have been greatest among junior high school students. Effects of marijuana use include decreased attention span, loss of motivation, poor school performance, lack of interest in usual activities, and withdrawal from friends who do not use drugs.

A survey that compared nutritional parameters of teenage males who used both alcohol and marijuana with nonusers did not show significant differences in biochemical measures, but abusers had lower intakes of milk, fruits, and vegetables and consumed more snack foods (Farrow et al, 1987).

Cocaine

Data from epidemiologic studies indicate that the use of cocaine is increasing among adolescents and young adults of all socioeconomic backgrounds (Schwartz et al, 1991; Fullilove et al, 1993). As with other substances, progression to use of harder drugs may be related to social and family relationships. There is a high degree of similarity in drug use among friends. For example, a study of junior and senior high school students found that those who used specific drugs in the last 30 days almost invariably had friends who also used those same drugs (Dinges & Detting, 1993).

pharmacologic tolerance—the dose level necessary to induce the desired effect increases

ischemia—lack of blood and therefore oxygen flow to a tissue

Cocaine has extremely potent euphoric effects, and users report preoccupation with thoughts of the drug and rapid loss of the ability to modulate drug use as well as development of pharmacologic tolerance (Schwartz et al, 1991). Cocaine elicits a number of effects such as euphoria and heightened self-confidence, but restlessness, irritability, insomnia, mistrust, and depression can also occur. Frequent use of cocaine can cause rapid and irregular heart beats, and even myocardial infarction, stroke, and intracerebral hemorrhage. Ischemic changes, which decrease blood flow, have been observed in the brains of cocaine abusers (Brown et al, 1992).

Role of Nutrition

Substance abuse compromises food intake and potentially impairs nutrition status. Smokers have lower body weights than non-smokers, and smoking cessation is associated with weight gain. Use of illicit drugs can create anorexia and reduce food intake as a result of impairments in eating behaviors associated with substance use. The use of cocaine lessens the desire for food. Therefore, weight loss is a common side effect. Many of the social and emotional factors that contribute to eating disorders are present in cocaine abusers, and many have coexisting anorexia or bulimia nervosa.

Abuse of drugs accelerates nutrition needs beyond normal so that even a well-balanced diet may be inadequate (American Dietetic Association, 1990). As substance use increases, its impact on dietary intake becomes greater. In addition, changes created by these substances may increase nutrition risk via decreased nutrient utilization due to the substances' effects on body metabolism. Nutrient deficiencies may be precipitated by the decreased intake, malabsorption of nutrients, increased nutritional requirements to metabolize the drug, poor utilization of nutrients in the body, inadequate storage or mobilization, and increased excretion in the urine or through diarrhea.

The negative effects of substance abuse on nutrition status depend on the frequency and intensity of use as well as use of other substances and the usual food habits. Any nutrition assessment of adolescents must include queries relative to use of alcohol, tobacco, and illegal drugs. Such information has to be obtained with a matter-of-fact approach in a non-threatening environment but will provide a basis for incorporation of nutrition into prevention and intervention efforts. Normalization of food habits is an essential component of any recovery program.

The dietitian is an integral member of the care team in addiction treatment centers. He must assess nutritional needs and plan intervention. Nutrition recovery is an important component of the physical foundation for rehabilitation that precedes recovery. An eating pattern that includes regular meals emphasizing complex carbohydrates, moderate amounts of protein, and conservative quantities of dietary fats with emphasis on balance, variety, and caloric appropriateness and regularity will be conducive to progress in recovery.

Preventing substance abuse is the major solution. Simply warning teenagers about the dangers of substance use, including the progression to abuse, will do little to keep them away. A family policy that gives adolescents a means or reason to avoid peer pressure, such as losing driving privileges, will add credibility to a decision not to participate. A potentially effective means within the community and school is programs or training to change "norms" among teenagers, making substance abuse less socially acceptable (Hansen and Graham, 1991).

Unfortunately, the best of intentions and programs do not always work. But, as illustrated with Mark, an even more difficult problem may be identifying abuse, getting the adolescent to acknowledge the problem, and initiating effective treatment programs. Early recognition is essential and can make the difference between a healthy, productive life and long-term emotional and physical compromise. The National Council on Alcoholism and Drug Dependence maintains a hopeline (1-800-NCA-CALL) that can provide information and referral to a local organization to assist with alcohol-related problems. The hopeline is open 24 hours a day, 7 days a week.

REFERENCES

American Dietetic Association. Position of the American Dietetic Association: Nutrition intervention in treatment and recovery from chemical dependency. J Am Diet Assoc 1990;90:1274.

American Medical Association. AMA white paper on adolescent health. Chicago: American Medical Association, 1986.

Bertrand LD, Abernathy TJ. Predicting cigarette smoking among adolescents using cross-sectional and longitudinal approaches. J Sch Health 1993;63:98.

Botvin GJ, et al. Factors promoting cigarette smoking among black youth; a causal modeling approach. Addict Behav 1992;18:397.

Brown E, et al. CNS complications of cocaine abuse: prevalence, pathophysiology and neuroradiology. Am J Roentgenol 1992;159:137.

Centers for Disease Control. Preventing tobacco use among young people. A report of the Surgeon General. MMWR 1994;43:2.

Centers for Disease Control. Selected tobacco-use behaviors, dietary patterns among high school students—United States, 1991. MMWR 1992;41:417.

Centers for Disease Control. Reducing the health consequences of smoking: 20 years of progress—a report of the Surgeon General. Rockville, MD: U.S. Department of Health and Human Services, Public Health Service, 1989. DHHS Publ. No. CDC 89–8411.

Cummings KM, et al. Trends in smoking initiation among adolescents and young adults. MMWR 1995;44:521.

Dinges MM, Detting ER. Similarity in drug use patterns between adolescents and their friends. Adolescence 1993;28:253.

Farrow JA, et al. Health, development and nutritional status of adolescent alcohol and marijuana abusers. Pediatrics 1987;79:218.

Foxcroft DR, Lowe G. Adolescent drinking behavior and family socialization factors: a meta-analysis. J Adolesc 1991;14:255.

Frezza M, et al. The role of decreased gastric alcohol dehydrogenase activity and first-pass metabolism. N Engl J Med 1990;322:95.

Fullilove MT, et al. Crack cocaine use and high risk behaviors among sexually active black adolescents. J Adolesc Health 1993;14:295.

Giraud DW, et al. Plasma and dietary vitamin C and E levels of tobacco chewers, smokers and nonusers. J Am Diet Assoc 1995;95;198.

Hansen WB, Graham JW. Preventing alcohol, marijuana, and cigarette use among adolescents: peer pressure resistance training versus establishing conservation norms. Prev Med 1991;20:414.

Johnston LE, et al. Drug use among American high school students, college students and other young adults: National trends through 1985. Rockville, MD: Department of Health and Human Services. DHHS Publication No. (ADM) 1986;86:1450.

Lee LL, et al. Changes in the patterns of initiation of cigarette smoking in the United States: 1950, 1965 and 1980. Cancer Epidemiology, Biomarkers Prevention 1993;2:593.

Martin CS, et al. Patterns of polydrug use in adolescent alcohol abusers. Am J Drug Alcohol Abuse 1993;19:511.

Myers MG, Brown SA. Smoking and health in substance-abusing adolescents: a two year follow-up. Pediatrics 1994;93:561.

Schwartz RH, et al. "Crack" use by American middle-class adolescent polydrug abusers. J Pediatr 1991;118:150.

Winkleby MA, et al. Cigarette smoking trends in adolescents and young adults: the Stanford Five-City Project. Prev Med 1993;22:325.

PART III

REPRODUCTION

CHAPTER 8

PREGNANCY

Melissa is a 24-year-old accountant. She is 165 cm (65 in) tall, physically active, and concerned about "being healthy." When her home pregnancy test was positive, Melissa immediately made an appointment at the obstetric clinic in her health care program.

Two weeks later, after a physical examination the obstetrician pronounced her "in excellent health" but at 52 kg (114 lb) a little underweight. When Melissa told her that she was having some difficulty with nausea and vomiting, the obstetrician reassured her that was normal and had the nurse give her a list of suggestions for controlling nausea. She gave Melissa a prescription for prenatal vitamins with iron and sent her to have some blood work done at a laboratory down the hall.

At her appointment the next month, Melissa's weight had dropped to 51 kg (112 lb). She said the nausea had subsided but that she didn't want to gain too much weight. Concerned, the physician made an appointment for her to see the dietitian, Amy Smith, the following week. When Melissa met with Amy she liked her right away. Amy measured her height, weight, and fatfolds, and they chatted about how Melissa felt and what she ate. Amy asked Melissa if she was taking the prenatal vitamin/iron supplement. Melissa assured her she was because she wants to do everything right for her baby. Amy then pointed out that Melissa should give as much attention to her weight gain so that the fetus will grow normally. She suggested that because Melissa was underweight (BMI 19) when she became pregnant, she should gain a total of 28 to 40 pounds. Amy gave Melissa a chart to monitor her weight gain, and using a Food Guide for pregnancy, they discussed foods she needed to eat to achieve that weight. Melissa met with Amy again the following month.

By the fifth month, Melissa had gained 5.5 kg (13 lb) and said she felt great. The blood tests were repeated, and a test was performed to screen for diabetes. Melissa felt well and she was gaining weight at about the rate Amy had suggested. At about 7 months, Melissa weighed 61.5 kg (135 lb). She and her husband attended prenatal classes, which helped prepare them for the labor and delivery. The classes included information about diet and exercise. They had a tour of the hospital labor and delivery areas. Soon Melissa was going for office visits every 2 weeks and then weekly. She called Amy about problems she was having with constipation and indigestion. Amy assured her that they were common during late pregnancy and made some suggestions about increasing the fiber and fluid content of her diet to relieve constipation and making some changes in her evening meal pattern to reduce heartburn. By the end of her pregnancy Melissa had gained 17 kg (37 lb), and her new baby daughter weighed 3.4 kg (7.5 lb).

The greatest assurance of a healthy start in life is to have a mother who has been well-nourished throughout her life as well as during pregnancy. Pregnancy is a critical period of rapid growth and development for the fetus, and high physiologic and metabolic demands are made on the mother. Nutrition deserves special consideration to make sure that it is not a limiting factor in maternal or infant health.

THE FEMALE REPRODUCTIVE CYCLE

■ Describe the sequence of changes in the menstrual cycle and the role they play in preparation for pregnancy.

■ What hormones regulate the follicular and luteal phases in the ovary and the proliferative and secretory stages in the uterus?

■ What is the premenstrual dysphoric disorder?

■ Can diet play a role in the treatment of PDD?

The onset of menarche, usually between 11 and 14 years of age in females living in developed countries, begins the female reproductive cycle, which continues until **menopause**. The female reproductive years are characterized by monthly cyclic changes in the secretion of the female hormones and corresponding changes in the ovaries and uterus. This pattern, called the menstrual cycle, usually lasts about 28 days. It is characterized by formation of a mature ovum that is released from one of the ovaries each month and a uterine **endometrium**, which is prepared for implantation of a fertilized ovum. If the ovum is released and fertilization does not occur, these preparations are discarded (menstruation) and the cycle repeats itself.

Hormones

The menstrual cycle is synchronized by the **gonadotropic hormones** from the anterior pituitary gland. The follicle-stimulating hormone (FSH) stimulates growth and maturation of follicles in the ovary, and luteinizing hormone (LH) stimulates development of the ruptured follicle into the corpus luteum and signals ovulation. Two other significant hormones, estrogen and **progesterone**, are produced by the ovary under the stimulation of FSH and LH.

Follicular/Proliferative Phase

Figure 8–1 depicts the various stages of the menstrual cycle in the ovaries and uterus. At the beginning of each cycle, the onset of menstruation, the concentrations of FSH and LH increase. These increases initiate acceler-ated growth of the cells in the ovarian follicles, ovum, and surrounding layers of cells (follicular phase). The ovum enlarges and develops into a mature follicle. Additional layers of cells develop around the ovum and secrete a fluid that contains a high concentration of estrogen. After approximately 12 days, the secretion of LH and FSH increases. LH causes some cells in the follicle to **luteinize** and increase secretion of progesterone. In this environment—rapid growth of the follicle during a prolonged phase of excessive estrogen, followed by diminishing estrogen secretion and increasing secretion of progesterone—**ovulation** occurs about 14 days after the onset of menstruation.

The cycle begins simultaneously in the uterus, with most of the uterine endometrium being shed during menstruation. Estrogen released from the ovarian follicle initiates the proliferative phase, which lasts for approximately 2 weeks and ceases with ovulation. This phase stimulates rapid cell proliferation of the uterine lining and endometrium. The endometrium thickens and develops an extensive vascular system in preparation for implantation of the ovum should fertilization occur.

Luteal/Secretory Phase

In the ovary, cells of the follicle that remained after expulsion of the ovum from the follicle undergo rapid physical and chemical change and become a **corpus luteum**. In this luteal phase of the cycle, the corpus luteum secretes progesterone and estrogen, which causes a feedback decrease in secretion of both FSH and LH. Therefore, during this period no new follicles begin to grow in the ovary. When the ovum is not fertilized, the corpus luteum **involutes**, and the lack of estrogen feedback suppression allows the anterior pituitary gland to secrete greater quantities of FSH and LH. The FSH and LH initiate growth of new follicles, and the next ovarian cycle begins.

The progesterone and estrogen secreted in large quantities by the corpus luteum during the luteal phase initiate the secretory phase in the uterus. This involves cellular proliferation, which results in swelling and increased secretion of the endometrium. These endometrial changes produce an endometrium containing large nutrient reserves that can provide favorable conditions for implantation of a fertilized ovum. If fertilization does not occur, approximately 2 days before the end of the monthly cycle the ovarian hormones estrogen and progesterone decrease sharply. Menstruation follows, and the cycle begins again.

Premenstrual Dysphoric Disorder (PDD)

Premenstrual **dysphoria** affects as many as 3% to 8% of American women in their reproductive years (Steiner et al,

1995). Headaches, mood swings, breast swelling, acne, depression, irritability, and food cravings—every month millions of women experience these symptoms, and more, just prior to their menstrual periods. Often referred to as premenstrual syndrome (PMS), the cluster of varied, nonspecific physical and/or psychological symptoms that appear during the luteal phase has been designated as premenstrual dysphoric disorder (PDD).

Overall, approximately 75% of women complain of some premenstrual symptoms but, only 3% to 8% of cycling women can be categorized with true PDD (Barnhart et al, 1995) according to the eleven criteria established by the American Psychiatric Association (Table 8–1). Diagnosis of PDD requires that five of the 11 symptoms must be severe premenstrually with postmenstrual remission, and the five must include at least one dysphoric symptom (irritability, mood swings, anxiety, or depression). Multiple physical symptoms are counted as one symptom.

The cause of the disorder is unknown, and over the last four decades at least 50 treatment options have been suggested to be effective. Nutrient metabolism and status may play a role in regulating normal menstrual cycles. Variations in energy intake, protein, fat, and carbohydrate have been correlated with the cycle phase. Interest currently centers on differences in tryptophan metabolism between follicular and luteal phases.

Premenstrual dysphoria shares many of the features of depression and anxiety states that have been linked to serotoninergic dysregulation. Deficiencies in serotonin-mediated brain neurotransmitters may be responsible, in part, for symptoms of dysphoria. In fact, treatment of premenstrual dysphoria with serotonin reuptake inhibitors reduces symptoms of tension, irritability, and dysphoria (Steiner et al, 1995).

Many women who suffer from PDD have cravings for sweets and increased consumption of carbohydrate-rich foods. A recent double-bind crossover study tested the effect of a high carbohydrate beverage and a placebo on PDD symptoms across three menstrual cycles (Sayegh et al, 1995). Compared to the placebo, the carbohydrate beverage decreased self-reported depression, anger, confusion, and carbohydrate craving and improved memory word recognition 90 to 180 minutes after ingestion. Results suggest that the psychological and affective symptoms of PMS can be relieved by consuming a carbohydrate-rich beverage known to increase serum tryptophan levels.

Because no specific cause has been identified for PMS, treatment has been difficult and controversial. More than 30% of affected women have shown improvement of symptoms when given a placebo. Serotonin uptake inhibitors (antidepressants) are becoming the therapy of choice for PMS because they are effective, easily tolerated, and free of major side effects (Barnhart et al, 1995). Other antidepressants are sometimes used. Treatment is often designed to improve or eliminate the symptoms. Tranquilizers may be useful to relieve anxiety; analgesics may relieve headaches; and diuretics may help with fluid retention.

For many women, an important part of coping with PDD is recognizing symptoms and changing lifestyles to minimize the effect of those symptoms. These changes include exercise, avoidance of tobacco and excess alcohol, relaxation training, psychotherapy, and proper nutrition. They are associated with an improvement in general health, which could make PDD more tolerable.

NUTRITION AND REPRODUCTION

■ How can prepregnancy nutrition intervention improve pregnancy outcome?

■ What is periconceptional nutrition?

■ What disorders can be treated before conception to improve pregnancy outcomes?

Periconceptional Nutrition

The birth, growth, and development of a healthy infant depends on a woman's general health and well-being before conception and the amount and quality of care provided during pregnancy. Preconceptual care is an organized, comprehensive program that identifies and reduces women's medical, psychological, social, and lifestyle reproductive risks before conception (Institute of Medicine, 1985; U.S. Public Health Service Expert Panel on the Content of Prenatal Care, 1989).

KEY TERMS

menopause: the span of time during which the menstrual cycle wanes and gradually stops, around age 50

endometrium: mucous membrane lining the uterus

gonadotropic hormone: hormone that has a stimulating effect on ovary and testis

progesterone: steroid hormone that causes changes in the endometrium preparatory to implantation

luteinize: the process after ovulation by which an ovarian follicle transforms into a corpus luteum

ovulation: process in which an ovum is discharged from an ovary

corpus luteum: mass formed in the ovary by a follicle after it has matured and lost the ovum. The corpus luteum secretes progesterone.

involute: regress

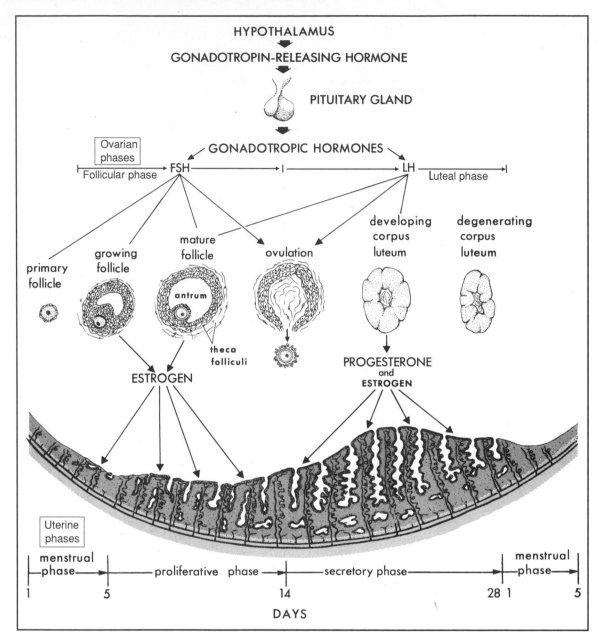

FIGURE 8–1. Hormones and phases of the menstrual cycle. The ovarian cycles are controlled by the pituitary gland, which in turn is controlled by gonadotropin-releasing hormone produced by neurosecretory cells in the hypothalamus of the brain. This schematic drawing illustrates the interrelations among the hypothalamus of the brain, the pituitary gland, the ovaries, and the endometrium of the uterus. One complete menstrual cycle is shown. Follicle-stimulating hormone (FSH) and luteinizing hormone (LH), which are released by the pituitary gland, stimulate the ovaries. Hormones from the ovaries (estrogen and progesterone) then promote changes in the structure and function of the endometrium. This process is called the menstrual cycle. Thus, the cyclical activity of the ovary is intimately linked with changes in the uterus. (Adapted from Moore KL, Persaud TVN. The developing human. 5th ed. Philadelphia: WB Saunders, 1993.)

Components of preconceptual care are essentially the same as those of the nutrition care process described in Chapter 2 and are often summarized as risk assessment, health promotion, and intervention to reduce risk. High-risk behaviors such as smoking and alcohol or substance abuse can be identified and counseling or treatment initi-ated. For some women, dietary changes before conception can reduce risk and have a positive influence on pregnancy outcome. Women with medical conditions such as diabetes mellitus or phenylketonuria have improved pregnancy outcomes with strict preconceptional metabolic control (Kuller and Laifer, 1994). Preconceptional modi-

TABLE 8–1 Criteria for Premenstrual Dysphoric Disorder

1. Markedly depressed mood, feelings of hopelessness, or self-deprecating thoughts
2. Marked anxiety, tension, feeling of being "keyed up" or "on edge"
3. Marked affective liability (e.g., feeling suddenly sad or tearful or feeling increased sensitivity to rejection)
4. Persistent and marked anger or irritability or increase in interpersonal conflicts
5. Decreased interest in usual activities (e.g., work, school, friends, hobbies)
6. Subjective sense of difficulty in concentrating
7. Lethargy, easy fatigability, or marked lack of energy
8. Marked change in appetite, overeating, or specific food cravings
9. Hypersomnia or insomnia
10. A subjective sense of being overwhelmed or out of control
11. Other physical symptoms, such as breast tenderness or swelling, headaches, joint or muscle pain, a sensation of bloating, weight gain

The disturbances *must* markedly interfere with work or school or with usual social activities and relationships with others (e.g., avoidance of social activities, decreased productivity and efficiency at work or school).

The disturbances *must not* be an exacerbation of the symptoms of another disorder (e.g., major depressive disorder, panic disorder, dysthymic disorder, or a personality disorder).

Reprinted with permission from the Diagnostic and Statistical Manual of Mental Disorders, Fourth Edition. Copyright 1994 American Psychiatric Association.

fication of exposure to medications or other substances known to be teratogens reduces the risk of anomalies in the newborn.

Preconceptional assessment of nutrition status also identifies conditions or practices such as bulimia, anorexia, pica, hypervitaminosis, vegetarianism, and extremes of body weight that may compromise nutrition status. Once identified, nutrition counseling and, in some cases, treatment of underlying conditions, can be initiated. Nutrient supplements may be recommended. For example multivitamins containing folate taken during the **periconceptional period** have been associated with a reduced recurrence of birth defects of the neural tube.

Effect of Nutrition on Reproduction

■ How is pregnancy outcome defined for mother and infant?

■ How can nutrition or diet influence pregnancy outcome?

Multiple Risk Factors

Although most experts agree that nutrition is a factor in successful reproduction, the accumulation of direct evidence of a correlation between nutrition and reproductive performance is complicated by variations in age, parity, socioeconomic and educational status of the mother, and her health and use of health care. Women most likely to be poorly nourished also have other risk factors for poor pregnancy outcome because of cultural, socioeconomic, or lifestyle factors. Although human studies on the effect of undernutrition on reproduction are limited, evidence has accumulated from observations of civilian populations subjected to semi-starvation during World War II and populations that have experienced famine. In the last two decades additional information has been contributed from studies of women at nutrition risk who received supplemental food and/or nutrition counseling. These include observations from several developing countries as well as the United States and Canada.

Undernutrition

Severe and acute undernutrition in previously well-nourished women is associated with a reversible decline in fertility rates (Stein, 1975). Severe undernutrition superimposed on previous marginal nutrition is associated with low fertility rates and an increase in **preterm births** and neonatal deaths (Winkvist et al, 1992).

Severe undernutrition at the time of conception and during early pregnancy can be manifested in birth defects. Although undernutrition that occurs later in **gestation**, is less likely to result in birth defects, infants are likely to experience **fetal growth restriction** and be of **low birth weight**. Mild to moderate malnutrition has less impact on fertility but may have far-reaching, and as yet undefined, effects on maternal and child health.

Intervention Studies

In developing countries, intervention studies of pregnant women that improved their diets or received nutrient

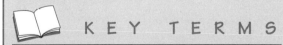

KEY TERMS

dysphoria: excessive disquiet, agitation, restlessness
periconceptional period: 1 to 3 months prior to pregnancy through the first 6 weeks after delivery
preterm birth: birth occurring after a gestation of less than 37 weeks
gestation: the period from conception to birth
fetal growth restriction: failure to grow at usual rate for time in the uterus; also called intrauterine growth retardation (IUGR)
low birth weight: a birth weight < 2500 g

RESEARCH UPDATE
Neural Tube Defects

Neural tube defects (NTDs) are the most common major birth defects world wide. Affecting 2500 infants in the U.S. annually, they contribute substantially to infant mortality and disability (Lynberg and Khoury, 1990). Neural tube defects include spina bifida and other malformations resulting from defective or delayed closure of the **neural tube** in the embryo. Spina bifida is an inclusive name for a group of congenital disorders associated with lack of bone encasement of the spine, which, in turn, often causes permanent damage to the spinal cord and spinal nerves. The result may be varying degrees of paralysis, loss of bladder and bowel control, and cognitive impairment. Anencephaly is a fatal malformation in which the brain lacks the cranial vault and cerebral hemispheres.

Mothers who have had an infant or fetus with a neural tube defect have a 2% to 3% risk of having another pregnancy resulting in a neural tube defect (Little and Elwood, 1991). Vitamin supplementation or nutrition counseling to improve nutrient intake in the periconcepual interval can reduce the recurrence of neural tube defects (Willett, 1992). In 1991, positive effects of folate supplementation were verified in a randomized controlled trial sponsored by the British Medical Research Council in 33 centers in seven countries (MRC Vitamin Study Research Group, 1991). All 1195 study participants were women who had had a previous pregnancy that resulted in a neural tube defect and who were planning a subsequent pregnancy. The women who received folate supplements (4 mg) had a 1.0% recurrence of offspring with NTD, compared to 3.5% of women who did not receive folate. Thus, daily folate supplementation before conception and during early pregnancy was associated with a 71% reduction in the recurrence of NTD. Recently, periconceptual use of multivitamins containing folate has been reported to be associated with decreased risks of orofacial clefts (Shaw et al, 1995) and congenital urinary tract abnormalities (Li et al, 1995).

Unusually high homocysteine levels have been observed in mothers of NTD offspring (Steegers-Theunissen, 1995). Because plasma homocysteine is a sensitive marker of folate status, it has been suggested that folate metabolism is abnormal in these mothers. Recently, van der Put and co-workers (1995) reported the isolation of a mutation in the gene for the enzyme 5,10-methylenetetrahydrofolate reductase, and reduced levels of the enzyme, suggesting defective folate metabolism in at least a subset of mothers with NTD offspring. It may be that folate administration overcomes the effects of reduced enzyme activity.

The Centers for Disease Control and Prevention (CDC) has published two recommendations for folate supplementation during the periconceptional interval to reduce the risk of NTDs. The first, 4 mg per day, is for women who have had a prior infant or fetus with NTD and plan another pregnancy (CDC, 1991a). The second is for 0.4 mg (400 μg) for all women of childbearing age who are capable of becoming pregnant (CDC, 1991b). This supplementation is to begin at least 4 weeks before conception and continue through the first trimester, when the neural tube is forming in the embryo.

It has been proposed that folic acid fortification of grain products would provide folate levels sufficient to reduce NTD risk in a cost-effective manner that would reach most women (Romano et al, 1995). Although the safety (especially the risk of masking Vitamin B_{12} deficiency) and effectiveness of this practice have been the subject of controversy (Crane, 1995), in 1996 the Food and Drug Administration (FDA) authorized the fortification of grain products with folic acid to reduce the incidence of NTD in the United States.

and/or caloric supplements have shown moderate improvements in birth weight, infant survival, and childhood growth and development. In developed countries the results of intervention programs have been mixed. The beneficial effect of food supplements on maternal weight gain and fetal growth appears to depend on the prior energy deficiency of the mother and the extent to which the supplement compensates for that deficit. In a program in Montreal, nutrition supplementation and counseling were shown to improve pregnancy outcome (Rush, 1981). Similarly, the Special Supplemental Food Program for Women, Infants and Children (WIC) has documented changes in pregnancy outcome in poor women at nutritional risk (see the Application at the end of Chapter 9). Although gains in infant birth weight have been lower than predicted from levels of supplementation, even modest changes in birth weight can have significant impact for reducing **perinatal** mortality and impairment (Susser, 1991).

Information regarding the effect of undernutrition on the male's reproductive role is limited. Malnutrition is associated with decreased libido and a reduction in the number, motility, and life span of sperm (Stein, 1975). Malnutrition during puberty can delay growth and development. For example, Prasad has demonstrated dwarfism, hypogonadism, and iron deficiency anemia in zinc-deficient males in Egypt and Iran (Prasad et al, 1988).

Factors Related to Pregnancy Outcome

A successful pregnancy can be defined in terms of many outcome measures, the most significant of which are perinatal mortality, infant birth weight, and gestational age (Wilcox and Skjerven, 1992). A number of nutritional factors are related to reproductive performance (Viteri et al, 1989). The nutrition status of a woman reflects her own birth status as well as her early nutrition and development. For example, there is a correlation between a mother's birth weight and the weight of her infant (Klebanoff and Yip, 1987). Maternal height also has been related to infant birth weight, and some researchers suggest this is a reflection of maternal growth and, indirectly, long-term nutritional adequacy (Parsons et al, 1991).

Maternal weight at the time of conception and gestational weight gain are the strongest predictors of infant birth weight (Abrams and Laros, 1986; Mitchell and Lerner, 1989a). Underweight women are more likely to have low-birthweight infants (Mitchell and Lerner, 1989b), higher fetal and neonatal mortality rates, and more complications (Nacye, 1979). Obese women have a greater risk of hypertension, diabetes, complications during labor and delivery, and **postterm births**. During pregnancy, inadequate dietary intakes and poor gestational weight gain increase the risk of an unfavorable outcome. In addition, diets that are low in energy are likely to be below recommended intake levels for other nutrients.

PREGNANCY

- Define ovulation, fertilization, and implantation.
- Describe the sequence and timing of critical phases of embryonic and fetal development.
- How are the embryo and the fetus nourished?
- What are the functions of the placenta?
- Outline the physiologic changes of pregnancy.
- How might maternal undernutrition influence these changes?

During pregnancy a single fertilized cell grows into millions of cells of complex tissues, organs, and systems in just 40 weeks. Such rapid growth makes the developing fetus vulnerable to nutritional inadequacies. Diet deserves special consideration during pregnancy to ensure that it is not a limiting factor in the growth and development of the fetus or the health of the mother.

Conception and Implantation

When ovulation occurs, the ovum, along with its attached cells, is expelled directly into the **peritoneal** cavity and enters one of the fallopian tubes (Fig. 8–2). Fertilization of the ovum normally takes place soon after the ovum enters the fallopian tube. Following fertilization, approximately 3 days are required for transport of the **zygote** through the tube into the uterus. Several stages of division occur before the zygote reaches the uterus. The first divisions produce a solid sphere of cells, the morula, but during subsequent divisions the cells pull away from the center and form a hollow cavity (Fig. 8–3). This is referred to as a blastocyst. The developing ovum remains in the uterine cavity 4 to 5 days before it implants in the endometrium. Therefore, implantation occurs 7 or 8 days after ovulation. During this time the nutrition needs of the ovum are met from the endometrial secretions.

Implantation is initiated by **trophoblastic** cells that develop over the surface of the blastocyst (Fig. 8–4). These cells secrete proteolytic enzymes that digest and liquefy the cells of the endometrium. Fluid and nutrients released from these cells are absorbed into the blastocyst via phagocytosis by the trophoblastic cells. These substances provide the sustenance for further growth. At the same time, additional trophoblastic cells form cords of cells that extend into deeper layers of the endometrium and attach. This is implantation. Once implantation has taken place, the trophoblastic and other cells proliferate rapidly and,

KEY TERMS

neural tube: tube formed in embryonic period from which the brain and spinal cord develop
perinatal: 28th week of gestation to 28 days after birth
postterm birth: birth occurring after a gestation of 42 or more weeks
peritoneal: space between the membranes lining the walls of the abdomen and pelvic cavities
zygote: fertilized ovum
trophoblast: *tropho*, food, nourishment; *blastic*, immature stage in cellular development

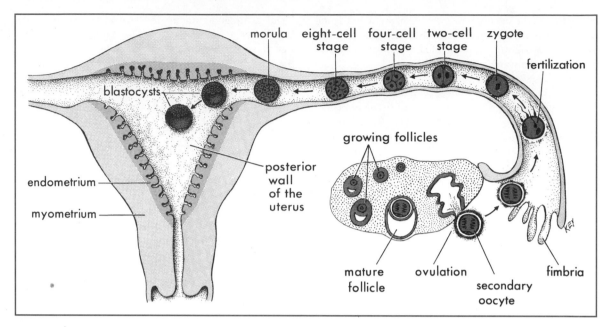

FIGURE 8–2. The beginning of human development: ovulation, conception, and blastocyst formation. Diagrammatic representation of ovulation, fertilization, and human development during the first week. Stage 1 of development begins with fertilization and ends when the zygote forms. Stage 2 (days 2 to 3) comprises the early stages of division, from 2 to about 6 cells of the morula. Stage 3 (days 4 to 5) consists of the free, unattached blastocyst. Stage 4 (days 5 to 6) is represented by the blastocyst attaching to the posterior wall of the uterus, a common site of implantation. The blastocysts have been sectioned to show their structure. (From Moore KL, Persaud TVN. The developing human. 5th ed. Philadelphia: WB Saunders, 1993.)

along with cells from the mother's endometrium, form the placenta and the various membranes of pregnancy.

As trophoblastic cells invade the endometrium, the stored nutrients are used by the **embryo** for growth and development. During the first week after implantation, the endometrium is the only source of nutrients to the embryo, and it continues to contribute a large measure of its nutrition for 8 to 12 weeks. During this time, the placenta grad-

ually begins to increase its efficiency in the transfer of nutrients from the mother.

The Placenta

While trophoblastic cords from the blastocyst are attaching to the uterus, blood capillaries from the vascular sys-

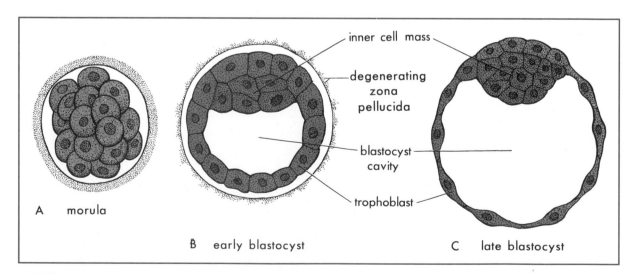

FIGURE 8–3. Formation of the embryoblast. The morula enters the uterus. The cells separate into two parts—an outer cell layer called the trophoblast and a group of centrally located cells mass on embryoblast. (From Moore KL, Persaud TVN. The developing human. 5th ed. Philadelphia: WB Saunders, 1993.)

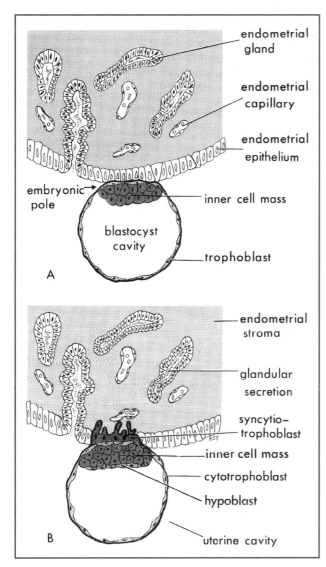

endometrial gland

endometrial capillary

endometrial epithelium

embryonic pole

inner cell mass

blastocyst cavity

trophoblast

A

endometrial stroma

glandular secretion

syncytio-trophoblast

inner cell mass

cytotrophoblast

hypoblast

uterine cavity

B

FIGURE 8–4. Attachment and implantation. Drawings of sections illustrating the attachment of the blastocyst to the endometrial epithelium and early stages of implantation. **(A)** 6 days: the trophoblast is attached to the endometrial epithelium. **(B)** 7 days: the syncytiotrophoblast has formed from the trophoblast and has penetrated the epithelium. (From Moore KL, Persaud TVN. The developing human. 5th ed. Philadelphia: WB Saunders, 1993.)

The major function of the placenta is to allow diffusion of oxygen and nutrients from the maternal blood across the placental membrane to the blood of the growing fetus and diffusion of carbon dioxide and metabolic excretory products such as urea, uric acid, and creatinine from the fetus back to the mother. The trophoblastic cells in the placental membrane can actively absorb certain nutrients such as amino acids, calcium, inorganic phosphate, and ascorbic acid, resulting in higher quantities in the fetal blood than in the maternal circulation. Early in the process human chorionic gonadotropin is synthesized by the placenta and appears to support implantation. The placenta is also a site of synthesis of estrogen, progesterone, and other hormones.

In the first few months of gestation the placenta grows much more rapidly than the fetus. During this time quantities of substrates including protein, calcium, and iron are stored in the placenta to be used later for fetal growth. This function of the placenta in early pregnancy has been compared to that of the liver in adults. Later in gestation these metabolic functions of the placenta become less important as the fetal liver progressively assumes this important role.

Physiologic Changes of Pregnancy

Many visible changes occur in a woman's body during pregnancy. Most women gain between 11 and 16 kg (25–35 lb). The dimensions of the uterus expand 150-fold, changing the woman's center of equilibrium, and the breasts enlarge in preparation for lactation. In late pregnancy water is retained, causing feet and ankles to swell. These changes are accompanied by a diversity of adaptations in the anatomic, biochemical, and physiologic functions of the mother, some of which are outlined in Table 8–2. In most instances physiologic activity is increased, but smooth muscle (urinary and gastrointestinal tracts) demonstrates decreased activity. Many of these changes occur during the first half of gestation to meet the metabolic demands of the placenta and fetus and prepare for future needs. Changes during the latter half of pregnancy meet increasing fetal requirements and prepare for labor, birth, and lactation.

tem of the embryo are growing into cords that will become part of the placenta. By the 16th day after fertilization, blood begins to flow. Simultaneously, blood **sinuses** supplied with blood from the mother develop between the surface of the uterine endometrium and the trophoblastic cords. Thus, the villi carrying fetal blood are surrounded by sinuses containing maternal blood (Fig. 8–5). Over time the fetal villi subdivide and form many branches, which will increase the exchange by providing a larger surface area. The fetus is surrounded by a fluid-filled sac called the amniotic sac. Within the sac the **umbilical cord** extends through the abdomen of the fetus to the placenta.

 K E Y   T E R M S

embryo: the developing organism from 1 week after conception to the eighth week of gestation.
sinus: cavity or hollow space
umbilical cord: structure through which fetal veins and arteries reach the placenta

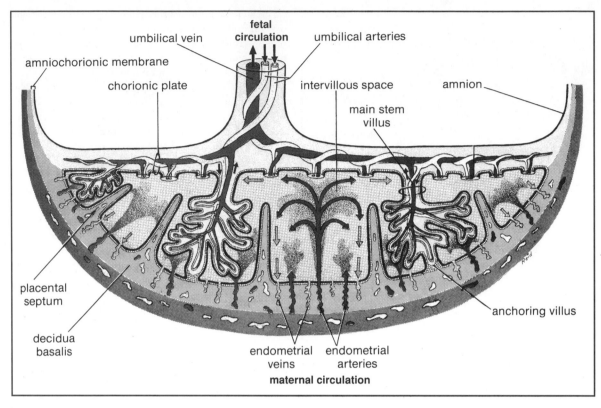

FIGURE 8–5. Schematic drawing of a section through a full-term placenta shows: (1) the relation of the villous chorion (fetal part of the placenta) to the decidua basalis (maternal part of placenta); (2) the fetal placental circulation; and (3) the maternal–placental circulation. Maternal blood flows into the intervillous space in funnel-shaped spurts, and exchanges occur with the fetal blood as the maternal blood flows around the branch villi (branches of stem villi). The main exchange of material between the mother and embryo/fetus occurs through the branch villi. The inflowing arterial blood pushes venous blood out into the endometrial veins, which are scattered over the entire surface of the decidua basalis. Note that the umbilical arteries carry poorly oxygenated fetal blood to the placenta and that the umbilical vein carries oxygenated blood to the fetus. (From Moore KL, Persaud TVN. The developing human. 5th ed. Philadelphia: WB Saunders, 1993.)

BODY COMPOSITION Many changes in body composition take place during pregnancy. An average weight gain of 12.5 kg associated with a typical 40-week pregnancy amounts to an approximate 20% increase in body weight. Most weight gain occurs during the last 20 weeks of gestation. About 40% of this weight gain is represented by the fetus, placenta, and amniotic fluid (Fig. 8–6), and 60% is the maternal weight change (Forbes, 1962). The 6 to 8 kg (13 to 18 lb) of maternal weight that accumulate, particularly in the last 20 weeks, include increased fluid volume, protein deposition, and fat stores. These changes are due to increased mammary, uterine, kidney, and heart tissue volume, as well as an increase in total fluid volume and body fat (Forbes, 1987). Changes in fat stores are somewhat more difficult to quantify. It has been estimated that approximately one-third of the total gestational weight gain is fat, i.e., 3 to 6 kg (6–13 lb) (Forsum et al, 1989). Based on densitometry, estimates of the increase in the percentage of body fat during gestation range from 2.6% to 8%. Women who gained more than 8.5

kg (19 lb) during pregnancy had greater fat accumulation than those who gained less weight.

BLOOD VOLUME Perhaps the most striking maternal physiologic alteration of pregnancy is the 45% to 50% increase in blood volume. Hypervolemia begins in the first trimester, increases rapidly in the second trimester, and plateaus at about the 30th week. The increase is needed to provide for extra blood flow to the uterus, extra metabolic needs of the fetus, and increased perfusion of other organs, especially the kidneys. The increase in blood volume is accompanied by a smaller increase in red cell volume and concentration of various blood proteins, lipids, and enzymes. Therefore, hemoglobin concentration falls during pregnancy until about the 30th week. This fall is the result of the relatively greater increase in plasma volume than of red cell volume, often referred to as hemodilution. Iron supplementation during pregnancy modifies but does not obliterate the usual fall in hemoglobin and hematocrit levels during pregnancy (Fig. 8–7).

TABLE 8–2 Physiologic Changes of Pregnancy

BLOOD COMPOSITION
Increase in body weight—15 to 40 pounds
Increase in maternal and fetal protein
Increase in maternal fat stores
Increase in body fluid

BLOOD VOLUME
Increase of about 50% in plasma volume
Increase of 18%–30% in red cell volume
Decrease in concentration of blood components, especially albumin, hemoglobin, hematocrit

CARDIOVASCULAR
Increase of 30% to 50% in cardiac output
Increase in stroke volume
Increase in pulse rate

RESPIRATION
Increase in tidal volume—amount of gases exchanged with each breath
Slight increase in respiratory rate; more efficient exchange of gases in alveoli

METABOLISM
Increase of about 15% in basal metabolic rate
Increase in oxygen-carrying capacity of the blood

KIDNEY
Increase in blood flow through the kidneys
Increase in glomerular filtration rate
Increase in excretion of glucose, amino acids, and water-soluble vitamins
Decrease in ability to excrete water, leading to edema of legs and ankles

GASTROINTESTINAL
Increase in appetite
Nausea and vomiting
Altered taste
Increase in absorption of nutrients
Decrease in emptying of the stomach; esophageal regurgitation and heartburn
Decrease in muscle tone, leading to increased water absorption from the colon, contributing to constipation

If the increases in blood volume are inadequate, there will be smaller increases in cardiac output, resulting in decreased blood flow to the placenta and reduced transfer of nutrients to the fetus. Such a series of events that compromise fetal growth can be due to a number of factors, including maternal undernutrition. In this case high levels of hemoglobin or hematocrit may be indicative of a reduction in volume expansion and increased fetal risk.

CARDIOVASCULAR During pregnancy, cardiac output increases approximately 40%, reaching maximum at 20 to 24 weeks and continuing at this level until term. There is little change in systolic blood pressure, but diastolic pressure declines somewhat. Peripheral resistance declines markedly, and there is increased blood flow to the uterus, placenta, and kidney.

METABOLISM As a consequence of the increased secretion of many different hormones during pregnancy, the basal metabolic rate of the mother increases about 15% during the latter half of pregnancy. Hormone changes also result in alterations in carbohydrates, protein, and fat utilization. Fat becomes the major source of fuel for maternal tissue, while the main source of fetal energy is glucose, which is transported across the placenta by facilitated diffusion. Late in the third trimester the fetus metabolizes about 7 g of protein, 35 g of glucose, and 1.7 g of fat each day (Rosso, 1983). If maternal blood glucose is low, the fetus will use more fatty acids.

RESPIRATION Because of the increase in basal metabolic rate and increased body size, the total amount of oxygen used by the mother increases, reaching approximately 20% above nonpregnant levels. The growing uterus presses upward against the diaphragm so that the total expansion of the diaphragm is decreased. Consequently, the respiratory rate is increased to maintain adequate ventilation.

KIDNEY FUNCTION The rate of filtration of blood by the kidney increases about 50% in early pregnancy, and the level remains high until term. Therefore, renal blood flow and clearance of waste products are increased, which tends to increase the loss of glucose, amino acids, and some water-soluble vitamins in the urine. Although the rate of urine formation is slightly increased, water is not excreted as well during pregnancy. This is a consequence of increased production of steroid hormones by the placenta and adrenal cortex, which enhance reabsorption of sodium, chlorine, and water by renal tubules. Hormones secreted during pregnancy have a direct effect on relaxing ureters, and the enlarging uterus displaces the urinary bladder upward, leading to increased urinary frequency.

GASTROINTESTINAL Gastrointestinal motility is reduced during gestation. Slowed gastric emptying and transit of food through the intestinal tract enhances absorption of some nutrients. Increased water absorption in the colon may lead to constipation. Esophageal peristalsis

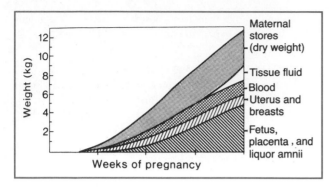

FIGURE 8–6. Components of gestational weight gain. (Reprinted with permission from *Maternal nutrition and the course of pregnancy.* Copyright 1970 by the National Academy of Sciences. Courtesy of the National Academy Press, Washington, DC.)

is decreased and gastric **reflux** is more prevalent because of slower gastric emptying time and relaxation of muscle between the esophagus and the stomach. Later in pregnancy this will be compounded by elevation of the stomach due to the enlarged uterus, possibly resulting in heartburn.

Embryonic Development

The development of the placenta and fetal membranes and amniotic sac allows the uterus to expand and support the growing embryo and fetus (Fig. 8–8). The embryonic period encompasses development from implantation of the fertilized ovum to the eighth week of gestation. Growth during this period results from an increase in cell number called hyperplasia. During this **critical period** of **organogenesis**, fetal tissue differentiates into three primitive cell layers, the endoderm, mesoderm, and ecto-

derm, which eventually become organs and tissues. The endoderm, the innermost layer of embryonic cells, develops into the gastrointestinal tract, lungs, and glandular organs. The middle layer, the mesoderm, forms into voluntary muscles, the skeleton, and the cardiovascular and renal systems. The ectoderm, the outside layer, evolves into the brain, nervous systems, hair, and skin. There is a specific timetable for development of each body organ or system (Fig. 8–9). Thus, specific tissues or organs have critical needs for specific nutrients at different periods. During such a period the organism is vulnerable to inadequate development or **congenital anomalies** if required nutrients are not available or if it is exposed to teratogenic substances such as drugs, alcohol, radiation, or excess vitamin A.

Embryosis is a period when a woman may not even be aware that she is pregnant and also a time when food intake may be reduced by the nausea common to early pregnancy. A mother who has adequate nutrient reserves at the time of conception will be at lesser risk during this period than one with poor or marginal status.

At the end of 4 weeks, the embryo weighs about 1 ounce and is less than 1 inch long. Many of the major organs have begun to develop and the heart has begun to beat. During this time nourishment is obtained from the degenerating cells of the wall of the uterus and, to some extent, from blood exchanges via the developing placenta. By week 8, placental exchange provides most nutritional needs, and all of the major organs and systems have been differentiated and organized. Cellular development of these structures will be completed in the following months.

Fetal Growth and Development

The remaining 7 months of gestation are known as the fetal growth period. The hyperplastic growth that characterized the embryonic period continues. In fact, the cells of most organs continue to divide after birth, but the rate varies. Fetal growth is also characterized by hypertrophy. At this time needs are high for both quantity and quality of

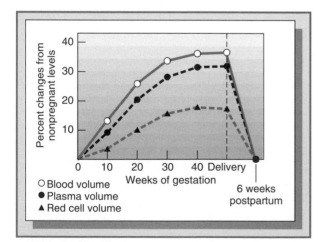

FIGURE 8–7. Changes in blood volume, plasma volume, and red cell volume during pregnancy. (From Peek TM, Arias F. Hematologic changes associated with pregnancy. Clin Obstet Gynecol 1979; 22:785.)

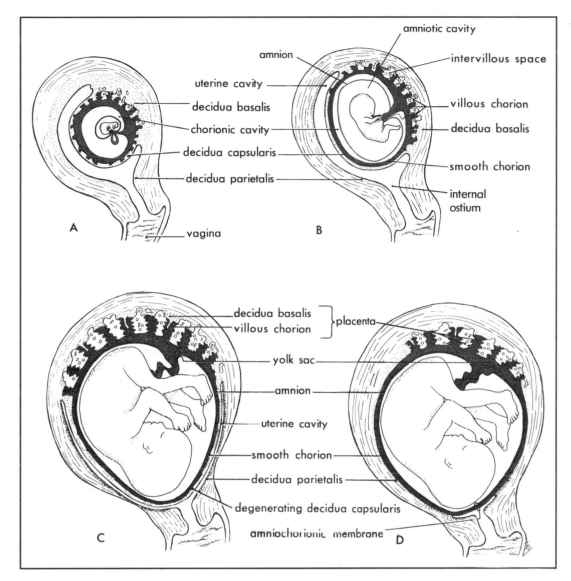

FIGURE 8–8. The fetus in amniotic sac showing the placenta and umbilical cord. Drawing illustrates development of the human placenta and fetal membranes. Sagittal sections of the gravid uterus from the fifth to the twenty-second weeks show the changing relations of the fetal membranes to the decidua. In **D**, the amnion and chorion are fused with each other and the decidua parietalis, thereby obliterating the uterine cavity. Note in **B** to **D** that chorionic villi persist only where the chorion is associated with the decidua basalis, i.e., where the placenta forms. (From Moore KL, Persaud TVN. The developing human. 5th ed. Philadelphia: WB Saunders, 1993.)

nutrients. A severe nutrient deficiency is less likely to result in a congenital defect than in the embryonic stage, but inadequate dietary intake can contribute to preterm birth or fetal growth restriction. During the third trimester the fetus gains more than two-thirds of its full-term birth weight. As much as 23 to 25 g accumulate daily in the final days of gestation. On average, the healthy term infant is about 51 cm (20 in) in length and weighs 3.4 kg (7.5 lb). Stages of development in fetal growth are shown in Fig. 8–9.

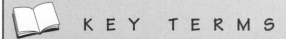

KEY TERMS

reflux: movement of some of the stomach contents back into the esophagus

critical period: a period during which specific development takes place and which, when passed, cannot be recovered

organogenesis: development of specific tissues, such as kidney, heart, lungs

congenital anomaly: birth defect

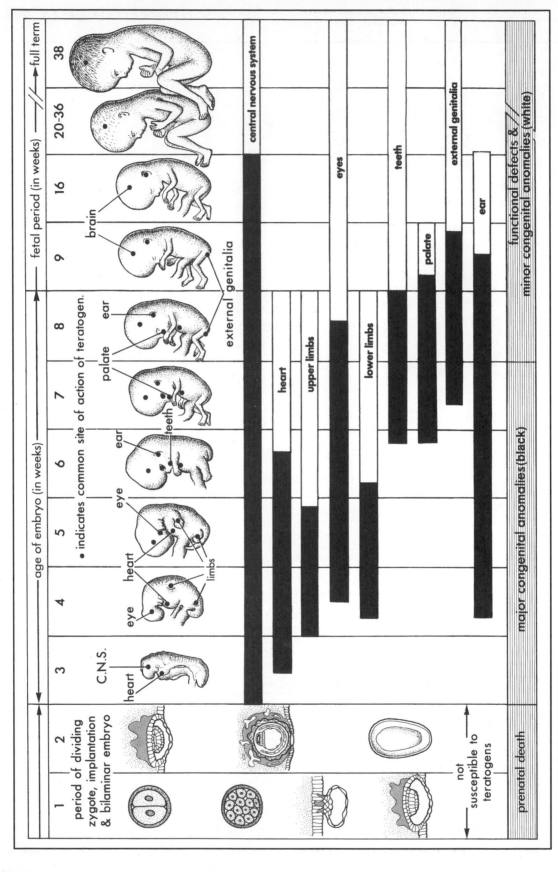

FIGURE 8–9. Schematic illustration of the critical periods in human development. During the first 2 weeks of development, the embryo is usually not susceptible to teratogens. During these pre-embryonic stages, a teratogen damages either all or most of the cells, resulting in the embryo's death, or damages only a few cells, allowing the conceptus to recover and the embryo to develop without birth defects. Black area denotes highly sensitive periods when major defects may be produced (e.g., absence of limbs). White area indicates stages that are less sensitive to teratogens when minor defects may be induced (e.g., hypoplastic thumbs). (From Moore KL, Persaud TVN. The developing human. 5th ed. Philadelphia: WB Saunders, 1993.)

ENERGY AND NUTRIENT REQUIREMENTS

■ How do energy needs increase during pregnancy?

■ For which nutrients do requirements increase during pregnancy?

■ What are appropriate pregnancy weight gains for underweight, normal weight, and overweight women?

■ Plan a menu that would be appropriate to meet the nutrient and energy needs of a normal weight pregnant woman.

■ What nutrient supplements are recommended during pregnancy?

Pregnancy is sometimes referred to as a hypermetabolic state because of the increased need for energy and nutrients to support growth of the fetus, the placenta and maternal tissue. There is substantial variation in nutrient requirements among individuals within a population (National Research Council, 1989). The RDAs for women and 19 to 24 years, women aged 25 to 50 years and pregnant appear in Table 8–3.

Energy

The increased energy cost of gestation includes a 25% increase in basal energy requirements—energy for growth of the fetus, accessory tissues, and maternal supporting tissue as well as the energy needed for the additional work of the mother required by her increased body weight. Estimates of total energy need for pregnancy range from 40,000 to 110,000 kilocalories. Energy recommendations from the NRC (1989) are based on the assumption that pregnancy costs 80,000 kcal for a mother who gains 12.5 kg (27.5 lb) and gives birth to an infant weighing 3.3 kg (7.5 lb). Daily caloric recommendations of an additional 300 kcal are determined by dividing the energy cost of gestation by the approximate duration of pregnancy (250 days) (National Research Council, 1989). For the normal weight woman, added energy intake is probably not required for the first trimester, and 300 kcal per day is an appropriate increase for the second and third trimesters.

Maternal Weight Gain

The components of gestational weight gain were shown in Figure 8–6. Less than half the weight gain is accounted for by the fetus, placenta, and amniotic fluid (Forbes, 1962). The remainder is found in maternal reproductive tissues, fluid, blood, and stores. The "maternal stores" are largely composed of body fat, although there is some increase in the lean body mass other than reproductive tissues. The pregnant woman who restricts weight gain to avoid accumulating body fat impairs, to some extent, nor-

mal fetal growth and development. Recommended weight gains are associated with infant birth weights between 3.5 and 4.0 kg, the birth weights with the lowest rates of infant mortality.

Gestational weight gain is often monitored as an indicator of the adequacy of the maternal diet. Over the last several decades, an appropriate weight gain during pregnancy has been much discussed. In 1970, the Food and Nutrition Board (National Research Council, 1970) recommended a gestational weight gain of 10 to 12 kg (22–27 lb). Since that time, it has been recognized that optimal pregnancy outcome reflects an interaction between gestational weight gain and the pregravid weight of the mother. A report from the Collaborative Perinatal Project of more

TABLE 8–3 Recommended Dietary Allowances for Reproduction

Nutrient	19–24 y	25–50 y	2nd and 3rd Trimester of Pregnancy
Energy (kcal)	2200	2200	+300
Protein (g)	46	50	60
Vitamin A (RE)*	800	800	800
Vitamin C (mg)	60	60	70
Vitamin D (μg)[†]	10	5	10
Vitamin E (mg)[††]	8	8	10
Vitamin K (μg)	60	65	65
Thiamin (mg)	1.1	1.1	1.5
Riboflavin (mg)	1.3	1.3	1.6
Niacin (mg)[§]	15	15	17
Vitamin B_6 (mg)	1.6	1.6	2.2
Vitamin B_{12} (μg)	2.0	2.0	2.2
Folate (μg)	180	180	400
Calcium	1200	800	1200
Phosphorus	150	800	1200
Magnesium	280	280	300
Iron	15	15	30
Iodine	150	150	175
Zinc	12	12	15
Selenium	55	55	65

* 1 RE (retinol equivalent) = 1 μg or 6 μg β-carotene.

[†] As cholecalciferol. 10 μg cholecalciferol = 400 IU of vitamin D.

[††] α-Tocopherol equivalents. 1 mg d-α = 1 α-TE.

[§] 1 NE (niacin equivalent) = 1 mg of niacin or 60 mg of dietary tryptophan.

Adapted with permission from Recommended dietary allowances, 10th ed. Copyright 1989 by the National Academy of Sciences. Courtesy of the National Academy Press, Washington, D.C.

than 50,000 pregnancies found that the relationship between gestational weight gain and perinatal mortality was strongly influenced by **pregravid** weight. As can be seen in Figure 8–10, mothers who were underweight prior to pregnancy had the lowest perinatal mortality when they gained at least 16 kg (30 lb), whereas for obese women the lowest perinatal mortality was seen when they gained only 7 kg (15–16 lb) (Naeye, 1979). Similar relationships between pregravid weight and antenatal weight gain have been observed for infant birthweight (Abrams and Laros, 1986; Mitchell and Lerner, 1989a). Low weight gains, especially in underweight women, are associated with increased risk of perinatal mortality and fetal growth restriction. High weight gains, particularly in obese women, are associated with increased birth weight and a greater likelihood of prolonged labor, complicated delivery, birth trauma, and **asphyxia**.

Healthy women who deliver full-term infants weighing between 3 and 4 kg (6.5–8.8 lb) have normal weight gains that range from 11 to 15 kg (25–35 lb). Current guidelines from the Institute of Medicine (1990) specify appropriate ranges for gestational weight gain based on maternal prepregnancy weight-for-height and age. Prepregnancy weight-for-height is categorized by body mass index (BMI) into underweight, normal weight, and overweight as a guide for suggested weight gain (Table 8–4). A chart incorporating these recommendations for underweight, normal weight, and overweight women is provided in Figure 8–11. It is characterized by a gradual steady increase over the second and third trimesters.

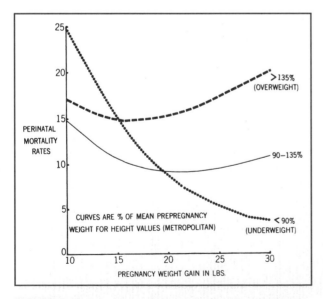

FIGURE 8–10. Perinatal mortality rates of overweight, normal weight, and underweight mothers as related to weight gain during pregnancy. (From Naeye RL. Weight gain and the outcome of pregnancy. Am J Obstet Gynecol 1979;135:3.)

Protein

The protein needs of a pregnant woman are superimposed on those of the non-pregnant woman and include increased maternal protein synthesis to support the expansion of blood volume and growth of the uterus and breasts, as well as synthesis of fetal and placental protein.

The RDA for protein has been based on calculation of total protein accumulated during gestation in the fetus, placenta, and maternal tissues, including blood. For a pregnancy with a maternal weight gain of 12.5 kg and an infant birth weight of 3.3 kg the total need is 925 g of protein or an RDA of an additional 10 g (total recommendation 60 g). Needs for synthesis of fetal proteins are small during the first trimester, but the maternal requirements for expanded blood volume and tissue growth are substantial. Over the second and third trimesters fetal demands accelerate, reaching as much as 10 g of protein per day in late pregnancy (Rosso, 1983). Many pregnant women consuming self-selected diets have protein intakes that exceed the RDA. The usual protein intake of women in the United States has been estimated to be 75 to 110 g per day (Rush, 1988).

Minerals

CALCIUM, PHOSPHORUS, AND MAGNESIUM
Calcium, phosphorus, and magnesium are accumulated by the fetus in substantial quantities, mainly during the last trimester. A total of approximately 30 g of calcium are deposited in fetal tissue. Daily accumulation increases across gestation and may reach 200 to 300 mg late in the third trimester. Calcium balance studies of pregnant women indicate that substantial increases in absorption and a positive calcium balance begin in the first trimester. This positive balance continues throughout gestation but does not increase substantially. Therefore, in late pregnancy the needs of the fetus must be met by increased calcium retained in early pregnancy or withdrawn from the skeleton of the mother.

The current RDA for calcium during pregnancy is 1200 mg per day. There is particular concern regarding calcium intake of women under 25 years of age because mineralization of their bones is probably still being completed. If calcium intakes of young women are low, dietary calcium should be increased, or, if that is not practical, a supplement of 600 mg of calcium should be given (Institute of Medicine, 1990). Individuals who cannot drink milk need to consume alternate sources of calcium or supplements.

The precise requirement for phosphorus is unknown. The current RDA sets the allowance for phosphorus at the same level as calcium, 1200 mg. Approximately 1 g of magnesium is accumulated by the fetus during gestation. In the last trimester magnesium is deposited at the rate of 6 mg per day. Assuming an absorption rate of 50%, the RDA is an additional 20 mg of magnesium per day.

IRON   Increased iron is needed throughout pregnancy for the synthesis of an expanded red cell mass, growth of placenta and fetus, and replacement of blood lost during delivery. Some iron is saved by the absence of losses through menstruation and enhanced absorption (Barrett et al, 1994), but the total iron requirement of pregnancy is estimated to be 1000 mg, or 3 mg per day over the 280 days of gestation. During pregnancy hemodilution and increased requirements cause a drop in hemoglobin levels in the first and second trimester and then a gradual increase during the third trimester. Iron supplementation is associated with a smaller decline in hemoglobin and hematocrit levels in early pregnancy and higher levels in the last trimester. The indications for and benefits of supplemented iron for mother and infant have been questioned recently.

A study of over 800 predominantly African-American women found that anemia diagnosed early in pregnancy was associated with a higher risk of preterm delivery and low birth weight (Scholl and Hediger, 1994). However, such associations could be influenced by confounding factors such as socioeconomic status, health status, and lifestyle, as well as difficulty in separating anemia from hemodilution. Other researchers have reported no statistical differences in pregnancy outcome between women who received routine iron supplementation and those who received it only for anemia (Hemminki and Merilainen, 1995).

Assuming an iron absorption of 10%, the Institute of Medicine (1990) recommends supplements of 30 mg of elemental iron during the second and third trimesters of pregnancy. It has been suggested that iron supplements are appropriate only for women with low iron status. It has been recommended that status be determined by measuring serum **ferritin** levels in addition to hemoglobin (Milman et al, 1995).

ZINC   The role of zinc in protein synthesis and cell development makes it essential for fetal growth. A recent study revealed that pregnant women with low blood zinc levels had a higher incidence of low-birthweight infants (Neggers et al, 1990). The fetal need for zinc is approximately 100 mg, with the daily accumulation increasing from about 0.1 mg per day during the first trimester to 0.7 g during the third trimester. The RDA for zinc has been set at 15 mg per day; usual intakes among American women appear to be 8.8 to 14.4 mg per day. Although the typical dietary intake may be below the RDA, zinc supplementation during pregnancy has not been recommended (Institute of Medicine, 1990).

IODINE   An increase of 25 μg per day in the allowance for iodine is recommended to cover the extra demands of the fetus.

SELENIUM   It is estimated that a total of 1.25 mg of selenium is deposited during pregnancy or that the average daily selenium accretion is 6.5 μg. Assuming an absorption rate of 80%, the average increase in dietary selenium recommended during pregnancy is 10 μg.

FLUORIDE   Fluoride accumulates in the external tooth enamel and provides protection against dental caries. Its effect appears to be greatest during the first 2 years after tooth eruption. Although fluoride in the mother's bloodstream can cross the placenta, maternal fluoride supplementation during pregnancy has not been recommended due to insufficient evidence of prenatal benefit (Institute of Medicine, 1990).

Fat-Soluble Vitamins

VITAMIN A   Vitamin A is required for growth, embryogenesis, and differentiation of epithelial tissue. The concentration of retinol in the fetal liver is low, and vitamin A supplements do not increase it appreciably. Fetal needs for vitamin A could easily be met by mobilization of less than 10% of usual maternal stores (Institute of Medicine, 1990); therefore, no increment in vitamin A intake is considered necessary for most women during pregnancy.

An excess intake of retinoids during pregnancy is a concern. Accutane or isoteretinoin (13-cis-retinoic acid), used in the treatment of severe acne, has been shown to be teratogenic in animals and humans, and its use in females who might become pregnant is contraindicated. Congenital defects include altered growth, central nervous system and cardiovascular abnormalities, and facial anomalies of the ear and palate (Lammer et al, 1995). A recent study of dietary and supplemental intake of vitamin A found that intake levels of approximately 10,000 IU (1 retinol equivalent = 50 IU) or more were associated with increased risk of birth defects (Rothman et al, 1995). Supplements above the RDA for vitamin A should be avoided. There is no evidence that high dietary intakes of carotenoids are toxic to mother or fetus, however.

VITAMIN D   No increased need for vitamin D during pregnancy has been established. However, since calcium is deposited in the growing fetus, an increase of 5 μg, or a total of 10 μg (1 μg vitamin D = 40 IU) per day has been recommended for women over 24 years of age. The RDA for vitamin D for women 24 years of age or younger is al-

K E Y   T E R M S

pregravid: before pregnancy
asphyxia: lack of oxygen in the body caused by interruption in breathing, which causes unconsciousness
ferritin: iron storage protein

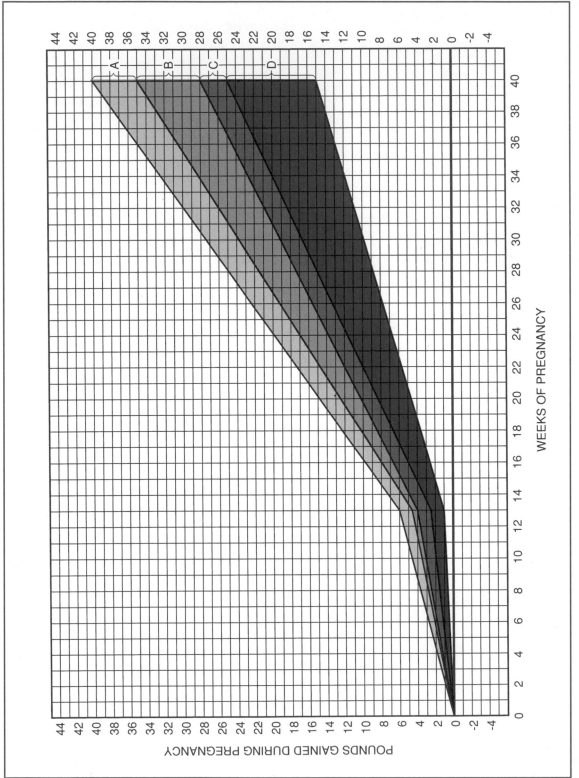

FIGURE 8–11. For a woman with a BMI between 19.8 and 26, weight gain should be in the B–C range (26–35 lb). For the underweight woman (BMI < 19.8) weight gain should be in the A–B range (28–40 lb). The overweight woman (BMI > 26) should gain in the D range (15–25 lb). (From The National Dairy Council. Great beginnings: the weighting game graph. Rosemont, IL: National Dairy Council, 1991. Courtesy of National Dairy Council. Adapted from the National Academy of Sciences. Nutrition during pregnancy. Washington, DC: National Academy Press, 1990.)

ready 10 μg. Fortified milk (400 IU of vitamin D per quart) is one of the few dietary sources of vitamin D, so women who avoid milk and have little exposure to sunlight may have low intakes. Supplements of 10 μg of vitamin D are recommended for women who follow a vegan diet, and 5 μg per day are recommended for pregnant women who consume little vitamin D–fortified milk. Supplements above the RDA should be avoided because of potential toxicity (Institute of Medicine, 1990).

VITAMIN E   Actual requirements for vitamin E during pregnancy have not been determined. Blood levels of tocopherol increase during pregnancy, and it is assumed that pregnant women require an increase of 2 mg per day in vitamin E to support fetal growth.

VITAMIN K   The transfer of vitamin K from mother to fetus appears to be minimal. The newborn has low blood levels of vitamin K and prothrombin and other vitamin K–dependent clotting factors regardless of maternal intake. Because prenatal supplementation with vitamin K does not appear to effectively increase fetal levels, no increase is recommended for pregnancy.

Water-Soluble Vitamins

VITAMIN C   It is believed that vitamin C is transported across the placenta. Fetal and infant blood levels of vitamin C are 50% higher than maternal levels. A daily increase of 10 mg of vitamin C is recommended to meet the increased demands on the mother's body pool.

THIAMIN, NIACIN, AND RIBOFLAVIN   Thiamin, niacin, and riboflavin function primarily in the release of energy from carbohydrate, lipid, and protein and are needed in increased amounts during pregnancy. The increase in the RDA for these vitamins is proportional to the 300 kcal increase recommended for pregnancy.

VITAMIN B$_6$ During pregnancy, blood levels of both vitamin B$_6$ and the active coenzyme pyridoxal phosphate are lower than those of nonpregnant women. These levels of vitamin B$_6$ may reflect either inadequate intake or normal physiologic changes of pregnancy. An increased intake of 0.6 mg is recommended. Vitamin B$_6$ is actively transported from maternal to fetal circulation, reducing the potential of a deficiency in the fetus.

FOLATE   Additional folate is required to support hematologic and growth needs of maternal and fetal tissue. Women with low intakes of folate, have a greater incidence of premature births and small-for-gestational age infants.

Assuming 50% absorption of folate from food, the RDA for folate during pregnancy is 400 μg—more than double non-pregnant levels. This level of folate can be obtained in a diet that includes fruits and vegetables and fortified or whole-grain cereals. For those at greatest risk of inadequate intake due to lack of knowledge or financial resources or due to abuse of alcohol, cigarettes, or drugs, supplementation may be appropriate. As discussed on page 196, 400 μg of folate are recommended for all women during the periconceptional period.

VITAMIN B$_{12}$ It is estimated that the fetal demands for vitamin B$_{12}$ are approximately 50 μg or 0.2 μg per day. Body stores of the adequately nourished mother are approximately 3000 μg so the drain of meeting the additional requirement for fetal needs is small. A woman who has followed a vegan diet for an extended period of time will have inadequate stores of vitamin B$_{12}$ and will require a supplement (Institute of Medicine, 1990).

ASSESSMENT OF NUTRITION STATUS

◼ How do parameters of nutrition assessment differ for pregnant women?

◼ What measurements or standards are unique to pregnancy?

Basic principles and techniques for nutrition assessment were presented in Chapter 2. This section addresses their application in pregnancy. Women who enter prenatal care early provide a unique opportunity to assess and monitor nutrition status and to provide nutrition education throughout the reproductive cycle. Nutrition education during this time may have long-term consequences for the mother, her infant, and her family. Unfortunately, many women who are at greatest nutritional risk do not enter prenatal care until late in pregnancy, if at all. Some actually appear for the first time when they are ready to deliver. Therefore, the effectiveness of nutrition assessment and intervention is contingent upon successful outreach programs to involve women in health care early in pregnancy.

Anthropometry

The only anthropometric measurements consistently available for pregnant women are height, prepregnancy weight, and a series of weight measurements during gestation. Prepregnant weight and antenatal weight gain are interrelated predictors of infant birth weight, and the pattern of gestational weight gain can have clinical value. Monitoring of weight changes during gestation is especially important for underweight and obese women, because their pregnancy outcome can be improved by achieving recommended weight gains (Table 8–4). Charts or grids for ges-

TABLE 8-4 Recommended Total Weight Gain Ranges for Pregnant Women, by Prepregnancy Body Mass Index (BMI)

Weight-for-Height Category	Recommended Total Gain*	
	kg	lb
Low (BMI† < 19.8)	12.5–18	28–40
Normal (BMI of 19.8–26.0)	11.5–16	25–35
High (BMI > 26.0–29.0)	7.0–11.5	15–25
Obese (BMI > 29.0)	≥6.0	15

*Young adolescents and African American women should strive for gains at the upper end of the recommended range. Short women (<157 cm [62 in]) should strive for gains at the lower end of the range.

†BMI is calculated in metric units.

Adapted from Institute of Medicine. Nutrition during lactation. Washington, DC: National Academy Press, 1991.

tational weight gain, as shown in Figure 8–8, can be helpful in tracking the pattern of weight gain.

It is difficult to obtain reproducible measurements of fat-fold thickness in the prenatal care setting. Even reliable measurements have limited usefulness because there are no reference standards for skinfold thickness measurements for pregnancy.

Biochemical

As blood volume expands during pregnancy, the fluid volume increases more than the cellular components. This hemodilution means that "normal" values for red blood cells, hemoglobin, and hematocrit are lower for pregnant women than for non-pregnant women (Table 8–5). It may be necessary to interpret levels of other nutrients and metabolites in this context as well.

Clinical

The initial prenatal visit provides the opportunity to identify factors that may increase the risk of an unfavorable outcome of pregnancy. Nutrition-related factors to be considered include anthropometric measures, age, signs of anemia, and chronic disease. During routine prenatal visits, urine is screened for sugar and protein. Blood pressure is measured and clinical signs of edema sought. These are useful in identifying women at risk for gestational diabetes or pregnancy-induced hypertension (see Chapter 5).

Dietary

Routine assessment of dietary practices is recommended for all pregnant women (Institute of Medicine, 1990). The typical pattern of intake can be determined effectively using a food frequency or dietary history questionnaire (see Chapter 2). Low intake of specific groups of foods, such as those rich in iron or calcium, can be identified quickly. Specific information that indicates risk of an inadequate diet includes the following:

- Low income and inadequate access to food
- Avoidance of a specific food group or groups due to intolerance, fad diets, or cultural practices
- Adherence to a diet that includes no animal tissue or products
- Consumption of substantial amounts of alcohol or use of tobacco or illicit drugs
- A lifestyle that is unlikely to support adequate acquisition, preparation, or consumption of food
- Diet restriction in an attempt to control weight
- Pica—consumption of nonfood substances such as clay or laundry starch
- Unhappiness with being pregnant

Identification of poor dietary practices should result in initiation of appropriate intervention via counseling, sup-

TABLE 8-5 Laboratory Values for Screening for Anemia in Women

Pregnancy Status	Nonsmokers		Smokers			
			0.5–1 pack/day		>1 pack/day	
	Hemoglobin (g/dL)	Hematocrit (%)	Hemoglobin (g/dL)	Hematocrit (%)	Hemoglobin (g/dL)	Hematocrit (%)
Non-pregnant	12.0	36	12.3	37	12.5	37.5
Pregnant						
First trimester	11.0	33	11.3	34	11.5	34.5
Second trimester	10.5	32	10.8	33	11.0	33.5
Third trimester	11.0	33	11.3	34	11.5	34.5

From Centers for Disease Control. CDC Criteria for anemia in children and childbearing-age women. MMWR 1989;38:400.

plementation, or referral to food assistance programs as appropriate.

A DIET PLAN FOR PREGNANCY

The requirements for energy and most nutrients increase during pregnancy. However, for the normal weight woman, the increase in energy needs is less than 15%, while the increased need for nutrients may range from none for vitamin A to 50% for iron to more than 200% for folate.

Food Guide

A diet plan based on the food pyramid that is appropriate for pregnant and lactating women appears in Figure 8–12. As in any food group plan, it is important to select the recommended number of servings from a variety of foods within each food group. Choices should emphasize foods low in fat and rich in complex carbohydrates to spare protein needed for growth. Inadequate energy intake restricts weight gain but may also compromise fetal growth and development as amino acids are mobilized to meet energy needs. Emphasis must be placed on sources of calcium, a mineral which even nonpregnant women have difficulty getting in sufficient amounts. The Healthy People 2000 (1990) goals include increasing calcium intake so that at least 50% of pregnant and lactating women consume three or more servings daily of foods rich in calcium.

Nutrient Supplements

Except for iron, the nutrient requirements of the pregnant woman can be met by a balanced, varied diet. A multivitamin and mineral supplement is *not* a substitute for a balanced diet. Supplements should be prescribed only when a deficiency is indicated or when it appears, after nutritional consultation, that dietary changes will not be made (Table 8–6). In addition, supplements may be recommended for complete vegetarians, women who are pregnant with twins, smokers, drinkers of alcoholic beverages, and drug abusers (Institute of Medicine, 1990).

DIET-RELATED CONCERNS DURING PREGNANCY

Nausea and Vomiting

The nausea and vomiting that frequently occur in the early months of pregnancy are referred to as "morning sickness," but they are not confined to the morning. Sickness usually begins about 6 weeks after the start of the last menstrual period and seems to disappear magically 6 to 8

weeks later. The cause of the nausea and vomiting of early pregnancy is unknown. Hormones that increase in early pregnancy have been implicated. Some studies have reported that women who experienced this discomfort during early pregnancy had higher blood levels of estrogen. Also, levels of human chorionic gonadotropin (hCG), produced by the corpus luteum, rise in the first trimester of pregnancy and then fall about the 14th or 15th week—just about the time the nausea and vomiting diminish for most women. Time seems to be the only cure, and treatment is **palliative**.

Approximately two-thirds of pregnant women experience some nausea during pregnancy, and about one-half of those also vomit. These unpleasant conditions may be a positive prognostic indicator for a favorable pregnancy outcome. In a study of 9098 pregnancies, researchers at the National Institutes of Health found that mothers who vomited had a 17% lower risk of a preterm delivery and a 30% lower risk of having a miscarriage or stillbirth than women who did not (Klebanoff et al, 1987).

The nausea of pregnancy is the only kind of nausea that improves with food on the stomach. Part of prevention is to keep the stomach filled but not overfilled. Other suggestions to reduce nausea include eating small frequent meals, separating consumption of fluids and solid foods, consuming easily digested carbohydrates, and avoiding highly seasoned or strong-flavored foods.

Although the nausea and vomiting of early pregnancy are usually mild and do not substantially reduce total food intake, excessive vomiting can cause an acute loss of fluid and electrolytes resulting in dehydration. If vomiting is prolonged, there is the potential for significant losses of protein and other nutrients, and medical intervention may be required.

Heartburn

The term "heartburn" is a misnomer, because it has nothing to do with the heart. Even so, the burning pain in the lower esophagus caused by the reflux of food and acid from the stomach can indeed feel like heart pain. Two factors contribute to heartburn during gestation. The hormone-mediated changes of pregnancy result in relaxation of the **lower esophageal sphincter**, while the growing

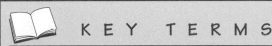

K E Y   T E R M S

palliative: reducing the severity of symptoms
lower esophageal sphincter: group of muscles located between the esophagus and stomach

Grain Products

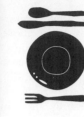

6 to 11 servings a day

- Grain products provide energy, vitamins and minerals.
- Whole grain products, like whole wheat breads, are good sources of **folic acid**.
- Limit pastries, doughnuts, and cookies because they are high in fat.

Choose these Grain Products

1 slice **whole grain bread**

3/4 cup ready-to-eat **enriched cereal**

1/2 cup oatmeal, grits, or cooked wheat

1 pancake or waffle

1/2 cup spaghetti or noodles

1/2 cup rice, enriched or brown

2 tortillas

1 pita

1 muffin or biscuit

4 soda-type crackers

2 rice cakes

Vegetables

3 to 5 servings a day

- Vegetables provide vitamins and minerals.
- Leafy green vegetables and beans are good sources of **folic acid**.
- Fresh vegetables are best, but frozen or canned vegetables are okay.
- Avoid fried vegetables like french fries.

Choose these Vegetables

1 cup brussels sprouts

1 cup **broccoli**

1/2 cup **spinach**

1/2 cup chopped green pepper

1 cup **collard greens, kale or cabbage**

1/2 cup carrots

1/2 cup squash

1/2 cup eggplant

1/2 cup **green beans**

1/2 cup **sweet peas**

1/2 baked potato

1 small sweet potato

1 medium tomato

4-6 medium spears **asparagus**

Fruits

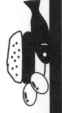

2 to 4 servings a day

- Fruits provide vitamins and minerals.
- Limit fruit drinks with added sugar. Real fruit juice has more of the vitamins you need.

Choose these Fruits

1 **orange**

1/2 cup orange or grapefruit juice

1-1/4 cups cubed watermelon

3/4 cup **strawberries**

1 small **banana**

1 apple

1 guava

1 mango

2 tablespoons dried fruit

Milk and Milk Products

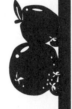

2 to 3 servings a day*

- Calcium builds bones and teeth.
- Limit non-dairy milk substitutes. Coffee creamers and condensed milk have low nutritional value.
- If you can't digest the sugar in milk, or are lactose-intolerant, there are special products in the dairy section you can buy.

Choose these Milk and Milk Products

1 cup milk: whole, lowfat, skim, powdered, or buttermilk

1 cup **yogurt**

1 cup cottage cheese

2 1" cubes cheese

1 cup pudding or custard

1-1/2 cups soup made with milk

1 cup ice milk or ice cream

*Women who are pregnant or breastfeeding, teenagers and young adults need 3 servings of milk and milk products daily.

Meat and Protein Foods

2 to 3 servings a day

- Protein builds strong muscles and blood.
- Liver is an excellent source of **folic acid**.
- Limit high fat and processed meats such as hot dogs, bologna, sausage, spare ribs, corned-beef hash, turkey wings and bacon.

Choose these Meat and Protein Foods

beef

lamb

pork

liver

chicken

turkey

fish

shellfish

2 eggs

1 cup canned baked beans

1 cup dried **peas/beans**

1 cup tofu

1/4 cup peanut butter

1/2 cup nuts

Sample Menus

Breakfast

Orange juice

Bran flakes with peaches

Muffin or biscuit

Milk

Lunch

Glass of vegetable juice

Egg salad on lettuce

Two slices of pumpernickel bread

Tomato slices

Dinner

Baked chicken

Mixed green salad

Baked sweet or white potato

Milk

Whole wheat roll

Apple

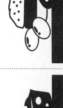

FIGURE 8-12. Good food guide. (From The March of Dimes. Eating for two: nutrition during pregnancy. White Plains, NY, 1992. Adapted from the Food Guide Pyramid.)

TABLE 8–6 Recommendations for Nutrient Supplements During Pregnancy

GENERAL POPULATION

30 mg ferrous iron daily during the second and third trimesters

This is equal to: 150 mg of ferrous sulfate
300 mg of ferrous gluconate
100 mg of ferrous furmarate

Take between meals or at bedtime on an empty stomach to facilitate iron absorption. Potential side effects: heartburn, nausea, upper abdominal discomfort, constipation, and diarrhea. The risk of side effects is proportional to the amount of elemental iron in various soluble ferrous iron compounds. Side effects are much less likely with 30 mg.

OTHER SUPPLEMENTS

Recommended only when assessment of dietary practices indicates inadequacies and when dietary intervention does not seem to be effective.

300 μg per day of folate when there are doubts about the adequacy of dietary folate, as in women who consume little fruit, juices, whole-grain or fortified cereals, or green vegetables.

Recommended for pregnant women who do not ordinarily consume an adequate diet and those in high-risk categories such as women carrying more than one fetus, heavy cigarette smokers, and alcohol and drug abusers. A multivitamin supplement should contain the following during the second and third trimester:

Iron	30 mg	Vitamin B_6	2 mg
Zinc	15 mg	Folate	300 μg
Copper	2 mg	Vitamin C	50 mg
Calcium	250 mg	Vitamin D	5 μg

Take between meals or at bedtime to promote absorption

IRON DEFICIENCY

If results of routine determination of hemoglobin and hematocrit at first prenatal visit indicate a deficiency:

60–120 mg of ferrous iron/day

When hemoglobin returns to normal: 30 mg/day

NUTRIENT SUPPLEMENTATION IN SPECIAL CIRCUMSTANCES

Vitamin D: 10 μg (400 IU) daily for complete vegetarians and others with a low intake of vitamin D–fortified milk. This is especially important for women who live at northern latitudes in winter and for others with minimal exposure to sunlight and, thus, reduced synthesis of vitamin D in the skin.

Calcium: 600 mg daily for women under age 25 whose daily dietary calcium is less than 600 mg. It should be taken at mealtime.

Vitamin B_{12}: 2.0 μg daily for complete vegetarians

Zinc and copper: When therapeutic levels of iron (>30 mg/day) are given to treat anemia, supplementation with 15 mg of zinc and 2 mg of copper is recommended because iron may interfere with the absorption and utilization of those trace minerals.

Adapted from Subcommittee on Dietary Intake and Nutrient Supplements During Pregnancy. Committee on Nutritional Status During Pregnancy and Lactation, Food and Nutrition Board, Institute of Medicine, National Academy of Sciences. Nutrition during pregnancy. Washington, DC: National Academy Press, 1990.

fetus puts increasing pressure on the stomach. Heartburn can be averted by eating small frequent meals, avoiding highly seasoned foods, and not lying down soon after meals. Occasionally discomfort can be relieved by antacids, if prescribed by the physician.

Constipation

Constipation is a common complaint of pregnancy, especially during the last trimester. This problem results from reduced intestinal motility, which slows passage of unabsorbed food residue through the large bowel, resulting in increased absorption of water. The feces become dry, hard, and difficult to expel. In addition, the enlarging uterus exerts pressure on the bowel. Decreased physical activity and a diet low in fiber also contribute to the problem. Measures to reduce constipation include adequate fluid intake and increased dietary fiber. For some women, the problem is persistent, and the physician may recommend bulking agents or stool softeners to facilitate laxation.

Cravings and Aversions of Pregnancy

A variety of dietary and lifestyle changes occur during pregnancy. Although many women make positive changes that will improve the nutritional quality of their diets, many dietary changes are based on alterations in taste or appetite, cultural patterns, or the mother's perceived value of specific dietary components.

Many women experience changes in food preferences during pregnancy. A mother's conscious choice not to consume certain foods or beverages during pregnancy is referred to as food *avoidance*. Food *aversions* are to foods or beverages that are normally consumed but that are not tolerated during pregnancy. Approximately one-half of pregnant women report an aversion to one or more foods or beverages, most frequently coffee, alcoholic beverages, highly seasoned foods, and fried foods.

Food cravings, which occur more frequently than food aversions, are not limited to any particular foods or food groups. They may range from the proverbial pickles to ice cream—although not necessarily together. The foods most frequently craved are sweets, chocolate, ice cream, cake, and candy. Other common cravings include spicy foods such as pizza or Mexican food and fruits and vegetables. There are few explanations for why cravings occur during pregnancy, but they are not due to nutrient deficiencies. Suggested causes are changes in senses of taste and smell, metabolic changes, and responses to increased physical needs. Food cravings and aversions may disappear in late pregnancy and are seldom experienced after delivery. They often reappear in a later pregnancy or may be replaced by a craving for or aversion to different foods or beverages.

POSTPARTUM

Basic nutrition concerns during the postpartum period are related to support for breast-feeding, replenishing of nutrient stores, and return to pregravid weight status. Nutrition services for pregnant women should be extended into this period. Breast-feeding is discussed in Chapter 10.

Replenishing Nutrient Stores

Nutrient stores, especially calcium, vitamin B_6, and folate, may be diminished during the gestational period. Continuation of prenatal multivitamin supplements for several weeks can assist in establishing nutrient reserves. Women who had multiple infants, are of low body weight, had poor gestational weight gain, smoke cigarettes, or use or abuse substances that may compromise nutrition status may benefit from continued nutrition counseling and use of supplements. Mothers whose diets are inadequate despite nutrition counseling should be encouraged to continue to take the multivitamin–mineral supplement that was prescribed during pregnancy.

Requirements for dietary iron decrease to nonpregnant levels after delivery unless there was excessive blood loss during delivery. As blood volume returns to pregravid levels, hemoglobin and hematocrit values rise. In part, iron salvaged from the breakdown of red blood cells can be recycled for synthesis of hemoglobin.

Postpartum Body Weight

Current gestational weight gain recommendations (7 to 18 kg) are associated with infants with birth weights between 3 and 4 kg and the lowest incidence of infant mortality. Average gestational weight gain is approximately 12.5 kg, and for most women all but 1 or 2 kg of this weight is lost by 6 to 12 months postpartum (Institute of Medicine, 1990). However, approximately 12% of the more than 50,000 women studied in the National Collaborative Perinatal Project were 6.8 kg or more above their prepregnancy weights 2 years after delivery (Greene et al, 1988). Some women have increased body weight following pregnancy, and one study of WIC participants found an association between antenatal weight gain, particularly during the first pregnancy, and retained weight in the postpartum period (Parker and Abrams, 1993). This was especially true for African-American women.

Approximately one-third (3.5 kg) of the average gestational weight gain is fat (Sadurskis et al, 1988). This increase in maternal body fat is not associated with increased birth weight, however, and may present a risk of retained excess body fat for the mother (Villar et al, 1992). Studies that have followed lactating postpartum women for up to 6 months have found that only 1 to 2 kg of body fat are mobilized during the period of breast-feeding (Forsum et al, 1989). It has been observed that 12 months after delivery as much as 2 kg of body fat deposited during pregnancy remained (Sohlstrom et al, 1995). Retention of gestational gains in weight and fat have the potential to contribute to long-term obesity in some women.

Interventions for weight reduction in the postpartum period may be important in prevention of long-term obesity

RESEARCH UPDATE
Pica During Pregnancy

Pica is the ingestion of non-food substances such as clay (geophagia) or laundry starch (amylophagia) (Institute of Medicine, 1990). A familiar example is the consumption of dirt or paint chips by young children. Pica is not limited to any one geographic area, race, gender, culture, or social status, but it does appear to have a predilection for underdeveloped areas and populations of low socioeconomic status.

The etiology of pica is poorly understood. Theories range from a learned pattern of behavior for relieving the nausea and vomiting of pregnancy to the body's instinctive search for a source of nutrients it is lacking. Pica is probably shaded by both cultural and physiologic bases, as it is associated with poor nutrition status, particularly deficiencies of iron and zinc, as well as culturally ingrained food preferences.

Although pica occurs often in iron deficiency, the substances the victims crave are rarely rich in iron. For example, people who eat tremendous quantities of ice (pagophagia) are often deficient in iron, but ice adds only water to their diets. In some cases, pica itself contributes to the deficiency. Some clays contain substances that bind with iron and decrease its absorption. A cause and effect relationship has not been established. In addition, not everyone with iron or zinc deficiency has pica, nor does everyone with pica have iron or zinc deficiency.

The most commonly reported pica in pregnant women in the United States involves the eating of dirt, clay, starch, or ice. Clay eating is especially common among Southern African-American women and may be a holdover from African culture. However, poverty and poor nutrition clearly aggravate the problem. The custom has followed the migration of the African-American population from the South, so that clays from a favorite "clay hole" may be mailed to relatives who have moved away. Clay consumption varies from a few lumps a day to a quart or more. Because the preferred clay is not often available in big cities, the craving is often transferred to laundry starch (cornstarch). Starch eating, like clay eating, interferes with iron absorption but can also add a great many calories to the diet. Consumption of a pound of starch each day, which contains about 1600 kilocalories, is not unusual.

There is no question that pica has the potential of having adverse effects on the mother and fetus. Pica may be associated with:

- Displacement of essential nutrients or kilocalories from food
- Reduced absorption of required nutrients
- Ingestion of toxins or parasites
- Intestinal obstruction or bowel perforation
- Weight gain due to excess calories from starch

The best defense against the negative effects of pica is to encourage a balanced, nutritious diet and to make pregnant women aware of the dangers of consuming large quantities of non-food substances.

in women. Few studies have investigated the role of dietary management or exercise in new mothers. There is evidence that nutrition counseling to reduce caloric intake can be effective in accomplishing weight loss without interfering with milk production (Dusdieker et al, 1994). Aerobic or weight training exercise has the potential to decrease body fat and protect lean body mass. It has been shown that aerobic exercise five times a week does not interfere with lactation (Dewey et al, 1994). It appears that a moderate physical activity program with moderation of dietary intake has the potential to assist postpartum women in losing body weight and fat.

Boardly and co-workers (1995), in studying WIC participants 7 to 12 months postpartum, found that energy intakes and activity levels were significant predictors of weight loss. Nutrition counseling in the postpartum period has been shown to facilitate weight loss (Caan et al, 1987). During pregnancy many women have marked changes in health norms and behaviors, including eating behaviors. Continuation of nutrition, exercise, and health programs after birth has the potential to improve the nutrition status of the mother and her infant. Additional efforts are needed, particularly culturally specific intervention strategies, in the postpartum period, to have an effect on the prevalence of overweight in at risk mothers.

CONCEPTS TO REMEMBER

▶ Periconceptional nutrition care is important in providing the mother with the best possible foundation for a favorable pregnancy outcome and successful lactation.

▶ Pregnancy outcome is influenced by the mother's growth patterns and nutrition status at conception as well as dietary intake during pregnancy.

▶ During the first 2 weeks after fertilization a blastocyst develops and is implanted in the uterine wall and the placenta begins to develop.

▶ The embryonic period from 2 to 8 weeks is critical for cell differentiation and organogenesis.

▶ The placenta synthesizes many important substances as well as providing an area for exchange of nutrients from mother to fetus and waste product from fetus to mother.

▶ Reproductive success is influenced by many factors.

▶ The rapid growth and development of the embryo and fetus create substantial physiologic and metabolic demands on the mother.

▶ Nutrition deserves special consideration during the reproductive interval to make sure that it is not a limiting factor in maternal or infant health.

▶ Early prenatal care and a varied, balanced diet and appropriate weight gain during pregnancy are important determinants of a favorable outcome.

▶ The physiologic changes of pregnancy involve almost every body system and support growth of maternal tissues as well as fetal growth and development.

▶ Prepregnancy weight and gestational weight gain, indirect indicators of nutrition status, are strong predictors of birth weight and, therefore, of infant mortality and morbidity.

▶ Current recommendations for weight gain during pregnancy, based on maternal pregravid weight, range from 6 kg for overweight women to 18 kg for underweight women.

▶ Caloric needs are estimated to be an additional 300 kcal per day over prepregnancy intake for the second and third trimesters.

▶ For pregnancy, the RDA increases for protein and most vitamins and minerals.

▶ Except for iron, nutritional needs can be met from dietary sources. An iron supplement of 30 mg ferrous iron is recommended for all pregnant women.

▶ Other supplements are indicated only when careful assessment of dietary intake indicates a major lack of one or more key nutrients.

References

Abrams BF, Laros RK. Pregnancy weight, weight gain, and birthweight. Am J Obstet Gynecol 1986;154:503.

American Psychiatric Association. Diagnostic and Statistical Manual of Mental Disorders. 4th ed. Washington, DC: American Psychiatric Association, 1994.

Barnhart KT, et al. A clinician's guide to the premenstrual syndrome. Office Gynecol 1995;6:1457.

Barrett JF, et al. Absorption of non-haem iron from food during normal pregnancy. BMJ 1994;309:79.

Boardley DJ, et al. The relationship between diet, activity, and other factors and post partum weight change by race. Obstet Gynecol 1995;86:834.

Caan B, et al. Benefits associated with WIC supplemental feeding during the interpregnancy interval. Am J Clin Nutr 1987;45:29.

Centers for Disease Control. Use of folic acid for prevention of spina bifida and other neural tube defects—1983–1991. MMWR 1991a;40:513.

Centers for Disease Control. Recommendations for the use of folic acid to reduce the number of cases of spina bifida and other neural tube defects. MMWR 1991b;41:1.

Crane NT, et al. Evaluating food fortification options: general principles revisited with folic acid. Am J Public Health 1995;85:600.

Dewey KG, et al. A randomized study of the effect of aerobic exercise by lactating women on breast-milk volume and composition. N Engl J Med 1994;330:449.

Dusdieker LB, et al. Is milk production impaired by dieting during lactation? Am J Clin Nutr 1994;59:833.

Forbes GB. Human body composition: growth, aging, nutrition and activity. New York: Springer-Verlag, 1987.

Forbes GB. Methods for determining body composition of the human body. Pediatrics 1962;29:477.

Forsum E, et al. Estimation of body fat in healthy Swedish women during pregnancy and lactation. Am J Clin Nutr 1989;50:465.

Greene GW, et al. Postpartum weight change: how much of the weight gained in pregnancy will be lost after delivery? Obstet Gynecol 1988;71:701.

Healthy People 2000: National Health Promotion and Disease Prevention Objectives. Conference Edition. Washington, DC: U.S. Dept of Health and Human Services, 1990.

Hemminki E, Merilainen J. Long-term follow-up of mothers and their infants in a randomized trial on iron prophylaxis during pregnancy. Am J Obstet Gynecol 1995;173:205.

Institute of Medicine. Nutrition during pregnancy: weight gain and nutrient supplements. Report of the Subcommittee on Nutritional Status and Weight Gain During Pregnancy, Subcommittee on Dietary Intake and Nutrient Supplements During Pregnancy, Committee on Nutritional

Status During Pregnancy and Lactation. Food and Nutrition Board. Washington, DC: National Academy Press, 1990.

Institute of Medicine. Preventing low birth weight. Washington, DC: National Academy Press, 1985.

Klebanoff MA, Yip R. Influence of maternal birth weight on rate of fetal growth and duration of gestation. J Pediatr 1987;111:287.

Kuller JA, Laifer SA. Preconceptional counseling and intervention. Arch Intern Med 1994;154:2273.

Lammer EJ, et al. Retinoic acid embryopathy. N Engl J Med 1995;313:837.

Li D, et al. Periconceptional multivitamin use in relation to the risk of congenital urinary tract anomalies. Epidemiology 1995;6:212.

Little J, Elwood JM. Epidemiology of neural tube defects. In: Kiley M (ed). Reproductive and perinatal epidemiology. Boca Raton, FL: CRC Press, 1991:251.

Lynberg MC, Khoury MJ. Contributions of birth defects to infant mortality among racial/ethnic minority groups, United States 1983. MMWR 1990:39:1.

Milman N, et al. Iron status markers and serum erythropoietin in 120 mothers and newborn infants. Acta Obstet Gynecol Scand 1995;73:200.

Mitchell MC, Lerner E. Weight gain and pregnancy outcome in underweight and normal weight women. J Am Diet Assoc 1989a;89:634.

Mitchell MC, Lerner E. A comparison of pregnancy outcome in overweight and normal weight women. J Am Coll Nutr 1989b;8:617.

MRC Vitamin Study Research Group. Prevention of neural tube defects: results of the Medical Research Council Vitamin Study. Lancet 1991;338:131.

Naeye RL. Weight gain and the outcome of pregnancy. Am J Obstet Gynecol 1979;135:3.

National Research Council. Recommended dietary allowances. 10th ed. Report of the Subcommittee, Food and Nutrition Board, Commission on Life Sciences. Washington, DC: National Academy Press, 1989.

National Research Council, Food and Nutrition Board. Maternal nutrition and the course of pregnancy. Washington, DC: National Academy of Sciences, 1970.

Neggers YH, et al. A positive association between maternal serum zinc concentration and birth weight. Am J Clin Nutr 1990;51:678.

Parker JD, Abrams B. Difference in postpartum weight retention between black and white mothers. Obstet Gynecol 1993;81:768.

Parsons MT, et al. Pregnancy outcomes in short women. J Reprod Med 1991;34:357.

Prasad AS. Zinc and growth development and the spectrum of human zinc deficiency. J Am Coll Nutr 1988;7:377.

Romano PS, et al. Folic acid fortification of grain: an economic analysis. Am J Public Health 1995;85:667.

Rosso P. Nutritional needs of the human fetus. Clin Nutr 1983;2:4.

Rothman KJ, et al. Teratogenicity of high vitamin A intake. N Engl J Med 1995;333:1369.

Rush D. Nutritional services during pregnancy and birthweight: a retrospective matched pair analysis. Can Med Assoc J 1981;125:567.

Rush D, et al. The National WIC Evaluation: Evaluation of the Special Supplemental Food Program for Women, Infants, and Children. V. Longitudinal study of pregnant women. Am J Clin Nutr 1988;48:439.

Sadurskis A, et al. Energy metabolism, body composition, and milk production in healthy Swedish women during lactation. Am J Clin Nutr 1988;48:44.

Sayegh R, et al. The effect of a carbohydrate-rich beverage on mood, appetite, and cognitive function in women with premenstrual syndrome. Obstet Gynecol 1995;86:520.

Scholl TO, Hediger ML. Anemia and iron-deficiency anemia: Compilation of data on pregnancy outcome. Am J Clin Nutr 1994;59:502S.

Shaw G, et al. Risks of orofacial clefts in children born to women using multivitamins containing folic acid periconceptionally. Lancet 1995;346:393.

Sohlstrom A, Forsum E. Changes in adipose tissue volume and distribution during reproduction in Swedish women as assessed by magnetic resonance imaging. Am J Clin Nutr 1995;61:287.

Steegers-Theunissen R, et al. Neural tube defects and elevated homocysteine levels in amniotic fluid. Am J Obstet Gynecol 1995;172:1436.

Stein Z, et al. Famine and human development: The Dutch hunger winter of 1944/1945. New York: Oxford University Press, 1975.

Steiner M, et al. Fluoxetine in the treatment of premenstrual dysphoria. N Engl J Med 1995;332:1529.

Susser M. Maternal weight gain, infant birth weight and diet: causal sequences. Am J Clin Nutr 1991;53:1384.

U.S. Public Health Service Expert Panel on the Content of Prenatal Care. Caring for Our Future. The Content of Prenatal Care. Washington, DC: U.S. Department of Health and Human Services, 1989.

van der Put NMJ, et al. Mutated methylenetetrahydrofolate reductase as a risk factor for spina bifida. Lancet 1995;346:1070.

Villar J, et al. Effect of fat and fat-free mass deposition during pregnancy on body weight. Am J Obstet Gynecol 1992;167:1344.

Viteri FE, et al. Maternal malnutrition and the fetus. Semi Perinatol 1989;13:236.

Wilcox AJ, Skjerven R. Birth weight and perinatal mortality: the effect of gestational age. Am J Public Health 1992;82:378.

Willett WC. Folic acid and neural tube defect: can't we come to closure? Am J Public Health 1992;82:666.

Winkvist A, et al. A new definition of maternal depletion syndrome. Am J Public Health 1992;82:691.

APPLICATION: Nutrition Care for Pregnant Women

The introduction to Chapter 8 illustrates nutrition care for a healthy woman during an uncomplicated pregnancy. Nutrition services (assessment, counseling, education and referral to programs and resources) are an essential component of health care across the reproductive interval (Institute of Medicine, 1992a). Basic client-centered, individualized nutrition care should be an integral part of the primary care provided to every woman (Institute of Medicine, 1992b). This is the responsibility of primary care providers such as physicians, midwives, and nurse practitioners, who may provide the nutrition care or delegate another member of the healthcare team. The dietitian provides nutrition counseling and education to clients and serves as a resource person for training and consultation for those who provide basic nutrition services or work directly with women.

The benefits of nutrition intervention are beginning to be documented. For example, in the National Maternal and Infant Health Survey, it was found that mothers who reported receiving nutrition advice, including information about weight gain, supplement use, avoidance of alcohol, and breast-feeding, had a significantly lower incidence of low-birthweight infants than did other mothers (Kogan et al, 1994). The cost of providing effective nutrition services to women can be offset by savings in infant and maternal medical care costs produced by these and other interventions (Buescher et al, 1993).

Characteristics of Care

Health care is structured for easy access.
Community providers are familiar with the cultural backgrounds and social circumstances of the clients.
Providers are aware of influences of their own culture on attitudes toward women and delivery of service.
Health care is centered on the woman's needs, preferences, culture, and resources.
Providers convey respect and concern for the woman.
The woman and the provider or team set goals jointly.

The characteristics of health care for women are outlined in the margin. Quality nutrition care, by definition, centers on the needs and concerns of the individual woman. Information from and about the woman is an essential basis for making decisions concerning nutritional care. Successful client-centered prenatal care depends on supportive networks of people within the health care system and in the community. Family members and friends are a significant source of support and may have a strong impact on the dietary habits and, therefore, nutritional well-being of the woman.

Continuity in nutritional care enhances its quality (Institute of Medicine, 1992). The progression of care should build on previous learning as the woman moves from the preconceptional period through pregnancy, the postpartum period, and breast-feeding. Consistency in the guidance provided by different members of the health care team is essential to minimize duplication of activities and avoid confusing the client.

Elements of Basic Nutrition Care

Basic nutrition care encompasses:
Early identification of nutritional risk factors
Provision of health maintenance activities such as education about pregnancy weight gain or breast-feeding
Implementation of common interventions

Basic nutrition care encompasses those services (outlined in the margin) that should be available to all women before, during, and after pregnancy.

Preconceptional Care

Conditions for early intervention:
Chronic disease
    Diabetes mellitus
    Hypertension
    HIV
    Tuberculosis
Dietary patterns
    Strict vegan diet
    Inadequate intake
Behaviors/habits
    Alcohol use
    Cigarette smoking
    Illicit drug use

For some conditions and nutrition-related behaviors the risk of an adverse pregnancy outcome can be reduced with early intervention. The overall objective of nutrition care during the preconceptional period is to assist women in achieving appropriate body weight for height and in following healthful dietary patterns that will optimize chances for a favorable pregnancy outcome. Such assessment before conception allows the woman to implement constructive actions to improve her health. This in turn, may decrease the likelihood or severity of adverse pregnancy outcomes. For situations that may require long-term changes or treatment, such as substance abuse or severe eating disorders, it is desirable to delay conception until nutrition status improves.

Prenatal Nutrition

The value of nutrition intervention in ensuring adequate dietary intakes and appropriate weight gains is well documented (Rush et al, 1988; Caan et al, 1987). The process begins with basic nutrition assessment, which encompasses measurement of stature and weight, determination of hemoglobin values, and assessment of dietary practices. Abnormal findings may indicate the need for nutrition education or counseling. In some instances, in-depth assessment and specialized nutrition care may be necessary.

Assessing Weight for Height

Extremes of maternal body weight increase the risk of an adverse pregnancy outcome. Recommendations for gestational weight gain are based on weight for height as determined by pregravid BMI. As described in Chapter 2, BMI can be calculated using the formula in the margin.

$BMI = weight\ (kg)/height^2\ (m)$

For example, Melissa was 165 cm (65 in) tall and weighed 52 kg (115 lb) before conception and had a prepregnancy BMI of 19. That value would be recorded on the prenatal weight gain chart (Fig. A8–1) at zero week of pregnancy. Because Melissa is somewhat underweight, her recommended weight gain (see Table 8–4) would be 28 to 40 lb. Throughout pregnancy Melissa's weight is plotted on the weight gain chart. Her pattern of weight gain should approximate that shown for underweight women along the dashed line at the top of the chart.

Laboratory Tests

Requirements for iron increase during pregnancy to support fetal and placental growth and expanded maternal blood volume. Daily supplementation with 30 mg of ferrous iron is recommended for all pregnant women by the 12th week of gestation. Analysis of hemoglobin or hematocrit is used routinely for screening for anemia (see Table 8–5). If those levels are low, a measurement of serum ferritin to confirm the diagnosis of anemia is appropriate. If anemia is present, supplements containing 60 to 120 mg of ferrous iron and copper and zinc are recommended until hematologic values return to acceptable levels.

Assessment of Dietary Patterns

Table A8–1 illustrates a nutrition questionnaire that can be completed by the woman before she meets with the health care provider. It addresses factors that affect the nutrition status of the mother, e.g., resources available to obtain an adequate diet and typical food intake and eating behaviors. Information gained from the questionnaire and a follow-up interview form the basis for dietary assessment.

If assessment of the woman's dietary pattern reveals major nutrient deficiencies, nutrition education or individualized counseling should be initiated (see Chapter 3). Nutrition counseling should build on the woman's strengths and reinforce the positive aspects of her diet while promoting small behavioral changes with positive reinforcement. Except for iron, nutritional needs can be met by selection of a variety of foods to meet the recommended servings consistent with the Good Food Guide (see Fig. 8–12). Women who have inadequate resources or skills to ensure an adequate diet should be referred to food assistance programs that provide improved access to food or assistance in learning basic food preparation practices. If, after counseling, the mother with inadequate nutrient intake is resistant to dietary changes, a multivitamin and mineral supplement may be prescribed (see Table 8–6). Women should be cautioned against taking self-prescribed supplements because that can create nutrient imbalances or excesses.

Follow-Up Visits

Follow-up prenatal visits are used to evaluate changes in behavior in response to nutrition counseling from previous visits, to address problems perceived by the client, and to reinforce principles of sound nutritional practices and establish new activities or goals. At each visit the woman is weighed and the weight recorded on the Prenatal Weight Gain Chart to assess her progress throughout pregnancy. If weight gain deviates substantially from that recommended, dietary assessment and counseling may need to be initiated or reinforced.

The Weighting Game Weight Graph

Your Beginning Weight _____ *lbs.*

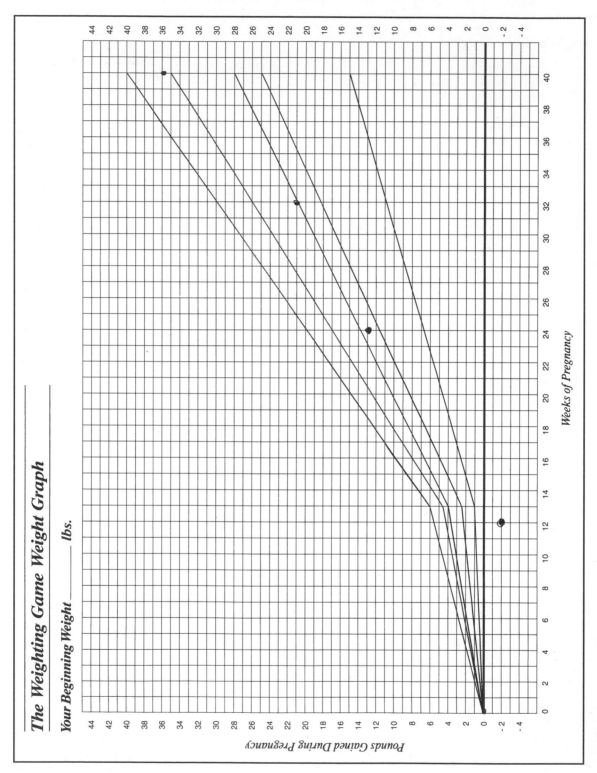

FIGURE A8–1. Prenatal weight gain chart showing Melissa's weight gains.

TABLE A8-1 Nutrition Questionnaire

What you eat and some of the lifestyle choices you make can affect your nutrition and health now and in the future. Your nutrition can also have an important effect on your baby's health. Please answer these questions by circling the answers that apply to you.

EATING BEHAVIOR

1. Are you frequently bothered by any of the following? (Circle all that apply)

    Nausea   Vomiting   Heartburn   Constipation

2. Do you skip meals at least 3 times a week?   No   Yes
3. Do you try to limit the amount or kind of food you eat to control your weight?   No   Yes
4. Are you on a special diet now?   No   Yes
5. Do you avoid any foods now for health or religious reasons?   No   Yes

FOOD RESOURCES

6. Do you have a working stove?   No   Yes

    Do you have a working refrigerator?   No   Yes

7. Do you sometimes run out of food before you are able to buy more?   No   Yes
8. Can you afford to eat the way you should?   No   Yes
9. Are you receiving any food assistance now?   No   Yes

    (Circle all that apply):

    Food stamps   School breakfast   School lunch

    WIC   Donated food/commodities   CSFP

10. Do you feel you need help in obtaining food?   No   Yes

FOOD AND DRINK

11. Which of these did you drink yesterday?

    (Circle all that apply):

Soft drinks	Coffee	Tea	Fruit drink
Orange Juice	Grapefruit juice	Other juices	Milk
Kool-Aid	Beer	Wine	Alcoholic drinks
Water	Other beverages (list) _____		

12. Which of these foods did you eat yesterday?

    (Circle all that apply):

Cheese	Pizza	Macaroni and cheese
Yogurt	Cereal with milk	

    Other foods made with cheese (such as tacos, enchiladas, lasagna, cheeseburgers)

Corn	Potatoes	Sweet potatoes	Green salad
Carrots	Collard greens	Spinach	Turnip greens
Broccoli	Green beans	Green peas	Other vegetables
Apples	Bananas	Berries	Grapefruit
Melon	Oranges	Peaches	Other fruit
Meat	Fish	Chicken	Eggs
Peanut butter	Nuts	Seeds	Dried beans
Cold cuts	Hot dog	Bacon	
Cake	Cookies	Doughnut	Sausage
Chips	French fries		Pastry

    Other deep-fried foods, such as fried chicken or egg rolls

Bread	Rolls	Rice	
Noodles	Spaghetti	Tortillas	Cereal

    Were any of these whole grain?   No   Yes

13. Is the way you ate yesterday the way you usually eat?   No   Yes

LIFESTYLE

14. Do you exercise for at least 30 minutes on a regular basis (3 times a week or more)?   No   Yes
15. Do you ever smoke cigarettes or use smokeless tobacco?   No   Yes
16. Do you ever drink beer, wine, liquor, or any other alcoholic beverages?   No   Yes
17. Which of these do you take?

    (Circle all that apply):

    Prescribed drugs or medications

    Over-the-counter products (such as aspirin, Tylenol, antacids, or vitamins)

    Street drugs (such as marijuana, speed, downers, crack, or heroin)

Reprinted with permission from Nutrition during pregnancy and lactation: an implementation guide. Copyright 1992 by the National Academy of Sciences. Courtesy of the National Academy Press, Washington, DC.

Postpartum Nutrition

The traditional emphasis of counseling in the postpartum period has been on breast-feeding. In addition, basic nutrition services for the postpartum woman should focus on replenishing nutrient stores and returning to prepregnant weight by promoting sound nutrition practices. Postpartum nutrition counseling and education can be a positive influence on the long-term food habits and health of the mother and her family. Establishment of healthy dietary practices is important in preparation for a later pregnancy.

Specialized Care

Special nutrition services may be necessary for some high-risk pregnancies. For a woman with a metabolic disorder such as diabetes mellitus or phenylketonuria, nutrition care may require detailed assessment, counseling for complex dietary modification, careful monitoring, and extended follow-up. Specialized nutrition care may also be necessary for women with health conditions that compromise dietary intake or nutrient utilization and those with poor intake. Lifestyle habits that include cigarette smoking and substance abuse increase nutrition risk, and women with such habits may require specialized nutrition care.

REFERENCES

Buescher PA, et al. Prenatal WIC participation can reduce low birth weight and newborn medical costs: a cost-benefit analysis of WIC participation in North Carolina. J Am Diet Assoc 1993;93:163.

Caan B, et al. Benefits associated with WIC supplemental feeding during the interpregnancy interval. Am J Clin Nutr 1987;45:29.

Institute of Medicine. Nutrition services in prenatal care. 2nd ed. Washington, DC: National Academy Press, 1992a.

Institute of Medicine. Nutrition during pregnancy and lactation: an implementation guide. Washington, DC: National Academy Press, 1992b.

Kogan MD, et al. Relation of the content of prenatal care to the risk of low birth weight. JAMA 1994;271: 1340.

Rush D, et al. Longitudinal study of pregnant women. Am J Clin Nutr 1988;48:439.

CHAPTER 9

HIGH-RISK PREGNANCY

Maternal Characteristics
Socioeconomic Status
Maternal Body Weight
Multiple Births

Health Conditions of the Mother
Substance Use and Abuse During Pregnancy
Concepts to Remember

Sue was looking forward to celebrating her "sweet 16" birthday. Not long ago she had such a good time at her best friend's sixteenth birthday party, where she met her boyfriend, Joe. But today she woke up feeling sick. She vomited all morning and had an upset stomach throughout the day. The party was no fun, her friends asked her what was wrong, and Joe remarked that she was "no fun to be with." After many more days of the same "puking feeling" she found out that she was pregnant. When the doctor told her, she couldn't believe it; after all, she had only "been" with Joe that one time! (Lifshitz et al, 1991).

In 1992, almost 40,000 babies born in the United States did not survive until their first birthday—approximately 10 deaths for every 1000 live births (MMWR, 1993). When babies die, it is most often because they are born prematurely and at a low birth weight. Preterm babies who are too small are 40 times more likely than full-term babies to die in the first month of life. Those who do survive are at increased risk of mental retardation, growth and developmental problems, visual and hearing defects, **cerebral palsy**, **epilepsy**, learning difficulties, chronic lung problems, and abuse and neglect.

The progression and outcome of pregnancy are described in Chapter 8. Pregnancy is usually a serene time in a woman's life. However, in some instances, maternal health status, psychosocial or economic factors, and lifestyle behaviors can complicate pregnancy. Each of the factors listed in Table 9–1 can constitute a risk for an adverse pregnancy outcome compromising embryonic development, fetal growth, and maternal health. When two or more factors occur together, the likelihood of a preterm birth, a low-birthweight infant, and other unfavorable outcomes increases. In the United States 10% to 20% of the

estimated 3.5 million pregnancies each year fall into the high-risk category.

Nutrition intervention through carefully planned nutrition care and monitoring can reduce the impact of these factors on pregnancy outcome. The high-risk pregnancies discussed in this chapter are those for which nutrition management is appropriate.

KEY TERMS

cerebral palsy: partial paralysis and lack of muscle coordination resulting from a malfunction of or damage to the brain
epilepsy: disorder of the nervous system resulting from a temporary disturbance of the nerve impulses that may be manifested in convulsive seizures

TABLE 9–1 Factors That Contribute to High-Risk Pregnancy

MATERNAL FACTORS
Age—adolescent, older gravida

Low socioeconomic status

Non-Caucasian race

Marital status

History of poor obstetric outcome

Short interpregnancy interval

High parity

BODY WEIGHT
Underweight

Obesity

PRENATAL—COMPLICATED PREGNANCY
Hyperemesis gravidarum

Gestational weight gain

Multiple fetuses

Anemia

MATERNAL HEALTH PROBLEMS
Maternal hyperphenylalaninemia

Hypertensive disorders of pregnancy

Diabetes mellitus

Anorexia nervosa, bulimia nervosa

Human immunodeficiency virus

MATERNAL BEHAVIORS
Cigarette smoking

Alcohol use/abuse

Illicit drugs

Caffeine

Restrictive dietary patterns, e.g., vegetarianism

MATERNAL CHARACTERISTICS

■ What are the risks of adolescent pregnancy for mother and infant?

■ What are the social, psychological, economic, and emotional concerns that influence nutrition status in adolescent gravida?

■ What steps can be taken to reduce the risks associated with adolescent pregnancy?

■ What are the maternal and fetal risks for gravida who are over 35 years of age?

■ How can interventions, including nutrition intervention, improve pregnancy outcome?

Maternal Age

Perinatal mortality, low birth weight, and preterm births occur more frequently at either end of the reproductive age spectrum. Very young adolescents (<15 years of age) or mothers over 35 years of age are more likely to have low gestational weight gains, a major contributor to low birth weight (National Center for Health Statistics, 1994). In addition, each age group has specific characteristics or factors that increase risk for an adverse pregnancy outcome.

Adolescence

Sue's story, which opened this chapter, is not unusual. In the United States approximately one million teenagers become pregnant each year, and almost one quarter are under 15 years of age (Alan Guttmacher Institute, 1994). Adolescent child-bearing rates are considerably higher in the United States than in many other developed countries. Approximately 12% of all births are to adolescents—4% to those under 18 years of age. Although the ability to conceive is determined by biologic maturation, adolescent pregnancy can have profound health, social, psychological, and vocational consequences for the teenager and her family (Committee on Adolescence, 1989). She is likely to be unmarried and poor and to have unstable peer group relations. Adolescents are more likely to enter prenatal care late, have lower prepregnancy weights, and have less adequate gestational weight gains than older women. Adolescent pregnancy is associated with reduced nutrition stores and inadequate intake (Story and Alton, 1995). In addition, early sexual activity is associated with a higher use of alcohol, tobacco, and drugs, which increases risk of a poor dietary intake, health problems, and inadequate health care.

RISKS   Because pregnancy in young adolescents is associated with numerous environmental and lifestyle risk factors, it is difficult to differentiate the effects of those factors from physiologic maturity. Frazer and co-workers (1995) examined the pregnancy outcomes of more than 134,000 singleton births of white primigravida between 13 and 24 years of age. After adjustment for marital status, education, and prenatal care, the younger groups (13–17 years and 18–19 years) had a significantly higher risk of preterm delivery and low-birthweight infants than mothers who were 20 to 24 years old.

Risks of early delivery in mothers 16 years of age or older can be reduced with early and continuing prenatal (including nutrition) care to ensure consumption of adequate energy and nutrients and attainment of recommended weight gains. In fact, for older adolescents, poor pregnancy outcome has a greater association with environmental and social conditions such as poverty, inadequate prenatal care, poor diet, and substance abuse than with young age. However, for the nearly 13,000 young adolescents (<15 years) who become pregnant each year, perinatal outcomes are poorer than those of older adolescents even when they receive adequate prenatal care (McArnarney, 1987, Zuckerman, 1984).

Adolescents of young **gynecologic age**, who have not completed their own development, have higher neonatal mortality rates and more preterm and low-birthweight infants than older women (Garn, 1986; Institute of Medicine, 1990). Preterm delivery is the underlying cause of low birth weight (Scholl et al, 1994a). Early childbearing is also associated with increased incidence of iron deficiency anemia and abruptio placentae and possibly increased **pregnancy-induced hypertension** (Scholl et al, 1994b).

MATERNAL GROWTH AND PREGNANCY   Although females gain substantial amounts of height and weight prior to menarche, growth continues for another 4 to 7 years. Estimates of gains in stature and weight after the onset of menses are from 4.3 to 10.6 cm (2–4 in) and 6–8 kg (13–18 lb) (Roche and Davilla, 1972). Thus, a pregnant teenager who is within 2 to 3 years of menarche may still be in a period of appreciable growth. Growth of pelvic girdle also continues after menarche, but at a slower rate. Early maturation associated with pregnancy may result in a smaller pelvis and more difficulties with pregnancy and delivery due to **cephalopelvic disproportion**.

Growth of young gravida may be masked by the tendency of women of all ages to measure slightly less in stature during pregnancy, probably as a result of weight gain and vertebral compression. Scholl and co-workers (1993) demonstrated continued maternal growth in 50% of young primiparas and multiparas by measuring increases in knee height. After controlling for other risk factors, girls who grew during pregnancy had infants 156 g lighter than those of teenagers who were not growing, despite a greater weight gain. Reduced infant birth weights of young, still growing, pregnant adolescents may result from competition for nutrients between the mother and fetus (Naeye, 1981; Garn et al, 1984; Scholl et al, 1994a) and ineffective transfer of nutrients due to lesser placental blood flow (Frisancho, 1985).

WEIGHT GAIN RECOMMENDATIONS   Adolescents who are underweight at the time of conception and who gain inadequate amounts of weight during pregnancy are at greatest risk for the delivery of low-birthweight or premature infants (Scholl et al, 1991). In fact, a young adolescent is more likely to have a small newborn than an older woman with a similar prepregnancy weight and gestational weight gain (Frisancho, 1985; Haiek and Lederman, 1988; Rosso, 1990). Recommended weight gains (based on pregravid BMI) for pregnant adolescents appear

TABLE 9–2 Recommended Gestational Weight Gains for Adolescents

BMI	Weight Gain	
	kg	lb
<19.8 (underweight)	14–18	35–40
19.8–26.0 (normal weight)	13–18	28–40
>26.0–29.0 (overweight)	8–11.5	18–25

Adapted from Institute of Medicine. Nutrition during pregnancy. Washington, DC: National Academy Press, 1990.

in Table 9–2. These levels represent the upper end of the ranges recommended for all women. Young mothers (gynecologic age <2 years) may require higher weight gains during pregnancy than older adolescents or adults to achieve optimum birth weights of 3.5 to 4.0 kg (Institute of Medicine, 1990).

The pattern of weight gain in young gravida also appears to be a significant factor in outcome. Infant birth weights of 3 to 4 kg in offspring of teenagers appear to be supported by a maternal weight gain of 1.4 to 2.3 kg (3 to 5 lb) during the first trimester, and increases of approximately 0.5 kg (1 lb) per week thereafter until term (Reese et al, 1992).

Maternal fat accretion usually occurs in the first two trimesters of pregnancy, and some of that fat is mobilized in the final trimester. In contrast, pregnant teenagers who are still growing (as measured by gains in knee height) continue to accumulate body fat after 28 weeks, resulting in larger weight gains. These gains appear to be related to failure to mobilize stored fat, as indicated by increased fat folds postpartum. This pattern of fat accretion has been associated with decreased fetal growth and lower infant birth weights (Hediger et al, 1990). In spite of this difference, these still-growing teens had caloric intakes comparable

K E Y   T E R M S

gynecologic age: current age minus age at menarche
pregnancy-induced hypertension: increased blood pressure with onset during pregnancy
cephalopelvic disproportion: maternal pelvic size/shape in relation to fetal head

with those of pregnant, non-growing adolescents and mature women (Scholl et al, 1994a).

ENERGY AND NUTRIENT NEEDS As discussed in Chapter 8, pregnancy increases the demand for energy, protein, and most vitamins and minerals. In young adolescents, this increased need is superimposed on the already high demands of pubertal growth. Specific guidelines for pregnant adolescents do not exist. Table 9–3 lists suggested energy and nutrient levels for pregnant adolescents based on the RDAs for pregnancy and baseline levels for adolescents. It may be assumed that the highest level of nutrient intake, or even somewhat higher, is appropriate for the pregnant adolescent. Energy needs depend on growth status, activity levels, body size, and the stage of gestation, and therefore will change throughout

TABLE 9–3 Recommended Dietary Intakes for Pregnant Adolescents

Nutrient	11–14 y	15–18 y
Energy (kcal)	2500	2500
Protein (g)	61	63
Vitamin A (RE)*	800	800
Vitamin C (mg)	70	70
Vitamin D (μg)[†]	10	10
Vitamin E (mg)[††]	10	10
Vitamin K (μg)	65	65
Thiamin (mg)	1.5	1.5
Riboflavin (mg)	1.6	1.6
Niacin (mg)[§]	17	17
Vitamin B_6 (mg)	2.2	2.2
Vitamin B_{12} (μg)	2.2	2.2
Folate (μg)	400	400
Calcium	1500	1200–1500
Phosphorus	1200	1200
Magnesium	300	300
Iron	30	30
Iodine	175	175
Zinc	15	15
Selenium	65	65

* 1 RE (retinol equivalent) = 1 μg or 6 μg β-carotene.

[†] As cholecalciferol. 10 μg cholecalciferol = 400 IU of vitamin D.

[††] α-Tocopherol equivalents. 1 mg d-α = 1 α-TE.

[§] 1 NE (niacin equivalent) = 1 mg of niacin or 60 mg of dietary tryptophan.

Adapted from Food and Nutrition Board, National Research Council, National Academy of Sciences. Recommended dietary allowances. 10th ed. Washington, DC: National Academy Press, 1989.

pregnancy. Levels greater than the additional 300 kcal per day for gestation may be required to support greater weight gains for adolescents who begin pregnancy underweight (Story and Alton, 1995). Increased protein requirements during gestation were discussed in Chapter 8. The RDA of approximately 46 or 48 g per day is increased by 15 g, to yield approximately 60 g per day. Dietary studies of pregnant adolescents indicate that most teens consume adequate protein (Institute of Medicine, 1990). However, adequate protein may be a concern for adolescents who have inadequate energy intakes or those who follow vegan diets.

Adolescence is associated with increased iron requirements to compensate for growth and menstrual losses. Gestational iron needs for adolescents include that required for maternal growth as well as that needed for fetal and placental tissue growth and increased red blood cell volume. According to the 1990 Nutrition Surveillance System data, the prevalence of iron deficiency anemia in adolescents was 11%, 16%, and 37% in the first, second and third terms of pregnancy, respectively, based on the criteria shown in Table 8–5 (Beard, 1994). Iron deficiency anemia is associated with increased risk of low birthweight and preterm birth (Allen, 1993; Scholl et al, 1992). As for adult gravida, the Institute of Medicine (1990) recommends iron supplementation with 30 mg of elemental iron daily during the second and third trimester of pregnancy. If iron deficiency anemia develops, supplementation of 60 to 120 mg per day is recommended until anemia is resolved. A multivitamin–mineral supplement supplying 15 mg of zinc and 2 mg of copper is also recommended to prevent the additional iron from decreasing body levels of those minerals due to impaired absorption (Institute of Medicine, 1990).

Calcium is transferred from the mother to the fetus at an average rate of 330 mg/day (Institute of Medicine, 1990). The National Institute of Health Consensus Development Conference on Optional Calcium Intakes (1994) recommended a daily calcium intake for adolescents of 1200 to 1500 mg to promote a higher peak bone mass. The need for calcium may be even higher for pregnant adolescents. An intake of 4 to 5 servings of dairy products or their equivalent has been shown to approach the level needed. The Institute of Medicine (1990) recommends a supplement of 600 mg of elemental calcium (1.5 g of calcium carbonate) for adolescents with dietary intakes below 600 mg per day.

Studies of the diets of pregnant adolescents have reported that intakes were most often below recommended levels for calcium, iron, zinc, magnesium, vitamin D, folate, and vitamin B_6 (Skinner et al, 1992; Schneck et al, 1990). If an adolescent does not consume a nutritionally adequate diet, despite nutrition counseling, a balanced vitamin and mineral supplement that provides the RDA is recommended (see Table 8–6). Supplementation is also indicated for adolescents who smoke heavily, use alcohol or drugs, or are strict vegetarians.

The American Dietetic Association (1994) emphasizes the importance of early, frequent, and continuous nutrition care in an interdisciplinary program specifically devoted to adolescents. Such care, which gives attention to the unique biologic, psychosocial, developmental, and economic needs of the teen mother will optimize the potential for a favorable pregnancy outcome.

Older Gravida

Concern about the **primigravida** 35 years or older has particular significance in the United States because the number of women aged 35 to 49 years is increasing and more women are electing to delay childbearing, increasing the number of older mothers. By the year 2000, approximately 10% of births in the United States will occur to women 35 to 49 years of age (National Center for Health Statistics, 1993).

Women 35 years and older have higher incidences of perinatal mortality and low-birthweight deliveries, of both preterm and small-for-gestational-age infants (Chattingius et al, 1992). Many medical conditions, such as cardiovascular and respiratory disorders, kidney disease, autoimmune disorders, obesity, **diabetes mellitus**, and tumors increase in frequency with advancing maternal age (Prysak et al, 1995). Increased maternal mortality with age is mostly a result of increases in these underlying illnesses, and a number of obstetric complications in older gravida may also be related to the increased incidence of chronic diseases. For example, the incidence of **placenta previa** and abruptio placentae increases with age and parity (Zhang and Savitz, 1993). These disorders may be related more to predisposing problems such as hypertension and smoking than to maternal age. Pregnant women 35 years and older, especially **nulliparas**, have more **macrosomic** infants and more frequent operative deliveries (cesarean section). These, too, may be related to an overall increase in disease, especially hypertension, obesity, and diabetes, all of which increase with advancing age (Newcombe et al, 1991; Hansen, 1986).

Studies of pregnancy outcome in older women have not been able to control for many important confounding variables such as substance abuse, lifestyle, cardiovascular fitness, obesity, or the use of medical care. Today's older mothers may have fewer risks than previous generations, however, because women who elect to delay childbearing tend to be better educated, to be in better general health, and to have more access to medical care (Berkowitz et al, 1990).

Preconceptional management, including nutrition care, of the underlying disorders that complicate pregnancy in older gravida and careful control throughout gestation can reduce the risk of adverse outcomes. This includes basic nutrition care (described in the Application at the end of Chapter 8) to ensure adequate dietary intakes to support fetal growth and maintenance of nutrition status, and spe-cialized nutrition care to normalize blood glucose levels or control of hypertension across the reproductive period.

SOCIOECONOMIC STATUS

■ What are the socioeconomic characteristics of a high-risk pregnancy?

■ How does a woman's socioeconomic status influence pregnancy outcome?

Infant mortality rates in the United States are higher than in many other developed countries. A number of interrelated socioeconomic factors contribute to the risk of an adverse pregnancy outcome. They include family income, social status, race, parental education, employment, marital status, and availability of health care and support systems.

Economically disadvantaged women have a higher incidence of low-birthweight and preterm infants than women of higher socioeconomic levels (Jonas et al, 1992; deSanjose and Roman, 1991). In fact, in multiparous women, low socioeconomic status (based on occupation) is a more important predictor of poor pregnancy outcome than parity (Seidman et al, 1991). Another confounding factor is marital status. Poor women are more likely to be unmarried, and the risk of an adverse outcome is greater for women who have never been married and for those who are divorced or separated (Melnikow et al, 1991).

Poor white women and poor African-American women are about equally likely to bear a low-birthweight infant. Overall, however, African-American infants are three times more likely to be of **very low birth weight** (Abrams et al, 1991). Among African-Americans, one in two babies is born in a family below the federal poverty level, and nearly two-thirds of all babies are born to unwed mothers—many of whom are teenagers. A similar pattern is ob-

KEY TERMS

primigravida: woman in her first pregnancy

diabetes mellitus: a chronic disorder of carbohydrate and fat metabolism that is characterized by a relative lack of insulin

placenta previa: the placenta is located in a lower position in the uterus than normal

nullipara: a woman who has never given birth to a viable infant

macrosomic: birth weight > 4000 g

very low birth weight: an infant birth weight of less than 1500 g (3.4 lb)

served for educational attainment of the mother and low-birthweight infants (Gould and LeRoy, 1988). A recent study found that for African-American women the lowest rates of fetal growth restriction occurred when weight gains exceeded those recommended (Hickey et al, 1993).

Almost 20% of mothers do not receive prenatal care during the first trimester. Among minority women, the rate is higher, close to 40%. Half a million of the women who give birth each year are not covered for maternity care by health insurance and do not have the money to pay for health care. Comprehensive prenatal care such as that provided by public health departments via Medicaid can reduce the number of low-birthweight infants (Buescher and Ward, 1992; Poland et al, 1991). (Programs for pregnant women and their offspring are discussed in the Application at the end of this chapter.) Unfortunately, women who are less likely to get prenatal care are those at greatest risk, because they tend to be poor, multiparous, less educated, young, and unmarried, and use tobacco, alcohol, and drugs (Melnikow et al, 1991). If all the women currently receiving inadequate prenatal care were to receive Medicaid-covered adequate care, there would be more than a two-to-one return in savings on the medical costs of caring for high-risk infants (Wilson et al, 1992).

MATERNAL BODY WEIGHT

■ What are the risks of maternal obesity or underweight to mother and fetus?

■ How does nutrition intervention modify the risks of pregravid body weight?

Women who are obese or extremely underweight at the time of conception are at risk of increased mortality and morbidity for themselves and their infants. Nutrition assessment and intervention, modifying dietary patterns, and weight gain can improve outcome.

Overweight and Obesity

Women who are overweight (BMI 26 to 29) or obese (BMI > 29) at the onset of pregnancy experience more complications than mothers of normal weight. The greatest risk occurs with maternal body weights that exceed 135% of the reference weight or a BMI >28 (Naeye, 1979; Perlow et al, 1992). The risks include hypertension, diabetes mellitus, and **thromboembolic** disease, labor abnormalities, and more induced labor and unscheduled cesarean sections (Ekbald and Grenman, 1992; Perlow, 1992; Johnson et al, 1992). Infants of heavy mothers are at increased risk for macrosomia, a condition associated with greater risk of **shoulder dystocia** and maternal or infant morbidity (Institute of Medicine, 1990).

Nutrition care of obese gravida must emphasize varied dietary intakes that are adequate in nutrients and provide sufficient energy to support fetal growth and sufficient carbohydrate to avoid ketosis. Weight reduction during pregnancy is not recommended under any circumstance. In obese mothers weight gains of approximately 6 kg are associated with the lowest rates of infant mortality and birth weights between 3 and 4 kg (Naeye, 1979).

Underweight

Underweight women (BMI < 19.8) have a greater risk of delivering a preterm or low-birthweight infant (Institute of Medicine, 1990); they also have a higher incidence of complications such as antepartum hemorrhage, **premature rupture of the membranes**, and anemia (Edwards et al, 1979). The level of maternal body weight that constitutes increased risk may vary. For example, an economically disadvantaged woman may have a higher risk of a low-birthweight infant, even though her body weight is greater than that of a middle-class woman (Mitchell and Lerner, 1989). Preconceptional and prenatal counseling, including referral to food assistance programs, can help the women reduce risk by normalizing body weight before conception. For underweight women, a weight gain of 12.5 to 18 kg (28 to 40 lb) is associated with improved birth weights and lower neonatal mortality rates (Naeye, 1979; Institute of Medicine, 1990).

MULTIPLE BIRTHS

■ What are the nutrition-related concerns for a pregnancy with multiple fetuses?

A pregnancy involving more than one fetus is associated with higher perinatal mortality rates. The greater the number of fetuses, the smaller the weight for each infant and the greater the risk of low birth weight (Fig. 9–1). Multiple-fetus pregnancies are less likely to go to term. For example, twin pregnancies are, on the average, 3 weeks shorter than singleton pregnancies and are associated with a 5- to 10-fold increase in preterm delivery and low birth weight (Luke and Keith, 1992).

It is obvious that multiple pregnancies increase requirements for energy and nutrients. Weight gain should exceed that of singleton pregnancies because there are greater increases in maternal, placental, and fetal tissue. A total weight gain of 16 to 20.5 kg (35 to 45 lb) has been recommended for twin pregnancies (Institute of Medicine, 1990). Pederson and co-workers (1989) found that a weight gain of 22 kg (44 lb) was associated with optimal pregnancy outcome (birth weight >2.5 kg and gestational age >37 wk) in twin pregnancies. A weekly weight gain of approximately 0.75 kg (1.5 lb) during the second and third trimesters of pregnancy is advisable for the mother

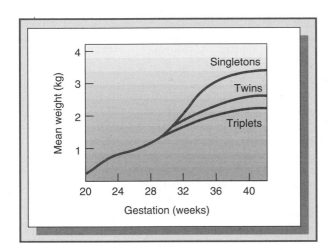

FIGURE 9–1. Mean fetal growth rates in singleton and multiple pregnancies. (From MacLennan AH. Multiple gestation: clinical characteristics and management. In: Creasy RK, Resnick R. (eds). Maternal-fetal medicine: principles and practice. Philadelphia: WB Saunders, 1994.)

who is carrying twins. There is evidence that intrauterine growth is achieved earlier for twins than for singletons (Luke et al, 1993) and that the lowest morbidity may occur with delivery between 35 and 37 weeks.

Appropriate weight gains for optimum growth of multiple fetuses and support of maternal health have not been defined. Recommendations for optimizing pregnancy outcome include liberalized weight gains, reduced physical effort, and early, comprehensive prenatal care (Ellings et al, 1993).

HEALTH CONDITIONS OF THE MOTHER

Hyperemesis Gravidarum

■ What are the implications of hyperemesis gravidarum for mother and fetus?

■ What are appropriate intervention strategies for severe cases of hyperemesis gravidarum?

As discussed in Chapter 8, many pregnant women experience some nausea and vomiting during early pregnancy. Hyperemesis gravidarum is a nutritionally debilitating condition characterized by **intractable** vomiting that develops in about 3.5 women per 1000 pregnancies (Barclay, 1990). The etiology of hyperemesis gravidarum is unknown, but suggested causes include elevated levels of progesterone, estrogens, sex hormone–binding globulin, and cortisol (Erick, 1995), increased levels of a trophoblastic factor, human chorionic gonadotropin (HCG), delayed gastric emptying, and immunologic or psychosomatic factors.

Hyperemesis gravidarum can result in weight loss, dehydration, electrolyte imbalance, and metabolic abnormalities. There are limited data relating this condition to pregnancy outcome. Loss of more than 5% of pregravid weight has been associated with significant fetal growth restriction in some (Gross et al, 1989) but not all studies. The hyperemetic woman who has little or no dietary intake because of nausea and vomiting must meet her energy needs by breaking down or metabolizing body fats and proteins. Utilization of fat in the absence of carbohydrate intake can result in the formation of ketone bodies, and high levels of ketonemia may impair neurologic development in the fetus.

Nutrition assessment and management are appropriate, particularly if nausea and vomiting persist beyond the first trimester. If fluid and electrolyte imbalances occur or if weight loss exceeds 5% or is accompanied by ketonemia, admission to the hospital may be indicated. Treatment includes intravenous (IV) fluid and electrolyte replacement, sedation, and **antiemetic** medication (Levine and Esser, 1988). When the acute phase of hyperemesis has passed and electrolyte balance has been restored, oral feeding begins with fluids. After tolerance of fluids has been established, oral intake is slowly introduced as small, frequent meals of foods low in fat and high in carbohydrate, with solid and liquid foods consumed at different times. Establishment of nutritional rehabilitation, including improved weight gain, may require extended hospitalization or outpatient nutrition management (Boyce, 1992).

For the small number of women who do not respond to the gradual progression to an oral diet, two alternatives have been reported to be effective. The first, total parenteral nutrition (TPN), which provides all energy and nutrient needs by intravenous infusion, has been successful in supporting maternal weight and fetal growth until oral intake can be resumed (Greenspoon et al, 1993). Duration of such therapy may be a few days or weeks, depending on the severity of the condition. A second option, enteral nu-

KEY TERMS

thromboembolic: a condition in which there is obstruction of a blood vessel by a blood clot
shoulder dystocia: difficulty in delivering the shoulders of the fetus through the birth canal after its head has emerged
premature rupture of the membranes: rupture of fetal membranes before the onset of labor
intractable: not easily managed
antiemetic: antinausea

trition, involves continuous infusion of a tube feeding product via a **nasogastric tube**. Enteral feeding is contraindicated in the acute phase of vomiting, but it can be initiated once intravenous rehydration has been achieved and vomiting has subsided, even if nausea is still present. Recently, Gulley and co-workers (1993) described women for whom nasogastric feeding was associated with complete resolution of hyperemesis.

Maternal Hyperphenylalaninemia

■ How does an elevated blood level of phenylalanine increase fetal risk?

■ Why is hyperphenylalaninemia a public health concern?

■ What is appropriate prenatal nutrition intervention for hyperphenylalaninemia?

Phenylketonuria (PKU), an inborn error of phenylalanine metabolism, is due to the absence of the enzyme phenylalanine hydroxylase, which is required for the first step in the catabolic pathway of phenylalanine (Fig. 9–2). The result is an increase in the level of phenylalanine in the blood, and the accumulation of other metabolites in body fluids and excreted in the urine. Restriction of dietary phenylalanine lowers blood levels and prevents mental retardation in infants and young children. If the enzyme block is mild and blood phenylalanine levels are only somewhat elevated, the individual is said to have hyperphenylalaninemia. Because blood levels are lower in mild cases, infants and children with this form of the disorder may not require restriction of dietary phenylalanine.

Ironically, improved diagnosis and successful treatment of PKU in infants have created new challenges in pregnancy and childbearing. There are approximately 2000 to 4000 females of childbearing age in the United States diagnosed with PKU or hyperphenylalaninemia, and it is estimated that there are more than two times that number of women with unknown hyperphenylalaninemia (Platt et al, 1992). During gestation, elevated blood phenylalanine levels constitute a risk of low birth weight, microcephaly, and even mental retardation and congenital heart disease in the infants. This has been referred to as maternal hyperphenylalaninemia (Lenke and Levy, 1990). Only 1 in 120 infants of these women actually have PKU, but when maternal blood levels increase the excess phenylalanine has teratogenic effects on the fetus (Platt et al, 1992; Thompson et al, 1991).

There is evidence that lowering blood phenylalanine levels prior to conception or in early gestation and throughout pregnancy reduces fetal abnormalities (Platt et al, 1992). Nutrition intervention is most effective if it occurs before conception (Luder and Greene, 1989). Nutrition management involves reducing dietary intake of phenylalanine to levels required for protein synthesis while maintaining normal blood levels of tyrosine. Guidelines for nutrition care appear in Table 9–4. The diet relies on a formula product for most of its protein. The formula, low in phenylalanine and complete in tyrosine and other nutrients, is supplemented in foods low in phenylalanine. The diet is highly restrictive, and the mother requires specialized nutrition care and follow-up. Dietary modification is monitored by measuring blood levels of phenylalanine and tracking gestational weight gain.

Hypertensive Disorders of Pregnancy

■ What is pregnancy-induced hypertension and what are its implications?

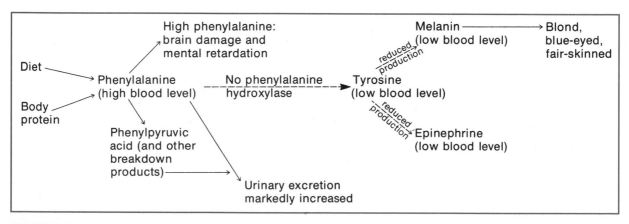

FIGURE 9–2. Structure and metabolic pathway of phenylalanine. (From Bolander. Basic nursing. 3rd ed. Philadelphia: WB Saunders, 1994:1089.)

TABLE 9–4 Guidelines for Prenatal Nutrition Care in Women with Hyperphenylalaninemia

Develop a diet plan to maintain serum phenylalanine levels between 2 and 6 mg/dL or lower prior to conception and throughout pregnancy.

Meet recommended levels for protein, phenylalanine, vitamins, and minerals.

Provide sufficient energy to maintain the recommended patterns of weight gain.

Limit intake of phenylalanine to an amount needed to maintain recommended serum levels using:
    Phenylalanine-free formula product
    Foods low in phenylalanine, to provide a minimum of 200 mg of phenylalanine as a baseline. Add additional foods to maintain blood levels

Provide sufficient tyrosine to maintain serum levels in the normal range.

Assist the mother in planning a diet to meet the dietary guidelines.

Assist the mother with food shopping, selection, and preparation.

Monitor blood levels of phenylalanine and tyrosine.

Monitor weight gain.

TABLE 9–5 Hypertensive Disorders of Pregnancy

Chronic hypertension
    Present in the nonpregnant state (blood pressure 140/90 mm Hg)
    Present before mid-gestation (blood pressure 140/90 mm Hg)
Pregnancy-induced hypertension (PIH)
    Preeclampsia
        Hypertension (blood pressure 140/90 mm Hg) after 20th week of pregnancy
        Proteinuria
        Edema
    Severe preeclampsia
        One or more of the following:
        Systolic blood pressure of 160 mm Hg or diastolic blood pressure of 110 mg Hg
        Proteinuria, edema
        Blurred vision, headache, altered consciousness
        Epigastric pain, impaired liver function
    Eclampsia
        Preeclampsia with seizure, occurs near time of labor
Chronic hypertension with preeclampsia
    Develops before the 30th week
    Same symptoms as preeclampsia
    Systolic blood pressure increase of 30 mm Hg
    Diastolic blood pressure increase of 15–20 mm Hg
    Often progresses rapidly to preeclampsia
Transient gestational hypertension
    Transient increase in blood pressure during labor or first 24 hours postpartum; no signs or symptoms of preeclampsia

From National High Blood Pressure Education Program Working Group Report on High Blood Pressure in Pregnancy. Am J Obstet Gynecol 1990;163:1691.

■ **What is the potential role of nutrition in pregnancy-induced hypertension?**

Hypertension occurs in approximately 7% to 10% of all pregnancies and is associated with increased maternal and perinatal morbidity and mortality (Naeye and Freidman, 1979). Hypertensive disorders of pregnancy include preexisting chronic hypertension, transient gestational hypertension, and pregnancy-induced hypertension (PIH) expressed as mild to severe preeclampsia or eclampsia and preeclampsia superimposed on chronic hypertension (National High Blood Pressure Education Program, 1993; Table 9–5).

In the majority of hypertensive pregnant women, hypertension is mild and the pregnancy is uncomplicated. The most severe form, preeclampsia, is associated with increased risk of abruptio placenta, maternal renal failure, and cerebral hemorrhage (Roberts and Redman, 1993). It is the major cause of fetal and maternal morbidity and mortality (National Center for Health Statistics, 1994).

Preeclampsia

Although the cause of preeclampsia is unknown, it occurs most often in primigravida, particularly black, low-income women who lack prenatal care and are younger than 20 or older than 35 years of age, or in women with chronic hypertension or kidney disease. Preeclampsia usually develops after 20 weeks gestation, often near term. It is characterized by a blood pressure of 140/90 mm Hg, **proteinuria**, edema, and one or more of the following: **hypovolemia**, **hypoalbuminemia**, and disturbances in

K E Y   T E R M S

nasogastric tube: tube placed into the stomach via the nasal cavity to be used for feeding
proteinuria: more than 5 g of protein in the urine in 24 hours
hypovolemia: low blood volume
hypoalbuminemia: low blood levels of the protein albumin

liver and/or kidney function or blood coagulation (Magann and Martin, 1995). Other signs and symptoms of preeclampsia may include upper abdominal pain, headache, visual disturbances, retinal hemorrhage, and fetal growth restriction (Cunningham and Lindheimer, 1992). Preeclampsia can progress rapidly to eclampsia, which is characterized by the above abnormalities accompanied by generalized convulsions.

MANAGEMENT OF PREECLAMPSIA The only cure for preeclampsia is the termination of pregnancy. If the diagnosis of preeclampsia is suspected, bed rest or hospitalization allows monitoring of mother and fetus and may reduce the likelihood of convulsions. Treatment of mild preeclampsia is aimed at relief of symptoms and prescription of drugs to regulate blood pressure and prevent convulsions. Delivery may be indicated, regardless of gestational age, if severe hypertension persists after 24–48 hours of treatment or if there is evidence of progressive kidney or liver dysfunction or signs of eclampsia.

ROLE OF DIET IN PREECLAMPSIA The diet for any pregnant woman must supply sufficient energy to achieve recommended weight gain and adequate amounts of protein, vitamins, and minerals. In preeclampsia, adequate dietary protein is essential due to protein loss in the urine and reduced levels of serum proteins. Restoration of serum protein levels is important in correction of hypovolemia.

Several epidemiologic studies have reported an association between low dietary calcium and a higher incidence of pregnancy-related hypertension (Marcoux et al, 1991). Women with preeclampsia excrete lower amounts of urinary calcium (Seely et al, 1992). Calcium supplementation has been reported to lower blood pressure in pregnant and nonpregnant women (Knight and Keith, 1992), particularly women who had low calcium losses suggesting variable levels of response (Belizan et al, 1991). In a review of six calcium supplementation trials during pregnancy, Guillermo and co-workers (1994) concluded that daily supplementation of 1.5 to 2.0 g was associated with a reduction of about 50% in pregnancy-induced hypertension. However, these results are from studies with small numbers of subjects and have not yet been confirmed in large well-controlled clinical trials.

Diabetes Mellitus

■ Why does diabetes mellitus increase the risk of an adverse pregnancy outcome?

■ How do pregestational and gestational diabetes differ?

■ What are the principles of nutrition care for diabetes during pregnancy?

Diabetes mellitus is a chronic disorder of carbohydrate and lipid metabolism in which blood levels of glucose and lipids are elevated. This abnormal metabolism results from a relative lack of insulin—either too little insulin is secreted or the insulin that is secreted is not effective. In addition, diabetes is associated with chronic systemic complications, which, over time, can affect the retina, kidneys, nerves, and cardiovascular system. The most common classifications of diabetes mellitus include type I, or insulin-dependent, diabetes mellitus (IDDM); type II, non–insulin-dependent diabetes mellitus (NIDDM); and gestational diabetes (GD), glucose intolerance that is first recognized in pregnancy. Treatment of diabetes requires a balance between the woman's dietary intake and the insulin produced by her pancreas or exogenous insulin, which must be administered to control blood glucose levels.

Diabetes that is detected during pregnancy may be pregestational or gestational. Pregestational diabetes, usually type I, is present prior to pregnancy and occurs in 0.2% to 0.8% of all pregnancies. Gestational diabetes, which occurs in 2% to 4% of all pregnancies, usually has an onset late in the second trimester. Carbohydrate tolerance is normal before gestation and usually returns to normal after delivery. Regardless of the form, diabetes that is untreated or poorly regulated during pregnancy increases the risk of maternal and fetal mortality and morbidity.

Metabolic Changes of Pregnancy

Maternal blood glucose concentration during pregnancy decreases about 20% compared to the nonpregnant state. Glucose is transported across the placenta to the fetus by **facilitated diffusion**. In order to spare glucose for fetal consumption, maternal metabolism increasingly uses alternative fuels. Several of the hormones that are synthesized by the placenta, such as human placental lactogen, estrogen, and progesterone, have anti-insulin activity and, therefore, can increase blood glucose levels. In addition, placental enzymes promote breakdown of insulin. Under normal circumstances the pancreas adapts to these changes by increasing insulin secretion. If the pancreas does not respond to the metabolic alterations with increased insulin release, gestational diabetes results (Jovanovic-Peterson and Peterson, 1996).

Pregestational Diabetes

The woman with type I diabetes requires exogenous insulin to control blood glucose levels, and the metabolic changes of gestation may increase insulin requirements. If insulin is not adequate, **hyperglycemia** and ketosis result. If the mother is hyperglycemic, greater amounts of glucose pass to the fetus, causing hyperglycemia, which stimulates fetal insulin secretion. The excess insulin increases protein synthesis and lipogenesis, promoting macrosomia, and may impair development of the lungs and cardiovascular and nervous systems (Jovanovic-Peterson and Peterson, 1996).

Adverse outcomes of pregnancy in mothers with diabetes are related to elevated blood glucose levels. Normalizing maternal glucose levels through diet and/or multiple insulin injections has produced significant improvement in infant mortality rates and other adverse outcomes (Coustan, 1992).

Preconceptional counseling is important to assist the mother with insulin-dependent diabetes in avoiding wide fluctuations in blood glucose levels before pregnancy and maintaining steady levels throughout gestation. Therefore, the goals of dietary management for the woman with type I diabetes are to maintain **normoglycemia** and to promote weight gain appropriate for pregravid BMI (see Table 8–4). The diet should consist of frequent small feedings designed to avoid **postprandial** hyperglycemia and preprandial fasting ketosis.

Three to five injections of insulin per day to coincide with food intake may be needed to maintain normoglycemia. The total amount of insulin administered daily is based on the week of gestation and the woman's pregnant body weight (Jovanovic-Peterson and Peterson, 1991).

Gestational Diabetes

The effects of gestational diabetes on pregnancy outcome are usually limited to those associated with hyperglycemia in the latter half of pregnancy. Women with gestational diabetes have a higher incidence of preeclampsia and operative delivery (Goldman et al, 1991) and an increased risk of developing of overt diabetes later in life (Damm et al, 1992). Infants of mothers whose pregnancies are complicated by gestational diabetes have a greater number of neonatal problems, including fetal macrosomia and associated birth injury and other neonatal morbidity, including **hypoglycemia**, **hyperbilirubinemia**, hypocalcemia, **polycythemia**, and major congenital anomalies (Hod et al, 1991). There is also a link between maternal gestational diabetes and macrosomia in the neonate and obesity and glucose intolerance in childhood and later life (Coustan, 1992).

SCREENING AND DIAGNOSIS All pregnant women should be screened for gestational diabetes at 24 to 28 weeks gestation, as outlined in Table 9–6. Rescreening at 32 weeks gestation is recommended for women at increased risk for development of diabetes.

TREATMENT AND MONITORING Women with gestational diabetes who are able to maintain normal blood glucose levels (fasting <105 mg/dL; postprandial <120 mg/dL) during the remainder of their pregnancy

TABLE 9–6 Screening for Gestational Diabetes

SCREENING FOR ALL PREGNANT WOMEN: 24–28 WEEKS
1. Administer 50 g oral glucose
2. After 1 h measure plasma glucose level
3. If plasma glucose >140 mg/dL, recommend diagnostic glucose tolerance test

DIAGNOSIS: GLUCOSE TOLERANCE TEST (GTT)
1. Measure plasma glucose
2. Administer 100 g oral glucose load
3. Measure plasma glucose at 1, 2, and 3 h
4. If two or more plasma glucose values exceed the following, a diagnosis of gestational diabetes is made.

Time/Plasma Glucose	Diagnostic of Diabetes Mellitus (mg/dL)
Fasting	105
75 or 100 g oral glucose	
1 h	190
2 h	165
3 h	145

From American Diabetes Association. Gestational diabetes mellitus. Diabetes Care 1996;16:5.

have mortality and complication rates approaching those of nondiabetic women (Coustan, 1992; Fagan et al, 1995).

Minimizing fluctuations in blood glucose concentration and ensuring adequate weight gain are imperative to assure favorable perinatal outcomes. This presents a challenge because energy and nutrient requirements change across pregnancy. All women with gestational diabetes

K E Y   T E R M S

facilitated diffusion: a carrier-mediated movement of gas, liquids, or solids across a membrane from a region of high concentration to one of lower concentration

hyperglycemia: high blood glucose levels

normoglycemia: blood glucose levels that remain within limits of persons with normal insulin function

postprandial: after eating

hypoglycemia: low blood glucose level

hyperbilirubinemia: hyper, increased; *bilirubin*, bile pigment from the breakdown of hemoglobin and other heme pigments; *emia*, in the blood

polycythemia: increase in the mass of red blood cells

should receive individualized nutrition counseling (American Diabetes Association, 1993). Nutrition intervention is the cornerstone of therapy. If dietary management alone does not maintain recommended glucose levels, insulin may be administered. Approximately 20% of women with gestational diabetes require insulin to maintain blood glucose levels (Goldman et al, 1991). The pattern of multiple insulin injections recommended for women with type 1 diabetes is appropriate for the woman with gestational diabetes. Self-monitoring of postprandial blood glucose allows the adjustment of insulin therapy, improving blood glucose values and glycemic control (deVeciana et al, 1995).

Human Immunodeficiency Virus Infection

◼ How can nutrition care influence the course and outcome of pregnancy in a woman with HIV infection?

The first case of **human immunodeficiency virus (HIV)** infection in a woman was reported in the United States in 1981. By mid-1993, acquired immunodeficiency syndrome (**AIDS**) was the fourth leading cause of death among women aged 15 to 44 years (U.S. Public Health Service, 1995). In 1990, approximately 11% of all AIDS cases occurred in women (Chu et al, 1990), and perinatal transmission of HIV resulted in an estimated 1800 HIV-infected infants (Nanda and Minkoff, 1992). These figures do not reflect the increasing prevalence of HIV and AIDS among women in the United States, however.

Basic concerns regarding HIV infection in pregnant women include transmission of the virus to the infant, the impact of HIV or AIDS on the outcome of pregnancy, and the effect of pregnancy on the progression of the disease. Studies available at this time indicate that, at least among asymptomatic women, HIV infection does not appear to have a major effect on pregnancy outcome. However, poor fetal outcomes appear to increase in pregnant women who manifest symptoms.

Due to biochemical and hormonal changes, pregnancy may be associated with a depression of **cell-mediated immunity**. However, based on studies currently available, pregnancy in women with HIV infection does not appear to accelerate the progression of disease. One study that followed HIV-positive women found no differences in the progression of the disease between pregnant and nonpregnant women after 12 to 15 months (Moreno and Minkoff, 1992).

Maternal transmission of HIV to the infant occurs in 15% to 35% of pregnancies in infected women (Mofenson, 1994). Transmission appears to occur through viral passage across the placenta, exposure to infected blood and vaginal secretions during labor and delivery, or in the postpartum period through breast-feeding. Infants and children who are infected are more likely to have mothers who have had the HIV infection longer and are also more likely to be symptomatic (Lindgren et al, 1991). Recently, older children and adolescents have been identified with late-onset perinatally acquired HIV infection (Grubman et al, 1995).

In 1994, it was demonstrated that treatment of HIV-infected pregnant women with the drug zidovudine (also referred to as AZT) from the 4th to the 34th week of pregnancy and during labor and delivery, and treatment of the newborn for 6 weeks reduced the percentage of HIV-infected infants (Connor et al, 1994). Therefore, early identification of pregnant women with HIV has become a major public health concern, because for optimal benefit the drug therapy must be begun during early pregnancy (U.S. Public Health Service, 1995).

The goal of treatment of the woman with HIV disease is to slow progression of the disease and ameliorate symptoms in order to improve or maintain the quality of life. Early aggressive nutrition care is essential to assure adequate intakes of kilocalories and nutrients, and to support weight gain appropriate for the mother's pregravid height and weight. Food intake must be carefully planned, with attention given to food preferences and tolerances. Multivitamin and mineral supplements may be necessary to achieve adequate intakes.

SUBSTANCE USE AND ABUSE DURING PREGNANCY

◼ Does caffeine consumption constitute a risk for pregnancy outcome? Why or why not?

◼ What are the fetal effects of maternal cigarette smoking? Does nutrition play a role?

◼ How does the amount and timing of alcohol use or abuse influence pregnancy outcome?

◼ What are the maternal and fetal effects of illicit drug use during pregnancy?

Maternal Smoking

Approximately 30% of women of child-bearing age are smokers. Although some pregnant women cease smoking and others decrease the number of cigarettes smoked each day, many women continue to smoke throughout pregnancy. It is difficult to define the effects of cigarette smoking during pregnancy because of the concurrence of other complicating risk factors including age, education, marital status, and use of alcohol and other drugs.

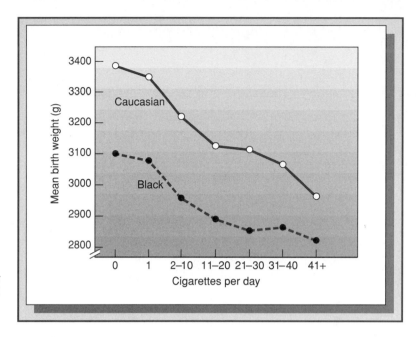

FIGURE 9–3. Dose effect of maternal cigarette use on infant birth weight. (From Niswander KR and Gordon M. The collaborative perinatal study of the National Institute of Neurological Diseases and Stroke: The women and their pregnancies. Philadelphia: WB Saunders, 1972.)

Pregnancy Outcome

Smoking during pregnancy has been linked to increased spontaneous abortions, particularly those that occur in the second trimester (Windham, 1992). Over the last few decades studies have documented a **dose-related** fetal growth restriction in offspring of mothers who smoke (Fig. 9–3). On average, the birth weights of infants born to smoking mothers are approximately 150 to 250 g lower than those of infants whose mothers did not smoke (Abell et al, 1991; Mitchell and Lerner, 1987). Smoking during pregnancy is also associated with a high incidence of preterm delivery and perinatal mortality (McDonald et al, 1992), probably due to the greater occurrence of placenta previa and abruptio placenta and premature rupture of the membranes in mothers who smoke (Williams et al, 1991; Williams et al, 1992). In addition, children of mothers who smoke during pregnancy may have slight but measurable deficits in long-term physical growth (Institute of Medicine, 1990), intellectual performance (Olds et al, 1994), and behavioral adjustment (Weitzman et al, 1992).

The mechanisms by which cigarette smoking causes fetal growth restriction have not been established, but it is generally assumed to be due to fetal **hypoxia** caused by increased carboxyhemoglobin levels. When carbon monoxide binds to the hemoglobin molecule, it is not readily displaced from that molecule, thereby decreasing available sites for oxygen binding. This is supported by observations that fetal body movements and fetal heart rate decrease 20 minutes after the mother has smoked a cigarette (Garcia et al, 1991).

Smoking is the single most important environmental in-

fluence on fetal growth and also the most readily modified. Mothers who smoke during one pregnancy but do not during a succeeding gestation give birth to an infant with a higher birth weight the second time. Women who stopped smoking during the first trimester had little or no greater risk of having a low-birthweight infant than did nonsmokers (McDonald et al, 1992). However, smoking cessation programs for pregnant women have had inconsistent results (Kindrick et al, 1995; Rush et al, 1992).

KEY TERMS

human immunodeficiency virus (HIV): virus that uses the T cells of the host's immune system to replicate itself
AIDS: a disorder of defective cell-mediated immunity associated with HIV infection. The victim becomes defenseless against numerous infections.
cell-mediated immunity: defense conferred by the reaction of T cells (lymphocytes that attack antigens) to an invading organism
diuresis: increased excretion of urine
dose-related: as the amount of use (e.g., number of cigarettes smoked) increases, the effect increases proportionately (e.g., decreased birth weight)
hypoxia: reduction of oxygen supply to tissues below physiologic levels

RESEARCH UPDATE
Caffeine

Caffeine, one of a group of compounds called methylxanthines, is found in coffee, tea, cola and cocoa beverages, and chocolate-containing foods. Tea and cocoa also contain large proportions of the methylxanthines theophylline and theobromine, respectively. Caffeine is listed in the Code of Federal Regulations as a multipurpose food substance that is generally recognized as safe (GRAS). It is a common additive in many nonprescription preparations such as cold tablets, allergy and analgesic preparations, appetite suppressants, and stimulants. Table 9–7 lists the caffeine content of common beverages, foods, and over-the-counter preparations.

Effects of Caffeine

Caffeine can stimulate catecholamine release, which, in turn, stimulates the central nervous system; increases gastric acid secretion, heart rate and basal metabolic rate; alters blood pressure; increases **diuresis**; and relaxes smooth muscle. Consumption of 500 to 750 mg of caffeine per day can result in restlessness, anxiety, irritability, agitation, muscle tremor, sensory disturbances (e.g., tinnitus), heart palpitations, nausea, or vomiting and diarrhea in some individuals.

For more than 30 years, scientists have investigated the potential effect of caffeine on pregnancy course and outcome. The fact that the structure of caffeine resembles that of bases (such as adenosine) in nucleic acids has led to speculation that excess caffeine could have teratogenic effects. This is a concern because caffeine readily crosses biologic membranes, including the placenta, but is not effectively metabolized by the fetus.

Fertility and Miscarriage

Several researchers have explored the relationship between caffeine and infertility or delayed conception. One study reported that women whose daily caffeine consumption exceeded the amount in one cup of coffee (or three cans of cola) were less likely to conceive than women who drank less caffeine. However, that study failed to control for age, frequency of intercourse, or lifestyle factors such as exercise, dietary habits, and stress. More recent studies have failed to establish a relationship between caffeine consumption and conception delay or infertility (Narod et al, 1991). Increased risk of first- and second-trimester spontaneous abortion in women consuming more than 150 mg caffeine per day has been reported (Srisuphan and Bracken, 1986), but this has not been confirmed by succeeding studies (Narod et al, 1991).

Teratogenic Effects

In 1980 the Food and Drug Administration issued a statement that warned pregnant women to avoid caffeine-containing foods and drugs or to consume them only sparingly (FDA, 1980). This warning was based on observations that offspring born to rats fed high doses of caffeine had an increased incidence of congenital anomalies. Subsequent research confirmed a caffeine–birth defect connection, but only when pregnant rats took enormous amounts of caffeine—equivalent to the amount in at least 18 cups of coffee a day. Since the FDA warning, a great deal of controversy and research on caffeine consumption during gestation has been generated. To date, there is no convincing evidence that caffeine is associated with birth defects in humans.

Infant Birth Weight

Caffeine and coffee consumption during pregnancy has been associated with a marginally increased risk of low infant birth weight (Caan and Goldhaber, 1989; Fenster et al, 1991). However, it is unclear if caffeine, coffee, or other characteristics of coffee drinkers are responsible for this effect (Godel et al, 1992).

Maternal Effects

Although coffee is the major source of caffeine in the American diet, consumption of large quantities of other substances, particularly cola beverages, can substantially increase caffeine intake. Caffeine may influence the nutrition status of the mother by increasing the urinary excretion of calcium and thiamin and decreasing zinc and iron absorption (Institute of Medicine, 1990). In addition, very large amounts of caffeine may produce tachycardia or increased blood pressure, interfere with normal sleep patterns, and cause gastric reflux associated with the heartburn common in late pregnancy.

Although data are insufficient to make a specific recommendation regarding caffeine intake, reducing or eliminating dietary caffeine cannot harm the mother or her unborn child.

TABLE 9–7 Caffeine Content of Selected Foods and Drugs

Substance	Caffeine (mg)
Coffee	
Brewed (cup)	85
Percolated (cup)	110
Instant (cup)	66
Instant, decaffeinated (cup)	3
Tea	
Brewed (cup)	46
Instant (teaspoon)	32
Carbonated beverages	
Cola (12 oz)	40–65
Chocolate	
Cocoa, dry (1 tbsp)	10
Hot chocolate (cup)	13
Milk chocolate (1 oz)	6
Semi-sweet chocolate (1 oz)	17
Dark chocolate (1 oz)	20
Chocolate powder for milk (1 tbsp)	10
Chocolate ice cream (cup)	8
Nonprescription drugs	
Anacin analgesic (tablet)	32
Dristan (tablet)	16
Excedrin (tablet)	65
Triamincin (tablet)	30

TABLE 9–8 Features of the Fetal Alcohol Syndrome and Alcohol-Related Birth Defects

Growth retardation
    Prenatal—low birth weight, microcephaly
    Postnatal
Neurologic—developmentally delayed
    Mental retardation
    Learning disabilities—poor school performance
    Behavioral disorders—hyperactivity, irritability, poor attention span
    Speech difficulties—slow development
    Sleep disorders—abnormal sleep/wake cycles
    Hypotonia, poor sucking reflex
    Tremor
Characteristic facial features
    Eyes—short palpebral fissures (eye openings)
    Nose—short and upturned in early childhood
    Midface—flattened, elongated
    Mouth—thin vermilion of upper lip, cleft lip, small teeth
    Ears—small, posterior rotation
Cardiac defects
    Atrial and ventricular septal defects
Genital abnormalities

Role of Nutrition

It has been suggested that the effect of smoking on infant birth weight is related to maternal nutrition status. Infants of obese mothers who smoke have birth weights similar to those of infants of normal-weight mothers who do not smoke. In addition, increased maternal weight gain during pregnancy counteracts the growth-retarding effects of smoking (Rush et al, 1992).

Reports of dietary intakes of pregnant smokers have produced conflicting results. Haste and co-workers (1991) reported that energy intakes were not significantly lower in smoking compared to non-smoking gravida, but intakes of protein, vitamins, and minerals were lower. Smoking lowers serum vitamin C levels, and additional vitamin C intakes are recommended for all smokers (National Research Council, 1989). Exposure to tobacco smoke may increase the requirements for iron, zinc, and folate and decrease the availability of some nutrients. Multivitamin–mineral supplements are recommended for heavy cigarette smokers (Institute of Medicine, 1990).

Alcohol Abuse

Alcohol has been recognized as a potent teratogen. The major adverse effects of maternal alcohol abuse during pregnancy are prenatal and postnatal growth retardation and morphological abnormalities especially facial **anomalies** and central nervous system impairment.

FETAL ALCOHOL SYNDROME The fetal alcohol syndrome (FAS), the most severe form of side effects of maternal alcohol abuse, is a cluster of these features observed in some offspring of women who abuse alcohol during pregnancy (Table 9–8). Figure 9–4 shows the typical facial appearance of FAS victims. FAS is estimated to affect 1 to 2 infants per 1000 live births and may account for as much as 20% of mental retardation in developed countries.

FAS was first described in 1973, and many cases have been documented in infants and young children. Follow-up of infants and children with FAS have described the long-term progression of the disorder into adulthood (Pykowicz et al, 1991; Spohr et al, 1993). Although characteristic facial features of FAS become less distinctive

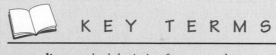

KEY TERMS

anomalies: marked deviation from normal, especially congenital defects

RESEARCH UPDATE
A Case of Fetal Alcohol Syndrome

Maryann is 13 years old, but when her parents go out she needs a babysitter. She does not get phone calls from friends inviting her to go to the mall or to parties or just hang out. She loves to buy new clothes like other 13-year-olds, but she knows she does not look like other girls and sometimes that really upsets her. When she gets frustrated, she yells at her parents that she is different and it's not fair.

Maryann's eyes are small and her ears are malformed. She has difficulty learning simple tasks, is poorly coordinated, and has a short attention span. Often her behavior is impulsive. Her mother says she is hyperactive and easily angered. According to her mother, she doesn't understand consequences and can't learn from her mistakes. She can repeat rules, such as don't go into the street, but she cannot remember or understand them. Maryann's life is the way it is because her birth mother abused alcohol both before and throughout her pregnancy.

Maryann was adopted when she was 5 months old. Her parents suspected something was wrong with her from the beginning. As a young infant she was very irrita-ble and couldn't be soothed. She had difficulty eating and seldom slept through the night. Her growth was slow— the 5th percentile on the growth charts for weight, height, and head circumference. By the time she was 3 years old, Maryann's short attention span and impulsive behavior had become more of a problem. She would repeatedly touch a hot stove, play with matches, or run into the street.

The diagnosis of fetal alcohol syndrome (FAS) was made shortly before her fifth birthday. In many cases, FAS is not formally diagnosed until the child enters school, when attention and learning problems become more apparent. If physical abnormalities are pronounced, and/or the maternal history of abuse is known, the diagnosis may be made much earlier. In Maryann's case the signs were more subtle.

Maryann attends a neighborhood school but is in a class for youngsters with severe behavioral handicaps. She has problems with learning, attention, memory, and problem solving. Education involves a lot of structure, repetition, and consistency. She does make slow progress, but backsliding is common.

with time, short stature and microcephaly persist. Mental retardation also persists, with no improvement in IQ with age. Maladaptive behaviors such as poor judgment, distractibility, and difficulty recognizing social cues are common and may present the greatest challenge to management of the adult with FAS.

Alcohol-Related Birth Defects

Alcohol-related birth defects (ARBD) is a partial syndrome that can result in central nervous system dysfunction and developmental difficulties in the absence of distinctive physical appearance. ARBD may be observed at birth or later in development. ARBD include microcephaly, malformations of the heart and lung, central nervous system problems such as tremors and decreased sucking, and minor physical abnormalities. As many as 36,000 infants may be born each year with these more subtle fetal alcohol effects.

Some infants exposed to alcohol during pregnancy do not show physical evidence of either FAS or ARBD at birth, but they may have a wide range of cognitive disturbances, which become apparent as they approach school age. These include shorter attention span and lower IQ than average, both of which have the potential for causing lasting learning and emotional problems (Smith and Eckardt, 1991; Autti-Ramo et al, 1992).

Amount and Timing of Alcohol Exposure

The mechanisms by which alcohol adversely affects fetal growth and **morphogenesis** have not been established. Alcohol readily crosses the placenta so that the embryo or fetus is exposed to the same blood alcohol levels as the mother. Because the fetal organs are immature, the fetus may not metabolize or detoxify the alcohol as rapidly, resulting in prolonged exposure to alcohol during critical growth periods. Overall, the fetal effects of alcohol are related to the quantity of alcohol consumed by the mother and her blood ethanol level. Approximately 4 drinks (one drink equals approximately 12 oz of beer, 4 oz of wine, or 1 cocktail) per day dramatically increases the risk of physical manifestation of FAS. Light drinking (1 to 2 drinks per day) has not been reported to increase harm to the fe-

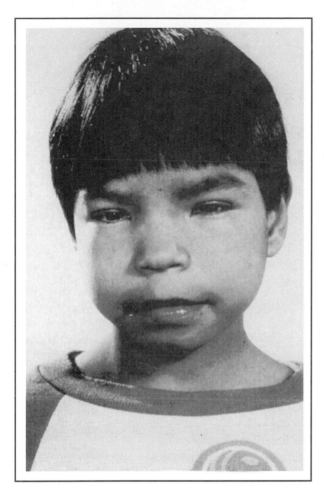

FIGURE 9–4. This 9-year-old boy has typical facial features of fetal alcohol syndrome (FAS). Note the widely spaced eyes, fat midface, short palpebral fissures, and thin upper lip. He has attention deficit disorder with hyperactivity and is mildly mentally retarded. (From Moore KL, Persaud TVN. The developing human. 5th ed. Philadelphia: WB Saunders, 1993. Courtesy of Dr. Albert E. Chaudley.)

tus (Knupfer, 1991). However, Jacobson and co-workers (1993) recently reported that 13-month-old infants whose mothers consumed an average of 7 drinks per week while pregnant had very poor cognitive performance scores twice as often as those whose mothers abstained. Because the occurrence of ARBD is related to maternal blood alcohol levels, a pattern of drinking several drinks on several separate occasions may constitute increased risk, depending on timing and the level of fetal exposure.

A critical time for development of malformations is during embryosis, often before recognition of pregnancy, when the woman may not even be aware of the risk. Effects of alcohol excess later in gestation are less severe, and Rossett and co-workers (1983) maintain that the outcome of pregnancy can be improved substantially if alcohol abusers reduce alcohol intake even after conception.

Safe Levels of Alcohol Consumption

A "safe" level of alcohol consumption during pregnancy cannot be defined because no one knows how much alcohol causes damage. The Food and Drug Administration recommends that pregnant women refrain from drinking alcoholic beverages during pregnancy. Many states require that warning notices regarding the risk of alcohol consumption during pregnancy be posted in establishments where alcoholic beverages are served. Warning labels are also required on containers of beer, wine, and hard liquor.

Role of Nutrition

Alcohol is directly toxic to the developing embryo and fetus. FAS and ARBD are completely preventable—if a pregnant woman does not drink. The mother who abuses alcohol may also be undernourished because alcohol (7 kcal/g) replaces food and its nutrients. In addition, alcohol reduces absorption and utilization of some nutrients. Undernutrition, especially in regard to protein and zinc, may enhance the effects of excess alcohol (Institute of Medicine, 1990). Nutrient supplements do not counteract the adverse effects of alcohol, but they may be needed to compensate for a poor diet and the effects of alcohol on nutrition status.

Use of Illicit Drugs

Use of licit and illicit drugs during pregnancy has important health implications for the mother and can have immediate and long-term effects on the infant. Infants born of women addicted to narcotics, cocaine, and alcohol often undergo a characteristic withdrawal syndrome and may have physical, behavioral, or neurologic abnormalities. Accurate determination of the impact of illicit drugs is difficult because of a combination of complex socioeconomic and lifestyle factors and polydrug use, cigarette smoking, and alcohol use (Thadani, 1995; Jacobson et al, 1994). Other factors that may complicate the problem include living arrangements, job stability, education, income, and marital status. In a drug-abusing population, pregnancy outcome has been shown to improve with five or more prenatal visits (Broekhuizen et al, 1992), but many drug users receive little or no prenatal care (Handler et al, 1991).

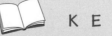

K E Y   T E R M S

morphogenesis: evolution and development of form as an organ or part of the body

Marijuana

According to a national survey conducted by the Department of Health and Human Services (1987), approximately 31% of American women under 30 years of age use marijuana. A study of prenatal drug use in a clinic population found that 27% of the mothers had used marijuana sometime during pregnancy (Zuckerman et al, 1989). Marijuana is the most common illicit drug chosen by adolescents, a population already at substantial risk for an adverse pregnancy outcome (Committee on Adolescence and Committee on Substance Abuse, 1991). Widespread use of marijuana by women in the reproductive years and during pregnancy raises important concerns about potential effects on fetal growth and development.

GENERAL EFFECTS The physiologic effects of marijuana use include a transient acceleration in heart rate and a small rise in blood pressure. There is an initial bronchodilation, but with chronic use the smoke particles can irritate the lungs and eventually cause airway obstruction. The immediate effects include euphoria, relaxation, and disinhibition, but marijuana can interfere with coordination; the ability to judge elapsed time, speed, and distance; the ability to track a moving object; and reaction time, as well as learning and memory.

PRENATAL EFFECTS The major active ingredient of marijuana, delta 9-tetrahydrocannabinol, can cross the placenta. Because marijuana is fat-soluble and is excreted slowly, maternal use may result in prolonged fetal exposure to the drug. Like tobacco smoking, marijuana smoking is associated with increased carboxyhemoglobin levels, potential fetal hypoxia, and, consequently, compromised fetal growth (Wu et al, 1988). This may be compounded by the increase in maternal heart rate and blood pressure, which could further reduce blood flow to the uterus and placental perfusion (Foltin et al, 1987).

PREGNANCY OUTCOME Although fetotoxic effects of marijuana have been reported in animals, information regarding the influence of marijuana smoking on pregnancy outcome in humans is inconsistent. Decreased birth weight and length as well as increased frequency of preterm delivery and altered neurobehavioral responses in neonates have been observed in infants of mothers who used marijuana during pregnancy (Zuckerman et al, 1989). Other studies, however, have reported no effect on birth weight or length of gestation or have produced equivocal results (Fried, 1991). Such inconsistencies may be related to difficulty in identifying and classifying marijuana use and difficulty in controlling for related factors, especially smoking, alcohol, and other drug use.

Cocaine

Cocaine is prepared from the leaves of the plant erythroxylon coca. It is available in two forms, cocaine hydrochloride and the highly purified more potent form known as free-base or "crack," because of the popping sound it makes as the crystals are heated. Cocaine hydrochloride is heat labile but water soluble and is generally administered orally, intravenously, or by nasal insufflation. Crack is heat stable but highly insoluble in water and is therefore generally administered by inhalation (smoking).

GENERAL EFFECTS Cocaine acts as a central nervous system stimulant that increases heart rate, causing hypertension and **vasoconstriction**. Cocaine can influence both the peripheral and central nervous systems. Many of its effects result from interference with the normal function of neurotransmitters. Cocaine impairs the reuptake of the neurotransmitters norepinephrine and epinephrine at the nerve synapses. These neurotransmitters activate the most dramatic acute effects of the drug, e.g., hypertension, **tachycardia**, and vasoconstrictions. Impaired reuptake of another neurotransmitter, dopamine, and its accumulation cause the sense of euphoria that follows the ingestion of cocaine. With long-term cocaine use, dopamine becomes depleted from the nerve endings, contributing to the dysphoria of withdrawal and to the subsequent craving for the drug (Volpe, 1992). Cocaine also impairs the normal metabolism of the neurotransmitter serotonin, which may account for the decreased need for sleep experienced by many users.

PRENATAL EFFECTS OF COCAINE Cocaine has become one of America's leading public health problems, and it is only logical to expect that its use would extend to pregnant women. Gomby and Shiono (1991) estimate that approximately 5% of infants born in 1991 were exposed to cocaine, but rates may vary substantially with socioeconomic status. One inner-city clinic reported that 18% of the women receiving prenatal care had used cocaine at least once during pregnancy (Zuckerman et al, 1989).

Because of its low molecular weight and solubility in water and lipids, cocaine readily crosses the placenta. Although the impact of intrauterine exposure to cocaine has been difficult to assess, there is evidence that its use throughout pregnancy is associated with an increased risk of abruptio placenta, stillbirth, prematurity, and fetal growth restriction (Frank et al, 1993; Young et al, 1992; Handler et al, 1991). Increased levels of catecholamines contribute to premature labor and delivery and increase uterine contractility and may also impair oxygen and nutrient transfer to the fetus, depleting nutrient stores. Vasoconstriction may result in fetal hypoxia by impairing placental blood flow (Woods et al, 1987).

POSTNATAL MANIFESTATIONS Infants of cocaine-abusing mothers have growth retardation, tremulousness, hyperirritability, and hypertoxicity. Cocaine-associated neonatal complications include congenital malformations, seizures, **cerebral infarction**, hemorrhage, auditory system deficits (Lester et al, 1991), sudden infant death syndrome (SIDS), cardiac abnormalities, and behavioral changes. The sudden infant death syndrome is three to seven times more common in offspring of cocaine-abusing mothers. It may be that cocaine exposure impairs the infant's regulation of respiration and arousal, contributing to SIDS. It has been suggested that the effects of the neonatal neurologic syndrome may be due to premature birth rather than cocaine (Coles et al, 1992). Data from other studies indicate inconsistent results regarding catch-up growth (Weathers et al, 1993). Children followed throughout the first year of life continue to show developmental delay and stunting in length but not weight, resulting in infants who are overweight (Harsham et al, 1994).

NEUROLOGIC AND COGNITIVE OUTCOMES

It is difficult to delineate the long-term effects of cocaine on pregnancy outcome because the neurologic and behavioral functions (attention, arousal, motivation, and social interaction) most likely to be affected by intrauterine cocaine exposure are not readily quantitated with conventional measures. Such behaviors and functions are crucial for effective adaptation to social and educational environments, and abnormalities have long-term consequences (Snodgrass, 1994). The relationship of diet to growth in drug-exposed infants is unknown. Based on adult data, it appears that supplementing the diet with additional nutrients may be beneficial (Harsham et al, 1994).

Determination of the effects of intrauterine cocaine exposure is also confounded by deleterious variables in the life of the fetus. As many as half of the pregnant women who use cocaine also abuse other illicit drugs (Handler et al, 1991). Many smoke cigarettes or marijuana, abuse alcohol, and transmit infections such as syphilis or human immunodeficiency virus infection to the fetus. All of this is compounded by the pregnant drug abuser's failure to seek prenatal care.

CONCEPTS TO REMEMBER

➡ A number of maternal characteristics, health conditions, and lifestyle factors, which may operate synergistically, can increase the risk of an adverse pregnancy outcome for infant and mother.

➡ Nutrition assessment and intervention can reduce or modify nutrition risk during the reproductive interval.

➡ Identification of risk and initiation of care before conception or early in pregnancy increase the effectiveness of nutrition intervention.

➡ Extremes of maternal age (particularly under 15 or over 35 years) increase the risk of an adverse pregnancy outcome.

➡ Many sociodemographic characteristics of the mother, including education, income, marital status, and access to health care, can increase reproductive risk.

➡ Maternal health conditions such as obesity, hyperphenylalaninemia, HIV infection, diabetes mellitus, and hypertension, which may contribute to an unfavorable pregnancy outcome, can be modified by nutrition care.

➡ Use or abuse of cigarettes, alcohol, and drugs is associated with adverse fetal outcomes.

References

Abell TD, et al. The effects of maternal smoking on infant birth weight. Fam Med 1991;23:103.

Abrams B, Newman V. Small-for-gestational-age birth: maternal predictors and comparison with risk factors of spontaneous preterm delivery in the same cohort. Am J Obstet Gynecol 1991;164:785.

Alan Guttmacher Institute. Sex and American teenagers. New York: 1994:1.

Allen LH. Iron-deficiency anemia increases risk of preterm delivery. Nutr Rev 1993;51:49.

American Diabetes Association. Gestational diabetes mellitus. Position statement. Diabetes Care 1996;16:5.

American Dietetic Association. Position of The American Dietetic Association: Nutrition care for pregnant adolescents. J Am Diet Assoc 1994;94:499.

Autti-Ramo I, et al. Mental development of 2-year-old children exposed to alcohol in utero. J Pediatr 1992;120:740.

Barclay BA. Experience with enteral nutrition in the treatment of hyperemesis gravidarum. Nutr Clin Proc 1990;5:153.

Beard JL. Iron deficiency: assessment during pregnancy and its importance in pregnant adolescents. Am J Clin Nutr 1994;59:502S.

Belizan JM, et al. Calcium supplementation to prevent hypertensive disorders of pregnancy. N Engl J Med 1991;325:1399.

Berkowitz GS, et al. Delayed childbearing and the outcome of pregnancy. N Engl J Med 1990;322:659.

KEY TERMS

vasoconstriction: decrease in the diameter of blood vessels

tachycardia: abnormally rapid heart rate

cerebral infarction: a clot in one of the blood vessels supplying the brain

Boyce RA. Enteral nutrition in hyperemesis gravidarum: a new development. J Am Diet Assoc 1992;92:733.

Broekhuizen FF, et al. Drug use or inadequate prenatal care? Adverse pregnancy outcome in an urban setting. Am J Obstet Gynecol 1992;166:1747.

Buescher PA, Ward NI. A comparison of low birth weight among Medicaid patients of public health departments and other providers of prenatal care in North Carolina and Kentucky. Public Health Rep 1992;107:54.

Caan BJ, Goldhaber MK. Caffeinated beverages and low birthweight: a case control study. Am J Public Health 1989;79:1299.

Chattingius S, et al. Delayed childbearing and risk of adverse perinatal outcome. A population based study. JAMA 1992;268:886.

Chu SY, et al. Impact of the human immunodeficiency virus epidemic on mortality in women of reproductive age, United States. JAMA 1990;264:225.

Coles CD, et al. Effects of cocaine and alcohol use in pregnancy on neonatal growth and neurobehavioral status. Neurotoxicol Teratol 1992;14:23.

Committee on Adolescence, American Academy of Pediatrics. Adolescent pregnancy. Pediatrics 1989;83:132.

Committee on Adolescence, Committee on Substance Abuse, American Academy of Pediatrics. Marijuana: a continuing concern for pediatricians. Pediatrics 1991;88:1070.

Connor EM, et al. Reduction in maternal-infant transmission of human immunodeficiency virus type I with zidovudine treatment. N Engl J Med 1994;331:1173.

Coustan DR. Gestational diabetes. Diabetes Care 1992;15:716.

Cunningham FG, Lindheimer MD. Hypertension in pregnancy. N Engl J Med 1992;326:927.

Damm P, et al. Predictive factors for the development of diabetes in women with previous gestational diabetes mellitus. Am J Obstet Gynecol 1992;167:607.

Department of Health and Human Services. National household survey on drug abuse: population estimates 1985. Department of Health and Human Services 1987;10 (DHHS publication No. 871539). Washington, DC.

deSanjose S, Roman E. Low birthweight, preterm, and small for gestational age babies in Scotland J Epidemiol Community Health. 1991;45:207.

deVeciana M, et al. Postprandial versus preprandial blood glucose monitoring in women with gestational diabetes mellitus requiring insulin therapy. N Engl J Med 1995;333:1237.

Edwards L, et al. Pregnancy in the underweight woman. Course, outcome and growth patterns of the infants. Am J Obstet Gynecol 1979;135:297.

Ekbald U, Grenman S. Maternal weight, weight gain during pregnancy and pregnancy outcome. Int J Gynaecol Obstet 1992;39:277.

Ellings JM. Reduction in very low birthweight deliveries and perinatal mortality in a specialized, multidisciplinary twin clinic. Obstet Gynecol 1993;81:387.

Erick M. Hyperolfaction and hyperemesis gravidarum: what is the relationship. Nutr Rev 1995;53:289.

Fagan C, et al. Nutrition management in women with gestational diabetes mellitus: a review by the ADA's Diabetes Care and Education dietetic practice group. J Am Diet Assoc 1995;95:40.

Fenster L, et al. Caffeine consumption during pregnancy and fetal growth. Am J Public Health 1991;81:458.

Foltin RW, et al. Marijuana and cocaine interactions in humans: cardiovascular consequences. Pharmacol Biochem Behav 1987;28:459.

Food and Drug Administration (FDA). Caffeine and pregnancy. FDA Drug Bull 1980;10:19.

Frank DA. Maternal cocaine use: impact on child health and development. Ann Pediatr 1993;40:65.

Frazer AM, et al. Association of young maternal age with adverse reproduction outcomes. N Engl J Med 1995;332:1113.

Fried PA. Marijuana use during pregnancy: consequences for offspring. Semin Perinatol 1991;15:280.

Frisancho AR. Developmental and nutritional determinants of pregnancy outcome among teenagers. Am J Phys Anthropol 1985;66:247.

Garcia LM, et al. Acute effects of maternal cigarette smoking on fetal heart rate and fetal body movements felt by the mother. J Perinat Med 1991;19:385.

Garn SM, et al. The biology of teenage pregnancy: the mother and child. In: Lancaster JB, Hamburg BA (eds). School-age pregnancy and parenthood: biosocial dimensions. New York: Aldine de Gruyter, 1986:77.

Garn SM, et al. Are pregnant teenagers still in rapid growth? Am J Dis Child 1984;138:32.

Godel JC, et al. Smoking and caffeine and alcohol intake during pregnancy in a northern population: effect on fetal growth. Can Med Assoc J 1992;147:181.

Goldman M, et al. Obstetric complications with GDM. Effects of maternal weight. Diabetes 1991;40(Suppl 2):79.

Gomby DS, Shiono PH. Estimating the number of substance-exposed infants. Future of children. 1991;1:17.

Gould J, LeRoy S. Socioeconomic status and low birth weight: a racial comparison. Pediatrics 1988;82:896.

Greenspoon JS, et al. Use of peripherally inserted central catheter for parenteral nutrition during pregnancy. Obstet Gynecol 1993;81:831.

Gross S, et al. Maternal weight loss associated with hyperemesis gravidarum: a predictor of fetal outcome. Am J Obstet Gynecol 1989;160:906.

Grubman S, et al. Older children and adolescents living with perinatally acquired human deficiency virus infection. Pediatrics 1995;95:657.

Guillermo C, et al. Calcium supplementation during pregnancy: a systematic review of randomized controlled trials. Br J Obstet Gynaecol 1994;101:753.

Gulley RM. The treatment of hyperemesis gravidarum with nasogastric feeding. Nutr Clin Pract 1993;8:33.

Haiek L, Lederman SA. The relationship between maternal weight for height and term birth weight in teens and adult women. J Adolesc Health Care 1988;10:16.

Handler A, et al. Cocaine use during pregnancy: perinatal outcomes. Am J Epidemiol 1991;7:270.

Hansen JP. Older maternal age and pregnancy outcome. A review of literature. Obstet Gynecol Surv 1986;41:726.

Harsham J, et al. Growth patterns of infants exposed to cocaine and other drugs in utero. J Am Diet Assoc 1994;94:909.

Haste FM, et al. The effect of nutritional intake on outcome of pregnancy in smokers and non-smokers. Br J Nutr 1991;65:347.

Hediger ML, et al. Rate and amount of weight gain during adolescent pregnancy: associations with maternal weight-for-height and birth weight. Am J Clin Nutr 1990;52:793.

Hickey CA, et al. Prenatal weight gain, term birth weight and fetal growth retardation among high-risk multiparous black women. Obstet Gynecol 1993;81:529.

Hod M, et al. Gestational diabetes mellitus. A survey of perinatal complications in the 1980s. Diabetes 1991;40(Suppl 2):74.

Institute of Medicine. Nutrition during pregnancy: weight gain and nutrient supplements. Report of the Subcommittee on Nutritional Status and Weight Gain During Pregnancy, Committee on Nutritional Status During Pregnancy and Lactation, Food and Nutrition Board. Washington, D.C.: National Academy Press, 1990.

Jacobson J, et al. Teratogenic effects of alcohol on infant development. Alcohol Clin Exp Res 1993;17:174.

Jacobson JL, et al. Effects of alcohol use, smoking and illicit drug use on fetal growth in black infants. J Pediatr 1994;124:757.

Johnson JWC, et al. Excessive maternal weight and pregnancy outcome. Am J Obstet Gynecol 1992;167:353.

Jonas O, et al. The association of maternal and socioeconomic characteristics in metropolitan Adelaide with medical, obstetric and labor complications and pregnancy outcomes. Aust NZ J Obstet Gynecol 1992;32:1

Jovanovic-Peterson L, Peterson CM. Pregnancy in the diabetic woman. Endocrinol Metab Clin North Am 1991;21:433.

Jovanovic-Peterson L, Peterson CM. Vitamin and mineral deficiencies which may predispose to glucose in tolerance in pregnancy. J Am Coll Nutr 1996;15:14.

Kindrick JS, et al. Integrating smoking cessation into routine public prenatal care: the Smoking Cessation in Pregnancy Project. Am J Public Health 1995;85:217.

Knight KB, Keith RE. Calcium supplementation on normotensive and hypertensive pregnant women. Am J Clin Nutr 1992;55:891.

Knupfer G. Abstaining for foetal health: the fiction that even light drinking is dangerous. Brit J Addict 1991;86:1063.

Lenke RR, Levy HL. Maternal phenylketonuria and hyperphenylalaninemia: An international survey of the outcome of treated and untreated pregnancies. N Engl J Med 1990;303:1202.

Lester BM, et al. Neurobehavioral syndromes in cocaine-exposed newborn infants. Child Dev 1991;62:694.

Levine MG, Esser D. Total parenteral nutrition for the treatment of severe hyperemesis gravidarum: maternal nutritional effects and fetal outcome. Obstet Gynecol 1988;72:102.

Lifshitz F, et al. Children's nutrition. Boston; Jones and Bartlett, 1991.

Lindgren S, et al. HIV and child-bearing: clinical outcome and aspects of mother-to-infant transmission. AIDS 1991;5:1111.

Luder AS, Greene CL. Maternal phenylketonuria and hyperphenylalaninemia: implications for medical practice in the United States. Am J Obstet Gynecol 1989;161:1102.

Luke B, Keith LG. The contribution of singletons, twins and triplets to low birth weight. J Reprod Med 1992;37:661.

Luke B, et al. The ideal twin pregnancy: patterns of weight gain and discordancy and length of gestation. Am J Obstet Gynecol 1993;169:588.

Magann EF, Martin JN. The laboratory evaluation of hypertensive gravida. Obstet Gynecol Surv 1995;50:138.

Marcoux S, et al. Calcium intake from dairy products and supplements and the risk of preeclampsia and gestational hypertension. Am J Epidemiol 1991;133:1266.

McAnarney ER. Young maternal age and adverse neonatal outcome. Am J Dis Child 1987;141:1053.

McDonald AD, et al. Cigarette, alcohol and coffee consumption and prematurity. Am J Public Health 1992;82:87.

Melnikow J, et al. Characteristics of inner-city women giving birth with little or no prenatal care: a case control study. J Fam Pract 1991;32:283.

Mitchell MC, Lerner E. Factors that influence the outcome of pregnancy in middle-class women. J Am Diet Assoc 1987;87:731.

Mitchell MC, Lerner E. Weight gain and pregnancy outcome in underweight and normal weight women. J Am Diet Assoc 1989;89:634.

Mofenson L. Epidemiology and determinants of vertical HIV transmission. Semin Pediatr Infect Dis 1994;5:252.

MMWR. Infant Mortality—United States. MMWR 1993;42:161.

Moreno JD, Minkoff H. Human immunodeficiency virus infection during pregnancy. Clin Obstet Gynecol 1992;35:813.

Naeye RL. Teenaged and pre-teenaged pregnancies: Consequences of the fetal-maternal competition for nutrients. Pediatrics 1981;67:146.

Naeye RL. Perinatal mortality rates of overweight, normal weight and underweight mothers as related to weight gain. Am J Obstet Gynecol 1979;135:3.

Naeye RL, Friedman EA. Causes of perinatal death associated with gestational hypertension and proteinuria. Am J Obstet Gynecol 1979;133:8.

Nanda D, Minkoff HL. Pregnancy and women at risk for HIV infection. Primary Care 1992;19:157.

Narod SA, et al. Coffee during pregnancy: a reproductive hazard? Am J Obstet Gynecol 1991;164:1109.

National Center for Health Statistics. Advance report of maternal and infant health data from the birth certificate. Monthly Vital Stat Rep 1994;42(no. 11S):1.

National Center for Health Statistics. Advance report of final natality statistics, 1991. Monthly Vital Stat Rep 1993;4:13 (Suppl).

National High Blood Pressure Education Program Working Group Report on High Blood Pressure in Pregnancy. Am J Obstet Gynecol 1993;163:1691.

National Institute of Health Consensus Development Conference on Optional Calcium Intakes. National Institutes of Health, Bethesda, MD, 1994.

National Research Council. Recommended Dietary Allowances. 10th ed. Report of the Subcommittee on the Tenth Edition of the RDAs. Food and Nutrition Board, Commission on Life Sciences. Washington DC: National Academy Press, 1989.

Newcombe WE, et al. Reproduction in the older gravida. A literature review. J Reprod Med 1991;36:839.

Olds DL, et al. Intellectual impairment in children of women who smoke cigarettes during pregnancy. Pediatrics 1994;93:221.

Pederson A, et al. Weight gain patterns during twin gestations. J Am Diet Assoc 1989;89.

Perlow JH. Perinatal outcome in pregnancy complicated by massive obesity. Am J Obstet Gynecol 1992;167:958.

Platt LD, et al. Maternal phenylketonuria collaborative study: obstetric aspects and outcome: the first six years. Am J Obstet Gynecol 1992;166:1150.

Poland ML, et al. Prenatal care: a path (not taken) to improved perinatal outcome. J Perinat Med 1991;19:427.

Prysak M, et al. Pregnancy outcome in nulliparous women 35 years and older. Obstet Gynecol 1995;85:65.

Pykowicz A, et al. Fetal alcohol syndrome in adolescents and adults. JAMA 1991;265:1961.

Reese JM, et al. Weight gain in adolescents during pregnancy: rate related to birth-weight outcome. Am J Clin Nutr 1992;56:868.

Roberts JM, Redman CWG. Pre-eclampsia: more than pregnancy-induced hypertension. Lancet 1993;341:1447.

Roche AR, Davilla GH. Late adolescent growth in stature. Pediatrics 1972;50:874.

Rossett HL, et al. Treatment experience with pregnant problem drinkers. JAMA 1983;249:2029.

Rosso P. Nutrition and metabolism in pregnancy. Mother and fetus. New York: Oxford University Press, 1990.

Rush D, et al. A trial of health education aimed to reduce cigarette smoking among pregnant women. Ped Perinat Epidemiol 1992;6:285.

Schneck ME, et al. Low-income pregnant adolescents and their infants: dietary findings and health outcomes. J Am Diet Assoc 1990;90:555.

Scholl TO, et al. Maternal growth during pregnancy and the competition for nutrients. Am J Clin Nutr 1994a;60:183.

Scholl TO, et al. Prenatal care and maternal health during adolescent pregnancy: a review and metanalysis. J Adolesc Health 1994b;15:444.

Scholl TO, Hediger ML. A review of the epidemiology of nutrition and adolescent pregnancy: maternal growth during pregnancy and its effect on the fetus. J Am Coll Nutr 1993;12:101.

Scholl TO, et al. Anemia vs. iron deficiency: increased risk of preterm delivery in a prospective study. Am J Clin Nutr 1992;55:985.

Scholl TO, et al. Maternal weight gain, diet and infant birth weight: correlations during adolescent pregnancy. J Clin Epidemiol 1991;44:423.

Seely EW, et al. Lower serum calcium and abnormal calciotropic hormone levels in preeclampsia. J Clin Endocrinol Metab 1992;74:1436.

Seidman DS, et al. The effects of high parity and socioeconomic status on obstetric and neonatal outcome. Arch Gynecol Obstet 1991;249:119.

Skinner JD, et al. Food and nutrient intake of white, pregnant adolescents. J Am Diet Assoc 1992;92:1127.

Smith KJ, Eckardt MJ. The effects of prenatal alcohol on the central nervous system. Recent Dev Alcohol 1991;9:151.

Snodgrass SR. Cocaine babies: a result of multiple teratogenic influences. J Child Neurol 1994;9:227.

Spohr HL, et al. Prenatal alcohol exposure and long-term developmental consequences. Lancet 1993;341:907.

Srisuphan W, Bracken MB. Caffeine consumption during pregnancy and association with late spontaneous abortion. Am J Obstet Gynecol 1986;154:14.

Story M, Alton I. Nutrition issues and adolescent pregnancy. Nutr Today 1995;30:142.

Thadani PV. Biological mechanisms and perinatal exposure to abused drugs. Synapse 1995;19:228

Thompson GN, et al. Pregnancy in phenylketonuria: dietary treatment aimed at normalizing maternal plasma phenylalanine concentration. Arch Dis Child 1991;66:1346.

U.S. Public Health Service. Recommendations for human immunodeficiency virus counseling and voluntary testing for pregnant women. MMWR 1995:44:1.

Volpe JJ. Effect of cocaine use on the fetus. N Engl J Med 1992;327:399.

Weathers WT, et al. Cocaine use in women from a defined population: prevalence at delivery and effects on growth in infants. Pediatrics 1993;91:350.

Weitzman M, et al. Maternal smoking and behavior problems of children. Pediatrics 1992;90:342.

Williams MA, et al. Cigarettes, coffee and preterm premature rupture of membranes. Am J Epidemiol 1992;135:895.

Williams MA, et al. Risk factors for abruptio placentae. Am J Epidemiol 1991;134:965.

Wilson AL, et al. Does prenatal care decrease the incidence and cost of neonatal intensive care admissions? Am J Perinatol 1992;9:281.

Windham GC, et al. Parental cigarette smoking and the risk of spontaneous abortion. Am J Epidemiol 1992;135:1394.

Woods JR Jr, et al. Effect of cocaine on uterine blood flow and fetal oxygenation. JAMA 1987;257:957.

Wu T-C, et al. Pulmonary hazards of smoking marijuana as compared with tobacco. N Engl J Med 1988;318:347.

Young SL, et al. Cocaine: its effects on maternal and child health. Pharmacotherapy 1992;12:2.

Zhang J, Savitz DA. Maternal age and placenta previa: A population-based, case-control study. Am J Obstet Gynecol 1993;168:641.

Zuckerman B, et al. Effects of maternal marijuana and cocaine use on fetal growth. N Engl J Med 1989;320:762.

Zuckerman B, et al. Adolescent pregnancy: behavioral determinants of outcome. J Pediatr 1984;105:857.

APPLICATION: Health Care and Nutrition Resources for Pregnant Women and Their Offspring

When Lori was 27 years old, she was the single mother of boys ages 2 and 4. Two years before, when Lori was divorced, she was awarded custody and child support of $100 per week. That was barely enough to pay her rent, much less feed her children. A social worker advised her to apply for Aid for Families with Dependent Children (AFDC). Qualifying for welfare also made her eligible for Medicaid, food stamps, and the Special Supplemental Food Program for Women, Infants and Children (WIC), which together allowed her to "get by" and make sure the children got enough food. Over time Lori became discouraged and wanted to "do something with her life." She applied for admission to a small community college and began to take classes one at a time. She was eligible for financial aid, and with some small scholarships and childcare allowances she was able to manage school and her children. Today is graduation. Lori will receive an associate degree and already has a part-time position. Because she won't make very much money at first she will continue to receive food stamps until she gets a full-time job. She can't wait to be on her own and is very grateful for the programs that made it possible.

Poverty creates a vulnerability that increases nutrition and health risk. Poor families are more likely to have inadequate diets than families with higher incomes (Kotch and Shackelfor, 1989). The primary goal of providing services for women is to improve their health and that of their children. Inadequate resources or skills may limit the ability of many women to obtain a sufficient quantity or quality of food or resources to access medical care. Government programs (Table A9–1) that help include general assistance programs that target individuals and families who live at or near the poverty level, and programs that have more liberal income criteria but are specifically designed for pregnant and lactating women and their infants and children who are considered at risk.

TABLE A9–1 Federal Programs That Assist Mothers and Their Offspring

Program	Recipients	Benefits
Medicaid	All individuals with incomes <133% of poverty level	Total health care
Healthy Start (Medicaid)	Pregnant women with incomes <185% of poverty level; special high risk pregnancies	Prenatal and postpartum care of infants and children
HEALTH CHEK (Medicaid)	Infants, children and adolescents through 21 years	Health screening—vision, hearing, dental checks, and health education
Food stamps	All individuals with incomes <133% of poverty level	Increased food buying power via stamps to be exchanged for food in food markets
Commodity distribution	Pregnant and postpartum women, infants and children < 6 years of age with household income ≤185% of federal poverty level	Monthly food package of fruits, vegetables, meats, infant formula, beans, and other foods as available
EFNEP*	Low income (≤125% of federal poverty level) households with children under 19 years of age	Nutrition aides provide nutrition education to homemakers
WIC†	Pregnant women, postpartum and lactating women, infants and children up to 5 years of age	Direct food supplements, nutrition education, referral to health services

* Expanded Food and Nutrition Education Program
† Special Supplemental Food Program for Women, Infants and Children

Health Care Programs

Medicaid

Medicaid is a healthcare program for low-income individuals of all ages who do not have the money or health insurance to pay for medical services. Eligibility criteria for Medicaid are determined by federal and state regulations. In general, a family is considered financially eligible if their monthly income after allowable deductions is below 133% of the federal poverty level for that family size. Medicaid is available to families who are on Aid for Families with Dependent Children (AFDC) and to low-income pregnant women and their young children. Other individuals eligible for Medicaid include low-income people 65 years of age or older, adults and children who are blind or disabled, and people in nursing facilities who do not have enough income or resources to pay for the cost of their care.

Applicants must complete an application and be interviewed by a case worker regarding the need for medical assistance. Applicants are required to provide Social Security numbers, birth certificates, proof of income and assets, medical bills, and information about medical treatment. The Medicaid recipient receives a medical assistance identification card, which is renewed monthly. A current ID card is necessary to get medical services. Pregnant women who are eligible for Medicaid can get Expedited Medicaid, which makes them eligible for Medicaid very quickly. They have 60 days to provide documentation to ensure continued eligibility.

If the healthcare service is covered under Medicaid, there is no charge to the client. Medicaid pays for doctors or clinic visits (up to 24 medical visits in a calendar year), laboratory services, and prescription drugs. Pregnancy-related visits and well child visits are not counted toward the 24-visit limitation. If a mother is already on Medicaid when she becomes pregnant, the medical care required during pregnancy, including regular checkups and the hospital stay during delivery, are covered. Medicaid is available to mothers who do not meet the eligibility requirements if the pregnancy is categorized as a high-risk. They can receive special services both prenatally and after the baby arrives.

Healthy Start

Healthy Start is a program established by Congress that extends Medicaid benefits to pregnant women with incomes up to 185% of the poverty level (Haas et al, 1993). Services provided include regular medical care during pregnancy and postpartum, delivery of the infant, regular check-ups for the new baby, medication prescribed for mother or child, vaccinations to prevent childhood disease, and routine care for the child. Coverage is extended to financially eligible pregnant mothers any time during their pregnancy until 60 days after delivery, and to their offspring up through 8 years of age.

Health Chek

HEALTH CHEK (EPSDT) is a preventive healthcare program for children and adolescents from birth through 21 years who are eligible for Medicaid. Four types of services are available through HEALTH CHEK—a complete screening physical examination including vision, hearing and dental checks; assessment of growth and development; immunizations (polio, whooping cough, measles, mumps, diphtheria, and tetanus); and health education. Tests for tuberculosis, lead poisoning, anemia, sickle cell anemia, and other problems are completed as needed. Those women who qualify for Medicaid are often eligible for other food or nutrition programs and, if so, are encouraged to participate.

Food Stamp Program

The Food Stamp Program, initiated in 1964, is the cornerstone of the nation's food assistance programs. It is designed to improve the diets of low-income families by helping them buy food. All low-income households that have resources (aside from income) of $2000 or less are eligible. Eligibility is determined after application and certification by

---

poverty level: defined by the federal government as a level below which people are at risk of being unable to obtain adequate food, shelter, and health care

Expedited Medicaid: eligibility for Medicaid card with only identification and proof of pregnancy

EPSDT: early and periodic screening, diagnosis and treatment

local public assistance or social services. The program increases the purchasing power of the eligible family by providing monthly allotments of coupons that can be used to purchase food at participating supermarkets. Monthly allotments are based on household size and income. The amount of coupons received is based on the cost of the Thrifty Food Plan. New programs are being developed in some states to allow electronic transfer of food stamp allotments, almost like credit cards to be used in the market, which will cut costs and decrease fraud (selling of food stamps) in the program.

Commodity Supplemental Food Program (CSFP)

The Commodity Supplemental Food Program was initiated to distribute surplus food commodities to individuals and federally supported organizations. Pregnant women, breast-feeding women, other postpartum women, infants and children (ages < 6 years) with a household income equal to or less than 185% of the federal poverty levels are eligible to receive food packages. The monthly benefits include fruits, vegetables, meats, infant formula, farina, beans and other foods as available.

There is a federally funded program (Food Distribution Program on Indian Reservations) for distribution of monthly food packages to American Indian households living on or near reservations. These packages contain a wide variety of canned or packaged foods. A third food distribution program is the Temporary Emergency Food Assistance Program (TEFAP), which provides emergency supplies of dairy products and grains once a month and other staples quarterly. These products are available to households whose incomes are equal to or below 150% of the federal poverty level.

Cooperative Extension—Expanded Food and Nutrition Education Program (EFNEP)

The EFNEP program was funded in 1969 through the USDA via the Agricultural Extension Service in each state. It is designed to teach low-income families the skills needed to select, purchase, and prepare a varied, adequate diet. Trained nutrition aides work directly with low-income homemakers (from households with incomes equal to or below 125% of the federal poverty level) and with children under 19 years of age who are considered at nutrition risk.

Special Supplemental Food Program for Women, Infants and Children (WIC)

The Special Supplemental Food Program for Women, Infants and Children (WIC) was authorized by Congress in 1972 (Public Law 92–433), which added a new section to the Child Nutrition Act of 1966. It was developed to improve the health of pregnant and postpartum women, infants, and children up to 5 years old by providing supplemental foods, nutrition education, and access to health services. Eligibility for the target population is determined by income level and residency requirements. Program benefits are directed toward pregnant women and their offspring who are at nutrition risk based on the criteria listed in the margin.

Supplemental Foods

By law, 80% of WIC funds must be expended on food benefits. Supplemental food is provided in the form of direct food deliveries to participants or as vouchers that can be exchanged for approved foods in a market. Food packages are tailored to meet the needs of the recipient, targeting specific nutrients frequently lacking in the diets of low-income individuals—protein, iron, calcium, and vitamins A and C. Except for infants, the food packages are provided to supplement the normal diet, not replace it.

To provide optimal nutrition and feeding for the infant, breast-feeding is promoted in the WIC program through education and support, but the mother is allowed to choose the feeding method. Breast-feeding women may receive benefits for up to 1 year postpartum, whereas non–breast-feeding women are eligible for only 6 months postpartum. Approx-

Thrifty Food Plan: a food plan prepared by the USDA that tests specific types and amounts of food needed to achieve a nutritionally adequate diet at minimal cost. Costs of such a diet are published quarterly.

surplus food commodities: food products purchased by the federal government as part of agricultural programs which are available for distribution

income criteria: 185% of the U.S. poverty level or below

residency criteria: the participant must live in the area served by the WIC clinic as specified by the local agency

evidence of nutrition risk:
Anemia
Extremes of leanness or obesity
Poor pregnancy history
Dietary risks resulting from inadequate dietary patterns

WIC packages consist of:
Iron-fortified infant formula
Milk and cheese, eggs
Iron-fortified adult and infant cereals
Fruit and vegetable juices rich in vitamin C
Dried peas or beans and peanut butter

WIC food packages for infants consist of:

0–3 months: 40 oz of concentrated liquid iron-fortified formula containing at least 10 mg iron/L and 67 kcal/100 mL

4–12 months: iron-fortified formula, iron-fortified infant cereal with a minimum of 45 mg of iron per 100 g of dry cereal, fruit or vegetable juice high in vitamin C.

imately one-third of WIC infants were being breast-fed at the time their mothers were discharged from the hospital compared with 64% of non-WIC infants.

The majority of the program's infants receive WIC food packages. The WIC program provides two separate food packages for infants, one for those up to 3 months of age and the other for those 4 to 12 months of age. The basic component of WIC food packages for infants is iron-fortified infant formula, which is a complete formula requiring only the addition of water before being fed. After 4 months additional foods are provided.

NUTRITION EDUCATION

Nutrition education, an integral component of the WIC program, became mandatory in 1975. Local agencies are required to spend at least 16% of WIC administrative funds on nutrition education and counseling. A minimum of two education sessions must be provided to the mother receiving WIC supplements in each 6-month certification period. However, participants cannot be denied food supplements if they do not attend the education sessions. The education component addresses dietary needs of the recipients and often focuses on preparing WIC foods and incorporating them into the diet.

REFERRALS TO HEALTH AND SOCIAL SERVICE AGENCIES

WIC funds are designated for foods and nutrition education. They may not be used to provide health care to participants. However, WIC providers must advise clients about available health care, accessible locations of healthcare facilities, how to receive health care, and why it is useful. In fact, a major benefit of the WIC program may be a general improvement in the health of mothers and their children due to increased health care obtained as a result of the referral.

EFFECTIVENESS OF THE PROGRAM

Since its inception in 1972, the WIC program has grown steadily. In the fiscal year 1991, an estimated 5.2 million women, infants, and children received benefits, at a cost of $2.3 billion. Because of the cost of the WIC program and the expectation that outcomes can be measured, much effort has been expended to document the effectiveness of the WIC program. The National WIC Evaluation (NWE) was a 5-year study (1979–1984) of pregnancy outcome of WIC participants compared to non-WIC women of similar backgrounds. Overall, WIC participants were found to have a greater mean duration of gestation (1.4 days longer) and an increase in mean birth weight of 23 g (Rush et al, 1988; Rush, 1986).

WIC is considered a cost-effective intervention program. The USDA estimates that, on average, every prenatal care dollar spent on WIC saves an average of $3 in later Medicaid costs (USDA, 1993). Numerous smaller studies have been conducted to evaluate the effect of WIC program participation on pregnancy outcome. Birth weight is considered the most significant predictor of subsequent short- and long-term health problems in neonates, such as respiratory difficulties and developmental disabilities. Most studies found a positive effect of prenatal participation in WIC on infant birth weight (Buescher et al, 1993; Kotelchuck et al, 1984). Only a few studies have examined the effect of WIC participation on infants and children, mainly because criteria for success are difficult to determine and measure. Studies have reported improved dietary intakes (Brown et al, 1986; Rush, 1986).

For millions of women, infants, and children, like Lori and her children, federal health and nutrition programs provide the safety net that decreases the risk of inadequate diets and promotes health. Increased referral of eligible pregnant women and their offspring to such programs will increase their effectiveness.

REFERENCES

Brown J, Tieman P. Effect of income and WIC on the dietary intake of preschoolers: results of a preliminary study. J Am Diet Assoc 1986;86:1189.

Buescher PA, et al. Prenatal WIC participation can reduce low birth weight and newborn medical costs: A cost-benefit analyses of WIC participation in North Carolina. J Am Diet Assoc 1993;93:163.

Haas JJ, et al. The effect of providing health coverage to poor uninsured pregnant women in Massachusetts. JAMA 1993;269:87.

Kotch J, Shackelfor J. The nutritional status of low-income preschool children in the United States: A review of the literature. Washington, DC: Food Research and Action Center, 1989.

Kotelchuck M, et al. WIC participation and pregnancy outcomes: Massachusetts statewide evaluation project. Am J Public Health 1994;74:1086.

Rush D, et al. National WIC Evaluation. Historical study of pregnancy outcomes. Am J Clin Nutr 1988;48:412.

Rush D. National Evaluation of the Special Supplemental Food Program for Women, Infants, and Children (WIC). Vol I. Summary. Washington, DC: US Dept. of Agriculture, 1986.

USDA. The Better Nutrition and Health for Children Act of 1993. The Federal Register 1993; S14841–S14855.

CHAPTER 10

LACTATION AND BREAST-FEEDING

Daren and Joyce are expecting their first child in 5 months. Amid discussions of possible names, nursery decor, and childcare possibilities they consider how to feed their infant. They learn that although both of them were bottle-fed, health experts now recommend breast-feeding. They wonder what breast-feeding is like. Is it easy or difficult? How will they be sure their infant is getting enough to eat? Can Joyce continue breast-feeding when she returns to work?

Many expectant parents wonder about breast-feeding, a natural relationship that has received increased medical interest as the unique composition and benefits of human milk have been discovered. To answer their questions parents look to family, friends, and health-care providers. Sometimes the information they receive is not complete or accurate. In the past, few health professionals were adequately prepared to discuss breast-feeding, and some discouraged it. Today the tide is changing. Health professionals are learning the benefits of and techniques for breast-feeding so they may better inform and aid concerned parents.

ADVANTAGES OF BREAST-FEEDING

■ What health advantages does breast-feeding provide to the infant?

■ What constituents in human milk help to provide health benefits for the infant?

■ What advantages does breast-feeding provide to the mother?

Breast-feeding is widely recognized as the optimal way to nourish a human infant. Experts on infant feeding recommend breast-feeding for all term infants, citing nutritional, immunologic, hygienic, and emotional benefits

(American Dietetic Association, 1993; Institute of Medicine, 1991). In addition, breast-feeding mothers benefit both in the immediate postpartum period and later in life.

In developing countries breast-feeding may mean the difference between life and death for the infant. Breast-feeding greatly reduces the incidence of diarrheal illness, particularly in environments with contaminated water and poor sanitation. Additionally, breast-feeding reduces the risk of respiratory illness, meningitis, and other serious infections. Researchers have repeatedly documented that artificially fed infants are 3 to 5 times more likely to die than breast-fed infants (Cunningham, 1991).

Even in industrialized countries where the use of hygienic, scientifically formulated commercial substitutes

Contributed by Kathryn Witt.

for human milk is commonplace, breast-fed infants are less likely to become ill and die. Breast-feeding is associated with reduced risks of gastrointestinal, respiratory, middle ear, and other infections as well as sudden infant death syndrome. Overall, breast-feeding is associated with a reduction in the infant mortality rate of 4 per 1000. Later in life, breast-fed infants are less likely to develop type I diabetes mellitus, food allergies, ulcerative colitis, and Crohn's disease (Cunningham, 1991).

The health benefits of breast milk are related to its unique composition. The nutrient content of human milk is ideally suited for rapidly developing human infants (Chapter 4 provides a description of the nutrient content of human milk). Moreover, several nutrients, including iron and zinc, have been shown to be better absorbed from human milk than from cow's milk or a commercial formula.

In addition to these nutritional advantages breast milk provides a complex array of cells and compounds that prevent infection, as well as enzymes, hormones, and growth factors (see Tables 4–8 and 4–9 in Chapter 4) (Institute of Medicine, 1991). The stomach of a newborn infant produces low amounts of acid and pepsin; thus, the beneficial substances in breast milk are able to survive digestion. They function largely on the mucosal surface of the gastrointestinal tract, but some also cross the mucosal barrier (Lawrence, 1994). These important nonnutritional benefits of breast milk are not available in commercial breast milk substitutes.

The benefits of breast-feeding are not confined to the infant. During the postpartum period the uterus shrinks back to its prepregnant size more quickly in breast-feeding mothers. Ovulation and menstruation are suppressed for a longer period in women who exclusively breast-feed, which lengthens the interval between births and conserves iron. When the infant is hungry, breast milk is readily available, eliminating the need to purchase and prepare formula and bottles. Additionally, the repeated intimate contact between mother and infant fosters **maternal–infant bonding**. A long-term benefit is that women who have breast-fed appear to be less likely to develop breast cancer and osteoporosis (American Dietetic Association, 1993).

BREAST-FEEDING RATES

■ How have breast-feeding rates in the United States changed in the past 2 to 3 decades?

■ What is the current rate of breast-feeding in the United States?

Breast-feeding in the United States declined after World War II to a low of about 25% of 1-week old infants in 1970. During the 1970s and early 1980s breast-feeding rates more than doubled, but then fell off slightly in the later 1980s. In 1989, 52% of new mothers initiated

breast-feeding and 18% were still breast-feeding at 6 months of age (Institute of Medicine, 1991; Ryan et al, 1991). In 1994 breast-feeding rates had increased somewhat, to 57.4% at discharge from the hospital and 19.7% at 6 months (Ross Products Division of Abbott Laboratories, 1995). The Healthy People 2000 goal for breast-feeding is to increase the incidence of breast-feeding to 75% at discharge from the hospital or other place of birth and 50% at 5 to 6 months (U.S. Department of Health and Human Services, 1990).

PHYSIOLOGY OF LACTATION

■ Describe the anatomy of the human breast.

■ What hormones control milk production?

■ How does infant suckling result in milk production and release?

■ How is milk production sustained?

The Mammary Gland

Anatomy

The human **mammary gland** consists of a system of 15 to 20 ducts surrounded by **alveoli** (Fig. 10–1). The nipple contains lactiferous ducts surrounded by firm muscular tissue. The circular pigmented skin area around the nipple, the areola, contains **sebaceous glands**, which are believed to release secretions that lubricate the nipple. The areolar tissues contain bundles of smooth muscle that can stiffen the nipple, allowing a better grasp by the suckling infant. The lactiferous ducts in the nipple expand back to form the short **lactiferous sinuses** in which milk may be stored. The lactiferous sinuses are continuations of the mammary ducts, which extend from the alveoli toward the nipple. Milk is produced in the alveoli and travels

K E Y   T E R M S

maternal–infant bonding: development of strong emotional ties between mother and infant
mammary glands: glands of the female breast that secrete milk
alveoli: small sac-like, milk-producing and secreting areas of the mammary glands
sebaceous glands: minute glands in the skin that secrete an oily, colorless, odorless fluid (sebum)
lactiferous sinus: a cavity or hollow space involved in transporting milk

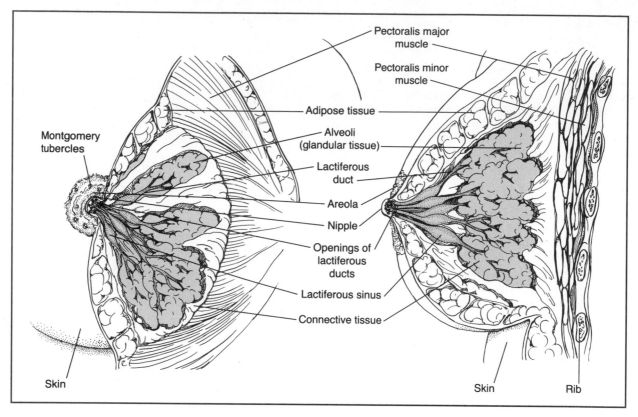

FIGURE 10–1. Anatomy of a mammary gland. (From Gorrie TM, McKinney ES, Murray SS. Foundations of National Newborn Nursing. Philadelphia: WB Saunders, 1994.)

down small ductules into larger ducts and finally into sinuses located beneath the areola.

Maturation

The breasts begin to develop at puberty, a process stimulated by estrogen. During pregnancy the hormones estrogen and progesterone stimulate proliferation of the ducts and alveoli. Although milk production begins during pregnancy, it is limited by the hormone prolactin inhibitory hormone (PIH), produced by the placenta. At delivery, the levels of estrogen, progesterone, and PIH decline dramatically, triggering the onset of lactation.

Milk Production

The process of milk production occurs in two distinct but closely related stages: production of milk and release of the milk for infant consumption. Production of milk involves the synthesis of the milk components and passage of the formed product into the alveolar **lumen**. The second stage, **let-down**, is the ejection of milk from the alveoli and ducts. Both of these processes are stimulated by the suckling of the infant.

Infant Sucking

Term human infants are born with reflexes that help them **latch-on** and suckle effectively. When an infant's cheek is lightly brushed, he will open his mouth and turn toward the touch. This **rooting reflex** enables a mother to position her infant so he is able to grasp the areolar area in its mouth and exert pressure on the lactiferous sinus located underneath the areola. When properly latched on, the infant's tongue and gums work together to push milk from the lactiferous sinus out through the nipple (Fig. 10–2). Sucking and swallowing reflexes work together. The tongue and jaw suck milk from the breast and swallowing follows.

Milk Production and Release

When an infant suckles, the hormones prolactin and oxytocin stimulate milk production and release (Fig. 10–3). **Prolactin**, secreted by the anterior pituitary, acts on mammary alveolar cells and promotes continued milk production and release. Milk is secreted continuously into the alveoli, but milk does not flow easily from the alveoli into

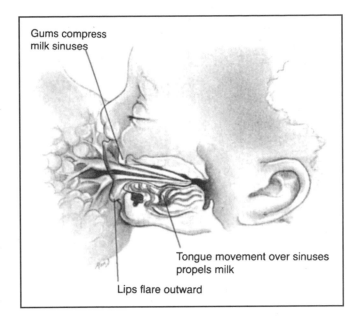

Gums compress
milk sinuses

Tongue movement over sinuses
propels milk

Lips flare outward

FIGURE 10–2. When the infant suckles, receptors in the nipple and areola send stimuli to the hypothalamus. The hypothalamus stimulates release of prolactin from the anterior pituitary which stimulates milk secretion and oxytocin from the posterior pituitary stimulates ejection of milk from the alveolus. (From Gorrie TM, McKinney ES, Murray SS. Foundations of National Newborn Nursing. Philadelphia: WB Saunders, 1994.)

the ductile system. The posterior pituitary secretes the hormone **oxytocin**, known as the "let-down hormone," which triggers ejection of milk from the breast. Oxytocin is carried in the bloodstream to the small muscle-like cells around the alveoli, causing them to contract. The muscle contraction pushes the milk out of the alveoli and along the duct system, where it is easily available to the nursing infant. The milk ejection or let-down reflex is sensitive to a variety of neurohormonal mechanisms. For example, milk ejection can become inhibited by anxiety, stress or fatigue in the mother. It can also become a conditioned response triggered by associations with nursing such as the infant's cry.

The fluid produced by the breasts changes during the course of lactation and within a feeding. Full lactation does not begin at **parturition**. During the first few days after birth the breasts secrete a small amount of **colostrum**. By the end of the first week postpartum colostrum is usually replaced by increasing amounts of mature milk. This transition occurs more slowly in women breast-feeding for the first time.

Mature milk varies in fat content during the course of a single feeding. The foremilk released when an infant initially latches on to a breast is lower in fat than the hindmilk available later. To receive adequate calories, infants need to nurse long enough to receive the rich hindmilk.

Maintenance of Lactation

If milk is not regularly removed from the mother's breasts, the ability to continue producing milk is lost in a week or two due to cessation of prolactin secretion. Suckling stimulation and breast emptying are the most effective

means of maintaining adequate milk volume (Dewey et al, 1991). Artificial sucking stimulation in the form of manual expression or use of a breast pump can maintain or increase milk production in the absence of the infant. A mother who returns to work after the birth of her baby can successfully maintain lactation by a combination of nursing and manual expression or pumping. Manually expressed milk can be refrigerated and given to the infant in the absence of the mother.

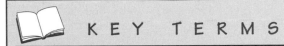

KEY TERMS

lumen: cavity or channel
let-down: movement of milk from the alveoli through the duct system and lactiferous sinuses to the nipple
latch-on: when the nursing infant grasps the nipple and a portion of the surrounding areola in its mouth, a good portion of the areola should be grasped for successful sucking
rooting reflex: a reflex in which an infant will turn and open its mouth toward the cheek that is brushed
prolactin: hormone from the anterior pituitary gland that stimulates milk production
oxytocin: hormone from the posterior pituitary gland that causes milk ejection and uterine contraction
parturition: process of giving birth
colostrum: a milk-like fluid produced by the breast during the first day or so after parturition; precedes mature milk production

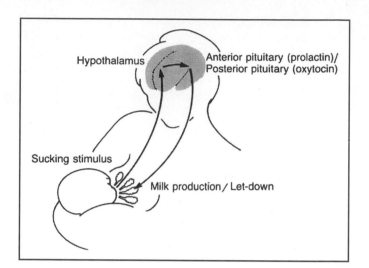

FIGURE 10–3. Proper latch-on draws the nipple and most of the areola into the infant's mouth. (From Mahan LK, Arlin MT. Krause's Food, Nutrition and Diet Therapy. 8th ed. Philadelphia: WB Saunders, 1992.)

ENERGY AND NUTRIENT NEEDS OF LACTATING WOMEN

■ What assumptions underlie the current recommendations regarding the nutrient needs of breast-feeding women?

■ How do maternal nutrient intake and body composition influence milk production?

■ Does breast-feeding influence maternal body composition?

■ How can adequate milk nutrient levels be maintained when dietary intake is low?

The production of human milk depends not only on the energy and nutrient intake of the mother, but also on her body reserves. Many women worry that the quality or quantity of their milk will be inadequate. It is reassuring to know that in the absence of severe malnutrition, the milk a mother produces will remain adequate for her infant's nutrition. In fact, many women successfully meet the nutritional needs of twins by breast-feeding. Attention to nutrition during lactation is important to maintain or replete maternal stores. Recommendations for energy and nutrient intakes during lactation appear in Table 10–1.

Energy

Energy Needs

The energy needs of lactation are proportional to the amount of milk produced. Human milk contains 67 to 70 kilocalories per 100 mL. Assuming that the conversion of maternal energy to milk energy is 80% efficient, the energy cost of producing 100 mL of milk is about 85 kcal. The recommended dietary allowance (RDA) for lactation

TABLE 10–1 Recommended Dietary Allowances for Lactation

Nutrient	Nonlactating Women (25–50 y)	Lactating Women 0–6 mo	Lactating Women 6–12 mo
Energy (kcal)	2200	2700	2700
Protein (g)	50	65	62
Vitamin A (RE)	800	1300	1200
Vitamin C (mg)	60	95	90
Vitamin D (μg)	5	10	10
Vitamin E (mg)	8	12	11
Vitamin K (μg)	65	65	65
Thiamin (mg)	1.1	1.6	1.6
Riboflavin (mg)	1.3	1.8	1.7
Niacin (mg)	15	20	20
Vitamin B_6 (mg)	1.6	2.1	2.1
Vitamin B_{12} (μg)	2.0	2.6	2.6
Folate (μg)	180	280	260
Calcium (mg)	800	1200	1200
Phosphorus (mg)	800	1200	1200
Magnesium (mg)	280	355	340
Iron (mg)	15	15	15
Iodine (μg)	150	200	200
Zinc (mg)	12	19	16
Selenium (μg)	55	75	75

Adapted with permission from Recommended dietary allowances, 10th ed. Copyright 1989 by the National Academy of Sciences. Courtesy of the National Academy Press, Washington, D.C.

is based on the assumption that average daily milk production is 750 mL during the first 6 months of lactation and 600 mL in the second 6 months (National Research Council, 1989). Thus, lactating women require an additional 640 kcal per day for the first 6 months and 510 for the second. This energy need can be met from the diet and from body stores. Current weight gain recommendations for pregnancy are associated with an increase of 2 to 3 kg of maternal fat stores, which normally are utilized during lactation (National Research Council, 1989). The RDAs for the lactating woman assume that in the first 6 months the 640 kcal/day cost of lactation will be met by 500 additional dietary kilocalories and 100 to 150 kcal/day from mobilization of accumulated fat stores. After 6 months the maternal fat stored during pregnancy is typically used up, and the 510 kcal needed for milk production must come from the diet. Therefore for both 0 to 6 and 7 to 12 months after the baby's birth the recommended increase in energy intake for lactation is 500 kcal/day, resulting in a total energy recommendation of 2700 kcal/day for lactating women (National Research Council, 1989).

Women in many parts of the world appear to maintain lactation on energy intakes much lower than those recommended. Studies of presumably well-nourished lactating women have revealed caloric intake levels of 1950 to 2350 kcal/day (Butte et al, 1984). These observations suggest that the caloric recommendations for lactating women may be higher than necessary. They also suggest that lactating women should lose weight more quickly than nonlactating postpartum women. This does not appear to be the case, suggesting that lactation may be associated with energy conservation. Although basal energy expenditure has not been reported to be different between lactating and nonlactating mothers (van Raaij et al, 1991), there do appear to be differences in the **thermic effect of food** (Motil et al, 1990) and energy expenditure for activity, which may contribute to this difference (van Raaij et al, 1991).

Although women seem to be able to maintain lactation on energy intakes lower than the current RDA, energy intakes that are too low may compromise milk production. When well-nourished mothers reduced their energy intakes to less than 1500 kcal/day for 1 week, a reduction in milk output occurred (Prentice and Prentice, 1988). To ensure adequate milk production energy intake should be at least 1800 kcal/day (Institute of Medicine, 1991).

Changes in Body Composition

Lactating women eating self-selected diets typically lose 0.5 to 1.0 kg/month during the first 4 to 6 months postpartum (Butte and Garza, 1986; Butte et al, 1984). The rate of weight loss appears to decline after 6 months. This weight loss does not appear to have deleterious effects on milk production. In well-nourished women, increased food intake is not associated with increased milk volume or energy content, nor are these measures related to maternal weight, height, or indices of fatness. In marginally-nourished women supplemental feeding trials have produced inconsistent results for milk volume, perhaps because adaptations in maternal energy expenditure maintain adequate milk production despite suboptimal energy intake (Institute of Medicine, 1991). Additionally, milk production appears to remain adequate even in very thin women (BMI < 18.5) (Prentice et al, 1994).

Weight loss in the immediate postpartum period is mainly fluid and is similar in lactating and nonlactating mothers. Following this is a period in which weight loss is greater for lactating women. However, by 12 months postpartum (after most women have stopped breast-feeding) the difference in weight loss between lactators and nonlactators is not significant (Dugdale and Eaton-Evans, 1989; Johnson, 1991). Although many postpartum women lose weight, not all do; some maintain weight and as many as one in five even gain weight (Potter et al, 1991).

Few studies have estimated changes in body composition during lactation. Changes in fatfolds are often small and variable. In fact, the triceps skinfold has been reported to remain the same or increase slightly in some populations (Butte et al, 1984) but increase dramatically in others (Forsum et al, 1989; Dugdale and Eaton-Evans, 1989). Subscapular skinfold and suprailiac skinfolds tend to decrease over the first 4 months postpartum (Butte et al, 1984). The long-term effects of pregnancy and lactation on body composition are unknown.

Protein

The protein requirements of the lactating woman are estimated from the composition of human milk, which contains about 1.1 g protein per 100 mL. Assuming that the average breast-feeding mother produces 750 mL of milk per day during the first 6 months of lactation and 600 mL during the second, the amount of protein secreted in milk is about 8 to 9 g/day in the first 6 months and 6 to 7 g/day in the second 6 months. Since the conversion of dietary protein to milk protein is about 70% efficient, the average increase in protein needs is about 12 g during the first 6 months and 10 g thereafter. These estimates are increased by 25% to account for population variability, resulting in an RDA of an additional 15 g of protein during the first 6 months of lactation and 12 grams for the second; a total intake of 65 and 62 g/day (National Research Council,

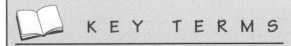

K E Y   T E R M S

thermic effect of food: the energy expended to digest and store or utilize ingested nutrients

1989). Except in clinically significant malnutrition, milk protein levels are relatively unaffected by maternal protein intake (Lawrence, 1994).

Vitamins and Minerals

Unfortunately, data on which to base estimates of vitamin and mineral needs during lactation are scarce. The RDAs for lactation are generally based on typical milk nutrient concentrations, milk volumes of 750 mL during the first 6 months of lactation and 600 mL during the second 6 months, a 25% increase to allow for intraindividual variations in milk production, and the efficiency with which a vitamin is absorbed and transferred to milk. The RDAs are listed as absolute figures rather than as additions to the RDAs for nonpregnant, nonlactating women (see Table 10–1).

Vitamins

The vitamin content of breast milk usually reflects maternal intake. However, the infant is protected to some extent from both maternal under- and over-consumption. When maternal intake is low, adequate vitamin levels in milk can be maintained at the expense of maternal reserves. When these reserves are depleted, however, inadequate vitamin content can result. On the other hand, the milk content of some, but not all, vitamins has been shown to plateau as maternal intake increases, protecting the infant from overdosing. Appropriate maternal vitamin intake ensures optimal milk vitamin levels and promotes adequate maternal reserves.

FAT-SOLUBLE VITAMINS Milk losses of retinol are typically 300 to 525 μg/day, amounting to 54 to 94 mg over the course of 6 months, or about 26% to 45% of the reserves of the average woman. To ensure the maintenance of maternal reserves, the RDA is increased by 500 μg RE for the first 6 months and 400 μg RE thereafter, resulting in totals of 1300 and 1200 μg RE, respectively. The vitamin A content of milk reflects maternal intake, but in vitamin A–depleted mothers, supplementation has had inconsistent effects (Institute of Medicine, 1991).

Vitamin D Vitamin D losses in milk parallel maternal vitamin D status, and are typically small (0.3 to 0.375 μg/day). The RDA for lactation is the same as that for pregnancy: 10 μg/day (National Research Council, 1989). The vitamin D content of milk from mothers with poor vitamin D status is inadequate. On the other hand, the vitamin D content may be raised to potentially harmful levels by pharmacologic supplementation (e.g., 2.5 mg of ergocalciferol) (Institute of Medicine, 1991; Greer et al, 1984).

The increase in the RDA for vitamin E during lactation is based on milk losses of 2.4 mg/day in the first 6 months and 1.9 mg/day in the second 6 months. An increase in the RDA of 4 mg TE during the first 6 months and 3 mg TE during the second 6 months results in recommendations of 12 and 11 mg TE (National Research Council, 1989). The vitamin E content of milk is influenced by maternal intake and possibly by maternal use of vitamin E–containing creams (Lawrence, 1994).

There is no increase in the RDA for vitamin K during lactation as milk losses are small (about 1.2 to 1.5 μg/day) and typical dietary intake appears sufficient (National Research Council, 1989; Institute of Medicine, 1991). Although the milk vitamin K levels of women with low vitamin K intakes are improved by supplementation, even the milk of supplemented women may not contain sufficient vitamin K to ensure adequate status of the neonate (Institute of Medicine, 1991).

VITAMIN C The RDA for vitamin C during lactation is based on milk losses of about 22 mg/day during the first 6 months and 18 mg/day during the second 6 months and an absorption efficiency of 85%. Altogether an additional 35 mg/day (95 mg total) is recommended during the first 6 months, and an additional 30 mg (90 mg total) is recommended during the second 6 months (National Research Council, 1989). Milk vitamin C levels increase as maternal intake increases, but plateau at maternal intakes above 100 mg/day (Institute of Medicine, 1991).

THIAMIN, RIBOFLAVIN, AND NIACIN The RDAs for thiamin and niacin during lactation are based on increased energy utilization as well as secretion in milk. Milk losses are approximately 0.2 mg/day for thiamin and 1.0 to 1.3 mg/day for niacin. The RDAs of 1.6 mg for thiamin and 20 mg niacin equivalent (NE) for niacin reflect increases of 0.5 mg and 5 mg NE, respectively (National Research Council, 1989). Maternal intake is reflected in the milk content of these vitamins, although the thiamin content of milk plateaus at higher levels of maternal intake (Institute of Medicine, 1991).

The RDA for niacin reflects milk losses of 0.26 mg/day and 0.21 mg/day during the first and second 6 months of lactation, and 70% efficiency in the utilization of riboflavin for milk production. The recommended intake is increased by 0.5 mg in the first 6 months to 1.8 mg/day and by 0.4 mg thereafter to 1.1 mg/day.

VITAMIN B$_6$ The increased need for vitamin B$_6$ during lactation reflects both secretion in milk (0.06 to 0.19 mg/day) and increased protein needs. Overall, the RDA committee recommends an increase of 0.5 mg/day to 2.1 mg/day during lactation (National Research Council, 1989). Milk B$_6$ levels are very responsive to maternal intake. Supplementation appears to increase milk B$_6$ levels and infant plasma pyridoxal 5-phosphate levels, but studies of the infants of unsupplemented mothers in the United

States have found no clinical signs of vitamin B_6 deficiency (Institute of Medicine, 1991).

FOLATE AND VITAMIN B_{12} The RDA for folate (280 μg/day during the first 6 months and 260 μg/day thereafter) is based on milk folate levels of 50 μg/L and 50% absorption (National Research Council, 1989). Improved analytical methods reveal an average milk folate content of 320 μg/day (Institute of Medicine, 1991). Additionally, the Centers for Disease Control recommends that all women of childbearing age consume 400 μg/day to reduce the risk of neural tube defects at birth (CDC, 1992). Milk folate levels are relatively unaffected by maternal folate intake, as milk concentrations are maintained at the expense of maternal reserves. However, supplemental folate increases milk folate levels of deficient women (Institute of Medicine, 1991).

Vitamin B_{12} losses in milk average about 0.45 μg/day. The RDA of 2.6 μg/day includes a 0.6 μg increase to account for variability in milk production (National Research Council, 1989). In general, milk B_{12} levels are not related to maternal B_{12} intake, although the milk B_{12} content of deficient mothers (for example, vegans) is inadequate (Institute of Medicine, 1991).

Minerals

The minerals secreted in breast milk may be obtained from both dietary intake and maternal reserves. For some minerals, including calcium, phosphorous, magnesium, sodium, potassium, iron, and zinc, body reserves and metabolic conservation allow adequate milk levels to be maintained regardless of dietary intake. However, the milk content of other minerals, such as manganese, selenium, iodine, and fluoride more readily reflects maternal intake. As for the vitamins, adequate maternal intake is important for both maternal and infant well-being.

CALCIUM AND PHOSPHORUS Calcium losses in milk average 240 mg/day, and an increased intake of 300 mg/day should replace milk losses in almost all women. Thus, the RDA is 1200 mg/day (National Research Council, 1989). More recently the National Institutes of Health Consensus Development Conference on Optimal Calcium Intake resulted in a recommendation of 1200 to 1500 mg/day for pregnant and lactating women (National Institute of Health, 1994). Women appear to be able to maintain adequate milk calcium even when calcium intake is very low by increasing the efficiency of calcium utilization and removing calcium from their bones. This raises concerns about the long-term effects of lactation on bone mineral mass. Currently available data suggest that lactation does not increase the risk of osteoporosis and may even be protective (Institute of Medicine, 1991), although the mechanisms involved are not clear.

The recommended dietary calcium phosphorus ration remains 1:1 during lactation. Thus, the RDA for phosphorus is 1200 mg/day (National Research Council, 1989).

MAGNESIUM The RDA for magnesium during lactation is based on losses of 24 to 40 mg/day in milk and 50% absorption. After accounting for intraindividual variability in milk production, increases of 75 mg/day in the first 6 months and 60 mg/day thereafter are recommended, leading to total recommendations of 355 mg/day and 340 mg/day, respectively (National Research Council, 1989). Magnesium intake appears to have little influence on maternal plasma or milk magnesium, although the long-term effect of low magnesium intake on maternal magnesium status is unclear (Institute of Medicine, 1991).

SODIUM AND POTASSIUM Milk losses of sodium and potassium are approximately 135 mg/day and 375 mg/day, respectively. These increases are easily met by usual dietary intake (National Research Council, 1989), and milk levels are not influenced by maternal intake (Institute of Medicine, 1991).

IRON AND ZINC Iron losses during lactation (0.13 to 0.3 mg/day) are smaller than menstrual iron losses (0.5 mg/day). Amenorrhea is typical in fully lactating women, so no increase in iron intake is recommended during lactation, and the RDA remains 15 mg/day (National Research Council, 1989). Maternal iron intake does not influence milk iron content (Institute of Medicine, 1991).

The zinc content of milk decreases over the course of lactation, resulting in average losses of 1.2 mg/day during the first 6 months and 0.6 mg/day thereafter. After accounting for intraindividual variability and 20% absorption, additional intakes of 7 and 4 mg/day were recommended for 0 to 6 months and 7 to 12 months, respectively. The resulting RDA is 19 mg/day and 16 mg/day (National Research Council, 1989). Zinc supplementation has little influence on milk zinc levels, although maternal plasma levels are affected (Krebs et al, 1995).

IODINE AND SELENIUM The iodine content of breast milk parallels maternal iodine intake. The RDA of 200 mg/day includes an increase of 50 μg. This increase is based on infant needs rather than maternal milk iodine content, which is greater than infant needs due to the high iodine intake of women in the United States (National Research Council, 1989).

The RDA for selenium is based on estimated milk losses of 13 μg/day, and 80% absorption efficiency. An additional 20 μg/day, for a total intake of 75 μg/day, is recommended (National Research Council, 1989). Milk selenium levels are influenced by maternal selenium intake, particularly at lower levels of intake (Institute of Medicine, 1991).

RESEARCH UPDATE
Adaptation in Calcium Metabolism During Lactation

Lactation creates a substantial drain of body calcium. In a nonpregnant, nonlactating adult obligatory calcium losses in urine, sweat and feces average 200 to 250 mg/day (National Research Council, 1989). During lactation 170 to 280 mg/day are secreted in milk (Institute of Medicine, 1991), potentially doubling daily calcium losses. When a lactating woman's calcium intake is low, calcium may be drawn from her bones to maintain adequate milk calcium levels. The calcium excreted in milk during 12 months of lactation represents 6% to 8% of total body calcium (Institute of Medicine, 1991).

Prolonged lactation combined with insufficient dietary calcium intake could place a woman at risk for reduced bone mineral mass and osteoporosis later in life. To prevent this, dietary recommendations from countries all over the world include increased calcium intake during lactation. The variation in the recommended increases (+100 to +825 mg/day) and total recommended calcium intakes during lactation (600 to 1425 mg/day) reflects differing dietary habits and the scarcity of data on which to base a recommendation (Prentice, 1995).

To more exactly define the calcium needs of lactating women, a better understanding of the effect of lactation on calcium metabolism is needed. More efficient calcium absorption, reduced urinary calcium losses during lactation, or both could reduce overall calcium needs and minimize the use of bone mineral for milk production. It appears that both of these adaptations occur to some extent.

Calcium Excretion

Several investigators have reported that urinary calcium excretion is reduced during lactation. Klein and colleagues found that the 24-hour urinary calcium excretion of a group of lactating women during the first 6 months postpartum averaged one-third lower than that of nonlactating postpartum and never pregnant women. Differences between the groups were most apparent during the first 2 months postpartum (Klein, 1995). Using a different approach, Cross and co-workers (1995) measured urinary calcium excretion in ten women before and during pregnancy, at 3 months postpartum while lactating, and at about 3 months postweaning. Urinary calcium excretion was not reduced during lactation (3 months postpartum) but was reduced after weaning. Finally, Specker and co-workers (1994) compared the urinary calcium excretion in six women when they were lactating and when they were not lactating. They also found reduced urinary calcium loss during lactation. These findings suggest that reductions in urinary calcium loss during lactation and after weaning help conserve body calcium.

Calcium Absorption

The percentage of dietary calcium absorbed appears to vary with habitual calcium intake. In the United States, where the average calcium intake is 740 mg/day, 30% to 40% of dietary calcium is absorbed (National Research Council, 1989). Fairweather-Tait and colleagues reported similar absorption (32%) in lactating British women consuming an average of 1170 mg calcium daily, but found higher absorption (52%) in lactating Gambian women accustomed to ingesting 300 mg/day (Fairweather-Tait, 1995).

Calcium absorption does appear to be influenced by lactation, but its effect is not apparent until after weaning or the resumption of menstruation. Neither Specker (1994) nor Kalkwarf and colleagues (1996) found evidence of increased efficiency of calcium absorption during lactation. However, Kalkwarf and co-workers (1996) found that the percentage of calcium absorbed about 3 months after weaning (37%) in 24 women who had breast-fed was greater than that in 24 women who had not breast-fed (32%). Additionally, lactating women who had resumed menstruation had higher calcium absorption than those who had not.

Bone Mineral Loss

Lactating women do lose bone mass initially, but it appears to be replaced after weaning. Cross and co-workers (1995) did not find a reduction in forearm bone mineral content in a small number of lactating women, although biochemical markers of bone turnover were increased. In a larger study, Prentice and colleagues (1995) detected a small (1%) reduction in forearm bone mineral content at 3 months of lactation, and Sowers and co-workers (1993) found a 5% reduction in spine and femoral bone mineral density after 6 months of lactation. In the women studied by Sowers and colleagues, who had an average calcium intake of >900 mg/day, bone mineral density increased back to the levels observed just after delivery by 12 months postpartum.

Conclusion

Although many unanswered questions remain, it appears that the increased calcium demands of lactation are met in part by reduced urinary calcium excretion and bone resorption during lactation, with increased calcium absorption, reduced urinary losses, and bone mineral deposition after weaning or the return of menstruation. In Gambian women, reduced breast milk calcium concentrations further reduce calcium needs during lactation (Prentice et al, 1995). Somewhat surprisingly, the adaptations in calcium absorption (Fairweather-Tait et al, 1995; Kalkwarf et al,

1996; Prentice et al, 1995), breast milk calcium concentration, and bone mineral metabolism (Fairweather-Tait et al, 1995) appear to be relatively unaffected by calcium supplementation during lactation, suggesting that they occur in response to the hormonal changes of lactation itself, not dietary inadequacy. Much more work needs to be done before calcium needs during lactation are fully understood. In the meantime, it is reassuring to note that epidemiologic investigations suggest that the risk of osteoporosis may be lessened, not increased, in women who have breast-fed (Institute of Medicine, 1991).

Fluid

Lactating mothers have been encouraged to drink 2 to 3 liters of fluid each day. Records of dietary intakes of lactating women indicate that total fluid intake, including food and beverages, is typically in this range (Stumbo et al, 1985). A number of investigators have demonstrated that milk output is unrelated to fluid consumption and that increased fluid consumption does not result in increased milk production. In fact, forced fluid consumption beyond thirst may reduce milk production (Institute of Medicine, 1991; Duskieker et al, 1985 and 1990). However, lactating women should be encouraged to be alert for and respond to thirst (Lawrence, 1994).

DIETARY RECOMMENDATIONS FOR LACTATING WOMEN

■ Which nutrients are likely to be low in the diets of lactating women in the United States?

■ Describe the recommended number of servings from each food group during lactation.

■ What guidelines for consumption of alcohol and caffeine, smoking, and physical activity are appropriate during lactation?

Adequacy of Typical United States Diets

The nutritional adequacy of a diet is related to both energy intake and nutrient density. A varied, balanced diet

that meets a woman's energy requirements usually provides adequate vitamins and minerals to support lactation. Women who consume a nutrient-dense diet and who meet the RDA for energy (2700 kcal) are likely to approach or meet the RDA for all nutrients. Careful attention must be given to sources rich in zinc and to the use of dairy products to ensure intake of 1200 mg of calcium.

As energy intake declines, vitamin and mineral intakes are less likely to be adequate. At caloric intake levels of approximately 2200 kcal/day (the average reported caloric intake of lactating women), nutrients that may be consumed in amounts less than the RDA are calcium, magnesium, zinc, vitamin B_6, and folate. When intake levels fall below 1800 kcal, predicted intakes fall short of the RDA for all the nutrients mentioned above and also for riboflavin, folate, phosphorus, and iron (Institute of Medicine, 1991). Because the RDAs are guidelines for intakes that include a wide margin of safety above requirements, it cannot be assumed that intake levels below the RDA are indications of deficiency. However, such levels consumed over time are associated with increased risk of deficiency. Careful attention to diet quality and quantity can help to ensure optimal nutrients for a mother and her infant.

Guidelines for Dietary Intake

Some women elect not to breast-feed because they do not wish to be subject to complicated dietary "rules" for breast-feeding. Because adequate milk quality and quantity is the result of maternal diet and maternal stores, dietary recommendations for breast-feeding can be applied with some flexibility in well-nourished women. General guidelines include consuming at least 1800 kcal/day, choosing nutrient-dense foods most of the time, and drinking when thirsty. More specific guidelines are given in Table 10–2. This food guide can be adapted to be acceptable to a variety of cultures (Table 10–3).

The nutritional needs of breast-feeding women should be met by a balanced, varied diet rather than by vitamin and mineral supplements. If dietary evaluation indicates a significant lack of important nutrient sources, mothers should be encouraged to select acceptable foods that will remedy the problem. If dietary counseling is not effective in improving intake, however, the guidelines for improving nutrient intake via supplementation described in Table 10–4 can be used.

Infant Reactions to Foods in the Mother's Diet

Some infants appear to be sensitive to certain foods in their mother's diet. Strong or spicy flavors such as garlic may alter the flavor of breast milk (Mennella and Beauchamp, 1991b). Occasionally, foods in the mother's diet appear to cause infant discomfort. Cow's milk, cruciferous vegetables, onion, and chocolate have been suggested to cause such discomfort (Lust et al, 1996), but there is no evidence that all nursing mothers need to avoid these foods. Sensitivity to any maternal dietary component must be documented by the reversal of the infant's symptoms when the food is removed from the diet, and confirmed with a repeat of symptoms when the food is reintroduced. When important nutrient sources must be removed from a mother's diet, an alternate source should be identified.

Maternal Behaviors

Caffeine and Alcohol

Maternal consumption of caffeine and alcohol may adversely affect the breast-feeding infant. When a breast-feeding mother consumes large doses of caffeine (6 to 8 cups of caffeine-containing beverages per day), caffeine can accumulate in the infant, causing irritability and wakefulness (Rivera-Calimim, 1987).

Alcohol is readily transferred to breast milk. Daily maternal intakes of more than 0.5 g ethanol per kg of body weight (about 24 oz beer, 9 oz wine, or 2 to 3 oz hard liquor for a 125-lb woman) can reduce infant consumption of breast milk and may partially interfere with the milk letdown (Mennella and Beauchamp, 1991a). Little and her co-workers (1989) found that consumption by breast-feeding mothers of one drink daily had no detrimental effects on mental development but did have a small negative effect on psychomotor development.

Smoking and Drug Abuse

In addition to its deleterious effects on maternal health, smoking hinders a woman's ability to breast-feed. Although no association between nicotine levels in the milk of heavy smokers and symptoms in nursing infants has been found (Luck and Nau, 1987), mothers who smoke have lower milk volume than nonsmoking mothers (Vio et al., 1991).

The American Academy of Pediatrics states that nicotine, amphetamine, cocaine, heroin, marijuana, and phencyclidine hydrochloride (PCP) are contraindicated during breast-feeding because these and other habit-forming drugs are hazardous to both mother and infant (American Academy of Pediatrics, 1994).

Rest and Physical Activity

Maternal fatigue is the most common cause of inadequate milk production (Lawrence, 1994). The demands of an infant, other family members, and social and job obligations may result in inadequate rest. This is especially detrimental in the first 4 to 6 weeks when breast-feeding is not yet fully established. Mothers should be encouraged to acknowledge fatigue and obtain help when needed.

Adequate physical activity is important for physical and psychological well-being. Although regular moderate exercise by physically fit women does not appear to hamper breast-feeding (Lovelady et al, 1990; Dewey et al, 1994), some mothers report that their infants fuss when they nurse soon after the mother has exercised strenuously (Lawrence, 1994). This response is the result of bitter-tasting lactic acid in the milk (Wallace et al, 1992). Breast-feeding mothers who exercise strenuously may need to avoid exercising just before feeding. If there are signs of infant discomfort, rinsing sweat off the breasts before nursing and expressing a small amount of milk before feeding may be helpful (Lawrence, 1994).

BREAST-FEEDING BASICS

■ Suggest guidelines for the successful initiation of breast-feeding.

■ What are some signs that breast-feeding is going well?

■ What difficulties occasionally complicate breast-feeding, and what can be done about them?

Initiating Breast-Feeding

Although the process of lactation is based on innate reflexes, breast-feeding behavior must be learned. Almost all healthy women who want to breast-feed can do so. Frequently the new mother and infant will need guidance to

TABLE 10–2 Daily Food Guide for Lactating Women

Food Group	One Serving Equals		Recommended Minimum Servings
PROTEIN FOODS Provide protein, iron, zinc, and B vitamins for growth of muscles, bone, blood, and nerves. Vegetable protein provides fiber to prevent constipation.	ANIMAL PROTEIN 1 oz cooked chicken or turkey 1 oz cooked lean beef, lamb, or pork 1 oz or $\frac{1}{4}$ c fish or other seafood 1 egg 2 fish sticks or hot dogs 2 slices luncheon meat	VEGETABLE PROTEIN $\frac{1}{2}$ c cooked dry beans, lentils, or split peas 3 oz tofu 1 oz or $\frac{1}{4}$ c peanuts, pumpkin, or sunflower seeds $1\frac{1}{2}$ oz or $\frac{1}{2}$ c other nuts 2 tbsp peanut butter	7 One serving of vegetable protein daily
MILK PRODUCTS Provide protein and calcium to build strong bones, teeth, healthy nerves and muscles, and to promote normal blood clotting.	8 oz milk 8 oz yogurt 1 c milk shake $1\frac{1}{2}$ c cream soup (made with milk) $1\frac{1}{2}$ oz or $\frac{1}{3}$ c grated cheese (like cheddar, monterey, mozzarella, or swiss)	$1\frac{1}{2}$–2 slices presliced American cheese 4 tbsp parmesan cheese 2 c cottage cheese 1 c pudding 1 c custard or flan $1\frac{1}{2}$ c ice milk, ice cream, or frozen yogurt	3
BREADS, CEREALS, GRAINS Provide carbohydrates and B vitamins for energy and healthy nerves. Also provide iron for healthy blood. Whole grains provide fiber to prevent constipation.	1 slice bread 1 dinner roll $\frac{1}{2}$ bun or bagel $\frac{1}{2}$ English muffin or pita 1 small tortilla $\frac{3}{4}$ c dry cereal $\frac{1}{2}$ c granola $\frac{1}{2}$ c cooked cereal	$\frac{1}{2}$ c rice $\frac{1}{2}$ c noodles or spaghetti $\frac{1}{4}$ c wheat germ 1 4-inch pancake or waffle 1 small muffin 8 medium crackers 4 graham cracker squares 3 c popcorn	7
VITAMIN C–RICH FRUITS AND VEGETABLES Provide vitamin C to prevent infection and to promote healing and iron absorption. Also provide fiber to prevent constipation.	6 oz orange, grapefruit, or fruit juice enriched with vitamin C 6 oz tomato juice or vegetable juice cocktail 1 orange, kiwi, mango $\frac{1}{2}$ grapefruit, cantaloupe $\frac{1}{2}$ c papaya 2 tangerines	$\frac{1}{2}$ c strawberries $\frac{1}{2}$ c cooked or 1 c raw cabbage $\frac{1}{2}$ c broccoli, Brussels sprouts, or cauliflower $\frac{1}{2}$ c snow peas, sweet peppers, or tomato puree 2 tomatoes	1
VITAMIN A–RICH FRUITS AND VEGETABLES Provide beta-carotene and vitamin A to prevent infection and to promote wound healing and night vision. Also provide fiber to prevent constipation.	6 oz apricot nectar or vegetable juice cocktail 3 raw or $\frac{1}{4}$ cup dried apricots $\frac{1}{4}$ cantaloupe or mango 1 small or $\frac{1}{2}$ c sliced carrots 2 tomatoes	$\frac{1}{2}$ c cooked or 1 c raw spinach $\frac{1}{2}$ c cooked greens (beet, chard, collards, dandelion, kale, mustard) $\frac{1}{2}$ c pumpkin, sweet potato, winter squash, or yams	1
OTHER FRUITS AND VEGETABLES Provide carbohydrates for energy and fiber to prevent constipation.	6 oz fruit juice (if not listed above) 1 medium or $\frac{1}{2}$ c sliced fruit (apple, banana, peach, pear) $\frac{1}{2}$ c berries (other than strawberries) $\frac{1}{2}$ c cherries or grapes $\frac{1}{2}$ c pineapple $\frac{1}{2}$ c watermelon	$\frac{1}{4}$ c dried fruit $\frac{1}{2}$ c sliced vegetable (asparagus, beets, green beans, celery, corn, eggplant, mushrooms, onion, peas, potato, summer squash, zucchini) $\frac{1}{2}$ artichoke 1 c lettuce	3
UNSATURATED FATS Provide vitamin E to protect tissue.	$\frac{1}{3}$ medium avocado 1 tsp margarine 1 tsp mayonnaise 1 tsp vegetable oil	2 tsp salad dressing (mayonnaise-based) 1 tbsp salad dressing (oil-based)	3

Adapted from California Department of Health Services. Nutrition during pregnancy and postpartum period: a manual for health care professionals. Sacramento, CA: Department of Health Services, 1990.

TABLE 10–3 Sample Menus to Meet the Daily Food Guide for Lactation

Mexican	African-American	Lacto-Ovo-Vegetarian	Protein	Milk	Grains	Vitamin C	Vitamin A	Other Fruits and Vegetables	Unsaturated Fat
BREAKFAST									
1 slice white toast	1 slice whole-grain toast	1 slice whole-wheat toast			1				
1 tsp margarine	1 tsp margarine	1 tsp margarine							1
½ c oatmeal	½ c grits	½ c Wheatena			1				
1 c lowfat milk	1 c whole milk	1 c nonfat milk		1					
Sugar*	Bacon*	Sugar*							
LUNCH									
TOSTADAS	CHILIBURGER	SOUP AND SALAD							
2 oz chicken breast	2 oz hamburger	1½ c lentil soup	2						
½ c refried beans	½ c chili beans	1 egg hard-boiled (in salad)	1						
2 corn tortillas	1 hamburger bun, white	2 whole-grain rolls			2				
fresh chili salsa: ½ tomato + ½ tbsp chili pepper	Cole slaw: ½ c cabbage ½ c french fries	Salad: 1 fresh tomato 1 c romaine lettuce				½		1	
2 corn tortillas	½ c whole milk	½ c nonfat milk		½					
¼ fresh mango	2 tsp salad dressing (mayonnaise-type)	1 tbsp Italian dressing							1
1 tsp corn oil (for frying)									
DINNER									
BISTEC RANCHERO	PORK CHOPS	STUFFED PITA							
3 oz chuck steak	3 oz pork chop	½ c kidney beans							
½ c kidney beans	½ c beans	6 oz tofu ½ c hummus	4						
½ c red potatoes	½ c mashed potato	½ c mushrooms						1	
Fresh chili salsa: ½ tomato + ½ tbsp chili pepper	½ medium orange	¼ c tomato puree				½			
2 corn tortillas	2 whole-grain rolls	1 pita, whole-wheat			2				
¼ fresh mango	½ c mustard greens	½ c carrots, raw					1		
1 tsp corn oil (for frying)	1 tsp margarine (on rolls)	1 tsp olive oil (in hummus)							1
SNACKS									
LICUADO		SMOOTHEE							
1 c lowfat milk	1 c fruit yogurt	4 oz nonfat milk + ½ c yogurt		1					
1 banana + sugar, vanilla*	½ c grapes	1 banana + honey*						1	
¾ c corn flakes	8 whole-wheat crackers	8 whole-wheat crackers			1				
½ c lowfat milk	¾ oz American cheese	¾ c frozen yogurt		½					
Totals			7	3	7	1	1	3	3

Each menu meets the minimum number of servings for all groups in the Daily Food Guide for Pregnant Women.

* Indicates foods that provide extra calories only or are used for seasoning.

Adapted from California Department of Health Services. Nutrition During Pregnancy and Postpartum Period: A Manual for Health Care Professionals. Sacramento, CA: Department of Health Services, 1990.

TABLE 10–4 Suggested Measures for Improving Nutrient Intake of Women with Restrictive Eating Patterns

Type of Restrictive Eating Pattern	Corrective Measures
Excessive restriction of food intake, i.e., ingestion of <1800 kcal of energy per day, which ordinarily leads to unsatisfactory intake of nutrients compared with the amounts needed by lactating women	Encourage increased intake of nutrient-rich foods to achieve an energy intake of at least 1800 kcal/day; if the mother insists on curbing food intake sharply, promote substitution of foods rich in vitamins, minerals, and protein for those lower in nutritive value; in individual cases, it may be advised to recommend a balanced multivitamin–mineral supplement; discourage use of liquid weight loss diets and appetite suppressants
Complete vegetarianism, i.e., avoidance of all animal foods, including meat, fish, dairy products, and eggs	Advise intake of a regular source of vitamin B_{12}, such as special vitamin B_{12}-containing plant food products or a 2.6-μg vitamin B_{12} supplement daily
Avoidance of milk, cheese, or other calcium-rich dairy products	Encourage increased intake of other culturally appropriate dietary calcium sources, such as collard greens for African Americans from the southeastern United States; provide information on the appropriate use of low-lactose dairy products if milk is being avoided because of lactose intolerance; if correction by diet cannot be achieved, it may be advisable to recommend 600 mg of elemental calcium per day taken with meals
Avoidance of vitamin D–fortified foods, such as fortified milk or cereal, combined with limited exposure to ultraviolet light	Recommend 10 μg of supplemental vitamin D per day

Reprinted with permission from Nutrition during lactation. Copyright 1991 by the National Academy of Sciences. Courtesy of the National Academy Press, Washington, DC.

ensure a successful breast-feeding experience. One of the most important opportunities for facilitating breast-feeding is assisting the mother in initiating latch-on (Neifert and Seacat, 1985).

Newborn infants are ready to breast-feed. In fact, they are especially alert, attentive, and able to begin breast-feeding the first hour after birth. Whenever possible, newborn infants should be allowed to nurse in the birthing room. A tranquil environment and reduced use of anesthesia during delivery facilitates a successful first feeding. Many hospitals and birthing centers have facilities and policies that promote this important first meeting whenever medically possible. However, if medical intervention requires rapid separation it should be remembered that early nursing is important but not essential for successful breast-feeding.

During the first feedings, a new mother learns how to position herself and her infant for comfortable, successful feeding. Nursing infants may be placed in one of several positions (Fig. 10–4). Nursing staff are usually available to help a new mother and her infant practice these. Alternating positions can help alleviate fatigue and the potential for sore nipples. For all positions, it is important that the baby's body and head face the same direction.

Once the infant is comfortably positioned, she can latch on to the breast. To help the infant latch on, the mother supports her breast and gently squeezes the area behind her areola using a palmar or scissor grasp (Fig. 10–5). Next she tickles the baby's lips with her nipple to stimulate the rooting reflex. When the infant opens her mouth wide, the mother pulls the baby in close so its tongue extends under the nipple and draws the nipple into her

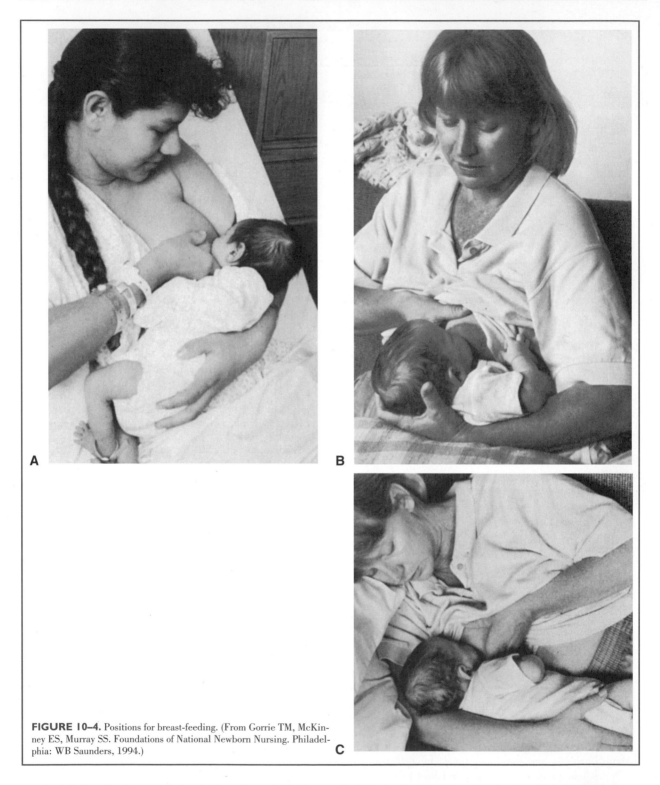

FIGURE 10–4. Positions for breast-feeding. (From Gorrie TM, McKinney ES, Murray SS. Foundations of National Newborn Nursing. Philadelphia: WB Saunders, 1994.)

mouth. A baby who is properly latched on draws both the nipple and much of the areola into her mouth.

When the infant is positioned and latched on correctly, the feeding experience should be pleasant. Occasionally the baby latches on to just the nipple, which results in very painful nursing. If the latch-on is not comfortable, the baby's suction must be broken before the nipple is removed. This is done by slipping a clean finger into the cor-

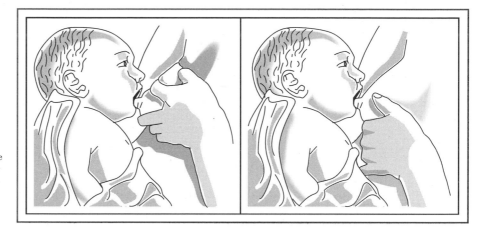

FIGURE 10–5. The breast may be supported using a palmar or scissor grasp. (From Lawrence RA. Breast-feeding: A Guide for the Medical Profession. St. Louis: Mosby–Year Book, 1994.)

ner of the baby's mouth. Most hospitals and birthing centers have a lactation consultant who can help with latch-on difficulties.

Once the baby is latched on and sucking, receptors in the nipple and areola send a neural message to the hypothalamus, which stimulates oxytocin release from the pituitary. Oxytocin stimulates milk "let-down," in which milk is pushed to the front of the breast where it is readily available to the infant. Oxytocin also stimulates uterine contractions. Let-down can be identified by the perception of uterine tightening, nipple tingling, and the infant's gulping. Anxiety and distraction interfere with this critical reflex. Therefore, every effort should be made to ensure that new mothers are comfortable, rested, and relaxed. Mothers having difficulty with let-down should alert the staff of the hospital or birthing center so the problem can be remedied before discharge. For most women, let-down is rapidly established and may occur in response to her infant's crying or other feeding cues.

Appropriate feeding intervals and durations stimulate abundant milk production. A newborn breast-fed infant typically nurses 10 to 14 times in 24 hours. The infant should nurse on each breast long enough to soften it, typically 10 to 20 minutes. When the first breast softens, the infant should be removed by breaking the suction gently and offered the other breast. Often, babies are gently burped between breasts. At the next feeding, the baby should be offered the fuller, heavier breast first (typically the second breast from the previous feeding). While the infant is sucking, prolactin release from the anterior pituitary along with breast emptying stimulates milk production.

Signs That Breast-Feeding Is Going Well

Mothers are often concerned that their infant's breast milk intake is adequate. Signs that breast-feeding is going well include softening of the breasts after nursing, observ-

ing that the baby gulps and slows its sucking pattern during the course of a feeding, a sleepy, relaxed feeling in the mother after feeding, and a content infant who has at least six wet diapers and one bowel movement per day after 4 days of age.

As the Infant Grows

As the infant grows and breast-feeding becomes well established, the interval between feedings increases and most infants need approximately six feedings per day. Periodically, however, an infant will appear to be constantly hungry and nurse very frequently. This is typically the result of a growth spurt. The frequent nursing stimulates the increased milk production needed to meet the needs of the growing infant. In a few days milk production will have increased to meet the baby's needs and the feeding pattern will return to normal.

Overcoming Difficulties

Many mothers have some concerns or difficulties related to breast-feeding after they leave the hospital. Most problems can be resolved while maintaining lactation. If minor difficulties are unattended, however, they may become major problems and result in lactation failure. It is important for new mothers to have someone to whom they can turn for assistance and support. A logical choice is the obstetrician or pediatrician—but neither has traditionally provided support for lactation. The best source is often a family member or friend who has breast-fed successfully. Many major hospitals have nurses on the maternity staff who provide assistance to new mothers and who are available by telephone after discharge. Support groups such as the La Leche League can provide information and moral support to a worried mother.

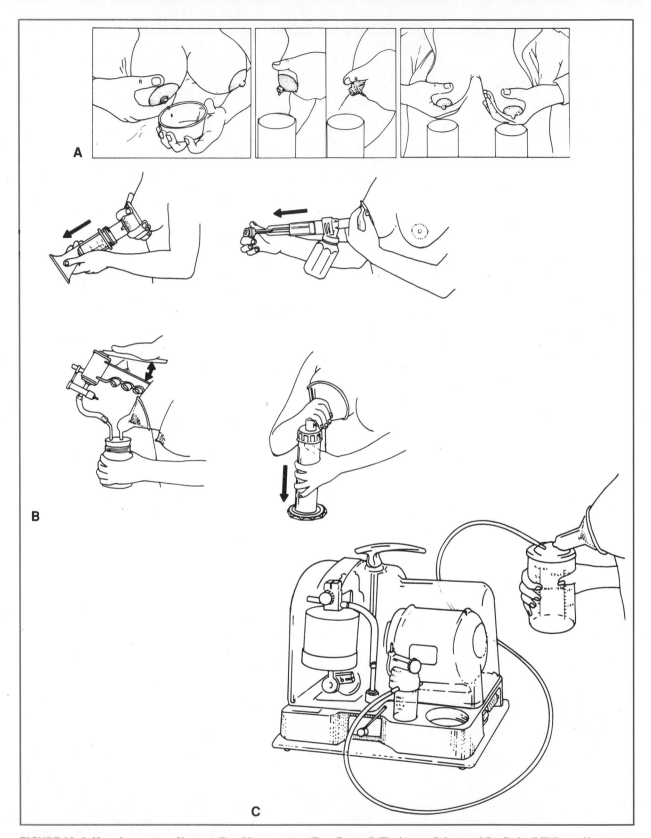

FIGURE 10–6. Manual expression of breast milk and breast pumps. (From Bonnie S. Worthington-Roberts and Sue Rodwell Williams. Nutrition in Pregnancy and Lactation. 4th edition. Copyright © 1989 The McGraw-Hill Companies, Inc. Reprinted by permission. All Rights Reserved.)

Sore Nipples

The best way to cope with the problem of sore nipples is to prevent them by careful attention to infant positioning in the early days of life. Many cases of sore nipples can be helped by correcting or changing feeding positions. Additional measures include eliminating the use of irritating or drying soaps and ointments, avoiding the use of plastic-backed breast pads, and the application of therapeutic ointments. If the nipple becomes cracked or damaged, healing can be aided by leaving a few drops of milk to dry in the nipple after feeding (Lawrence, 1994). Sore nipples may also be due to infection, so a healthcare provider familiar with breast-feeding should be consulted for severe or persistently sore nipples.

Engorgement

When colostrum is replaced by mature milk the breasts may become temporarily swollen. It is often difficult for the infant to latch on to the enlarged breasts. This results in a hungry, frustrated infant and painfully engorged breasts. **Engorgement** can be minimized by frequent nursing. When it occurs, applying cold packs to the breasts helps to provide some relief. Additionally, softening the breasts by a warm shower or by expressing or pumping a small amount of milk so the baby can latch on is helpful. Engorgement is more likely in primiparas and usually resolves within a few days.

Separation

When mother and infant cannot be together, lactation can be maintained by manual expression or pumping of breast milk (Fig. 10–6). The infant can be fed breast milk that has been expressed or pumped on previous occasions or commercial formula. Initially, it may take several pumping sessions to produce the volume of milk required for a feeding. Breast milk can be refrigerated for 1 to 2 days or frozen for 3 to 4 months. Mothers who work can pump their milk at work so the infant can receive it in a bottle the next day. Alternatively, the infant may receive commercial formula while its mother is at work and breast-feed while they are together.

Nipple Confusion

Some infants have difficulty switching back and forth between human and artificial nipples. Artificial nipples are less flexible, and the tongue movements used to control milk flow from a bottle are different from those used in breast-feeding. To avoid nipple confusion it is best to avoid the use of artificial nipples in the first month of an infant's life, when breast-feeding is becoming established. If bottle feeding is needed after that time most infants learn to switch back and forth successfully. If an infant re-

jects the artificial nipple, it may help if a caregiver other than the mother introduces the bottle.

Slow Growth

Occasionally breast-feeding gets off to a slow start. This is more likely with primiparas and may be due to a variety of causes, including fatigue, stress, misinformation about appropriate breast-feeding practices, or a small, sleepy infant. Inadequate breast milk is a significant concern as it can rapidly result in life-threatening dehydration of the infant. Women and their infants are often discharged before their breast-feeding knowledge and skill can be thoroughly evaluated; thus, it is important that breast-fed infants be evaluated several days after discharge to ensure that all is well and provide guidance for questions and uncertainties. When breast-feeding is not progressing adequately, medical intervention is warranted. Usually, instructing a mother to rest and nurse frequently and long enough resolves the problem in a few days. In more severe cases, a mother may be instructed to pump her breasts after her baby has finished nursing to provide additional stimulation for milk production.

Providing supplements of bottled commercial formula to the infant ensures an adequate intake but often hampers breast-feeding. When an infant receives supplemental bottles, he nurses less frequently, reducing the sucking stimulation necessary to increase milk production. Nipple confusion may also result. If supplemental feedings are necessary, use of a supplemental nursing system (Fig. 10–7) ensures adequate infant nutrition and promotes milk production without introducing nipple confusion. Supplemental nursing systems can be used to induce lactation in adoptive mothers or birth mothers who initially choose not to breast-feed.

Plugged Ducts/Mastitis

Tenderness in one area of the breasts may indicate a plugged or blocked collecting duct. Application of warm, moist heat, breast emptying, and gentle massage of the tender area usually resolve the problem. If tenderness persists, the use of overly restrictive bras or clothing should be considered as a cause. If the tenderness is joined by redness, swelling, or fever, **mastitis** should be suspected and a physician should be contacted.

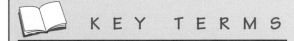

K E Y   T E R M S

engorgement: temporary swelling of the breasts that occurs as mature milk secretion begins
mastitis: infection of the breast

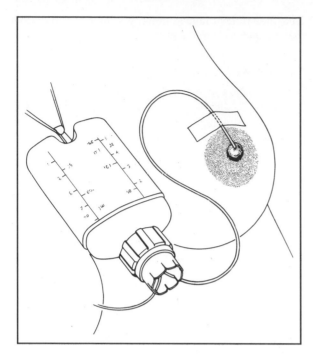

FIGURE 10–7. A supplemental nursing system helps stimulate milk production while providing nourishment to the infant. (From Lawrence RA. Breastfeeding: A Guide for the Medical Profession. St. Louis: Mosby–Year Book, 1994.)

Leaking Milk

Leaking milk can be a source of embarrassment or discomfort. Soft, breathable, washable, or disposable bra pads are available to absorb leaked milk. If let-down occurs in response to an infant's crying at a time other than feeding, gentle pressure on the nipples reduces the flow. This can be accomplished inconspicuously by crossing the arms across the chest.

CONTRAINDICATIONS TO BREAST-FEEDING

■ Describe the circumstances in which breast-feeding may be contraindicated.

There are a few circumstances in which breast-feeding is contraindicated. These are related to maternal health, medications, and personal habits that may influence the safety, composition, or availability of breast milk, and to some disorders in the infant. Newborns with some inborn errors of metabolism, such as **phenylketonuria, galactosemia,** or **primary lactase deficiency,** cannot digest or metabolize one of the nutrients in human or cow's milk, and require full or partial feeding of specialized formula or specially treated breast milk. Breast-feeding is con-

traindicated by some cancer treatments in the mother and some communicable diseases such as active tuberculosis. For women with chronic diseases such as diabetes mellitus, renal disease, and hypertension, the decision to breast-feed must be assessed with the physician on a risk-to-benefit ratio. Many women with these conditions do successfully breast-feed their infants.

The human immunodeficiency virus (HIV) can be transmitted from mother to child in utero or perinatally. Recently, transmission of HIV through breast-feeding has been described (Ruff et al, 1992). However, the prevalence and viability of HIV has not been defined. It has been shown that IgA and IgM antibodies to HIV occur in breast milk of **seropositive** women (Van de Perre et al, 1993), and there is evidence that immunoglobulins in human milk interfere with the binding of HIV to its target on the T cell (Belec et al, 1990; Newburg et al, 1992). Currently, recommendations regarding breast-feeding by HIV-1–seropositive women reflect assumptions about risks and benefits. The Centers for Disease Control recommends that women seropositive for HIV-1 should not breast-feed (CDC, 1985). In developing countries where safe and effective alternatives to breast-feeding are not available, the World Health Organization recommends that breast-feeding should be initiated regardless of HIV-1 serologic status of the mother (WHO, 1987).

Prescription medications must be evaluated when the mother makes the decision to breast-feed. There are few prescription drugs that are contraindicated during lactation because of possible negative effects on the infant. Some medications may not be transferred via breast-milk but might influence milk production or release. For example, some oral contraceptives contain sufficiently high levels of estrogen to reduce milk volume and affect the let-down reflex. In many instances, safer, alternative drugs may be prescribed (American Academy of Pediatrics Committee on Drugs, 1994; Lawrence, 1994).

Environmental pollutants such as DDT and PCBs (polychlorinated biphenols) and toxic metals such as lead or mercury have been found in breast milk. The toxicity of these agents to the breast-fed infant has not yet been determined. Women at high risk for these contaminants must carefully weigh the potential risk against the benefits of breast-feeding.

WEANING

■ At what ages are children typically weaned?

■ How should weaning be accomplished?

Weaning, the transition from exclusive breast-feeding to other sources of nourishment, is typically a gradual process. Children are weaned for varying reasons and at varying times. In many developing countries children are normally breast-fed for 2 to 3 years. In fact, the average worldwide age for weaning is 4.2 years (Lawrence, 1994). In the United States, the Healthy People 2000 goals include the recommendation that infants be breast-fed for at least 6 months (U.S. Department of Health and Human Services, 1990). In infants under 1 year of age, commercial formula should be used if breast-feeding is discontinued. The guidelines for adding solid foods to a breast-fed infant's diet are the same as those for a formula-fed infant (see Chapter 4).

When an infant is weaned, decreasing breast-feeding slowly allows mother and infant to adjust to the change. Generally, one feeding at a time is eliminated. After adaptation to the change an additional feeding is stopped, usually during another part of the day. Eventually, one morning and one evening feeding remain. These feedings may be continued to provide nourishment and comfort if desired, or they too may be phased out. After breast-feeding has stopped, the breasts continue to be partially functional for about 1 month (Lawrence, 1994).

PROMOTING BREAST-FEEDING

■ What maternal characteristics and medical practices are associated with higher breast-feeding rates?

■ When do parents decide whether or not to breast-feed?

In spite of universal recommendations for breast-feeding, only half of American mothers initiate breast-feeding. The typical woman who breast-feeds her infant is white, married, middle or upper income, and college educated. She decided to breast-feed during pregnancy and has support from family members. Maternal employment does not seem to be a detriment to the initiation of breast-feeding, but at 6 months, the overall rate of breast-feeding in mothers working full time (14%) is lower than the breast-feeding rate in mothers who are not working or who are working part time (24%) (Ross Laboratories, 1995).

In promoting breast-feeding, attention must be given to cultural, social, and family acceptance factors as well as the mother's perceived value of breast versus bottle feeding. Subtle differences in the care and counseling of the new mother and even hospital procedures may influence her decision. For example, breast-feeding is more successful if it is initiated within 6 hours of delivery (Kurinij and Shiono, 1991). Additionally, new mothers are more likely to continue breast-feeding after hospital discharge if the packets sent home with them contain breast pumps rather than samples of infant formula (Dungy et al, 1992). Successful breast-feeding requires support from family, friends, and the healthcare system.

TABLE 10–5 National and International Organizations Promoting Breast-Feeding

NATIONAL

American Academy of Pediatrics
141 NW Point Blvd.
Elk Grove Village, IL 6009-0927
(800) 433-9016

Best Start Inc.
3500 E. Fletcher Ave., Suite 308
Tampa, FL 33613
(813) 971-2119

National Center for Education in Maternal and Child Health
2000 15th St. N., Suite 701
Arlington, VA 22201-2617
(703) 524-7802

INTERNATIONAL

INFACT Canada (Infant Feeding Action Coalition)
10 Trinity Square
Toronto, Ontario M5G 1B1
CANADA
(416) 595-9819

La Leche League International, Inc.
1400 North Meacham Rd.
Schaumburg, IL 60173-4840
(800) LA-LECHE

UNICEF
UNICEF House
3 United Nations Plaza
New York, NY 10017
(212) 326-7000

Wellstart, Inc.
4062 First Avenue
San Diego, CA 92103

Prenatal Counseling

Most parents make the decision regarding breast-feeding during pregnancy. Therefore, it is important that health care professionals provide complete information about breast-feeding during prenatal visits. Prenatal health care

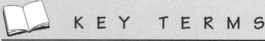

KEY TERMS

phenylketonuria: a metabolic error in which the infant lacks an enzyme required to metabolize phenylalanine
galactosemia: lack of an enzyme required to convert galactose to glucose
primary lactase deficiency: genetic lack of the enzyme that digests lactose
seropositive: having a blood test positive for HIV

should include education about the benefits of and techniques for breast-feeding, and evaluation of breast anatomy. Before the popularity of bottle feeding in the 1950s and 1960s, know-how was passed from one generation to the next, and children grew up watching their mothers and relatives breast-feed. Today's mothers lack social support for breast-feeding, may be uncertain about technique, and are frequently misled by myths and misinformation.

Resources for Breast-Feeding Promotion

Many governmental and non-profit organizations have joined to provide women the information and support they need to breast-feed successfully. Several national and international resources are listed in Table 10–5. Regional resources include state and local health departments, WIC offices, La Leche League chapters, and hospital-based breast-feeding consultants. Recently the Woman, Infants, and Children (WIC) program has placed a strong emphasis on breast-feeding, including a new food package for exclusively breast-feeding mothers. Many WIC clients have no experience or exposure to breast-feeding and need education and counseling to prepare for and sustain this practice. WIC staff are trained to provide the needed information and social support. However, some critics have pointed out that the free formula available to WIC participants encourages artificial feeding.

CONCEPTS TO REMEMBER

▶ Lactation, the process by which the mammary gland produces and releases milk for the infant, is the natural extension of pregnancy. Successful lactation involves learning breast-feeding behaviors.

▶ Breast milk offers immunologic, nutritional, and psychological advantages, yet only half of mothers in the United States choose to breast-feed.

▶ Breast-feeding mothers require more energy, nutrients, and fluid than their non-nursing peers. When nutrient intake is less than requirements, nutrients are usually removed from maternal stores to ensure adequate nutrition for the infant. To protect maternal stores and nourish the infant, a breast-feeding mother's diet should be rather nutrient dense, and she should be careful to drink when thirsty.

▶ Mothers are more likely to breast-feed successfully when they have accurate information, support from family, friends, and health professionals, and help with breast-feeding basics soon after the baby is born.

▶ Many breast-feeding difficulties can be prevented when breast-feeding is started in the delivery room, mothers nurse their infants frequently and long enough, and careful attention is paid to positioning and latch-on.

References

American Academy of Pediatrics Committee on Drugs. The transfer of drugs and other chemicals into human breast milk. Pediatrics 1994;93: 137.

American Dietetic Association. Position of the American Dietetic Association: Promotion and support of breast-feeding. J Am Diet Assc 1993;93:467.

Belec L, et al. Antibodies to human immunodeficiency virus in the breast milk of healthy seropositive women. Pediatrics 1990;85:1022.

Butte NF, et al. Effect of maternal diet and body composition on lactational performance. Am J Clin Nutr 1984;39:296.

Butte NF, Garza C. Anthropometry in the appraisal of lactation performance among well-nourished women. In: Hamosh M, Goldman AS (eds.), Human lactation 2: maternal environmental factors. New York: Plenum Press, 1986:61.

Centers for Disease Control. Recommendations for assisting in the prevention of perinatal transmission of human T-lymphotropic virus and acquired immunodeficiency syndrome. MMWR 1985;34:721.

Centers for Disease Control. Recommendations for the use of folic acid to reduce the number of cases of spina bifida and other neural tube defects. MMWR 1992;41:1.

Cross NA, et al. Calcium homeostasis and bone metabolism during pregnancy, lactation, and postweaning: a longitudinal study. Am J Clin Nutr 1995;61:514.

Cunningham AS, et al. Breastfeeding and health in the 1980s: a global epidemiologic review. J Peds 1991;118:659.

Dewey K, et al. Maternal vs. infant factors related to breast milk intake and residual milk volume: The Darling Study. Pediatrics 1991;87:829.

Dewey KG, et al. A randomized study of the effects of aerobic exercise by lactating women on breastmilk volume and composition. N Engl J Med 1994;330:449.

Dugdale AE, Eaton-Evans J. The effect of lactation and other factors on post-partum changes in body-weight and triceps skinfold thickness. Br J Nutr 1989;61:149.

Dungy CL, et al. Effect of discharge samples on duration of breast-feeding. Pediatrics 1992;90:233.

Duskieker LB, et al. Effect of supplemental fluids on human milk production. J Pediatr 1985;106:207.

Duskieker LB, et al. Prolonged maternal fluid supplementation in breast feeding. Pediatrics 1990;86:737.

Fairweather-Tait S, et al. Effect of calcium supplements and stage of lactation on the calcium absorption efficiency of lactating women accustomed to low calcium intakes. Am J Clin Nutr 1995;62:1188.

Forsum E, et al. Estimation of body fat in healthy Swedish women during pregnancy and lactation. Am J Clin Nutr 1989;50:465.

Greer FR, et al. High concentrations of vitamin D_2 in human milk associated with pharmacologic doses of vitamin D_2. J Pediatr 1984;105:61.

Institute of Medicine, Food and Nutrition Board. Nutrition during lactation (Report of the Subcommittee on Lactation, Committee on Nutritional Status During Pregnancy and Lactation). Washington, DC: National Academy Press, 1991.

Johnson EM. Weight changes during pregnancy and the postpartum period. Progressive Food Nutrition Science 1991;15:117.

Kalkwarf HJ, et al. Intestinal calcium absorption of women during lactation and after weaning. Am J Clin Nutr 1996;63:526.

Klein CJ, et al. A longitudinal study of urinary calcium, magnesium, and zinc excretion in lactating and nonlactating postpartum women. Am J Clin Nutr 1995;61:779.

Krebs NF, et al. Zinc supplementation during lactation: effects on maternal status and milk zinc concentrations. Am J Clin Nutr 1995;61:1030.

Kurinij N, Shiono PH. Early formula supplementation of breast-feeding. Pediatrics 1991;88:745.

Lawrence RA. Breastfeeding: a guide for the medical profession. St. Louis: Mosby–Year Book, 1994.

Little RE, et al. Maternal alcohol use during breast-feeding and infant mental and motor development at one year. N Engl J Med 1989;321:425.

Lovelady CA, et al. Lactation performance of exercising women. Am J Clin Nutr 1990;52:103.

Luck W, Nau H. Nicotine and continine concentration in the milk of smoking mothers: influence of cigarette consumption and diurnal variation. Eur J Pediatr 1987;146:21.

Lust KA, et al. Maternal intake of cruciferous vegetables and other foods and colic symptoms in exclusively breastfed infants. J Am Diet Assoc 1996;96:47.

Mennella JA, Beauchamp GK. The transfer of alcohol to human milk: effects in flavor and the infants behavior. N Engl J Med 1991a;325:981.

Mennella JA, Beauchamp GK. Maternal diet alters the sensory qualities of human milk and the behavior of the nursing. Pediatrics 1991b;88:737.

Motil KJ, et al. Basal and postprandial metabolic rates in lactating and nonlactating women. Am J Clin Nutr 1990;52:610.

National Institutes of Health. Optimal calcium intake. NIH Consensus Statement 1994;12:1.

National Research Council, Food and Nutrition Board, Commission on Life Sciences. Recommended Dietary Allowances. 10th ed. (Report of the Subcommittee on the Tenth Edition of the RDAs.) Washington, DC: National Academy Press, 1989.

Neifert MR, Seacat JM. Contemporary breastfeeding management. Clinical Perinatol 1985;12:319.

Newburg DS, et al. A human milk factor inhibits binding of human immunodeficiency virus to the CD4 receptor. Pediatric Research 1992;31:22.

Potter S, et al. Does infant feeding method influence postpartum weight? J Am Diet Assoc 1991;91:441.

Prentice AM, Prentice A. Energy costs of lactation. Annu Rev Nutr 1988;8:63.

Prentice AM, et al. Body mass index and lactation performance. Eur J Clin Nutr 1994;48:578.

Prentice A. Maternal calcium requirements during pregnancy and lactation. Am J Clin Nutr 1995;61:514.

Prentice A, et al. Calcium requirements of lactating Gambian mothers: effects of a calcium supplement on breast-milk calcium concentration, maternal bone mineral content, and urinary calcium excretion. Am J Clin Nutr 1995;62:58.

Rivera-Calimlim L. The significance of drugs in breast milk. Clinical Perinatol 1987;14:51.

Ross Products Division of Abbott Laboratories. Mother's Survey, 1995.

Ruff AJ, et al. Breast-feeding and maternal-infant transmission of human immunodeficiency virus type 1. J Pediatr 1992;121:325.

Ryan AS, et al. Recent declines in breast-feeding in the United States, 1984 through 1989. Pediatrics 1991;88:719.

Sowers MF, et al. Changes in bone density with lactation. JAMA 1993;269:3130.

Specker BL, et al. Calcium kinetics in lactating women with low and high calcium intakes. Am J Clin Nutr 1994;59:593.

Stumbo PJ, et al. Water intakes of lactating women. Am J Clin Nutr 1985;42:870.

U.S. Department of Health and Human Services. Healthy People 2000: National Health Promotion and Disease Prevention Objectives (Conference Edition). Washington, DC: Public Health Service, 1990.

Van de Perre P, et al. Infective and anti-infective properties of breast milk from HIV-1 infected women. Lancet 1993;341:914.

van Raaij JMA, et al. Energy cost of lactation and energy balances of well-nourished Dutch lactating women: Reappraised of the extra energy requirements of lactation. Am J Clin Nutr 1991;53:612.

Vio F, et al. Smoking during pregnancy and lactation and its effects on breast-milk volume. Am J Clin Nutr 1991;54:1011.

Wallace JP, Inbar G, Ernsthausen K. Infant acceptance of postexercise breast milk. Pediatrics 1992;89:1245.

World Health Organization. Breast-feeding/breast milk and human immunodeficiency virus HIV. Weekly Epidemiological Record 1987;62:245.

Additional Resources

Eiger MS, Olds SW. The complete book of breastfeeding. New York: Workman, 1972.

Huggins K. The nursing mother's companion. Boston: Harvard Common Press, 1986.

Journal of human lactation. New York: Human Sciences Press.

Lawrence RA. Practices and attitudes toward breast-feeding among medical professionals. Pediatrics 1982;70:912.

Tully MR, Overfield ML. Breastfeeding: a special relationship (video). Raleigh: Eagle Video Productions, 1991.

APPLICATION: Counseling for Breast-Feeding Success

In the early days and weeks of lactation, mother and baby learn the art of breast-feeding. Many new mothers need support or knowledge to help this process go well, and occasionally infants have physical traits or behaviors that hamper progress. Therefore, many hospitals and health clinics employ a lactation specialist. The lactation specialist is typically a health professional with interest and expertise in breast-feeding. Lactation specialists promote breast-feeding, and provide assistance and support for nursing mothers and their babies. Their knowledge and skill can make the difference between a successful breast-feeding experience and lactation failure. In the following story, Traci, a lactation specialist in a WIC clinic, helps Laurie, a client, establish a healthy breast-feeding relationship with her first child, Mark. Our story begins as the phone rings in Traci's office.

TRACI: Madison County WIC, may I help you?

LAURIE: Traci, this is Laurie. You talked to me about breast-feeding when I was in the clinic last month. I think there is something wrong with my milk. What should I do?

TRACI: Tell me what you're experiencing.

LAURIE: My baby, Mark, was born 4 days ago. Things went fine in the hospital, a nurse showed me how to hold him and help him latch on. He seemed very content and slept a lot. This morning when I got up my breasts were large and hurt. They feel awful. It hurts when I try to feed Mark and he cries and won't eat.

TRACI: How often did Mark nurse yesterday?

LAURIE: He slept a lot. I guess I fed him 6 or 7 times.

TRACI: Do you have a fever?

LAURIE: No, but my breasts feel like bricks! Do you know what is wrong?

TRACI: From what you are describing it sounds like your milk has come in. New moms often experience some temporary fullness or engorgement when this happens. When your breasts become too full it is difficult for Mark to latch on properly. He may be sucking on only your nipple. That hurts you and he won't get much milk so he cries.

LAURIE: So I shouldn't nurse him?

TRACI: No, the way to get over this problem is to get a little bit of the milk out of your breasts so he can latch on, then nurse him frequently so your breasts won't become so full. The problem usually clears up within a few days.

LAURIE: My breasts really hurt. What should I do?

TRACI: Try taking a warm shower, then express or pump a little milk out to soften your breasts. Do you have a pump?

LAURIE: Yes, I got one at the hospital.

TRACI: After you pump a little milk out, see if Mark can nurse. Remember to get some of the dark area around your nipple into his mouth—not just your nipple. Try feeding him every 2 to 3 hours during the day. You can put ice on your breasts between feedings to help reduce the swelling and help you feel more comfortable.

LAURIE: Ice? I'll try it.

TRACI: Good. Would you call me this afternoon when it is convenient for you to let me know how things are going?

LAURIE: Yes, I'll try. Bye, I'm going to go find the pump.

TRACI: Goodbye, talk to you later.

That afternoon Laurie called back.

TRACI: Hi Laurie. Thanks for calling back. How are you doing?

LAURIE: Not great but better. Mark was able to nurse after I pumped a little milk out. My breasts are still sore but they're not as bad as this morning. Mark has nursed every 2 hours today. I don't like the ice but it helps.

TRACI: It sounds like you are coping well. It might be a good idea to nurse once or twice during the night. That way your breasts won't get too full for Mark to latch on again.

LAURIE: OK, I sure don't want that to happen again.

TRACI: You'll be glad to know that engorgement doesn't last long. I think you'll feel better tomorrow. Will you call me again?

LAURIE: Yes. Thanks. Bye.

The next day Laurie called.

TRACI: Laurie, thanks for calling. How are you and Mark doing today?

LAURIE: Well, I had to pump a bit this morning but it's not nearly as bad. I don't think I'll need the ice today.

TRACI: Great. I'd continue to nurse at least every 3 hours during the day and once at night for a few days. You're over the hump!

The next week Laurie stopped in at the clinic.

TRACI: Hi, Laurie. Good to see you.

LAURIE: Hi, Mark just had his first check-up and I stopped to say thanks. I also have a question. The doctor said he has gained 4 ounces. That doesn't sound like much to me for 10 days and my breasts don't feel so full anymore. Do you think that I have enough milk?

TRACI: Four ounces is a good weight gain for a 10-day-old. Babies lose a little weight after they are born. They usually are back up to their birth weight by about one week. Mark seems to be right on track. It's normal for the breasts to feel softer once you and Mark have gotten a feeding routine down. I'm glad you are both doing well.

LAURIE: Me too. I was afraid I couldn't breast-feed, but now I feel like I can.

TRACI: Great. See you at Mark's next check-up.

PART IV

THE ADULT YEARS

CHAPTER 11

ADULTHOOD

Physiologic Changes
Psychosocial Development
Nutrition Assessment
Energy and Nutrient Needs

Chronic Health Concerns of Adults
Nutrition and Health Concerns of Women
Promoting Health and Well-Being
Concepts to Remember

Andrew, a 42-year-old office manager, lives in a suburb of a large New England city with his wife, Betty, a daughter, and two sons. The boys are in elementary school and his daughter has just begun high school. To make ends meet and to plan for college expenses, Betty got a job at a nearby school district and Andrew took a part-time job selling real estate. The children are busy with sports, church, and school activities. Andrew and Betty try to attend as many of the children's activities as they can, but their busy schedules mean they are on the go all the time.

Betty is a good cook and Andrew helps out in the kitchen. They try to have dinner together as a family each evening but it is often at odd hours. In the morning, everyone makes his or her own breakfast—usually fruit or fruit juice and cereal with milk. There is always toast and sometimes muffins and donuts. The children eat school lunch most days but sometimes pack a lunch from home. Betty always packs a sandwich and fruit for lunch. Andrew eats in the cafeteria in his building or at a fast-food restaurant down the street.

Andrew is 188 cm (74 in) tall and weighs 105 kg (230 pounds). He has a bit of a "gut" and could afford to lose some weight. He knows that he should exercise on a consistent basis, but he has difficulty finding time. Betty gave him an exercise bicycle for Christmas but he uses it only once or twice a week. Andrew doesn't like "feeling fat," especially around his midsection, and wants to eat better to "live longer and healthier" but doesn't know where to begin.

Andrew does most of the family grocery shopping. He is interested in nutrition and checks the Nutrition Facts label, particularly for calories and fat content. He tries to control his weight by avoiding snacks, especially cakes, cookies, and chips and dip. He tends to categorize these as "bad" and many of the foods he eats less often as "good" because they are "good for him." When Andrew gets the urge for something sweet, he'll eat as many as a dozen cookies at one sitting and then will avoid them for weeks.

Andrew really wants to make improvements in his diet but he gets confused about what to do and frustrated at his apparent lack of progress. He reports eating more "good" foods, fruits, and vegetables than he used to. Despite these efforts, in the last 3 days he has had only two 4-ounce glasses of orange juice, a half cup of stir-fried broccoli and mushrooms, two lettuce leaves, and half a tomato. Andrew wonders if he should take a supplement of some kind to improve his diet.

Last month Andrew wasn't feeling very well and went to see his family physician. The doctor treated him for a throat infection but insisted that he come back in 2 weeks for a complete physical examination and some blood work. When the laboratory results came back, the physician told Andrew that his total blood cholesterol and LDL cholesterol were too high and that his HDL levels were a little low. He recommended that Andrew make some changes in his diet and get more exercise and also suggested he needed to lose a few pounds. He said this was particularly important because of Andrew's family history of diabetes mellitus and heart disease.

Andrew's situation is representative of the many nutrition-related concerns facing adults as they approach middle age. With maturation and the first discernible stages of aging, adulthood focuses on nutrition for promoting lifelong health. This includes physical fitness and optimum dietary intakes to minimize the progression of chronic diseases and their impact on quality of life.

Physiologically, adulthood begins with the attainment of sexual maturity and the completion of growth; the former occurs in the late teen years and the latter well into the third decade of life. Emotionally, it is often associated with significant life events such as completion of education, getting the first job, getting a credit card, or reaching the age of eligibility to vote or buy (legally) alcoholic beverages. Typically, young adulthood begins at 18 years and encompasses at least the next two decades. Middle age remains one of the least studied phases of life. It is uncharted territory in human development without set stages or transition points. By conventional definition, middle age starts at age 40. However, as life gets longer, it becomes more difficult to define middle life. Individuals who are called middle-aged today are very different from those of a generation ago. The "baby boomers" (those born between 1946 and 1964) have not been referred to as middle-aged until they turned 50. In fact, it has been suggested that this group seems to be "programmed to never get old," and many of them will not confront old age until well into their seventies (Chernoff, 1995). As in the growth years, there is a great diversity in individual responses to maturation and aging. Although the rate of change is determined by genetics, it is influenced by growth during early life as well as by adult lifestyles (McGill et al, 1996).

PHYSIOLOGIC CHANGES

■ What are the physiologic changes that occur across adulthood?

■ How do body weight and composition change as an individual moves from adolescence through adulthood?

■ What is menopause, and what are the long-term health implications? What are the advantages and disadvantages of hormone replacement therapy?

There are no dramatic markers in physical development in the adult. Physiologic maturity is defined as the completion of skeletal growth, as characterized by the achievement of maximum height and the formation of peak bone mass. Most body systems reach their peak efficiency and optimum functioning before age 30. The human body is a dynamic organism, and stability is the major physiologic characteristic of adulthood. In general, the cells of most tissues are catabolized and replaced at approximately the same rate. With time, catabolism slightly exceeds anabolism and there are small changes in function or performance. Most of these changes accelerate after middle age and are discussed in greater detail in Chapter 12.

Musculoskeletal

Approximately 5 years after maximum height is attained, an adult reaches maximum strength, endurance, and agility. From this point there is a gradual but steady decline. Bone mass increases well into the third decade. In young adult women, this increase is positively influenced by physical activity, dietary calcium, and use of oral contraceptives (Recker et al, 1992). Data from cross-sectional studies indicate that, beginning in the third decade, there is a continuous loss of trabecular bone mineral density in men and women. For females the marked decrease in estrogen and progesterone production of menopause is associated with an acceleration in loss of cortical bone.

Muscle mass increases into the third decade and then declines. Because the decrease is gradual, these changes may not become apparent for more than a decade. Physical activity, especially resistance training, may attenuate or prevent the bone and muscle mass loss associated with aging (Vuori, 1996).

Oral Health

Although the process of tooth decay can continue beyond childhood, tooth loss during the adult years most frequently is due to **periodontal disease**. Periodontal disease is promoted by the same factors that contribute to dental caries. Accumulation of bacteria-containing plaque can cause the gums around the teeth to become inflamed and bleed easily, a condition called gingivitis. If the symptoms are ignored, the gingiva become scarred and bacteria work their way below the gumline and into the jawbone.

The ensuing infection results in destruction of the bone that holds in the teeth, resulting in tooth loss.

Menopause

During a woman's childbearing years, the ovaries produce estrogen and progesterone that signal the **endometrium** to grow and thicken. One of the ovaries releases an ovum each month. If the ovum is not fertilized, it moves to the uterus and is absorbed. Consequently, hormone levels decline and the endometrial tissue breaks up and is discharged during menstruation. The normal menstrual cycle is discussed in Chapter 8.

Menopause occurs toward the end of a woman's reproductive period (about age 50) when there is a progressive decline in estrogen secretion. In the years just before menopause, the menstrual cycle may become irregular, and menstrual flow is usually lighter and of shorter duration. Eventually ovulation ceases and menstruation ends. A woman is not completely without estrogen even after menopause, but levels are severely diminished.

Hormone Replacement Therapy

For many women a variety of symptoms are associated with menopause, ranging from mild discomfort to "hot flashes" with extreme flushing of the skin, vaginal dryness, fatigue, anxiety, sleep disturbances, and many others (Wiklund et al, 1993). For over 30 years, hormone replacement therapy (HRT) has been used to mitigate the acute symptoms of menopause. Now, HRT is prescribed to reduce the risks of some chronic diseases, e.g., osteoporosis and cardiovascular disease, that accelerate after menopause.

ESTROGEN REPLACEMENT THERAPY (ERT)
Conjugated estrogen (a mixture of several forms of the hormone) may be available as pills and as estrogen patches from which **estradiol** is absorbed **transdermally**. Taking estrogen reduces a woman's risk of developing coronary artery disease by lowering low-density-lipoprotein cholesterol (LDL-C), the form most readily incorporated into arterial deposits, and by raising HDL cholesterol, the type responsible for preventing LDL-C from being deposited on blood vessel walls (Vaziri et al, 1993). Replacing estrogen decreases the average lifetime risk of osteoporosis, reducing the risk of hip fracture. There have been some reports that estrogen helps alleviate wrinkling by stimulating the production of collagen, a major protein of the skin. Others have suggested that estrogen improves mood, memory, and mental agility, but data are far from conclusive.

Estrogen stimulates the growth of the endometrium and thus increases the risk of endometrial cancer. There is no evidence that short-term ERT is associated with the oc-

currence of breast cancer, but risk is elevated with more than 8 years of therapy. The potential for development of gallstones is greater in women who take oral estrogen, presumably because the hormone stimulates the liver to increase the cholesterol content of bile.

ESTROGEN PLUS PROGESTERONE (HRT)
Because ERT alone increases the risk for endometrial cancer in menopausal women, progestins (synthetic progesterone) are added to estrogens for HRT. Use of progestin counters estrogen's effect on endometrial growth but does not appear to negate the other positive effects of estrogen (Writing Group for the PEPI Trial, 1996). However, adding progestin may increase such side effects as breast tenderness, bloating, irritability, depression, monthly vaginal bleeding, and irregular bleeding, which usually subside within the first year of treatment.

It has been suggested that postmenopausal women who received HRT tended to gain less weight or develop less abdominal fat than women who received a placebo, but other studies have provided inconsistent results. A recent 5-year prospective and cross-sectional cohort study of 6871 postmenopausal women found that intermittent or continuous HRT was not associated with any differences in the central obesity commonly observed in postmenopausal women (Kirtz-Silverstein, 1996).

Metabolism

During adulthood the resting energy expenditure (REE) decreases gradually at first and then at an accelerating rate as muscle mass declines. Diminished resting energy expenditure translates into reduced caloric requirements. Failure to adjust levels of dietary intake and physical activity to compensate for this decline in energy expenditure has the potential to promote excess gains of body weight and fat.

Body Weight

In the United States average body weight increases throughout the seventh decade in both sexes. Not all adult

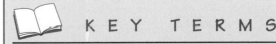

K E Y T E R M S

periodontal disease: a disease of tissues supporting the teeth—gingiva, ligaments, and bone
endometrium: lining of the uterus
estradiol: the most potent naturally occurring form of estrogen
transdermally: through the skin

Americans gain weight, though—by the age of 50 years, those who lose weight are as prevalent as those who gain weight, but gainers gain more than losers lose, and averages climb (Garn, 1996).

Middle-aged spread is not a myth. Weight gain begins as early as the 20s and 30s and accelerates with age, especially after menopause for women. Extra pounds often tend to settle around the midsection. As waistlines increase, so do health risks. A 3-year prospective study among 29,122 men, aged 40 to 75 years, found that weight gain was associated with increased risk of coronary heart disease (Rimm et al, 1995). Similarly, a prospective study that followed more than 100,000 registered nurses over 14 years found that among women of normal weight, gains of 5 kg or more after 18 years of age increased the risk of both fatal coronary heart disease and non-fatal **myocardial infarction** (Willett et al, 1995). In addition, women who gained 5 kg or more experienced increased risk of diabetes mellitus (Colditz et al, 1995). Women who lost 5 kg or more, however, had a decreased risk of diabetes. These researchers suggest that the long-held assumption that it is normal for body weight to increase with age is erroneous

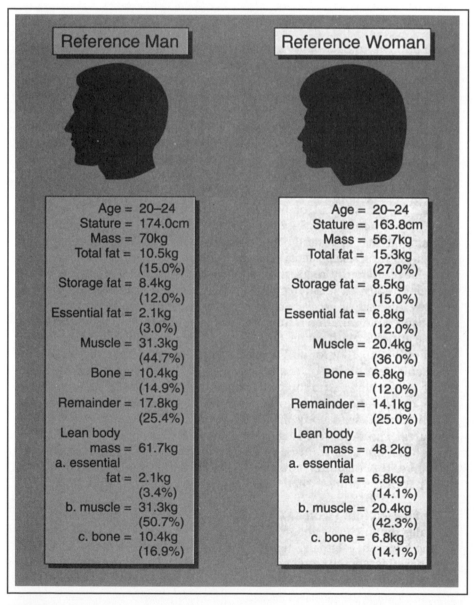

FIGURE 11–1. Body Composition of reference man and reference woman. (From Katch FI, McArdle WD. Introduction to nutrition, exercise and health. 4th ed. Philadelphia: Lea & Febiger, 1993.)

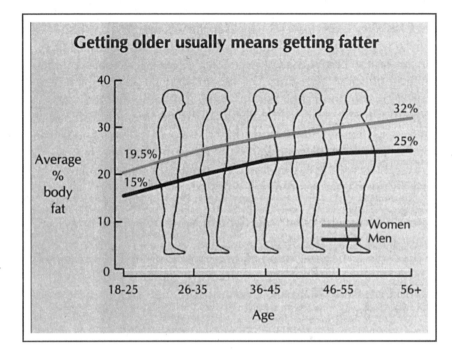

FIGURE 11–2. Average body fat increases with age. Average body fat for young men is about 15 percent. For young women, the average range is 18 to 23 percent. With age, the amount of muscle tends to drop, and fat accounts for a greater percentage of weight. By age 60, body fat gradually increases to about 25 percent in men and 32 percent in women. (From Medical Essay. Supplement to Mayo Clinic Health Letter. Rochester, MN: Mayo Foundation for Medical Education and Research; June, 1994.)

and that maintenance of the weight of early adulthood is an appropriate lifetime goal.

Body Composition

At a genetically determined point, overall growth is achieved and an adult pattern of body composition is established. The major structural components of the human body are muscle, fat, and bone. Figure 11–1 summarizes body composition for a "reference man" and "reference woman" 20 to 24 years of age. These standards are not considered ideal or average but are a frame of reference to which individuals may be compared (Katch and McArdle, 1993). In these models, essential fat refers to that stored in the marrow of bones; in the heart, liver, spleen, kidneys, intestines, and muscles; and in the central nervous system. The storage fat is the most variable component of body composition.

At entry to adulthood, women have a larger body fat mass and lower lean body mass than men. Over time, body composition changes. As illustrated in Figure 11–2, the average percentage of body weight that is fat mass increases. This is accompanied by a decline in lean mass in both men and women. During the middle adult years, these changes are reflected in increased skinfold thicknesses for both males and females, but body fat is greater and fluctuates more in women. Increased body fatness is associated with increased risk of diabetes mellitus, coronary heart disease, and hypertension.

Blood Lipid Levels

Serum total cholesterol (TC) levels increase in men until about 50 years of age. This pattern differs markedly from that observed in women, who have significantly lower levels, which increase after menopause from 50 to 65 years of age and then remain steady or slightly decline into old age. Throughout adulthood males have a much greater ratio of TC to high-density-lipoprotein cholesterol (HDL-C), but after age 50 this ratio is similar in males and females.

PSYCHOSOCIAL DEVELOPMENT

■ What are the psychosocial changes associated with the adult years?

■ How do stress and social and psychological issues influence dietary patterns?

Psychosocial development of adulthood is characterized by changing patterns as societal roles develop and evolve.

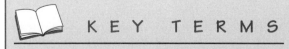

KEY TERMS

myocardial infarction: an area of tissue necrosis in the heart muscle due to obstruction of circulation

The early adult years are characterized by the formation of personal relationships, career development, establishment of home, rearing of young children, and assumption of a role within the community. Gradual changes to middle adulthood are accompanied by adaptation to growing of families, greater economic responsibilities, stable careers, and greater identity of self. Many of today's middle agers find themselves sandwiched between generations, caring for aging parents and, because of delayed childbearing, raising young children. As their children mature and leave home the transitions of middle-aged adults are accompanied by less demanding family responsibilities, preparation for retirement, and renewed opportunities for personal development.

Physiologic needs form the foundation for health and nutrition status, but overall dietary patterns probably are more influenced by social and psychological factors. Psychological well-being is a multifaceted phenomenon that comprises both emotional functioning and satisfaction with life (Stewart and Ware, 1992). Psychological well-being has been equated with the absence of anxiety and depression, the presence of positive affect, high levels of self esteem, the capacity to deal with daily stresses, and positive ratings of satisfaction with personal life circumstances (Gauvin and Spence, 1996).

A combination of psychological stress, social pressures, and sedentary lifestyle can contribute to poor dietary and activity patterns with negative health implications. As discussed in Chapter 3, the challenge is to motivate adults to make modest changes, primarily in food habits and exercise patterns, to improve their well-being and reduce the risk of disease. An understanding of the individual's lifestyle and psychosocial behaviors is central to monitoring and improving nutrition status.

NUTRITION ASSESSMENT

■ What tools are used for assessment of nutrition status of adults?

■ Why is it appropriate to include identifiers of chronic disease in nutrition assessment?

■ How are risks of chronic disease measured and monitored?

The anthropometric, biochemical, clinical, and dietary techniques of nutrition screening and assessment are discussed in Chapter 2. Particular attention is given to identification of individuals at risk of undernutrition. In this chapter, additional measurements used for assessment of risk for nutrition-related chronic diseases are presented. Such information is essential for early intervention and for monitoring the effectiveness of nutrition care. Of particular importance are those diseases related to major causes of death and disability: obesity, diabetes mellitus, hypertension, and cardiovascular disease.

Excess Body Weight

Traditionally overweight and obesity are defined by comparison of an individual's weight for height to a reference standard such as the Metropolitan relative weight (MRW) or body mass index (BMI). In the past the reference weight has been designated as "ideal" or "desirable." Such terms are misleading because there is no single appropriate weight for all individuals. Reference weights can be useful when they are associated with decreased health risks.

Recently the American Health Foundation (a nonprofit organization dedicated to finding preventive strategies to reduce chronic diseases) convened an Expert Panel that identified a healthy weight as one associated with the lowest morbidity (Meisler and St. Jeor, 1996). A BMI of less than 25 was considered the upper limit beyond which morbidities of obesity are identifiable and weight-related disease risks become a concern. These data, converted to weight for height, regardless of gender, are illustrated in Table 11–1.

Fatfold measurements increase and decrease with body fat. Values can be compared with the percentiles of reference data from the National Health and Nutrition Examination Survey (NHANES) (Appendices 3A and 3B). Deposition of increased body weight as abdominal fat during adulthood is a risk factor for hypertension and diabetes mellitus, and, thus, coronary heart disease, beyond that of excess weight alone (Croft et al, 1995). To identify increased risk due to an accumulation of abdominal fat, routine measurement of the circumferences of waist and hips is recommended to determine the waist:hip ratio (WHR). A WHR greater than 0.80 in women and greater than 0.95 in men indicates that a high proportion of abdominal fat is likely to be present. This is associated with a significant health risk.

Screening for Diabetes Mellitus

Diabetes mellitus is characterized by an abnormal metabolism of glucose that results from an absolute or relative lack of the hormone insulin. Type II or non–insulin-dependent diabetes mellitus (NIDDM) is more common in obesity. Screening and diagnostic testing is particularly important when the individual is obese, has a family history of diabetes mellitus, or has symptoms that suggest the presence of the disease. Screening for diabetes mellitus is based on plasma glucose levels.

When urine is tested as part of a routine physical examination, diabetes may be detected by the presence of glucose. A random plasma glucose level above 200 mg/dL is suggestive of the presence of diabetes. While neither glucose in the urine nor a single elevated blood glucose is diagnostic for diabetes mellitus, an elevated level in the presence of symptoms or a family history of diabetes melli-

TABLE 11-1 Healthy-Weight Target for Adults Regardless of Sex, as Derived from a Body Mass Index of 25

Height		Maximum Weight	
cm	in	kg	lb
147	58	54	119
150	59	56	124
152	60	58	128
155	61	60	132
157	62	62	136
160	63	64	141
163	64	66	145
165	65	68	150
168	66	70	155
170	67	72	159
173	68	75	164
175	69	77	169
178	70	79	174
180	71	81	179
183	72	84	184
185	73	86	189
188	74	88	194
190	75	91	200
193	76	93	205

From Meisler JG, St Jeor S. Summary and recommendations from the American Health Foundation Panel on Healthy Weight. Am J Clin Nutr 1996;63(Suppl):476S. © Am J Clin Nutr. American Society for Clinical Nutrition.

TABLE 11-2 Blood Glucose Values Associated with Diabetes Mellitus

Blood Glucose	Normal Value (mg/dL)	Diagnostic for Diabetes Mellitus (mg/dL)
Random glucose	<200	≥200 with signs and symptoms of diabetes mellitus
Fasting glucose	115	≥140 on at least two occasions
GLUCOSE TOLERANCE TEST Glucose Load		
After 60 minutes	200	>200
After 120 minutes	140	200

tus is an indicator for a glucose tolerance test (GTT) for diagnosis. A GTT involves the measurement of fasting blood glucose levels, administration of a glucose "load" (a solution containing 75 to 100 g glucose), and measurement of plasma glucose levels up to 5 hours later to determine **glucose tolerance**. There are several variations of the glucose tolerance test. The values in Table 11–2 are representative of "normal" plasma glucose levels in response to a glucose load and those that would be considered to confirm the diagnosis of diabetes mellitus. Specific values may vary somewhat due to the measurement used and the laboratory completing the analysis.

Hypertension

Chronic hypertension is a major risk factor for coronary heart disease, cerebrovascular disease, and renal insuffi-

ciency. Blood pressure is measured in millimeters of mercury (mm Hg), a standard unit for the measurement of pressure.

Hypertension, a major public health problem, is defined as blood pressure exceeding the upper limit of normality; the upper limit is generally accepted as **systolic pressure** greater than 140 mm Hg and **diastolic pressure** greater than 90 mm Hg (Joint National Committee on Detection, Evaluation and Treatment of High Blood Pressure, 1993).

Serum Lipids and Lipoproteins

Elevated levels of serum total cholesterol (TC) and low-density-lipoprotein cholesterol (LDL-C) and low levels of high-density-lipoprotein cholesterol (HDL-C) have been correlated with increased rates of coronary heart disease. They are used routinely for assessment of risk and monitoring of intervention. Approximately 7% of the body's cholesterol circulates in the blood. Because lipids such as cholesterol and triglycerides are fat soluble, they must be transported in the bloodstream from sites of absorption or

K E Y   T E R M S

glucose tolerance: efficiency with which the body can clear a bolus of glucose from the blood
systolic pressure: pressure that occurs with the contraction of the heart muscle
diastolic pressure: the pressure during relaxation of the ventricles

synthesis to sites of storage or metabolism on lipoproteins. Lipoproteins are spherical macromolecular complexes of lipids (triglycerides, cholesterol, cholesterol ester, and phospholipids) and special proteins known as apoproteins. The apoprotein portions control the interaction and metabolic fate of lipoproteins. They activate enzymes that modify the composition and structure of lipoproteins, are involved in the binding and uptake of lipoproteins by cells, and participate in the exchange of lipids between lipoprotein of different classes. Major transport lipoproteins are chylomicrons, high-density lipoproteins (HDL), very-low-density lipoproteins (VLDL), and low-density lipoproteins (LDL).

Chylomicrons, synthesized in the small intestine, transport dietary triglyceride from small intestine to adipose tissue, muscle, and the liver. They are 90% triglyceride. The dietary cholesterol they carry is taken up by the liver for production of bile acids or later incorporated in VLDL. Chylomicrons are found in the serum in the postprandial state.

VLDL are 60% triglyceride by weight and contain 10% to 15% of the serum's total cholesterol. Synthesized in the liver, VLDL carry triglycerides to the cells for storage and metabolism. When triglycerides are removed from VLDL the remaining smaller and denser lipoprotein particles are known as intermediate density lipoprotein (IDL) because the density of IDL falls between that of VLDL and LDL. Approximately half the IDL is catabolized by the liver, and the remaining IDL undergoes changes that transform it into LDL.

LDL contains approximately 70% of the serum total cholesterol. Its primary role is to transport cholesterol to various cells of the body. LDL is considered the most atherogenic lipoprotein. About 70% to 80% of LDL is removed from the serum by LDL receptors located on the plasma membranes of hepatic and peripheral cells. The remaining 20% to 30% are degraded by **macrophages**.

Most clinical laboratories do not measure LDL-C directly. Instead, it is calculated based on measurements of TC, HDL-C, and triglycerides. In this procedure, VLDL-cholesterol is estimated by dividing triglycerides by 5.

The following equation for calculating LDL-C is recommended by the National Cholesterol Education Program (1993):

$$LDL\text{-}C = TC - HDL\text{-}C - (Triglyceride/5)$$

This formula cannot be used when the triglyceride level is greater than 400 mg/dL.

HDL is the smallest and most dense of the lipoproteins. Secreted by the liver and small intestine in a disc-shaped form, HDL eventually assumes a spherical shape as it takes up phospholipids and cholesterol from other lipoproteins and body cells. It appears that HDL picks up cholesterol from the bloodstream, other lipoproteins, and various cells of the body and transports it to the liver where it is excreted in the bile, converted to bile acids, or reprocessed into VLDL. This reverse transport process is thought to be at least part of the explanation for the strong inverse relationship between serum HDL-C and CHD risk.

In 1985, the National Institutes of Health (NIH) founded the National Cholesterol Education Program (NCEP) to encourage Americans to modify their diets to reduce the risk of coronary heart disease. The NCEP guidelines define risk status according to serum cholesterol levels, including HDL and LDL, in conjunction with other coronary heart disease risk factors. Blood lipid levels are classified as desirable, borderline high, and high (Table 11–3). Accurate cholesterol testing is needed to provide guidelines for treatment.

ENERGY AND NUTRIENT NEEDS

■ What are the Recommended Dietary Allowances?

■ How do energy and nutrient needs change across adulthood?

■ For which nutrients are there concerns about adequate intakes?

During the adult years, excluding pregnancy and lactation, nutrients are used for body repair and maintenance. The 1989 Recommended Dietary Allowances (RDAs) are

TABLE 11–3 Risk Status According to Serum Cholesterol and Lipoprotein Status

Lipid	Desirable	Borderline	Risk
Serum total cholesterol	<200 mg/dL	200–239 mg/dL	>240 mg/dL
Low-density-lipoprotein cholesterol	<130 mg/dL	130–159 mg/dL	≥16 mg/dL
High-density-lipoprotein cholesterol	≥35 mg/dL	—	≤35 mg/dL

From Second Report of the National Cholesterol Education Program (NCEP) Panel on Detection, Evaluation and Treatment of High Blood Cholesterol in Adults (Adult Treatment Panel II). Bethesda, MD: National Heart and Blood Institute. National Institutes of Health, 1993.

TABLE 11–4 Recommended Dietary Allowances for Adults by Age in Years

	19–24		25–50		50+	
	Males	Females	Males	Females	Males	Females
Weight (kg)	72	58	79	63	77	65
Height (cm)	177	164	176	163	173	160
Energy (kcal)	2900	2200	2900	2200	2300	1900
Protein (g)	58	46	63	50	63	50
FAT-SOLUBLE VITAMINS						
Vitamin A (μg RE)*	1000	800	1000	800	1000	800
Vitamin D (μg)†	10	10	5	5	5	5
Vitamin E (mg α-TE)††	10	8	10	8	10	8
Vitamin K (μg)	70	60	80	65	80	65
WATER-SOLUBLE VITAMINS						
Vitamin C (mg)	60	60	60	60	60	60
Thiamin (mg)	1.5	1.1	1.5	1.1	1.2	1.0
Riboflavin (mg)	1.7	1.3	1.7	1.3	1.4	1.2
Niacin (mg NE)§	19	15	19	15	15	13
Vitamin B_6 (mg)	2.0	1.5	2.0	1.6	2.0	1.6
Folate (μg)	200	180	200	180	200	180
Vitamin B_{12} (μg)	2.0	2.0	2.0	2.0	2.0	2.0
MINERALS						
Calcium (mg)	1200	1200	800	800	800	800
Phosphorus (mg)	1200	1200	800	800	800	800
Magnesium (mg)	350	300	350	280	350	280
Iron (mg)	10	15	10	15	10	10
Zinc (mg)	15	12	15	12	15	12
Iodine (μg)	150	150	150	150	150	150
Selenium (μg)	70	50	70	55	70	55

* 1 RE (retinol equivalent) = 1 μg or 6 μg β-carotene.
† As cholecalciferol. 10 μg cholecalciferol = 400 IU of vitamin D.
†† α-Tocopherol equivalents. 1 mg d-α = 1 α-TE.
§ 1 NE (niacin equivalent) = 1 mg of niacin or 60 mg of dietary tryptophan.

levels of essential nutrients that are considered to adequately meet the needs of practically all healthy persons (Food and Nutrition Board, 1989). For adults, the recommended levels are divided into the age groups 19 to 24 years, 25 to 50 years, and older than 50 years (Table 11–4). The heights and weights of the reference male and female for these age groups are designated in order to quantify daily levels. Obviously, actual levels needed or consumed by healthy adults vary with individual age, body size, and activity level. As discussed in Chapter 1, the Recommended Dietary Allowances are currently under review, and it is reasonable to expect that some values and the manner in which they are presented will change in a future edition.

Data from the 1989 Continuing Survey of Food Intakes by Individuals suggest that, on the average, both men and women in the United States meet the 1989 Recommended Dietary Allowances for the majority of nutrients. Men met the RDAs for more nutrients than women because they

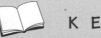

K E Y   T E R M S

macrophages: large phagocytic cells located within connective tissue

TABLE 11–5 Recommended Energy Intakes for Adults

Age (y)	Weight (kg)	kcal/day	kcal/kg
MALES			
19–24	72	2900	40
25–50	79	2900	37
51+	77	2300	30
FEMALES			
19–24	58	2200	38
25–50	63	2200	35
51+	65	1900	30

tend to eat larger quantities of food (USDA, 1993). However, levels of several nutrients fell short of the RDA, and a substantial portion of the population failed to achieve recommended levels (Kant et al, 1994), especially as the quantity of nutrient-poor food consumed increased. For example, a study from the National Cancer Institute using the same USDA data found that the mean intake of fruits and vegetables was 4.3 servings per day, but only 32% of American adults met the Healthy People 2000 Objective of 5 or more servings (Krebs-Smith et al, 1995).

The nutrients discussed in this section are those for which there is evidence that current recommended levels should be modified or about which there are concerns regarding adequate intake.

Energy

The energy need of an individual is the level required to balance that utilized for resting energy expenditure (REE), physical activity, and the thermic effect of food. For most adults, the REE represents the largest component of total energy used each day and, as mentioned previously, it is highly correlated with lean body mass. Hence, males have higher REEs than females, and lean individuals have higher levels than those with greater proportions of body fat. Except in individuals who engage in vigorous physical activity, daily energy expenditure for physical activity is less than that for REE.

Energy needs vary widely. They are determined, to some extent, by age, gender, body size and composition, genetic factors, energy intake, activity level, and ambient temperature. The RDA for energy assumes that an individual's body size and composition and level of physical activity are consistent with long-term good health. The RDAs reflect average needs of individuals based on median heights and weights (see Table 1–4 in Chapter 1). The RDA for adults, expressed as kilocalories per kilogram of body weight, appear in Table 11–5. Energy recommendations range from 40 kcal/kg for the "reference" 72-kg male, aged 19 to 24 years, to 37 kcal/kg at age 25 to 50 years, to 30 kcal/kg for those older than 50 years. Energy levels for females of equivalent ages are 38, 35, and 30 kcal/kg body weight respectively.

Mean daily total food energy intakes of adults aged 20 to 59 years participating in the Third National Health and Nutrition Examination Survey (NHANES III) appear in Table 11–6. It is apparent that energy intakes decline with

TABLE 11–6 Mean Daily Total Food-Energy Intake (TFEI) and Percentages of TFEI from Total Dietary Fat and from Saturated Fat, by Age Group and Sex

Age Group	Sample Size	Daily TFEI	TFEI from Total Dietary Fat (%)	TFEI from Saturated Fat (%)
MALES				
20–29	844	3025	34.0	12.0
30–39	735	2872	34.6	11.9
40–49	626	2545	33.9	11.4
50–59	473	2341	35.7	11.8
FEMALES				
20–29	838	1957	34.0	11.9
30–39	791	1883	34.2	11.9
40–49	602	1764	34.9	11.8
50–59	456	1629	33.8	11.4

From Third National Health and Nutrition Examination Survey, Phase I, 1988–91, MMWR 1994:116.

age for both men and women. It is important to note that for females of all ages and males 40 to 49 years mean food energy intakes are consistently below the RDA. In spite of this, the prevalence of overweight Americans has increased in the last decade (Kuczmarski et al, 1994). Such observations have led to concerns about the nutrient adequacy of American diets with levels below recommended amounts and reduced energy output via physical activity. Any nutrition recommendation to support health must be based on this consideration.

Protein

Recommended protein intakes of 0.8 g/kg body weight per day for adult men and women assume that a diet of mixed sources of protein is consumed. Mean protein intakes in NHANES III were 15% of kilocalories, a level adequate for most individuals (McDowell et al, 1994). If an individual restricts his or her total food intake or of some protein foods, careful dietary planning is required to achieve the recommended allowance. Equally important, the recommendations for protein are based on the assumption that the individual consumes an adequate amount of energy to spare dietary protein for protein synthesis. If energy intake is below maintenance levels, additional protein is required to compensate for that used to meet energy needs.

Lipids

Total fat consumption among Americans has decreased from approximately 41% of energy intake in the late 1970s to 36% in the mid-1980s to 33% in 1994 (Agricultural Research Service, 1996). However, only one-third of adults met the recommendation of 30% or less of kilocalories of fat. Preliminary data from NHANES III indicate that saturated fat constitutes a mean of 12% of kilocalories in the diets of Americans (McDowell et al, 1994). The National Health and Nutrition Examination Survey (NHANES) I Epidemiologic Follow-Up Survey (NHEFS) found that from the survey in 1971–74 to a decade later, the percentage of energy intake from fat and weight change were inversely related in women but positively associated in men (Kant et al, 1995).

Fat-Soluble Vitamins

VITAMIN A Vitamin A plays many roles in the body, particularly in vision and maintenance of epithelial tissue. In addition to its role as an antioxidant there has been substantial interest in the use of creams containing retinoic acid (traditionally a medication to treat acne) to prevent wrinkling or diminish the brown age spots that begin to appear on the skin of some individuals in middle age.

VITAMIN D There is an RDA for vitamin D for adults, but most adults are likely to get sufficient exposure to sunlight to meet it. As discussed in Chapter 12, to minimize the effects of osteoporosis, sufficient vitamin D must be available to facilitate calcium absorption and bone formation. If an individual has little exposure to sunlight and does not consume vitamin D–fortified milk, a supplemental source should be considered.

VITAMIN K Vitamin K is required for normal blood coagulation. Adequacy of status is assessed by maintenance of plasma prothrombin concentrations. Anticoagulant drugs function by interfering with the utilization of vitamin K in the process of blood coagulation. Individuals who are treated with these drugs should have their vitamin K status monitored carefully. Treatment of individuals with broad-spectrum antibiotics may reduce gastrointestinal absorption of vitamin K and make them susceptible to deficiency.

Water-Soluble Vitamins

VITAMIN C The recommended allowance for vitamin C for adults (60 mg) is a level considered sufficient to provide an average body pool of 1500 mg and a margin of sufficiency because vitamin C is poorly retained in the body. It is well recognized that cigarette smoking increases the destruction of vitamin C, and the Food and Nutrition Board (1989) recommends higher intake levels (100 mg/day) for individuals who smoke tobacco.

VITAMIN B_6 Vitamin B_6 is required for a variety of metabolic reactions, particularly those in protein metabolism. Because of its central role in protein metabolism, the allowance for vitamin B_6 has been set at a level that appears to maintain adequate blood values for most indices of vitamin B_6 status. The recommended levels are higher than those in many countries around the world because they reflect the fact that protein intake levels in the United States may be as high as two times the RDA.

FOLATE Current dietary allowances for folate reflect levels that maintain adequate folate status and liver stores. The allowance, 3 μg per kg body weight, is an amount within the range of typical consumption levels by healthy adults in the United States and Canada. Folate appears to be critical in embryonic development. Recent evidence from clinical intervention studies indicates that intakes of folate above the RDA during the period prior to conception and during early pregnancy can reduce significantly the recurrence of neural tube defects in newborns (see page 196). The U.S. Public Health Service (Centers for Disease Control and Prevention, 1992) recommends that

Homocysteine: Is Vitamin Status a Risk Factor for Atherosclerosis?

Homocysteine is a sulfur-containing amino acid that is an intermediary product in the metabolism of methionine (Fig. 11–3). The transfer of the methyl group (CH₃) from methionine is an important step in the metabolism of nucleic acids, fats, and high-energy bonds. When methionine donates its methyl group, homocysteine is formed. In normal metabolism the majority of homocysteine is recycled into methionine by a transmethylation reaction requiring methyltetrahydrofolate and vitamin B_{12} as a coenzyme. Another pathway, the condensation of serine to homocysteine, forms cysteine in the first reaction of the transsulfuration pathway, which requires vitamin B_6. Plasma folate, vitamin B_{12}, and vitamin B_6 concentrations are inversely related to plasma homocysteine values, and supplementation with folate, in particular, has been shown to reduce homocysteine concentrations (Ubbink et al, 1994; Chasan-Taber et al, 1996).

Although hyperhomocysteinemia has been associated with major cardiovascular risk factors (smoking, high blood pressure, elevated cholesterol levels, and lack of exercise) (Nygard et al, 1995), it is an independent risk factor for peripheral vascular, cerebrovascular, and coronary heart disease (Pancharuniti et al, 1994; Boushey et al, 1995). Hyperhomocysteinemia can arise from multiple causes. The most common may be heterozygote deficiencies of enzymes required for homocysteine metabolism and from deficiencies of folate, vitamin B_6, or vitamin B_{12}.

Mechanisms for a role of homocysteine in the etiology of atherogenic processes have been postulated (Stamler and Silvka, 1996). One leading hypothesis is that homocysteine and its metabolites have a toxic effect on vascular endothelium, resulting in hyperplasia, fraying, and fibrosis. Another possible mechanism is that homocysteine stimulates the proliferation of smooth-muscle cells, a key component in atherogenesis. End products of cholesterol and cysteine metabolism are cholic acid and taurine, which are excreted in bile acids. Impairment of the conversion of homocysteine to cysteine could decrease the efficiency of cholesterol metabolism, resulting in higher blood levels. Homocysteine can also act as a **thrombogenic** agent by inducing or inhibiting factors involved in blood coagulation.

Selhub and co-workers (1995), in studying over 1000 male and female survivors of the Framingham Study, found that as blood and dietary folate levels decreased, plasma homocysteine and **stenosis** of the **carotid arteries** increased. In fact, they actually demonstrated a graded increase in the prevalence of carotid artery stenosis with increasing plasma levels of homocysteine. Similar findings have been observed for coronary artery stenosis, myocardial infarction, and death due to cardiac disease (Stampfer and Malinow, 1995). A meta-analysis of more than 20 **case control** and cross-sectional studies involving over 2000 subjects concluded that because of the consistency of data from studies by different investigators, using different methods in different populations, there is strong evidence for a role of homocysteine in the pathogenesis of vascular disease (Boushey et al, 1995).

Although cross-sectional and case control studies cannot rule out the possibility that vascular disease itself may have altered homocysteine levels, similar results have been observed in large prospective studies in which blood was drawn before cardiovascular disease was diagnosed. In the Physicians' Health Study, men who later had myocardial infarctions had significantly higher mean baseline levels of homocysteine than matched controls who remained free of infarction (Stampfer et al, 1992). Even after adjustment for other coronary risk factors, men with the highest homocysteine levels had a threefold greater risk than those with lower levels.

Mean homocysteine levels reached a stable low level only with folate intakes of approximately 400 μg per day or above (Stampfer and Malinow, 1995) (the current RDA for folate is 180 and 200 μg for adult females and males, respectively). It has been suggested that as much as 40% of the adult population is not consuming enough folate to keep homocysteine levels low (Selhub et al, 1993). Folate supplements in the range of 1 to 2 mg per day have been recommended to normalize high homocysteine levels even if the elevation is not due to folate deficiency (Selhub et al, 1993). Although such a recommendation may be considered premature, Stampfer and Malinow (1995) maintain that epidemiologic data linking high blood homocysteine levels with vascular disease are consistent, and plausible biologic mechanisms have been described. They consider folate supplements a safe, inexpensive, and effective intervention. Concerns that folate supplements might mask cobalamin deficiency could be lessened by adding 1 mg of cobalamin to folic acid supplements. Alternatively, concerns about homocysteine can be alleviated by increasing dietary folate levels by consuming more fruits and vegetables and grain fortification.

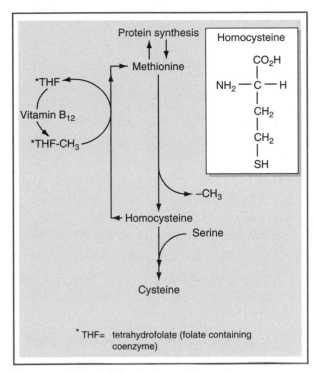

* THF= tetrahydrofolate (folate containing coenzyme)

FIGURE 11–3. Metabolism of homocysteine.

TABLE 11-7 **Optimal Calcium Requirements for Adults**

Age Group	Optimal Daily Intake (mg)
11–24 years	1200–1500
MEN	
25–65 years	1000
Over 65 years	1500
WOMEN	
25–65 years	1000
Over 50 years (postmenopausal)	
On estrogens	1000
Not on estrogens	1500
Over 65 years	1500

From National Institutes of Health, Office of the Director. Optimal calcium intake. NIH Consensus Statement. June 6–8, 1994, 12(4):1–31.

women of childbearing age consume at least 400 μg of folic acid daily to reduce their risk of having a pregnancy in which the child is affected with spina bifida or other neural tube defect. In order to significantly increase the daily folate intake, the Food and Drug Administration (FDA) has mandated that effective January 1, 1998, folate must be added to most enriched flour, breads, corn meals, rice, noodles, macaroni, and other grain products (Federal Register, 1996). Fortification of grains to improve folate intake will improve intake levels for the whole population, which has the potential of having a positive impact on cardiovascular disease by reducing elevated blood levels of homocysteine, a recognized independent risk factor for coronary heart disease (see Research Update).

VITAMIN B$_{12}$ The Vitamin B$_{12}$ allowance for adult males and females is based on levels that will sustain metabolic functions, maintain normal serum concentrations, and promote accumulation or maintenance of substantial body stores (Food and Nutrition Board, 1989).

Minerals

CALCIUM   The recommendation for calcium is 1200 mg per day for men and women up to 25 years of age to promote development of maximum peak bone mass and, potentially, to reduce the risk of osteoporosis in later life

(Food and Nutrition Board, 1989). The current RDA for calcium for adults (800 mg) does not address the possible need for greater amounts of calcium to prevent or treat osteoporosis, however. As discussed in Chapter 12, several studies suggest that increased calcium intake may reduce the risk of progressive osteoporosis, especially in women. Indeed, the National Institutes of Health (1994) sets optimal calcium requirements at between 1000 and 1500 mg per for adults (Table 11–7).

IRON   The recommended allowances for iron are based on amounts required to replace daily iron losses, which are estimated to be 1 mg for men and postmenopausal women and 1.5 mg in menstruating women. Assuming an overall absorption of 10% for dietary iron,

K E Y   T E R M S

thrombogenic: promoting the formation of a blood clot (thrombosis)
stenosis: constriction of the diameter
carotid arteries: the two chief arteries that pass up the neck to supply the brain
case control: a research technique to identify factors related to a disease in which a subject with a disease, such as heart disease, is matched to an individual of the same background or exposure but who does not have the disease

the RDA for iron is 10 mg for men and postmenopausal women and 15 mg for premenopausal women.

Adult men have an iron store of about 1 g; menstruating women have a store of about 300 mg. When total body iron is increased 5- to 10-fold, clinical manifestations of damaging effects of iron occur (Lynch, 1995). Experimental data from animal studies and epidemiologic research suggest that increased iron storage status may be a pathogenic factor in several disorders, including infections, ischemic heart disease, and various types of cancer.

Iron can mediate the production of free radicals, which lead to tissue damage. Evidence suggests that oxidation of LDL within the arterial wall may depend on the presence of iron or copper. Salonen and co-workers (1992) found a strong association between high serum ferritin concentrations and the risk for acute myocardial infarction in men, particularly those with elevated serum LDL concentrations, but results of other studies have been inconsistent. A major difficulty with current epidemiologic surveys is dependence on a single measure of iron status (Sempos et al, 1994). A second limitation is the absence of reports of vascular damage in patients with hereditary disorders of severe iron overload. An association between increased iron stores and the prevalence of cancer has also been postulated on the basis of recent epidemiologic studies (Knekt et al, 1994), but, again, iron storage status has not been adequately characterized in these studies.

Other Vitamins and Minerals

Recommended levels of other vitamins and minerals are presented in Table 11–4. Estimated minimum requirements for sodium, chloride and potassium and estimated safe and adequate daily dietary intakes of the vitamins and minerals appear in Appendices 1A and 1B. Specific levels of nutrients recommended for adults are only guides for positive nutrition. The recommended levels of nutrients are based on the assumption that the diet contains adequate energy to maintain a healthy weight and includes recommended servings from all food groups. The potential benefits of eating a variety of foods include preventing excesses or deficiencies of micronutrients, promoting balance among nutrients, limiting exposure to any one type of food and, thereby, to any associated contaminants, and the less tangible advantages of increased personal choices and enjoyment of eating (Krebs-Smith et al, 1987). However, a single value or group of values must be considered in the context of the overall diet, which contains foods from all food groups. As will become apparent in the following section, the potential role of specific nutrients in prevention or treatment of chronic disease is an area of great interest. If future research does support such a benefit, however, the levels required are likely to be higher than the RDA.

CHRONIC HEALTH CONCERNS OF ADULTS

Coronary Heart Disease

■ How does atherosclerosis develop and progress?

■ What are the major risk factors for coronary heart disease?

■ What effect does excess body fatness and its distribution have on risk of chronic disease?

■ How do dietary factors influence levels of blood lipids, lipoproteins, and platelet aggregation?

■ What dietary recommendations are appropriate to prevent coronary heart disease for all Americans and individuals at risk?

■ Why are diabetes mellitus and hypertension risk factors for coronary heart disease?

■ Can nutrition intervention for diabetes mellitus influence the development of coronary heart disease?

■ What are the roles of excess body weight and dietary intake in development and control of hypertension?

Despite a decline of more than 50% in the death rate from coronary heart disease (CHD) since 1950, CHD is the single largest cause of death of American males and females. Coronary heart disease results when the coronary arteries supplying the heart with oxygen and nutrients become narrowed and inelastic because of atherosclerosis. Atherosclerosis begins with the deposition of fatty streaks in macrophages and smooth muscle cells within the inner lining of large elastic and muscular arteries. High levels of low-density lipoproteins (LDL) are atherogenic. Evidence supports the hypothesis that LDL undergoes oxidative modification that targets it for uptake by macrophages. Lipoprotein-loaded macrophages (foam cells) accumulate in fatty streaks, which are the earliest identifiable lesions in atherogenesis. Foam cells may become nonfunctional and die, releasing cytotoxic contents that damage the overlying endothelium. These early lesions do not substantially diminish blood flow in the affected artery. Eventually, however, more lipid accumulates and a **fibrous plaque** develops that projects into the channel or lumen of the artery, resulting in ischemia, or impaired blood flow. Ischemia within the myocardium can result in **angina pectoris**. If the impairment of blood flow is severe, the tissues nourished by the obstructed artery may die. When this process affects the coronary arteries, a myocardial infarction occurs; in cerebral arteries, a stroke results. Atherosclerotic changes within other arteries can result in peripheral vascular disease.

An individual's risk of developing CHD and the rate at which atherosclerosis progresses are influenced by many factors (Table 11–8). They include some that cannot be modified, such as age, gender, and family history of premature CHD. Others, such as body weight, cigarette smoking, blood pressure, blood lipid levels, and diabetes mellitus may be modified to reduce the risk of myocardial infarction or death.

Risk Factors for Coronary Heart Disease

Overweight and Regional Adiposity

Overweight constitutes a substantial burden because it leads to a worsening of all the elements of the cardiovascular risk profile (Garrison and Kannel, 1993). Systolic and diastolic blood pressures are higher, serum total cholesterol and LDL cholesterol are increased, and concentrations of sugar in the blood are moderately greater. Furthermore, there is a graded relation so that risk is proportional to the degree of adiposity (Hubert et al, 1983). Reduction of weight has the potential to reduce the incidence of many risk factors. For example, a recent followup of data from the Framingham Study showed improvement in blood pressure and plasma cholesterol with weight loss (Kannel et al, 1996).

The Expert Panel of the American Health Foundation has defined healthier weight goals for adults as a reasonable upper limit for body weight that would offer a reduction in disease risk for most overweight adults (Table 11–9). These appropriate weight loss goals, which, if

achieved, will improve health risks for chronic diseases, are within reach for most overweight adults (Meisler and St. Jeor, 1996).

Regional obesity appears to be an independent contributor to cardiovascular disease. For men under the age of 65 years, obesity, regardless of fat distribution, is a risk factor for CHD (Rimm et al, 1995). For older men, the waist-to-hip ratio is the best predictor of risk. Central obesity is associated with a greater risk of developing diabetes than is adiposity per se (Haffner et al, 1991). Reduction of body fat has the potential to reduce each of these diseases.

Blood Lipid Levels

The risk factors most directly associated with CHD are elevated serum TC and LDL-C and reduced HDL-C. Guidelines for classifying total cholesterol and HDL-C levels in adults appear in Table 11–3. Figure 11–4 shows the distribution of serum TC in the United States population as reported in data from NHANES II and III (Phase I). As can be seen, using the cutoff point of 240 mg/dL, the percentage of individuals at risk has declined to approximately 20% of the population since 1976–80. It has been demonstrated in controlled prospective studies that lowering TC and LDL-C with diet (Schaefer et al, 1995) or drug therapy (Gotto, 1995; Brown et al, 1990), halts the progression of atherosclerotic lesions and may stabilize the rupture-prone lesions that are present, thereby reducing the subsequent risk of CHD morbidity and mortality (Gould et al, 1995).

The National Cholesterol Education Program (NCEP) sponsored by the National Heart, Lung and Blood Institute began in 1985 to provide guidelines for physicians and individuals in reducing levels of TC and LDL-C in order to reduce the risk of heart attacks and the associated mortality. Revised guidelines developed by the Expert Panel on Detection, Evaluation and Treatment of High Blood Cholesterol in Adults, Adult Treatment Panel II (1993) contain a two-step plan of dietary recommendations outlined in Table 11–10. The Step 1 diet was originally designated for people with borderline high and high LDL-C, but over time it has come to be used as general recommendations for everyone. Sample menus based on the Step 1 diet

---

TABLE II–8 Major Risk Factors for Coronary Heart Disease

LDL cholesterol $\geq$ 160 mg/dL

Male gender, age 45 years or older

Female gender, age 55 years or older, or with premature menopause and not on estrogen replacement therapy

HDL cholesterol $\leq$ 35 mg/dL

Hypertension—diastolic pressure $\geq$ 90 mm Hg

Smoking

Diabetes mellitus

Family history of heart attacks or sudden death before age 55 in a male parent or sibling or before age 65 in a female parent or sibling

Subtract 1 risk factor if HDL cholesterol $\geq$ 60 mg/dL

From National Cholesterol Education Program: Second report of the expert panel on detection, evaluation and treatment of high blood cholesterol in adults (Adult Treatment Panel II). NIH Publication No. 93-3095. Washington, DC: National Institutes of Health. National Heart, Lung and Blood Institute, 1993.

K E Y   T E R M S

fibrous plaque: the lesion of atherosclerosis that bulges into the lumen. It is composed of lipid, cell debris, smooth muscle cells, and collagen.

angina pectoris: chest pain caused by insufficient blood flow to the heart

TABLE 11-9 Healthier-Weight Goals for Adults Who Are Above the Healthy-Weight Target for a Given Height, Regardless of Sex, as Derived from Two-Unit Equivalents of the Body Mass Index

Height		Weight Loss	
cm	in	kg	lb
147	58	4.5	10
150	59	4.5	10
152	60	4.5	10
155	61	5	11
157	62	5	11
160	63	5	11
163	64	5.5	12
165	65	5.5	12
168	66	5.5	12
170	67	6	13
173	68	6	13
175	69	6.5	14
178	70	6.5	14
180	71	6.5	14
183	72	7	15
185	73	7	15
188	74	7.5	16
190	75	7.5	16
193	76	7.5	16

From Meisler JG, St Jeor S. Summary and recommendations from the American Health Foundation Panel on Healthy Weight. Am J Clin Nutr 1996;63(suppl):476S. © Am J Clin Nutr. American Society for Clinical Nutrition.

for a traditional American diet and various other food patterns appear in Table 11–11. If implementation of the Step 1 diet does not lower TC, the Step 2 diet, lower in saturated fat and cholesterol, is recommended. Individuals who do not respond to nutrition therapy and those considered to be high risk are candidates for drug therapy. High risk is defined as those with LDL cholesterol values at or above 190 mg/dL, 160 mg/dL in the presence of two or more CHD risk factors, or 130 mg/dL in the presence of CHD.

Medications for lowering cholesterol include bile acid sequestering agents, which reduce body cholesterol by binding bile acids in the gut, thereby increasing fecal excretion, and fibric acid derivatives, which increase the breakdown of lipoproteins and excretion of sterols, including cholesterol. Drugs that inhibit the enzyme 3-hydroxy-3 methylglutaryl-coenzyme A (HMGCoA) reductase decrease hepatic cholesterol synthesis, thereby stimulating the synthesis of LDL receptors and the uptake of LDLs, decreasing blood cholesterol. Niacin (nicotinic acid), in doses many times the RDA, lowers blood cholesterol levels by mechanisms that are not entirely understood but that appear to interfere with lipoprotein formation.

Fatty Acids

In 1994, Americans consumed approximately 33% of kilocalories from fat, higher than the 30% recommended in the Healthy People 2000 goals. Although total dietary fat has been linked to several chronic diseases, the effects of individual fatty acids are just beginning to be explored. There is a growing body of evidence that individual fatty acids can affect TC and LDL-C levels and that the fatty acid composition of the LDL particle can influence lipoprotein oxidation, the key factor in the atherogenic effects of the LDL particle (Jonnalagadda et al, 1996). Overall it has been recognized that saturated fatty acids (SFA) tend to increase TC and are significantly correlated with carotid artery wall thickness (Folsom et al, 1993) and 5-year incidence of CHD (Keys, 1970). Myristic, palmitic, and lauric acids increase serum TC, and stearic acid appears to be neutral (Yu et al, 1995). It has been suggested, however, that palmitic acid may play a role in improving LDL/HDL ratio. Monounsaturated fatty acids, which can be obtained from both plant and animal sources, appear to lower TC and LDL cholesterol levels when substituted for saturated fatty acids.

Among the polyunsaturated fatty acids, it is well established that the omega-6 fatty acids (linoleic acid) lower TC and LDL-C levels. Monounsaturated fatty acids (MUFA) elicit a neutral effect or are hypocholesterolemic but less potent than polyunsaturated fatty acids (PUFA). Omega-3 fatty acids lower blood triglyceride levels. A statistically significant inverse relationship between omega-3 fatty acids and death from CHD and all-cause mortality has been observed (Nordoy and Goodnight, 1990).

Studies have demonstrated the antithrombotic effects of omega-3 PUFA or fish oil. In general, subjects given omega-3 PUFAs consistently show a mild prolongation of the bleeding time and decreased reactivity to platelet aggregation (Nordoy and Goodnight, 1990). By substituting for arachidonic acid and reducing the precursor available for **thromboxane** synthesis, these fatty acids also reduce blood platelet aggregation and decrease interactions of the platelets within the vessel wall, thereby reducing the tendency for blood to clot.

Trans fatty acids have been the topic of much debate among nutrition scientists. They are byproducts of hydrogenation of liquid vegetable oils in the manufacture of margarines and hydrogenated fats to formulate commercially prepared baked goods and fried foods (Lichtenstein, 1995). (See page 25). The average per capita consumption in the United States is estimated to be approximately 12.5 g/day, approximately 8% of total fat intake (Hunter and Applewhite, 1991).

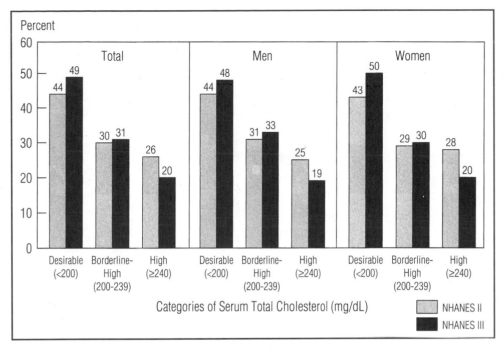

FIGURE 11–4. Distribution of serum total cholesterol values for U.S. adults (20–74 years) by sex for NHANES II and NHANES III. (From NHANES II [1976–80], NHANES III [Phase I, 1988–91.])

Two studies in adults have reported a positive relationship between *trans* fatty acids and risk of coronary heart disease or myocardial infarction (Willett et al, 1993; Aschcrio et al, 1994). In both studies, however, the lowest

TABLE 11–10 National Cholesterol Education Program, Adult Treatment Panel II Dietary Recommendations

	Step I Diet ATP II	Step II Diet ATP II
Total fat	≤30%*	≤30%
Saturated fat	<10%	<7%
Monounsaturated fat	5–15%	5–15%
Polyunsaturated fat	<10%	<10%
Carbohydrate	50–70%	50–70%
Protein	10–20%	10 20%
Cholesterol	<300 mg/day	<200 mg/day
Calories	To maintain optimal body weight	

* Percent indicates percentage of kilocalories.

From National Cholesterol Education Program: Second report of the expert panel on detection, evaluation and treatment of high blood cholesterol in adults (Adult Treatment Panel II). NIH Publication No. 93-3095. Washington, DC: National Institutes of Health. National Heart, Lung and Blood Institute, 1993.

risk for coronary heart disease was for subjects in the middle quintile (one fifth) of *trans* fatty acid intake (Jonnalagadda et al, 1996). Other studies have failed to find a relationship between *trans* fatty acid intake and coronary heart disease (Kris-Etherton and Nicolosi, 1995).

The concern regarding *trans* fatty acids has centered around feeding studies that have demonstrated decreases in HDL-C and increases in LDL-C concentrations (Judd et al, 1994; Katan et al, 1995). However, elevations of the LDL-C concentrations shown with *trans* fatty acids are less than those that would occur with consumption of highly saturated fats such as butter or palm oil. In 1995, the Expert Panel on *Trans* Fatty Acids and Coronary Heart Disease concluded that evidence for a link between *trans* fatty acids in the diet and coronary heart disease risk is weak and inconsistent.

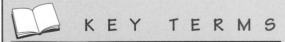

KEY TERMS

thromboxane: a compound of released endothelial cells and platelets following activation of thrombin. It interacts with a variety of molecules to induce platelet aggregation (clotting).

TABLE 11–11 Heart Healthy Sample Menus for Step I Diets for Various Food Patterns

Traditional American Cuisine	Mexican-American Cuisine	Asian-American Cuisine	Lacto-Ovo-Vegetarian Cuisine
BREAKFAST			
Bagel, plain	Cantaloupe	Banana	Orange
Low-fat cream cheese	*Farina prepared with 1% milk	Whole wheat bread	*Pancakes made w/1% milk and egg whites
Cereal, shredded wheat	White bread	Margarine	Pancake syrup
Banana	Margarine	Orange juice	Margarine
Milk, 1%	Jelly	Milk, 1%	Milk, 1%
Orange juice	Orange juice		Coffee
Coffee	Hot cocoa prepared with 1% milk		Milk, 1%
Milk, 1%			
LUNCH			
Minestrone soup, canned, low sodium	Beef enchilada	Beef noodle soup, canned, low sodium	Vegetable soup, canned, low sodium
Roast beef sandwich	Tortilla, corn	*Chinese noodle and beef salad	Bagel
Whole wheat bread	*Lean roast beef	Sirloin steak	Processed American cheese, low fat, low sodium
*Lean roast beef, unseasoned	Vegetable oil	Peanut oil	
American cheese, low fat, low sodium	Cheddar cheese, low fat, low sodium	Soy sauce, low sodium	Spinach salad
Lettuce	Onion	Carrots	Spinach
Tomato	Tomato	Squash	Mushrooms
Mayonnaise, low fat, low sodium	Lettuce	Onion	*Olive oil dressing, regular calorie
Apple	Chili peppers	Chinese noodles, soft type	Apple
Water	*Refried beans prepared with vegetable oil	*Steamed white rice	Iced tea
	Carrots	Apple	
	Celery	Tea, unsweetened	
	Milk, 1%		
DINNER			
*Salmon	Chicken taco	Pork stirfry with vegetables	*Omelette
Vegetable oil	Tortilla, corn	*Pork cutlet	Egg whites
*Baked potato	*Chicken breast without skin	Peanut oil	Green pepper
Margarine	Vegetable oil	Peanuts, unsalted	Onion
*Green beans seasoned with margarine	Cheddar cheese, low fat, low sodium	Soy sauce, low sodium	Mozzarella cheese made from part 1% milk
*Carrots seasoned with margarine	Guacamole	Broccoli	Vegetable oil
*White dinner roll	Salsa	Carrots	*Brown rice seasoned with margarine
Margarine	*Corn, seasoned with margarine	Mushrooms	*Carrots, seasoned with margarine
Ice milk	*Spanish rice prepared with margarine	*Steamed white rice	Whole wheat bread
Iced tea, unsweetened	Banana	Milk, 1%	Margarine
	Coffee	Tea, unsweetened	Fig bar cookies
	Milk, 1%		Tea
			Honey
SNACK			
*Popcorn	*Popcorn	Wonton soup prepared with low-sodium broth	Corn flake cereal
Margarine	Margarine		Milk, 1%
		Tea, unsweetened	

* No salt is added in recipe preparation or as seasoning. All margarine is low sodium.

From National Cholesterol Education Program: Second report of the expert panel on detection, evaluation and treatment of high blood cholesterol in adults (Adult Treatment Panel II). NIH Publication No. 93-3095. Washington, DC: National Institutes of Health. National Heart, Lung and Blood Institute, 1993.

Alcohol

Alcohol appears to plays several roles in relation to cardiovascular disease. A 10-year follow-up of subjects in NHANES I and II reported that moderate drinkers had a life span 3% to 4% longer than that of nondrinkers or light drinkers (Coate, 1993). There is evidence that drinking in moderation (1 to 2 drinks a day) can be beneficial in reducing the risk of heart attack. However, three or more drinks a day increase blood pressure. The most significant benefit of moderate alcohol intake appears to be that it raises HDL cholesterol, which clears cholesterol from the blood thus avoiding the build-up of deposits along the artery walls (Linn et al, 1993).

Alcohol appears to help render **platelets** less "sticky" and therefore less likely to aggregate and form a clot that could result in a myocardial infarction. This may occur because endothelial cells exposed to alcohol increase the production of endogenous **tissue plasminogen activator** (t-PA). In participants in the Physicians' Health Study a direct association was observed between moderate alcohol intake and plasma levels of endogenous t-PA that was independent of HDL levels (Ricker et al, 1994).

Diabetes Mellitus

Diabetes mellitus is a major cause of morbidity and premature mortality. Individuals with non–insulin-dependent diabetes mellitus (NIDDM) experience significant complications associated with atherosclerosis. Their blood lipid profiles are consistent with high risk of coronary heart disease and are usually associated with poor control of blood glucose levels. Obesity increases insulin resistance (Pi-Sunyer, 1996). In data from the second National Health and Nutrition Examination Survey, the relative risk of developing diabetes was 2.9 times greater for obese persons than persons of normal weight (van Itallie, 1985).

Weight reduction improves blood glucose control in diabetics. Actually, the effect of energy restriction due to reduced energy intake improves glucose control very quickly even before much weight loss occurs (Pi-Sunyer, 1996). As weight is lost, the concentration of **glycosylated hemoglobin** drops. Some individuals are able to cease or reduce taking insulin and can even be managed without hypoglycemic agents. Even a 5% loss of weight can decrease blood glucose concentration by improving insulin sensitivity and glucose uptake into muscle and adipose tissue. Nutrition therapy consisting of foods that are low-fat and high in complex carbohydrate accompanied by daily aerobic exercise can improve glycemic control and reduce serum lipid levels.

Hypertension

Because hypertension is generally asymptomatic, it often is referred to as the silent disease. Its implications are significant, however. Elevated blood pressure can accelerate aging of the circulatory system and is a major risk factor for coronary heart disease, cerebrovascular disease, renal insufficiency, and vascular disease. The atherosclerotic process, in which the arteries lose their elasticity, increases hypertension.

Burt and co-workers (1995) estimated that 24% of American adults—approximately 43 million individuals—have hypertension. The incidence increases with age, occurring in 50% or more of those above age 55 years and 63% of those aged 65 to 74 years. The prevalence is greater in African-Americans (Working Group on Hypertension, 1986).

Most causes of hypertension are unknown, and it is probable that causes are multiple and interrelated. In epidemiologic studies, elevated systolic and diastolic pressures have been associated with diets high in calories, sodium, simple sugars, and saturated fat and low in calcium, iron, potassium, fiber, and complex carbohydrates (Preuss et al, 1996).

Numerous population studies have associated hypertension with salt (sodium) intake, and there is evidence that decreasing body sodium via dietary restriction or diuretics reduces blood pressure for some individuals. Some researchers recommend that all Americans should reduce daily salt consumption, from 9 g/day to 6 g (2.4 mg sodium) or less per person/day (Stamler, 1995). Others maintain that reanalysis of data from early studies on sodium and the results of more recent studies raise questions regarding the effectiveness of sodium restriction in treating hypertension (Stern, 1995). This point of view is supported by the fact that there are no data on the impact of sodium restriction on cardiovascular disease morbidity or mortality. Nevertheless, salt consumption by Americans far exceeds the physiologic sodium requirement, and a moderate reduction is not harmful and may be beneficial, at least for some individuals.

The impact of sodium restriction is modest compared to the robust effect of weight loss both in lowering blood pressure and in decreasing the risks of other chronic diseases (Dyer and Elliot, 1989). Mechanisms that contribute to the relation between body weight and blood pressure include elevated cardiac output with expanded intravascu-

---

KEY TERMS

platelet: a disk-shaped structure found in blood, which lacks a nucleus and DNA; known chiefly for its role in coagulation

tissue plasminogen activator: an enzyme secreted by endothelial cells that plays a central role in the regulation of intravascular fibrinolysis

glycosylated hemoglobin: hemoglobin with glucose attached to the terminal of the amino acid chain. The amount of glucose increases in hyperglycemia (uncontrolled diabetes mellitus).

TABLE 11–12 Risk Implications for Major Forms of Cancer by Consumption of Foods in Major Groups; Intake of Energy-Generating Nutrients, Alcohol, and Salt; and Nutrition-Related Indicators

	Oral Cavity	Nasopharynx	Esophagus	Stomach	Large Bowel	Liver	Larynx	Lung	Breast	Endometrium	Ovary	Prostate	Urinary Bladder
MAJOR FOOD GROUPS													
Cereals				Increase?									
Vegetables	Reduce		Reduce	Reduce	Reduce.	Reduce?	Reduce	Reduce	Reduce?	Reduce?	Reduce?	Reduce?	Reduce
Fruits	Reduce		Reduce	Reduce	Reduce	Reduce?	Reduce	Reduce	Reduce?	Reduce?	Reduce?		Reduce
Red Meat					Increase								
Fish													
Milk and milk products													
Eggs and egg products				Increae?									
Sugars					Increase?								
MACRO-NUTRIENTS													
Animal proteins				Increase?	Increase?					Increase?			
Carbohydrates (total)				Increase?									
Fiber					Reduce?								
Saturated fat (as animal)					Increase?			Increase?	Neutral	Increase?		Increase	
Mono-unsaturated fat									Reduce?				
Poly-unsaturated fat					Neutral?				Neutral?				
NONNUTRIENTS													
Alcohol	Increase		Increase		Increase				Increase				
Salt (NaCl)		Increase		Increase									
NUTRITIONAL COVARIATES													
Height					Increase?				Increase			Increase?	
Obesity					Increase				Both	Increase			
Physical activity					Reduce				Reduce	Reduce?		Reduce?	
Hot drinks			Increase										

From Willett WC, Trichopoulos D. Nutrition and cancer: a summary of the evidence. Cancer Causes Control 1996;7:178. Reprinted by permission of Rapid Science Publishers.

lar and cardiopulmonary volume in the presence of a normal peripheral resistance. A positive correlation between peripheral insulin concentrations and arterial pressure in overweight hypertensive individuals suggests that the metabolic disturbances of obesity are related to the blood pressure elevation (McCarron and Reusser, 1996).

Numerous clinical intervention trials have documented the effectiveness of weight loss in lowering blood pressure. One national multicenter program of nonpharmacologic interventions on blood pressure involving more than 2000 men and women with high-normal blood pressure found that weight loss was the single most effective means of lowering blood pressure (Trials of Hypertension Prevention Collaborative Research Group, 1992). Modest reductions in weight (3 to 5 kg) can improve blood pressure in both those who are hypertensive and those who are normotensive, regardless of sodium intake (McCarron and Reusser, 1996). Changes in blood pressure were found to be proportional to weight loss among overweight men and women who had had mild hypertension for 5 years (Davis et al, 1993). For almost 25% of the participants, weight loss lowered blood pressure to the normal range and kept it there. For others, weight loss significantly reduced the requirement for antihypertensive medication.

Epidemiologic studies have documented an inverse relationship between calcium intake and systolic and diastolic pressure (McCarron et al, 1990; Pryer et al, 1995). However, the range of values is large, and substantial differences exist among population subgroups (sex, age, and ethnicity). It appears that a portion of individuals with hypertension respond to increased calcium intake, supporting calcium insufficiency as one of the contributors to this multifactorial disorder (Morris and Reusser, 1995). Because many adults consume calcium at levels well below those recommended, encouraging adequate calcium intake has important benefits for hypertension. A meta-analysis of pooled data from 2412 subjects in 33 randomized controlled trials of calcium supplementation showed a reduction in systolic blood pressure (but not diastolic blood pressure) with calcium supplementation (Bucher et al, 1996).

Cancer

- Why is it difficult to identify nutrition or dietary components that may promote or prevent cancer?

- For which cancers might nutrition be a contributing factor?

- What dietary recommendations are appropriate for cancer prevention?

Cancer is the second leading cause of death in the United States. During the 1970s large-scale **ecologic** studies observed substantial international differences in the prevalence of cancer rates, suggesting correlations with environmental factors, including diet (Armstrong and

Doll, 1975). Evidence for environmental influences including diet in cancer causation is supported by observations that migrating populations adopted, sooner or later, the cancer rates of their new host population.

In the most general terms, **carcinogenesis** can be thought of as requiring one or more **genotoxic** events, resulting in a **mutation** and the proliferation of mutated cells. Early research focused on possible mutagens, such as those occurring naturally in many foods or produced by cooking food at high temperatures. Current research also focuses on the likelihood that protective factors may alter the metabolism of potential mutagens or act as antioxidants or cofactors for antioxidant enzymes.

Nutrition could contribute to the causation and prevention of cancer in many ways. Dietary factors influence the rate at which cells multiply through the availability of energy and essential nutrients. Some dietary components have hormonal effects or act indirectly by influencing the endogenous synthesis or metabolism of hormones. Some nutrients have physiologic roles in regulating gene expression (e.g., vitamin A) or in the normal regulation of cell differentiation and proliferation (e.g., folate) and thus may also affect the likelihood that a mutation is reproduced.

While evidence of a diet–cancer connection does not establish a cause and effect relationship, there is substantial epidemiologic (Block et al, 1992) and experimental evidence in animal models to suggest that some dietary components may increase or decrease the risk of particular cancers. A variety of approaches are being used to explore the significance of dietary factors. Case control and **cohort** epidemiologic studies provide the opportunity to study the effects of specific dietary factors with much greater capacity to control for confounding variables than in the early general comparisons of populations. However, the effects of specific dietary factors may be difficult to disentangle when they exist together in foods such as vitamin A and carotene. Table 11–12 summarizes current evidence in relation to major food groups, energy-generating

K E Y   T E R M S

ecologic: studies across populations, usually international

carcinogenesis: production of a malignant new growth made up of epithelial cells tending to infiltrate surrounding tissue

genotoxic: damaging to DNA

mutation: permanent transmissible change in genetic material, usually of a single gene

cohort: group of individuals sharing a characteristic (such as date of birth or exposure to asbestos) who are used in epidemiologic studies

nutrients, salt, alcohol, and indicators of energy balance to various cancers. The following discussion summarizes some of the most pronounced relationships between dietary factors and cancer.

ORAL AND LARYNGEAL CANCER   Oral and laryngeal cancer are marked by two risk factors that appear far more powerful than nutrition—tobacco use and alcohol consumption. Case control evidence indicates that a diet that emphasizes fruits and vegetables may protect against oral cancer even after statistical adjustment for alcohol and tobacco use (Marshall and Boyle, 1996). For laryngeal cancer, available studies provide no estimate of risk of the role of diet in subjects not exposed to tobacco and alcohol (Riboli et al, 1996).

ESOPHAGEAL CANCER   A protective effect of fruit and vegetable consumption is supported by a large body of evidence, especially from case control studies. Recent intervention studies in areas of China with a high incidence of esophageal cancer suggest that micronutrient supplements may have a modest effect in reducing risk (Cheng and Day, 1996), but the implication of these results is uncertain.

STOMACH CANCER   There is substantial ecologic evidence for a role of dietary factors in determining the risk of stomach cancer. High salt intake has been associated with an increased risk in many case control studies and limited cohort studies. There has been a consistent **negative association** with consumption of fresh vegetables and fruits in numerous case control studies in different populations (Kono and Hirohata, 1996). Both epidemiologic and experimental data suggest that vitamin C intake is inversely related to stomach cancer mortality (Ocke et al, 1995). Evidence is sparse and inconsistent with reference to protective effects of carotene, vitamin E, or selenium, however.

LUNG CANCER   Lung cancer is the leading cause of cancer death in men and women. Cigarette smoking has been established as the dominant risk factor in lung cancer deaths in men and women. Diet may be of particular importance, because prevention is considered the only viable strategy for reducing lung cancer mortality. Early detection of lung cancer has not been successful, because symptoms often do not appear until the disease is advanced and, therefore, treatment is not very effective.

Prospective and retrospective studies suggest strongly that increased vegetable and fruit intake is associated with reduced risk in men and women, in smokers, ex-smokers, and never-smokers, and for all types of lung cancer (Ziegler et al, 1996). Some prospective studies have observed that blood levels of beta-carotene (a biomarker of vegetable and fruit intake) are consistently related to

lower risk of cancer (van Poppel and Goldbohm, 1995). Conversely, in a 25-year follow-up of the participants in the Seven Countries Study, average intake of vitamin C, alpha or beta-carotene, or alpha tocopherol showed no relationship to mortality from lung cancer (Ocke et al, 1995).

COLORECTAL CANCER   Inheritance and numerous environmental and lifestyle factors such as diet, low levels of physical activity (Glynn et al, 1996), and obesity (Lee et al, 1991) have been implicated in carcinogenesis of the colon (Shike, 1996).

There is strong evidence from epidemiologic studies and experimental studies in animals that a diet high in fat and energy and low in fruits, vegetables, and dietary fiber strongly predisposes to the development of colon cancer (Ziegler, 1991; Wynder et al, 1996). Furthermore, as meat consumption rises so does risk, but this is not explained solely by the fat content of meat (Potter, 1996). Mutagenic compounds, particularly heterocyclic amines, produced when protein is cooked plausibly explain the meat association.

Many **phytochemicals** in vegetables and fruits prevent cancer in experimental animals. The results of clinical trials to test the ability of antioxidant vitamins to prevent colorectal adenomas have been inconsistent. Also, high dietary fiber intake is associated with lower risk, but fiber alone does not account for this association.

Data from epidemiologic studies suggest that dietary calcium may have a protective role for colon and rectal cancer (Garland et al, 1991). Recent clinical trials in individuals at high risk for development of **adenomas** have reported a reduction in hyperproliferation of epithelial cells in the **colonic crypts** when calcium is added to the diet (Bostick et al, 1995; Alberts et al, 1996) and no improvement in mucosal cell proliferation in similar patients given 1200 mg of calcium/day for 6 to 9 months (Baron et al, 1995). A recent double-blind, placebo-controlled study of calcium in families with hereditary colorectal cancer did not find any increase in epithelial cell proliferation with calcium supplementation (Cate et al, 1995).

BREAST CANCER   Breast cancer is the second leading cause of cancer mortality in women. The incidence of breast cancer increases with age and adiposity. But factors that predict risk of breast cancer in premenopausal women are different from those for postmenopausal women. For example, obese women appear to be at decreased risk for developing premenopausal breast cancer but increased risk of developing and dying from postmenopausal breast cancer (Ballard-Barbash and Swanson, 1996).

A role for dietary fat in breast cancer development has been hypothesized for more than 30 years. Ecologic evidence shows a positive correlation between fat consumption and breast cancer rates (Whittemore and Henderson, 1993). Nonetheless, these observations are not supported by results from large prospective cohort studies of pre- and postmenopausal women (Willett et al, 1992; Jones et al, 1987). It may be that if fat intake is relevant to breast cancer, the relationship is to intakes during early life. This is consistent with an emerging hypothesis that higher energy intake and growth rate in childhood and adolescence increases risk (Hunter and Willett, 1996).

Considerable evidence suggests that low intakes of vegetables modestly increase the risk of breast cancer; however, the dietary components responsible remain elusive (Fredudenheim et al, 1996). In a 3-year prospective study of 2569 women, Negri and co-workers (1996) found an inverse relationship between risk of breast cancer and dietary levels of beta carotene, vitamin E, and calcium, but not of vitamin C. Such observations raise important questions regarding components of fruits, vegetables, and grains, and other food components that may impact on cancer risk.

Phytoestrogens, a group of phytochemicals that are weaker versions of human estrogen, are of particular interest in the areas of breast and prostate cancer. Phytoestrogens of dietary origin, lignans and isoflavinoids, occur in more than 300 plants, but major amounts are found in soybean and whole-grain products and various seeds. Evidence for positive effects of phytoestrogens relates to observations that in areas where large amounts of soy products are consumed, such as Japan, China, and Korea, symptoms of menopause, breast cancer rates, and death from prostate cancer are much lower than in the West.

It appears that the effects of phytoestrogens may vary with menopausal status. It is speculated that prior to menopause, phytoestrogens act as antiestrogens, staving off breast cancer by blocking the action of some of the body's naturally occurring estrogens. After menopause, when production of endogenous estrogen dramatically declines, phytoestrogens may provide some hormone activity without raising breast cancer risk. In men, phytoestrogens appear to act as a blocker of testosterone, the male hormone that can spur the growth of prostate tumors (Adlecreutz, 1995).

EXPLORING NUTRIENT RELATIONSHIPS

On the basis of epidemiologic observations and studies in laboratory animals, antioxidants, particularly beta carotene and vitamin A, have attracted wide interest as agents to prevent cancer. It is difficult to determine from observational studies whether the apparent benefits of fruit and vegetable consumption are due to beta carotene, other substances in those foods, other dietary habits, or other nondietary lifestyle characteristics (Hennekens and Buring, 1993).

In principle, **randomized clinical trials** are the most powerful tool in determining the effects of dietary factors on cancer risk.

Three large, randomized, placebo-controlled trials in well-nourished populations were designed to validate the protective effects of beta carotene. The first, The Alpha-Tocopherol, Beta Carotene (ATBC) Cancer Prevention Study (1994), assigned 29,000 Finnish male smokers to receive beta carotene, vitamin E, both active agents, or neither, for an average of 6 years. There were no benefits of supplementation in terms of the incidence of cancer or cancer or cardiovascular death; indeed, rates of lung cancer were somewhat higher among the subjects given beta carotene. The second clinical trial, The Beta-Carotene and Retinol Efficacy Trial (CARET), was designed to assess the chemopreventive efficacy and safety of beta carotene and retinyl palmitate in 18,314 smokers, former smokers, and workers exposed to asbestos (Omenn et al, 1996). For heavy smokers receiving beta carotene, the risk of lung cancer was higher than the placebo group. These two studies raised the possibility that not only was beta carotene not effective in preventing cancer but that it may be harmful to smokers.

The Physicians' Health Study, a randomized double-blind, placebo-controlled trial, tested aspirin and beta carotene in primary prevention of cardiovascular disease and cancer in 22,071 male physicians (40 to 84 years of age at enrollment) in the United States (Hennekens et al, 1996). Average duration of treatment was 12 years. In this largely nonsmoking population, supplementation with beta carotene did not increase or reduce the incidence of cancer, cardiovascular disease, or death from all causes.

None of the studies showed a benefit from supplementation with beta carotene, and the estimated excess risks in smokers were small. It remains unclear whether beta

KEY TERMS

negative association: as one variable increases (fruit and vegetable consumption), the other decreases (cancer risk)

phytochemicals: substances derived from naturally occurring ingredients that may have health-promoting potential

adenoma: benign epithelial tumor

colonic crypts: deep indentations or pits in the lining of the colon

randomized clinical trials: a research technique in which subjects are assigned randomly to experimental (treatment) or control groups

carotene was truly harmful or whether it might prove to be beneficial over a longer period. The **induction period** for cancers is often unknown and may be decades long (Willett and Tridropoulos, 1996). Because the duration of these studies was relatively short, they leave open the possibility that benefit, especially in terms of cancer risk reduction, would become evident with longer treatment and follow-up. In addition, the nutrition factors that influence cancer development may interrelate with each other and may differ with the type of cancer.

Regardless of the results of these studies related to beta carotene, there is substantial evidence that diets that include moderate energy and fat; abundant vegetables, fruits, and grains; and adequate calcium can provide important practical guidance for cancer prevention.

NUTRITION AND HEALTH CONCERNS OF WOMEN

■ What are the major issues of women's health that have nutrition implications?

■ What is the Women's Health Initiative?

Throughout the life span, females have nutrition needs or concerns that are unique from those of men. Lifelong physiologic, psychological, and environmental influences on women elicit a set of behaviors and biologic responses distinct from those of men that create unique health and nutrition needs or concerns. Throughout this chapter and this book, the nutrition concerns of women have been stressed, particularly in reference to excess body weight, coronary heart disease, diabetes mellitus, cancer, and osteoporosis.

Awareness of issues in women's health is, however, a relatively new occurrence. Historically, the health concerns of women have received little attention. Women were not included in major clinical and preventive research trials for various reasons, such as the potential confounding effect of variable menstrual cycles, potential risks to fetuses, and the assumption that many health risks were less prominent in woman than in men. As a result, research into many chronic diseases that affect both men and women often included only male participants. Over time the results from these studies have been applied to women as well. Only recently have health concerns of women been given consideration in research and as issues for nutrition intervention and care, particularly with reference to chronic disease. Political, medical, and scientific commitment to women's health is being reflected in one major national research effort in the form of the Women's Health Initiative (WHI).

In 1993 the National Institutes of Health launched WHI, the largest and most complex epidemiologic intervention study ever undertaken in the United States. It involves 40 clinical centers and approximately 163,000 postmenopausal women in a major study of outcomes related to heart disease, breast and colorectal cancers, and osteoporosis. A three-component clinical trial (hormone replacement therapy [HRT], calcium and vitamin D supplements, and dietary modification) includes more than 60,000 women, and the observational study includes more than twice that number. The clinical trials and observational study will continue to monitor participants for 9 years, with close-out visits to be completed in 2005.

The primary hypothesis of the HRT component is that estrogen replacement in postmenopausal women reduces the risk of coronary heart disease, the leading cause of death in women. A secondary hypothesis is that HRT reduces the risk of osteoporotic hip fractures.

The primary hypothesis of the calcium and vitamin D component is that calcium and vitamin D supplementation reduces the risk of osteoporosis and hip fractures in postmenopausal women. A secondary hypothesis is that colorectal cancer is reduced with calcium and vitamin D supplementation. In the double-blinded design, women randomized into the intervention group receive 1000 mg elemental calcium (from calcium carbonate) daily plus 400 IU vitamin D daily. Women randomized to the control group receive a placebo.

The primary hypothesis of the dietary modification (DM) component is that a low-fat dietary pattern (20% of energy from fat, with 7% from saturated fat) with increased intake of fruits and vegetables (five servings daily) and grains (six servings daily) reduces the risk of breast and colorectal cancers in postmenopausal women. A secondary hypothesis of DM is that the risk of coronary heart disease is reduced with low-fat, high fruit, high vegetable, and high grain interventions.

Participants in DM are randomized into one of two groups: control (comparison) or intervention. Sixty percent of the women are randomly assigned to the comparison group and receive no dietary intervention; 40% of the women are randomly assigned to the dietary change group. Women in the comparison group receive a copy of the Dietary Guidelines for Americans plus other health-related materials and are not asked to make dietary changes. Women in the dietary change group receive nutritionist-facilitated group instruction on changing their food-related behaviors (e.g., decreasing total fat intake, and increasing intake of fruits, vegetables, and grains).

Women have been neglected in the current health care system. In fact, many of the diseases and disorders affecting adult women are preventable or their impact on well-being can be reduced through early diagnosis and intervention. Improved health care for women will affect the health of the whole population as nutrition prevention and intervention are implemented.

PROMOTING HEALTH AND WELL-BEING

Health has traditionally been defined as the absence of disease or illness. Major strides in medicine (particularly the control of infection), food safety, and public health have resulted in increased life span (and expectancy). As individuals live longer, the advances that prolong life should be employed to ensure that the additional years are healthy, quality years.

Because of these changes, today health is viewed as a complex concept that encompasses physical, mental, emotional, social, and spiritual well-being. This broad definition of health focuses on the individual and his or her needs and abilities to attain optimum health. Obviously, nutrition is an integral part of each of the components of health.

Health Promotion

Health promotion is an exciting opportunity to improve and maintain the health status of individuals and families and communities. It is integrated into health care, but emphasis is on prevention of disease in community or worksite settings. The purpose of health promotion is to improve the health status of individuals by facilitating permanent changes in lifestyle that will promote **wellness** behaviors. Wellness encompasses day-to-day habits, including food eaten, exercise taken, sleep patterns, and management of stress. As described in Chapter 3, this depends on the individual's knowledge of what constitutes good health behaviors and development of techniques needed to apply that knowledge in modifying current behaviors and developing new behaviors and life styles. In addition, health promotion is most effective in a family, work, or community environment that supports wellness behaviors.

Promoting Nutrition Health

Nutrition is a critical part of all aspects of health. The role of nutrition is complex and is integrated with other health behaviors. Healthy People 2000, developed by the U.S. Public Health Service, outlines national health promotion and disease prevention objectives for Americans with a goal for achievement by the year 2000 (see Table 1–11 in Chapter 1). One of the three broad goals is to "increase the span of healthy life for Americans." Obviously, nutrition is a component of this goal, and there are 21 nutrition-related objectives.

Promotion of nutrition health begins with the Food Guide Pyramid (see Fig. 1–6 in Chapter 1). This foundation will allow individuals to develop basic understanding and practice in positive eating behaviors to meet nutrition needs. An important component of wellness is prevention of disease. The Nine Dietary Guidelines from the National Academy of Sciences (Table 1–5 in Chapter 1) and the Dietary Guidelines for Americans from the U.S. Departments of Agriculture and Health and Human Services (see Fig. 1–1 in Chapter 1) can provide guidance for food

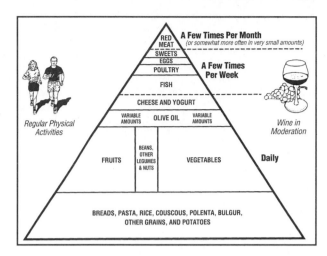

FIGURE 11–5. The traditional healthy Mediterranean diet pyramid. (© 1994, Oldways Preservation & Exchange Trust. From Practical Practice 1995 [Winter].)

choices that will minimize nutrition health risks as they are currently perceived. The most recent edition of the Dietary Guidelines emphasizes the importance of diet and exercise in the maintenance of body weight. This reflects a trend toward using the synergy between diet and physical activity to create the greatest health benefit (Blair, 1995; Eaton et al, 1993; Paffenbarger et al, 1993). The NIH Consensus Development Panel on Physical Activity and Cardiovascular Health (1996) and the American College of Sports Medicine (1995) recommend that every adult should accumulate at least 30 minutes of moderate-intensity physical activity over the course of most, preferably all, days of the week.

It has been known for decades that, compared with North America, populations living in other regions of the world have low rates of chronic disease, especially CHD, and increased life expectancies (Willett et al, 1995). The Mediterranean Food Pyramid (Fig. 11–5) characterizes the diet of populations living in the regions surrounding the Mediterranean Sea. In many ways the Mediterranean Diet is similar to the U.S. Food Guide Pyramid. At the base of the pyramid are a variety of grains (including many that are unknown or are just becoming popular in the

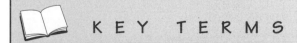

KEY TERMS

induction period: the period it takes for specific cellular changes to occur
health promotion: strategies to increase the level of health of individuals
wellness: a lifestyle that enhances the level of health

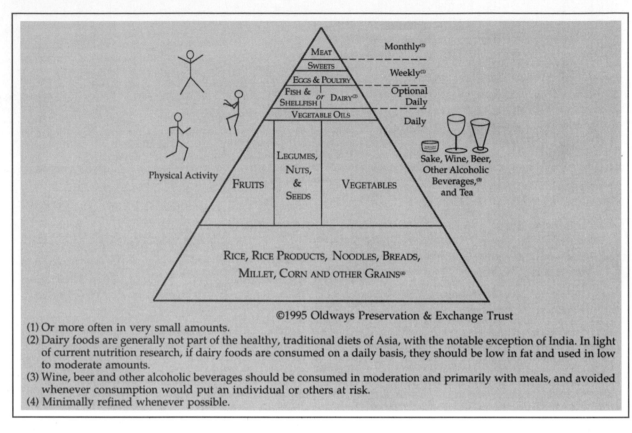

Physical Activity

MEAT — Monthly[1]

SWEETS — Weekly[1]

EGGS & POULTRY — Weekly[1]

FISH & SHELLFISH *or* DAIRY[2] — Optional Daily

VEGETABLE OILS — Daily

LEGUMES, NUTS, & SEEDS   FRUITS   VEGETABLES

Sake, Wine, Beer, Other Alcoholic Beverages,[3] and Tea

RICE, RICE PRODUCTS, NOODLES, BREADS, MILLET, CORN AND OTHER GRAINS[4]

©1995 Oldways Preservation & Exchange Trust

(1) Or more often in very small amounts.
(2) Dairy foods are generally not part of the healthy, traditional diets of Asia, with the notable exception of India. In light of current nutrition research, if dairy foods are consumed on a daily basis, they should be low in fat and used in low to moderate amounts.
(3) Wine, beer and other alcoholic beverages should be consumed in moderation and primarily with meals, and avoided whenever consumption would put an individual or others at risk.
(4) Minimally refined whenever possible.

FIGURE 11–6. The traditional Asian diet pyramid: preliminary concept. (© 1995, Oldways Preservation & Exchange Trust. From Nutr Today 1996;31:4.)

United States, such as couscous, polenta, bulgur, and others), fruits, and vegetables. However, the Mediterranean guide includes a fruit/vegetable subsection of beans, other legumes, and nuts. Use of olive oil, the only recommended fat, is encouraged, but no limits are suggested. Cheese and yogurt are specified as preferred dairy products, but no recommendations are made relative to fat content. Fish, poultry, and eggs are consumed only a few times a week rather than daily, and red meat only a few times a month. A major difference is that the guide encourages wine, in moderation, and regular physical activity.

A preliminary concept of a traditional Asian Diet Pyramid appears in Figure 11–6. It too has grains and grain products at its base and a subsection for legumes, nuts, and seeds. Meats, eggs, and poultry are at the top, with suggestions of monthly and weekly consumption, respectively. The major difference between the two pyramids is that the Asian diet includes little use of dairy products. Attention would need to be paid to consuming adequate calcium sources.

These models for healthy eating are already used by many Americans because the models reflect their cultural

backgrounds or because they are willing to explore and enjoy consuming healthy diet alternatives. They are two examples of acceptable and health-promoting dietary patterns.

CONCEPTS TO REMEMBER

▶ Adulthood begins with the completion of growth and is a period of physiologic homeostasis characterized by gradual changes of aging.

▶ For women, menopause and declining estrogen levels have implications for increased risk of coronary heart disease, osteoporosis, and cerebrovascular disease.

▶ Hormone replacement therapy can be used during menopause and to reduce risk of osteoporosis and heart disease.

▶ Resting energy expenditure decreases with age and may contribute to a gradual increase in body weight

➧ Nutrition assessment for adults includes screening the body weight and risk factors for chronic disease.

➧ Energy and nutrient needs are relatively stable during adulthood, but caloric intakes tend to vary widely.

➧ Homocysteine is a nutrition-related risk factor for coronary artery disease.

➧ Nutrition plays a role in the development or progression of chronic diseases.

➧ Dietary changes, particularly of energy and fat intake, may have health benefits for cardiovascular disease, diabetes mellitus, hypertension, and cancer.

➧ Exercise is an important adjunct to dietary interventions for disease.

➧ Reductions in dietary fat and changes in the type of fat can reduce blood TC and LDL-C.

➧ There is substantial evidence linking consumption of certain food groups with the occurrence of some chronic diseases.

➧ There is much speculation, but little evidence, linking specific nutrients to the occurrence or progression of chronic disease.

➧ The unique health concerns of women may require specific nutrition modifications.

References

Adlecreutz H. Phytoestrogens: epidemiology and a possible role in cancer protection. Environ Health Perspect 1995;103:103.

Agricultural Research Service. Continuing Survey of Food Intakes by Individuals. U.S. Department of Agriculture. Riverdale, MD:1996

Alberts DS, et al. Randomized, double-blinded, placebo-controlled study of effect of wheat bran fiber and calcium on fecal bile acids in patients with resected adenomatous colon polyps. J Natl Cancer Inst 1996; 88:81.

American College of Sports Medicine. ACSM position stand on osteoporosis and exercise. Med Sci Sports Exec 1995;27:1.

Armstrong B, Doll R. Environmental factors and cancer incidence and mortality in different countries, with special reference to dietary practices. Int J Cancer 1975;15:617.

Ascherio A, et al. Trans fatty acids intake and risk of myocardial infarction. Circulation 1994;89:94.

Ballard-Barbash R, Swanson CA. Body weight: estimation of risk for breast and endometrial cancers. Am J Clin Nutr 1996;63:437S.

Baron JA, et al. Calcium supplementation and rectal mucosal proliferation: a randomized controlled trial. J Natl Cancer Inst 1995;87:1303.

Blair SN. Diet and activity: the synergistic merger. Nutr Today 1995;30:108.

Block G, et al. Fruit, vegetables, and cancer prevention: a review of the epidemiological evidence. Nutr Cancer 1992;18:1.

Bostick RM, et al. Calcium and colorectal epithelial cell proliferation in sporadic adenoma patients: a randomized, double-blinded, placebo-controlled clinical trial. J Natl Cancer Inst 1995;87:1307.

Boushey CJ, et al. A quantitative assessment of plasma homocysteine as a risk factor for vascular disease. Probable benefits of increasing folic acid intakes. JAMA 1995;274:1049.

Brown G, et al. Regression of coronary artery disease as a result of intensive lipid-lowering therapy in men with high levels of apoprotein B. N Engl J Med 1990;323:1289.

Bucher H, et al. Effects of dietary calcium supplementation on blood pressure. A meta-analysis of randomized controlled trials. JAMA 1996;275:1016.

Burt VL, et al. Prevalence of hypertension in the U.S. population. Results from the Third National Health and Nutrition Examination Survey 1988–1991. Hypertension 1995;25:308.

Cate A, et al. Randomized, double-blinded, placebo-controlled intervention study with supplemental calcium in families with hereditary nonpolyposis colorectal cancer. J Natl Cancer Inst 1995;87:598.

Centers for Disease Control and Prevention. Recommendations for the use of folic acid to reduce the number of cases of spina bifida and other neural tube defects. MMWR 1992;44:1.

Chasan-Taber L, et al. A prospective study of folate and vitamin B_6 and risk of myocardial infarction in U.S. physicians. J Am Coll Nutr 1996;15:136.

Cheng KK, Day NE. Nutrition and esophageal cancer. Cancer Causes and Control 1996;7:33.

Chernoff R. Baby boomers come of age: nutrition in the 21st century. J Am Diet Assoc 1995;95:650.

Coate D. Moderate drinking and coronary heart disease mortality: evidence from NHANES I and the NHANES II follow-up. Am J Publ Health 1993;83:888.

Colditz GA, et al. Weight gain as a risk factor for clinical diabetes in women. Ann Intern Med 1995;122:481.

Croft JB, et al. Waist-to-hip ratio in a biracial population: measurement, implications, and cautions for using guidelines to define high risk for cardiovascular disease. J Am Diet Assoc 1995;95:60.

Davis BR, et al. Reduction in long-term antihypertensive medication requirements: effects of weight reduction by dietary intervention in overweight persons with mild hypertension. Arch Int Med 1993;153:1773.

Dyer AR, Elliott P. The Intersalt Study: relations of body mass index on blood pressure. J Hum Hypertens 1989;3:299.

Eaton CB, et al. Self-reported physical activity predicts long-term coronary heart disease and all-cause mortalities. Arch Fam Med 1993;4:323.

Expert Panel on Detection, Evaluation, and Treatment of High Blood Cholesterol in Adults. Summary of the Second Report of the National Cholesterol Education Program (NCEP). (Adult Treatment Panel II). JAMA 1993;269:3015.

Federal Register. Folic acid fortification. March 5, 1996;61:8781.

Folsom AR, et al. Association of hemostatic variables with prevalent cardiovascular disease and asymptomatic carotid artery atherosclerosis (The Atherosclerosis Risk in Communities [ARIC] Study). Arterioscler Thromb 1993;13:1829.

Food and Nutrition Board, National Research Council. Recommended dietary allowances. 10th ed. Washington, DC: National Academy of Sciences, 1989.

Fredudenheim JL, et al. Premenopausal breast cancer risk and intake of vegetables, fruits and related nutrients. J Natl Cancer Inst 1996;88:340.

Garland CG, et al. Can colon cancer incidence and death rates be reduced with calcium and vitamin D? Am J Clin Nutr 1991;54:193S.

Garn SM. Fractionating healthy weight. Am J Clin Nutr 1996;63:412S.

Garrison RJ, Kannel WB. A new approach for estimating healthy body weights. Int J Obesity 1993;17:417.

Gauvin L, Spence JC. Physical activity and psychological well-being: knowledge base, current issues and caveats. Nutr Rev 1996;54:S53.

Glynn SA, et al. Alcohol consumption and risk of colorectal cancer in cohort of Finnish men. Cancer Causes and Control 1996;7:214.

Gotto AM. Lipid risk factors and the regression of atherosclerosis. Am J Cardiol 1995;76:3A.

Gould AL, et al. Cholesterol reduction yields clinical benefit: a new look at old data. Circulation 1995;91:2274.

Haffner S, et al. Greater influence of central distribution of adipose tissue in incidence of non-insulin dependent diabetes in women than men. Am J Clin Nutr 1991;53:1312.

Hennekens CH, et al. Lack of effect of long-term supplementation with beta carotene on the incidence of malignant neoplasms and cardiovascular disease. N Engl J Med 1996;334:1145.

Hennekens CH, Buring JE. Observational evidence. Ann NY Acad Sci 1993;703:18.

Hubert HB, et al. Obesity as an independent risk factor for cardiovascular disease: a 26-year follow-up of participants in the Framingham Heart Study. Circulation 1983;61:968.

Hunter DJ, et al. Cohort studies of fat intake and risk of breast cancer—a pooled analysis. N Engl J Med 1996;334:356.

Hunter DJ, Willett WC. Nutrition and breast cancer. Cancer Causes and Control 1996;7:56.

Hunter JE, Applewhite TH. Reassessment of *trans* fatty acid availability in the US diet. Am J Clin Nutr 1991;54:363.

Joint National Committee on the Detection, Evaluation and Treatment of High Blood Pressure: Fifth Report. (JNC V). Arch Intern Med 1993;153:149.

Jones DY, et al. Dietary fat and breast cancer in the National Health and Nutrition Examination Survey I. Epidemiologic Follow-up Study. J Natl Cancer Inst 1987;79:465.

Jonnalagadda S, et al. Effects of individual fatty acids on chronic diseases. Nutr Today 1996;31:90.

Judd JF, et al. Dietary *trans* fatty acids: effects on plasma lipids and lipoproteins of healthy men and women. Am J Clin Nutr 1994;59:861.

Kannel WB, et al. Effect of weight on cardiovascular disease. Am J Clin Nutr 1996;63:419S.

Kant AK, et al. Consumption of energy-dense, nutrient-poor foods by the US population: Effect of nutrient profiles. J Am Coll Nutr 1994;13:285.

Kant AK, et al. Proportion of energy intake from fat and subsequent weight change in the NHANES I Epidemiologic Follow-up Study. Am J Clin Nutr 1995;61:11.

Katan MB, et al. *Trans* fatty acids and their effects on lipoproteins in humans. Ann Rev Nutr 1995;15:473.

Katch FI, McArdle WD. Introduction to nutrition, exercise, and health. 4th ed. Philadelphia: Lea & Febiger, 1993.

Keys A. Coronary heart disease in seven countries. Circulation 1970;41:1S.

Kirtz-Silverstein D, Barrett-Connor E. Long-term postmenopausal hormone use, obesity, and fat distribution in older women. JAMA 1996;275:46.

Knekt P, et al. Body iron stores and risk of cancer. Int J Cancer 1994;56:379.

Kono S, Hirohata T. Nutrition and stomach cancer. Cancer Causes and Control 1996;7:41.

Krebs-Smith SM, et al. US adults' fruit and vegetable intakes, 1989 to 1991: A revised baseline for the Healthy People 2000 Objectives. Am J Publ Health 1995;85:1623.

Krebs-Smith SM, et al. The effect of variety in food choices on dietary quality. J Am Diet Assoc 1987;87:897.

Kris-Etherton PM, Nicolosi RJ. *Trans* fatty acids and coronary heart disease risk. International Life Sciences Institute, Technical Committee on Fatty Acids. Washington, DC: ILSI Press, 1995.

Kuczmarski RJ, et al. Increasing prevalence of overweight among US adults. The National Health and Nutrition Examination Surveys 1960 to 1991. JAMA 1994;272:205.

Lee I-M, et al. Physical activity and risk of developing colorectal cancer among college alumni. J Natl Cancer Inst 1991;83:1324.

Lichtenstein AH. Trans fatty acids and hydrogenated fat—what do we know? Nutr Today 1995;30:102.

Linn S, et al. High-density lipoprotein cholesterol and alcohol consumption in US white and black adults: Date from NHANES II. Am J Publ Health 1993;83:811.

Lynch SR. Iron overload: prevalence and impact on health. Nutr Rev 1995;53:255.

Marshall JR, Boyle P. Nutrition and oral cancer. Cancer Causes and Control 1996;7:101.

McCarron DA, Reusser ME. Body weight and blood pressure regulation. Am J Clin Nutr 1996;63:423S.

McCarron DA, et al. Dietary calcium and chronic diseases. Med Hypotheses 1990;31:265.

McDowell M, et al. Energy and macronutrient intakes of persons ages 2 months and over in the United States: Third National Health and Nutrition Examination Survey, Phase I, 1989–1991. Advance Data No. 225, page 1. Oct 24, 1994.

McGill HC, et al. Early determinants of adult metabolic regulation: effects of infant nutrition on adult lipid and lipoprotein metabolism. Nutr Rev 1996;54:S31.

Meisler JG, St Jeor S. Summary and recommendations from the American Health Foundation's Expert Panel on Healthy Weight. Am J Clin Nutr 1996;63:474S.

Morris CD, Reusser ME. Calcium intake and blood pressure: epidemiology revisited. Semin Nephrol 1995;15:490.

National Institutes of Health. Optimal calcium intake. NIH Consensus Statement, Bethesda, MD:1994.

National Institutes of Health Consensus Development Panel on Physical Activity and Cardiovascular Health. Physical activity and cardiovascular health. JAMA 1996;276:241.

Negri E, et al. Intake of selected micronutrients and the risk of breast cancer. Int J Cancer 1996;65:140.

Nordoy A, Goodnight SH. Dietary lipids and thrombosis. Relationships to atherosclerosis. Atherosclerosis 1990;10:149.

Nygard O, et al. Total plasma homocysteine and cardiovascular risk profile. The Hordaland Homocysteine Study. JAMA 1995;274:1526.

Ocke MC, et al. Average intake of anti-oxidant (pro) vitamins and subsequent cancer mortality in the 16 cohorts of the Seven Countries Study. Int J Cancer 1995;61:480.

Omenn GS, et al. Effects of a combination of beta carotene and vitamin A on lung cancer and cardiovascular disease. N Engl J Med 1996;334:1150.

Paffenbarger RS, et al. The association of changes in physical activity and other lifestyle characteristics with mortality among men. N Engl J Med 1993;328:538.

Pancharuniti N, et al. Plasma homocysteine, folate, and vitamin B_{12} concentrations and risk for early-onset coronary artery disease. Am J Clin Nutr 1994;59:940.

Pi-Sunyer FX. Weight and non-insulin-dependent diabetes mellitus. Am J Clin Nutr 1996;63:426S.

Potter JD. Nutrition and colorectal cancer. Cancer Causes and Control 1996;7:127.

Preuss HG, et al. Association of macronutrients and energy intake with hypertension. J Am Coll Nutr 1996;15:21.

Pryer J, et al. Dietary calcium and blood pressure: a review of the observational studies. J Hum Hypertens 1995;9:597.

Recker RR, et al. Bone gain in young adult women. JAMA 1992;268:2403.

Riboli E, et al. Nutrition and laryngeal cancer. Cancer Causes and Control 1996;7:147.

Ricker PM, et al. Association of moderate alcohol consumption and plasma concentration of endogenous tissue-type plasminogen activator. JAMA 1994;272:929.

Rimm EB, et al. Body size and fat distribution as predictors of coronary heart disease among middle-aged and older US men. Am J Epidemiol 1995;14:1117.

Salonen JT, et al. High stored iron levels are associated with excess risk of myocardial infarction in Eastern Finnish men. Circulation 1992;86:803.

Schaefer EJ, et al. Body weight and low-density lipoprotein cholesterol changes after consumption of ad libitum diet. JAMA 1995;274:1450.

Selhub J, et al. Association between plasma homocysteine concentrations and extracranial carotid-artery disease. N Engl J Med 1995;332:286.

Selhub J, et al. Vitamin status and intake a primary determinant of homocysteinemia in an elderly population. JAMA 1993;270:2693.

Sempos CT, et al. Body iron stores and the risk of coronary heart disease. N Engl J Med 1994;330:1119.

Shike M. Body weight and colon cancer. Am J Clin Nutr 1996;63:442S.

Stamler J. Adverse effects of habitual high dietary salt in health and longevity. Prespect Appl Nutr 1995;3:116.

Stamler JJ, Slivka A. Biological chemistry of thiols in the vasculature and in vascular-related disease. Nutr Rev 1996;54:1.

Stampfer MJ, Malinow MR. Can lowering homocysteine levels reduce cardiovascular risk? [editorial] N Engl J Med 1995;332:328.

Stampfer MJ, et al. A prospective study of plasma homocysteine and risk of myocardial infarction in US physicians. JAMA 1992;268:877.

Stern JS. Perspectives on Sodium. Perspect Appl Nutr 1993;3:127.

Stewart AL, Ware JE (eds). Measuring functioning and well-being: the Medical Outcomes Study Approach. Durham, NC: Duke University Press, 1992.

The ATBC Cancer Prevention Study Group. The effect of vitamin E and beta carotene on the incidence of lung cancer and other cancers in male smokers. N Engl J Med 1994;330:1029.

Trials of Hypertension Prevention Collaborative Research Group. The effects of nonpharmacologic interventions on blood pressure of persons with high normal levels. Results of the Trials of Hypertension Prevention, Phase I. JAMA 1992;267:1213.

Ubbink JB, et al. Vitamin requirements for the treatment of hyperhomocysteinemia in humans. J Nutr 1994;124:1927.

USDA, Human Nutrition Information Service. Continuing Survey of Food Intake by Individuals, 1989–90. Washington, DC: US Department of Agriculture, 1993.

van Itallie T. Health implications of overweight and obesity in the United Stated. Ann Intern Med 1985;103:983.

van Poppel G, Goldbohm RA. Epidemiologic evidence for beta carotene and cancer prevention. Am J Clin Nutr 1995;62:1393S.

Vaziri SM. The impact of female hormone usage on the lipid profile. The Framingham Offspring Study. Arch Intern Med 1993;153:2200.

Vuori I. Peak bone mass and physical activity: a short review. Nutr Rev 1996;54:S11.

Whittemore AS, Henderson BE. Dietary fat and breast cancer: Where are we? J Natl Cancer Inst 1993;85:762.

Wiklund I, et al. Quality of life of postmenopausal women on a regimen of transdermal estradiol therapy: a double-blind placebo-controlled study. Am J Obstet Gynecol 1993;168:824.

Willett WC, et al. Weight, weight change, and coronary heart disease in women. JAMA 1995;273:461.

Willett WC, et al. Intake of *trans* fatty acid and risk of coronary heart disease among women. Lancet 1993;341:581.

Willett WC, et al. Dietary fat and fiber in relation to risk of breast cancer. JAMA 1992;268:2034.

Willett WC, Trichopoulos D. Nutrition and cancer: a summary of the evidence. Cancer Causes and Control 1996;7:178.

Working Group on Hypertension in the Elderly. Statement on hypertension in the elderly. JAMA 1986;256:70.

Writing Group for the PEPI Trial. Effects of hormone replacement therapy on endometrial histology in postmenopausal women. JAMA 1996;275:370.

Wynder EL, et al. High fiber intake: indicator of a healthy lifestyle. JAMA 1996;275:488.

Yu S, et al. Plasma cholesterol-predictive equations demonstrate that stearic acid is neutral and monounsaturated fatty acids are hypocholesterolemic. Am J Clin Nutr 1995;61:1129.

Ziegler RG, et al. Nutrition and lung cancer. Cancer Causes and Control 1996;7:157.

Ziegler RG. Vegetables, fruits and carotenoids and the risk of cancer. Am J Clin Nutr 1991;53:251S.

APPLICATION: Foods, Supplements, Herbs?

Abby is a 36-year-old wife and mother of two sons, 2 and 3 years of age. Her husband is a salesman. She contributes to the family income by teaching aerobic dance classes two evenings a week, but she says they always have difficulty making ends meet.

Abby is very concerned about her health and appearance. She is 165 cm (65 in) and she weighs 60 kg (132 lb). In addition to teaching aerobic dance classes, she walks 2 miles with a neighbor, three to four times a week, and works out at least twice a week using a set of weights she purchased at a garage sale. Abby says she doesn't want to "get old" like her mother did.

Abby is convinced that nutrition is an important component of her "stay young" campaign. She tries to eat a balanced diet but feels she needs supplements to help her feel and look better. Abby drinks ginseng tea with every meal and takes the following supplements, which she buys at the health food store or by mail from a catalogue:

1 mineral supplement
1 multivitamin supplement with trace minerals
1 vitamin supplement of "antioxidants" (vitamins A, E, C and beta-carotene)
2 melatonin capsules
3 garlic tablets

ginseng—the root of the Chinese shrub Panax ginseng, which contains compounds called saponins that interact with neurotransmitters in the body

melatonin—a hormone that is secreted mostly at night by the pineal gland, which regulates many cyclical body functions, such as sleep and fertility. Natural levels in the body decrease with age.

carpal tunnel syndrome—a complex of symptoms resulting from compression of the nerves in the wrist, which causes pain, burning, or tingling in the fingers and hand

antioxidants—substances that prevent tissue damage by trapping organic free radicals and/or deactivating excited oxygen molecules, which occur as a byproduct of many metabolic reactions

in vitro—observable in the laboratory

As illustrated by Abby's story, dietary supplements can be varied. Figures from national surveys reveal that 30% to 60% of adults take one supplement product or another on a regular basis (Park et al, 1991; Subar and Block, 1990; Kim et al, 1993). Supplement users tend to be healthy people, and often their diets are more likely to provide recommended nutrient intake levels than those of non–supplement users. While the most commonly used supplements are multivitamins, supplements of single nutrients and small groups of nutrients are gaining in popularity. In 1992 the nutritional supplement market in the United States amounted to approximately $4 billion (Time, November 1, 1993:73). Of that amount, $123 million was spent for vitamin E alone and $22 million for beta-carotene (Crowley, 1994).

Traditionally, nutrient supplements, defined as vitamins and minerals, were used to replace nutrient deficits due to poor dietary intake. Over time the concept of supplements has evolved from "insurance" of nutrient adequacy to "protection" in improvement of health and prevention of disease. Although there has been considerable controversy regarding the use of nutrient supplements at levels above the recommended dietary allowances (RDA), supplements have been shown to be beneficial in certain circumstances. There is evidence that supplements of vitamin B_6 may prevent the onset of carpal tunnel syndrome, nicotinic acid lowers blood total cholesterol (Reynolds, 1994), folate prior to and during early pregnancy helps prevent neural tube defects (Keen and Zidenberg-Cherr, 1994), and calcium and vitamin D aid in the prevention of osteoporosis (National Institutes of Health, 1994).

Supplemental vitamins to prevent disease have become a major commercial enterprise. Many epidemiologic studies have observed a relationship between foods containing antioxidants (vitamins C and E and carotenes) and risk of cancer or cardiovascular disease, the two major causes of mortality in adults. A chief limitation of observational studies is their inability to control for all factors that might independently affect health risk. To use a specific example, current evidence indicates that oxidatively modified low-density lipoproteins (LDLs) promote atherogenesis and in vitro studies suggest ascorbate is an effective antioxidant against plasma lipid peroxidation.

A 4-year prospective study of almost 40,000 male health professionals did not find a significant association between lower risk of coronary heart disease and high intakes of vitamin C or beta carotene but did find such an association for vitamin E (Rimm et al, 1993). Randomized placebo-controlled trials with varying levels of vitamin E demonstrated that vitamin E supplements were associated with decreased susceptibility of LDL to oxidation (Jialal et al, 1995) and reduced coronary artery lesion progression as measured by angiography (Hodis et al, 1995), supporting a link between vitamin E and coronary artery disease. In response, sales of vitamin E supplements have increased dramatically (Crowley, 1994), but there is still much to be learned about the relationship between vitamin E and the progression of coronary artery disease.

Currently, millions of dollars are invested in beta carotene supplements each year on the assumption that it will reduce cancer risk. However, several recent randomized clinical trials have failed to find any benefit from beta carotene in cancer incidence or mortality (Greenberg et al, 1996; Omenn et al, 1996; Hennekens et al, 1996). This illustrates that it is difficult to identify compounds that may have protective effects from other dietary components. It may be that the positive effects of fruits and vegetables on cancer are due to other substances in the foods and interactions among food components.

It should be remembered that the origin of these observations between nutrition and disease is the diet. Obviously, food is more than the sum of its nutrients and there is the possibility that taking supplements in large doses may have detrimental effects on nutrition status and health due to direct toxicity of the supplemented nutrient or interference with other nutrients (Thomas, 1996). Therefore, it is appropriate to emphasize the importance of food sources by recommending eating a wide variety of foods as the best way to obtain essential nutrients and disease prevention factors.

Scientific research has begun to identify specific components in foods that have health benefits beyond meeting nutrient needs. Confusion exists about how to describe this newly evolving area of food and food components. Numerous interchangeble names such as herbals, medicinals in food, phytochemical, phytomedicinals, nutraceuticals, and functional food have been used. Common to all these terms is the assumption that the food or components have a potential beneficial role in prevention and treatment of disease (ADA, 1995). The Dietary Supplement Health and Education Act of 1994 (see page 15) includes these substances as dietary supplements, defined as a new category of foods that includes vitamins and minerals as well as herbal or other botanical ingredients (often referred to as phytochemicals), amino acids, and dietary substances used to increase total dietary intake. By definition this includes the ginseng tea, garlic tablets, and melatonin taken by Abby, as well as her vitamin and mineral supplements.

It is estimated that with the new regulations thousands of new products will appear on the market to promote health. Pharmaceutical companies will be motivated to isolate components in foods and to package them as pills and supplements for their health benefits (Reynolds, 1994).

An important effect of the DSHEA is that, in contrast to foods and drugs, for dietary supplements FDA has the legal burden of proving that a supplement product is unsafe rather than the manufacturer having to prove it is safe. Products may be marketed if there is a history of use or other evidence of safety establishing that the product is reasonably expected to be safe when used under the conditions recommended or suggested in its labeling. In general, as long as a product is labeled as a dietary supplement and is not represented as a traditional food, claims may be made on the labels under one of four conditions listed in the margin.

Claims on the labels of dietary supplements do not have to be approved by FDA before they are made, but manufacturers must have substantiation that their marketing statements are truthful and not misleading and must notify the FDA of the claim within 30 days of its appearance on the label. Furthermore, the label of products bearing such claims must prominently display in boldface type the disclaimer, "This statement has not been evaluated by the Food and Drug Administration. This product is not intended to diagnose, treat, cure or prevent any disease."

The Office of Dietary Supplements Research, a division of the National Institutes of Health, has been established recently and is responsible for regulating herbs and other dietary supplements and for deciding whether to allow manufacturers' claims for the products. The FDA will be called in if the ODSR decides that a product presents a danger to public health.

Sometimes supplements are promoted by commercial and other forces on the basis of incomplete or preliminary evidence. As the number of these dietary supplements appearing on the shelves increases, it becomes essential that consumers be assisted in

herbal—plant used to produce a desired effect on the body

nutraceutical—any substance (food or part of food) that provides medical or health benefit

functional food—any modified food or ingredient that may provide a health benefit beyond the traditional nutrients it contains

garlic has been shown to lower blood total cholesterol small amounts and may have other beneficial effects

Conditions for Claims on Labels of Supplements
*The statement claims a benefit to a classical nutrient deficiency disease and discloses the prevalence of such disease in the United States
*describes the role of a nutrient or dietary ingredient intended to affect the structure or function in humans
*characterizes the documented mechanism by which a nutrient or dietary ingredient acts to maintain such structure or function
*describes general well-being from consumption of a nutrient or dietary ingredient

making careful selections (McNutt, 1995). Because dietary supplements are not sold in standardized doses and do not come with the FDA-required list of possible adverse responses, consumers may be unaware of the side effects that could result from taking the products. Thus, recommendations to use dietary supplements should be based on well accepted scientific evidence (American Dietetic Association, 1996), keeping in mind that although most are not likely to be harmful, "natural" is not a synonym for "safe."

Nutrients and other dietary substances relevant to health are readily available in familiar and attractive packages called fruits, vegetables, legumes, grains, and animal products. And they come in concentrations and in combinations with which humans have had long cultural familiarity (Thomas, 1996).

REFERENCES

American Dietetic Association. Position of The American Dietetic Association: Vitamin and mineral supplementation. J Am Diet Assoc 1996;96:73.

American Dietetic Association. Position of The American Dietetic Association: Phytochemicals and functional food. J Am Diet Assoc 1995;95:493.

Crowley G. Are supplements still worth taking? Newsweek, April 25, 1994, p 47.

Greenberg ER, et al. Mortality associated with low plasma concentration of beta carotene and the effect of oral supplementation. JAMA 1996;275:699.

Hennekens CH, et al. Lack of effect of long-term supplementation with beta carotene on the incidence of malignant neoplasms and cardiovascular disease. N Engl J Med 1996;334:1145.

Hodis HN, et al. Serial coronary angiographic evidence that antioxidant vitamin intake reduces progression of coronary artery atherosclerosis. JAMA 1995;273:1849.

Jialal I, et al. The effect of alpha-tocopherol supplementation on LDL oxidation. A dose-response study. Arterioscler Thromb Vasc Biol 1995;15:190.

Keen CL, Zidenberg-Cherr S. Should vitamin-mineral supplements be recommended for all women with childbearing potential? Am J Clin Nutr 1994;59:532S.

Kim I, et al. Vitamin and mineral supplement use and mortality in a US cohort. Am J Public Health 1993;83:546.

McNutt K. Medicinals in food. Part II. What's new and what's not. Nutr Today 1995;30:261.

National Institutes of Health Consensus Development Panel. Optimal calcium intake. JAMA 1994; 272:1942.

Omenn GS, et al. Effects of a combination of beta carotene and vitamin A on lung cancer and cardiovascular disease. N Engl J Med 1996;334:1150.

Park YK, et al. Characteristics of vitamin and mineral supplement products in the United States. Am J Clin Nutr 1991;54:750.

Reynolds RD. Vitamin supplements: current controversy. J Am Coll Nutr 1994;13:118.

Rimm EB, et al. Vitamin E consumption and the risk of coronary disease in men. N Engl J Med 1993;328:1450.

Subar AE, Block G. Use of vitamin and mineral supplements: demographics and the amounts of nutrient consumed. Am J Epidemiol 1990;132:1091.

Thomas PR. Food for thought about dietary supplements. Nutr Today 1996;31:46.

CHAPTER 12

AGING AND OLDER ADULTS

Aging
Physiologic Changes of Aging
Physical, Economic, Psychosocial, and Health
  Factors Associated with Aging
Energy and Nutrient Needs

Dietary Intakes of Older Adults
Assessment of Nutrition Status
Promoting Nutrition for Older Adults
Chronic Health Concerns
Concepts to Remember

Martha is a 75-year-old widow. She married in her late 30s and had no children, but does have a niece and nephew close by. She worked intermittently during her life but has not been employed for the last two decades. Her husband owned extensive property and had a moderate pension so she has few financial concerns. She had smoked two plus packages of cigarettes each day since her early twenties, but she stopped about 2 years ago because she began to have difficulty breathing. Approximately a year ago Martha was hospitalized for emphysema and returned home on oxygen and medication. Several weeks later she was moved to an extended care facility. Her activities consist of bathing, dressing, and watching television. She dresses each day but refuses to go to the dining room for meals and has to be coaxed to walk occasionally in the halls. Martha is frequently curt with the staff and refuses to interact with the other patients. She complains little and does not indicate that she wants to be anywhere else but she doesn't seem very happy and isn't responsive to the staff or visitors.

    Jane is also 75 years of age and she is also a widowed housewife who was employed only a short time before her marriage. Her husband died 12 years ago and left her sufficient income to maintain her current lifestyle. Jane has one daughter and a granddaughter who live in another city and whom she sees 3 or 4 times a year. Jane's home is a small apartment in a Midwestern city, but she spends 5 months during the winter in southern Florida. She owns a station wagon and drives south in November and north in April. Jane lives alone and is active in church and community organizations. She is also physically active. Three or four days a week she walks 3 to 4 miles or plays 18 holes of golf walking the course and pulling her clubs on a small cart. She would play golf more frequently but her other activities keep her too busy.

The process of aging converts healthy adults into frail ones with diminished physiologic reserves and increased vulnerability to disease. Yet, as seen in these two women, there is marked variety among older adults and the ways in which they age.

  Jane might be considered an example of what has been termed "successful" aging with a gradual progressive

functional decline. Increased morbidity with aging is usually associated with progressive illness and rapid functional decline or a catastrophic event such as a stroke or a hip fracture with some degree of improvement after rehabilitation (Vellas et al, 1992). In Martha's case, quality of life is compromised by health problems associated with a lifetime of poor health habits (Gray-Donald, 1995). Due to

TABLE 12–1 Factors Associated with the Ability to Function at an Advanced Age

Genetic potential for longevity

Intelligence, motivation, curiosity

Well-developed sense of humor

Pursuit of active challenges

Stimulating, highly organized, complex daily life

Social contacts maintained

Capacity to adapt to changing events

Religious conviction

Financial independence

Living arrangements—independence, convenience, safety, contact with younger people, preferably family

Responsibility

Family integrity—strong family bonds

Intimacy—marriage, intimate friendships, love and mutual understanding

Moderate body size—improves agility and decreases risk of systemic disease

Life habits of moderation—avoidance of substance abuse (alcohol, smoking, drugs); prudent diet (i.e., avoidance of excess)

Availability of community health care

Relative freedom from accidents

such factors, she is frail and requires assistance with the basic activities of living. What makes the difference in their lives? Genetics, environment, health, lifestyle, nutrition? All of the above.

The physiologic and psychological changes of aging influence an individual's ability to function independently and determine his or her quality of life. Researchers in **gerontology** have identified some characteristics common to individuals who are able to function actively at an advanced age (Table 12–1).

AGING

■ How old is old?

■ What are the characteristics of the older adult population?

■ What are some of the theories of why we age?

The most apparent consequences of aging are gray hair, wrinkles, age spots, changes in physique, decreased strength and endurance, and declines in the acuity of taste and smell. The overall process is more complex, however, encompassing molecular, cellular, physiologic, and psy-

chological changes that are influenced by genetics and socioeconomic environment.

Being old is less a chronologic age than a state of mind and physical status. No two people age in exactly the same way, and older adults are a remarkably diverse group. Older adulthood is often defined as beginning at age 65 years because that is the age at which eligibility for Medicare and Social Security benefits begins. However, many people choose to retire while still in their 50s whereas others continue to work and lead active lives into their 70s and beyond.

The Aging Population

Since 1900, life expectancy in the United States has increased by approximately 25 years. A female born today can expect to live 79 years, which is 6.9 years longer than her male counterpart (Bureau of the Census, 1995). Increased life expectancy due to control of infections and improved treatment of chronic diseases has contributed to the graying of America.

At the beginning of the 20th century, only 4% of the population of the United States was over 65 years of age. In 1994, 12.7% (33.2 million) of Americans were 65 or older, and the number increases at the rate of 5,500 per day (Bureau of the Census, 1995). Of that group, almost one-third (10.8 million) are between 75 and 84 years and 3.4 million are the "oldest old," those 85 and over. It is estimated that by the year 2030, one in five individuals will be over 65, and 17% of that group will be over 85 (Fig. 12–1). In fact, the most rapidly growing segment of United States society is that consisting of people over 85. In 1994, 1 in 10 older persons was of a race other than white. By 2030, minorities will represent 25% of the population of older adults, with the largest increases in Hispanics and Asians.

The majority of older adults are free-living active individuals (Fig. 12–2). In 1992, three of every four community-dwelling persons between 65 and 74 years and two of three people 75 years or older considered their health to be good. Overall, only 5% of older adults are in long-term care facilities, and less than 17% require assistance with the day-to-day activities of living. On the other hand, with increasing age, chronic illnesses and health conditions result in greater dependency on others for performing activities of daily living. The percentage of older adults who require assistance with everyday activities increases from 9% of those 65 to 75 years of age to 50% of individuals older than 85 (Bureau of the Census, 1994).

Theories of Aging

Gerontologists have documented many changes of the gradual process of aging, but the fundamental processes

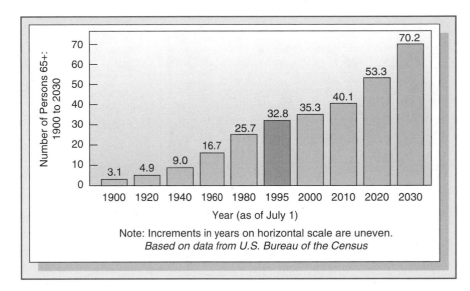

FIGURE 12–1. Predicted increases in the number of persons 65 years and older by the year 2030.

that control the rate at which people age and how **senescence** leads to the diseases of aging are essentially unknown (Miller, 1994). The majority of theories of aging suggest that an intracellular molecule, cell, or organ that loses function over time triggers age-dependent changes in a whole range of body organs and cells. Most current theories relate to some form of impairment of DNA replication, but no single theory explains all of the facts known about aging. The theories currently receiving the greatest attention are discussed in this section. No doubt others will emerge in the near future.

Free Radical Damage

Free radicals are formed in oxidation metabolism by the splitting of a **covalent bond** in a molecule so that each atom joined by the bond retains an electron from the shared pair. Formation of these free radicals is common in normal cell physiology, and most are handled by the body's antioxidant defenses. The free radical theory of aging hypothesizes that free radicals, such as superoxide and hydroxyl, cause changes in DNA resulting in dysfunctional molecules that interfere with cellular function (Morley and Solomon, 1994). In spite of evidence supporting a free radial theory of aging, supplementary antioxidants do not appear to lengthen the maximum life span of mammals appreciably.

Glycation Theory

The glycation theory suggests that elevated blood and tissue glucose levels of aging result in linkages between the excess glucose and proteins and other macromolecules, resulting in cellular dysfunction (Lee and Ce-

rami, 1992). Glycation may also play a role in decreased DNA function, resulting in changes in body proteins such as collagen.

Repair of Ultraviolet Light Damage

Exposure to ultraviolet light damages cellular DNA, and it has been observed that there are differences among species in the rate of repair of this damage in **fibroblasts**. Fibroblasts from species with long maximum life spans showed a greater rate of DNA repair compared to those with shorter life spans. Although some forms of DNA damage do seem to accumulate with age, in general they seem to involve large-scale chromosomal rearrangements rather than smaller-scale changes ordinarily associated with repair of damage induced by ultraviolet light. The extent to which these differences reflect alteration in the repair mechanisms themselves and the relevance to age-related changes in tissues that are not exposed to ultraviolet light has not been explored.

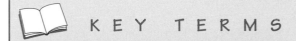

KEY TERMS

gerontology: the scientific study of all aspects of aging
senescence: the process or condition of growing old
covalent bond: a chemical bond between two atoms formed by sharing a pair of electrons
fibroblasts: connective tissue cells that differentiate to form various fibrous tissues in the body

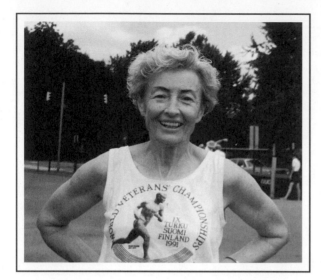

FIGURE 12–2. Most older adults are active, involved individuals. This 67-year-old woman competes in track events all over the world.

TABLE 12–2 Age-Related Changes in Physiologic Function at 70 Years as a Percentage of That Function at Age 30	
CARDIOVASCULAR SYSTEM	
Cardiac output	70
Maximum heart rate	75
RESPIRATORY SYSTEM	
Vital capacity	60
Residual volume	130–150
Maximum O_2 uptake	40
MUSCULOSKELETAL	
Muscle mass	70
Hand grip, flexibility	70
Bone mineralization	70–80
Renal Function	60
NERVOUS SYSTEM	
Conduction velocity	85
Resting glucose uptake	100
Taste and smell	10
METABOLISM	
Fasting blood glucose	100
Basal metabolic rate	85

From Berry EM. Undernutrition in the elderly: a physiological and pathological process? In: Munro H., Schlierf A, (eds). Nutrition of the elderly. Nestle Workshop Series Vol 29. Nestle Ltd. New York: Vervey/Raven Press, 1992.

Mitochondrial DNA

Of particular interest has been the theory that mutations in the DNA in the **mitochondria** may play a major role in aging and the degenerative diseases associated with aging. That is because DNA in the mitochondria has a much greater mutation role than DNA found in the nucleus. This has been supported by observations of increases in mitochondrial DNA mutations in human brains and hearts with advancing age and in some chronic diseases (Morley and Solomon, 1994).

PHYSIOLOGIC CHANGES OF AGING

■ How does body composition change with aging?

■ Describe the major age-related changes that occur in the senses and body systems.

■ What is the impact of the physiologic changes of aging on function and quality of life?

Changes in body and organ function occur throughout adult life, making old age the culmination of diverse processes that began at earlier ages. Overall, in the absence of disease, physical function is maintained by older adults, but **reserve capacity** diminishes with time. With aging, there are declines in the number of active cells and in organ size and function. Table 12–2 lists the age-related changes in several physiologic functions between ages 30 and 70. Aging is associated with a loss of strength,

flexibility, and cardiovascular fitness, which leads to a further decrease in activity. Table 12–3 summarizes many of the age-related changes in physiologic systems.

Body Composition

Aging is associated with slow declines in weight, bone mass, and lean body mass, and gains in adipose tissue. In general, adults gain weight until the sixth decade, after which there is a gradual decline, typically 10% between 70 and 80 years (Flynn et al, 1992). Extremes in body weight are associated with a greater risk of functional impairment in older adults (Galanos et al, 1994).

There is an almost linear decline in muscle mass, approximately 2–3% per decade (Fontera et al, 1991; Fig. 12–3). As lean body mass decreases, the percentage of body fat increases. In addition, there is a shift from subcutaneous to central or truncal body fat, with fat deposited in the abdomen and on the thighs and buttocks.

Resistance training exercise can preserve fat-free mass

and increase muscle strength in the aged. In a recent study, 100 elderly nursing home residents who completed a program of resistance training had improved muscle strength and gait velocity as well as enhanced thigh muscle area, stair climbing power, and levels of spontaneous activity (Fiatarone et al, 1994).

Basal Metabolic Rate

As lean body mass declines after age 30, there is a gradual but accelerating decrease in the basal metabolic rate (BMR). Early in the process the decrease in energy output may contribute to weight gain and obesity. However, over time dietary intakes appear to diminish and underweight becomes more common. The decrease in weight further reduces lean body mass and, therefore, the BMR declines even more. With lower energy intakes, it becomes difficult for older persons to satisfy all of their nutrient needs.

The Senses

Vision

Age-related reductions in visual acuity vary widely from person to person. The central area of the **retina** is the most sensitive site of visual perception, and it tends to degenerate with age. There is a loss of ability to focus on near objects (presbyopia) due to the inability of the aging lens to change in curvature in response to needs of near vision. An increase in lens size and a narrowing of the angle between the **cornea** and the **iris** may impair drainage of fluid present in the anterior chamber of the eye, leading to a buildup of interior or intraocular pressure and impaired vision, referred to as glaucoma.

Cataract can reduce visual acuity. In the early stages, there is reduced night vision. Later there is progressive loss of vision, which can be relieved by surgical extraction of the lens. A growing body of evidence suggests that development of cataracts can be retarded by avoidance of smoking and excessive light exposure. In addition, adequate levels of antioxidant nutrients in and around the lens of the eye may have a protective effect (Taylor, 1992). This protection has been reported with increasing levels of the antioxidants vitamins C and E and beta carotene in the diet and in the circulation (Vitale et al, 1993).

Macular degeneration, a slow insidious atrophy of the photoreceptors on the retinal pigment epithelium, is the most common irreversible cause of blindness in older adults. Macular degeneration affects almost 30% of Americans over the age of 65, and the proportion increases with age. Evidence is also accumulating for a protective effect

of antioxidant nutrients from macular degeneration (Seddon et al, 1994).

Hearing

Age-related hearing loss disorders result from impaired function of the inner ear (cochlea) and/or the connections of the auditory nerve close to or within the brain. These changes may result from several factors but are most commonly related to genetics, occupational noise exposure, chronic middle ear disease, or atherosclerosis.

Taste and Smell

The diminished senses of taste (hypogeusia) and smell (hyposemia) common with advancing age can contribute to inadequate food intake and to compromised nutrition status. The losses reach statistical significance at approximately 60 years of age and become increasingly severe after 70.

The receptor cells for taste are arranged in buds located on the surface of the tongue, the roof of the mouth, the passage between the mouth and the windpipe, and the upper third of the esophagus. Signals from taste buds are transmitted via the cranial nerves. The cells in taste buds have an average turnover time of about ten days. Some age-related losses in taste are caused by interruption of turnover of taste cells.

The receptor or olfactory cells of the sense of smell are located in the upper part of the nasal cavity. Like taste cells, they are in a constant state of flux, turning over about every 30 days. Olfactory cells project to the olfactory bulbs, which contain groups of cells called glomeruli. During the aging process the number of glomeruli decreases. Olfactory information is processed by the limbic system of the brain, which also is the emotional seat of the brain. Therefore, stimulation of olfactory bulbs can affect emotions as well as the ability to perceive odor.

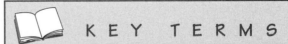

KEY TERMS

mitochondria: the organelle within the cell where most of the energy is generated
reserve capacity: the ability to respond to stress
retina: innermost layers of the eyeball
cornea: transparent structure forming the anterior portion of the eye
iris: the circular pigmented membrane behind the cornea
cataract: an opacity of the crystalline lens of the eye

TABLE 12–3 **Physiologic Changes Associated with Aging**	
System/Function	**Physiologic Change**
Basal metabolic rate	Decrease of 20% between 20 and 90 years that accelerates with age
Senses	General decline
Taste	Decreased taste buds and papillae on tongue; loss of ability to detect salt and sweet
Smell	Decrease in olfactory nerve endings
Hearing	Bilateral symmetric hearing loss
Sight	Decreases in dark adaptation, distance vision, visual acuity; thickening and loss of elasticity of crystalline lens; cataracts
Gastrointestinal oral cavity	Reduced saliva flow; thinning of gum tissue, shrinking of connective tissue; periodontal disease causing loss of teeth
Eosphageal function and swallowing	Minor changes, including disordered contractions
Gastric function	Decreased secretion of hydrochloric acid, intrinsic factor, and pepsin (atrophic gastritis); increased pH in small intestine may contribute to bacterial overgrowth; decreased bioavailability of some minerals and vitamins
Liver and biliary function	Decreased liver size, reduced blood flow to liver; decreased rate of albumin synthesis; reduced activity of drug metabolizing enzymes
Pancreatic secretion	Slightly reduced output of bicarbonate and enzymes
Small intestine	Decreased absorption of calcium and vitamin B_{12}
Laxation	Decreased motility; delayed transit; retention of feces within rectum, constipation common
Respiratory function	Linear decline from ages of 20 to 80, decreased vital capacity
Cardiovascular	Decreased heart size; increased rigidity of arterial walls causes a decrease of blood flow to tissues; decreased contractibility; general loss of tolerance for physical stress
Skin	Dryness, wrinkling, mottled pigmentation, loss of elasticity; changes acelerated by exposure to sunlight; increased water loss from surface; decrease in sebaceous gland activity
Hair	Graying, hair loss
Nails	Slow growth, thickening
Neuromuscular	Progressive loss of cells, neuromuscular loss (decline in number of nerve fibers and contractile process), motor function and muscle strength decline; 15% decrease in nerve conduction velocity; decrease in muscle mass
Skeletal system	Decrease in bone mass
Kidneys	Fewer nephrons after age 40 years; glomerular filtration rate declines about 50% at age 80, decreased ability to concentrate or dilute urine
Endocrine	Decreased response of beta cells of pancreas to glucose; reduced glucose tolerance and production of insulin, slight changes in other endocrine secretions; large decreases in estrogen, some decrease in activity of testosterone
Immune system	Decline in size and function of immune system, especially cell-mediated

The Gastrointestinal Tract

Oral Cavity

Age-related changes in teeth include abrasion or wearing down of crowns. On the other hand, there is an increased resistance to tooth decay because of maturation of enamel and dentin. However, the gums deteriorate with age, causing loss of teeth and gum (periodontal) disease, which afflicts up to 90% of adults over the age of 65. Older adults often have missing teeth or poor fitting-dentures that impair mastication resulting in reduced food intake. Masticatory efficiency is also compromised by loss of mobility of the mandibular (lower jaw) joint often caused by

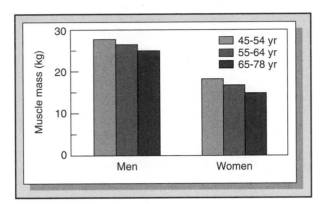

FIGURE 12–3. Declining muscle mass with age. (Redrawn after Frontera WR, et al. A cross-sectional study of muscle strength and mass in 45- to 78-year-old men and women. J Appl Physiol 1991;71:644.)

osteoarthritis (a noninflammatory joint disease occurring chiefly in older persons).

In a healthy mouth, copious amounts of saliva containing essential electrolytes, glycoproteins, and antimicrobial enzymes continually lubricate and protect the teeth and oral mucosa. Aging is associated with decreased salivary flow, which can cause the healthy mouth to become susceptible to painful deterioration. **Xerostomia** is particularly prevalent among the aged. Inadequate lubrication and moisture within the mouth, lack of ability to taste, food sticking to the tongue, and difficulty swallowing are among the most devastating manifestations of xerostomia in older adults, and xerostomia is a major contributor to geriatric malnutrition in the United States (Rhodus and Brown, 1990).

Xerostomia is a potential side effect of many drugs widely used in **geriatrics**. Treatment is aimed at increasing the flow of saliva when possible or providing oral moisture by other means.

Esophagus, Stomach, and Small Intestine

Older people report gastrointestinal complaints more frequently than younger adults, and some disorders, such as diverticulosis, occur primarily in the elderly. Older adults also take more medications, which may affect gastrointestinal function as well as food intake. Overall, age-related changes in the anatomy and physiology of the digestive tract are small.

There is a slight decline in gastrointestinal motility and a general reduction in secretory ability of digestive glands, resulting in lower levels of enzymes, especially amylase, pepsin, and trypsin. In the stomach gastric **atrophy** and **atrophic gastritis** increase significantly with age. Reduced hydrochloric acid secretion may result in decreased bioavailabilty of calcium, iron, folate, and vitamins B_6 and B_{12}, as well as increased risk of bacterial overgrowth of the small intestine. At typical intake levels, absorption of carbohydrate, lipid, and protein appears unaffected by age in healthy elderly persons. However, high fat diets (>100 g/day) are less well tolerated (Holt and Balint, 1993).

Colon

Age-related alterations in motility of the colon may contribute to the retention of feces and constipation. Constipation is more common in older adults, partially due to decreased activity, limited fluid intake, low-fiber diets, and, possibly, medications used. With low fiber intakes, increased intraluminal pressure and greater muscle contraction is required to move the digestive contents through the colon. The resulting weakening of the muscle wall may result in "outpouching," or the formation of small pouches in the wall of the colon, a condition known as diverticulosis.

Pancreas and Liver

Although there are morphologic changes in the liver and pancreas, digestive function appears to be adequate on usual intakes. The liver is the major site of drug metabolism in the body. The rate at which drugs are metabolized and detoxified is slower in older than in younger persons, causing drugs to remain in the body longer and to exert their effects over a longer time.

Anorexia of Aging

"Anorexia of aging" is a term used to describe the decline in appetite and loss of weight that are common with advancing age. Many factors contribute to anorexia and weight loss (Table 12–4). Depression and side effects of medication are the two most common treatable causes of weight loss in older persons. In addition, restricted diets

KEY TERMS

xerostomia: the feeling of dry mouth caused by a severe reduction in the flow of saliva

geriatrics: branch of medicine that treats problems particular to old age and the aging process

atrophy: diminution in size of cell tissue or organ

atrophic gastritis: chronic inflammation of the stomach with decreased thickness of the mucosa and disappearance of gastric and pyloric glands

TABLE 12–4 Factors That May Contribute to Anorexia of Aging

Hypothalmic control: decreased opioid feeding drive

Senses: decreased sense of taste and smell

Food ingestion: chewing difficulties due to endentulous problems, xerostemia

Gastrointestinal: delayed gastric emptying—early satiety, difficulties in swallowing; increased cholecystokinin—increased satiety; abdominal angina (pain)

Chronic constipation

Psychosocial: poverty, depression, dementia; social isolation

Physical: impaired mobility

Disease states: cancer; chronic obstructive pulmonary disease

Medications: digoxin, psychotropic and analgesic/anti-inflamatory drugs, other medications

with limited taste appeal, such as those low in cholesterol or salt, often precipitate weight loss.

Respiratory System

With aging there is a reduction in surface area of the alveoli (air sacs), which is accompanied by deterioration of the elastic properties of lung tissue. These decreases are almost linear between ages of 20 and 80 years, and by age 80 the level is approximately 30% of maximal young adult values. Because of these changes, the lungs become stiffer and alveolar tissue less distensible and less permeable to respiratory gases; therefore, gas exchange is lowered. **Vital capacity** decreases with age, and the ability to exercise is reduced.

Cardiovascular System

Cardiac output may decline with aging by as much as 30%. This change is due to increased rigidity of arterial walls, decreased blood flow to tissues, and decreased oxygen uptake, all of which contribute to age-related changes in other tissues such as the kidney.

There is an overall decrease in the size of the heart muscle as well as the size of the cavity of the ventricle (lower chamber of the heart) and an increase in the size of the left atrium (chamber). The heart valves become more rigid due to thickening from increased collagen, and there is calcification in aortic valve. Hypertrophy (enlargement) of individual muscle fibers of myocardium apparently occurs to compensate for other muscle fibers that are lost. The ag-

ing heart tolerates physical stress less well, which means there is reduced tolerance of strenuous exercise and, possibly, increased systolic blood pressure.

Skin, Hair, and Nails

The **collagen** content of the body increases with age, resulting in changes in skin and the loss of elasticity of blood vessels. The many age-related changes in the skin include dryness, wrinkling, enlarged sebaceous glands (but decreased sebaceous gland activity), mottled pigmentation, loss of elasticity, dilation of capillaries, and senile purpura (bleeding into skin in response to minor trauma). Chronic exposure to sunlight causes premature aging of these tissues.

There are also the changes of graying of hair and more hair loss. The nails grow more slowly and may be thicker.

Neuromuscular System

Generalized age-related muscle weakness is related to a decline in the number of functioning muscle fibers, a general loss of muscle mass, and a decrease in the contractile process itself (Carmeli and Reznich, 1994). Because there is some loss of peripheral motor neurons, muscle response to nerve stimulation declines. The extent of these age-related changes varies from muscle to muscle.

There is progressive age-associated loss of brain cells, particularly in the cortex, the area responsible for higher mental function, movement perception, and behavioral reactions. Therefore, memory may decline, but the degree varies greatly. Although loss of memory affects ability to learn and retain information, there is evidence that intellectually active and socially stimulated individuals are less likely to show severe impairment.

It is possible that subclinical vitamin deficiencies play a role in the pathogenesis of declining neurocognitive function with aging. Attention has focused on vitamins C, B_6, B_{12} and folate (Rosenberg and Miller, 1992). Administration of vitamin B_{12} has been shown to reverse both cognitive and peripheral nervous system deficits in older adults who have no evidence of the hematologic abnormalities of vitamin B_{12} deficiency (Lindenbaum et al, 1994).

Skeletal Tissue

Bone mass increases rapidly during growth, especially at sites composed largely of cortical bone. Gains continue into the third decade of life, and then plateau. The bone loss that begins in the fourth or fifth decades of life is proportionately less for men than women. Among women, bone loss accelerates with decreased estrogen secretion after menopause; then, after a time, the rate of loss slows.

The clinical importance of low bone mass is the increased risk of subsequent fractures. Osteoporosis, accelerated bone loss, is discussed on page 331.

Kidney Function

Kidney function deteriorates with age. There is a net loss of **nephrons** and decreased blood flow through the kidney. As a result, the rate at which blood is filtered through the kidney (the glomerular filtration rate) declines so that the rate of blood filtration at age 80 years is approximately 50% of that at age 25 years. The ability to concentrate or dilute urine is also decreased. This reduces the ability of the kidneys to deal with large fluctuations in the workload so that, for instance, it takes longer to excrete a large amount of dietary sodium from a food or meal high in salt.

Endocrine System

Aging is associated with a myriad of changes in the endocrine system. The most prominent may be the decline in the production of insulin in response to an oral load of glucose. Reduced insulin levels are thought to contribute to adiposity, especially abdominal obesity (Parker et al, 1993), and are associated with an increased incidence of non–insulin-dependent diabetes mellitus (NIDDM) with age. For women, the dramatic decline in estrogen production at menopause has substantial implications for bone mass and osteoporosis.

Immune System

Throughout adult life there is a decline in the mass of immune tissue, with loss of immune function, and an increased incidence of infections, cancer, and autoimmune disorders (Makinodan, 1995). Some immune cell functions decrease rapidly, while others resist change or are even disproportionately elevated.

Nutrition can influence both immune function and the aging process. In fact, most age-related changes of the immune system parallel those observed in protein energy undernutrition (PEU) (Chandra, 1995). Specific nutrient deficiencies have been shown to produce some impairments of immune function in older people. These include short- and long-term supplementation with vitamin E (Meydani, 1995), and low-dose multivitamin and mineral supplements as well as supplements of vitamins A, B_6, C, and E and zinc (Bogden et al, 1994; Rosenberg and Miller, 1992). However, megadoses of some nutrients may also suppress the immune system. More studies are needed before specific recommendations can be made.

PHYSICAL, ECONOMIC, PSYCHOSOCIAL, AND HEALTH FACTORS ASSOCIATED WITH AGING

■ Describe the kinds of nonphysiologic factors that influence health and nutrition status in older adults.

■ How do economic factors influence dietary intake?

■ What are ADL and IADL, and what is their significance in determining quality of life and nutrition health?

■ How is social isolation related to health and nutrition status in older adults?

■ What are the effects of cigarette smoking and alcohol consumption on the health of older adults?

Although age-related physiologic changes reduce the ability of the older person to respond to stress, many other factors influence the health, well-being, and quality of life of older adults. For example, being poor, being a member of a minority, and living alone and in poor health are factors which reduce social integration and can lead to social alienation, isolation and powerlessness. Table 12–5 summarizes physical, economic, psychosocial, health and dietary factors that interact to influence the process of aging and nutrition status.

Physical

Physical mobility determines the level of independence and, thus, the quality of life, for all individuals but particularly for the older generation. Increasing infirmity, **osteoarthritis,** and failing eyesight are common with aging, and reduce mobility. Simple things, such as not being able to read labels or prices while shopping or the inability to stand or move about for cooking and cleaning up after eating can compromise quality of life and reduce food intake.

 K E Y   T E R M S

vital capacity: the volume of gas that can be expelled from the lungs after full inspiration
collagen: protein substance of white fibers of the skin, tendon, bone, cartilage, and other connective tissue
nephron: functional unit in the kidney for filtering blood
osteoarthritis: a noninflammatory degenerative joint disease accompanied by pain and stiffness

TABLE 12–5 Physical, Economic, Psychosocial, and Health Factors Associated with Aging

TABLE 12–5 Physical, Economic, Psychosocial, and Health Factors Associated with Aging

PHYSICAL

Functional status

Activities of daily living

Instrumental activities of daily living

Disabling conditions
   Immobility
   Inactivity

Inability to obtain and prepare food

ECONOMIC

Limited income

Inadequate housing

Limited access to medical care

Access to economic assistance programs

Access to food

Medical expenses

SOCIAL STATUS

Social isolation

Support systems—family, friends

Living arrangements

Access to community services/transportation

PSYCHOLOGICAL

Depression

Dementia

Alzheimer's disease

Cognitive impairment

Emotional impairment

FOOD INTAKE

Frequency of food consumption

Quantity

Quality

Dietary modifications

Use of supplements

Use of alcohol/tobacco

Food quackery

HEALTH CONDITIONS

Underweight or overweight

Alcohol or tobacco abuse

Oral health

CHRONIC DISEASES

Cardiovascular

Cerebrovascular

Diabetes mellitus

Rheumatoid arthritis

Cancer

CHRONIC MEDICATION USE

Control

Polypharmacy

centages needing help were greater in women than men and increased sharply with age for both genders, especially after 85 years.

Physically impaired older adults are likely to have poor dietary intakes due to inability to perform one or more daily activities related to eating, food procurement, or food preparation. This inability serves as a warning sign of increased nutritional risk. Preventable factors that have been associated with functional decline include smoking, frequent alcohol use, lack of regular physical activity, and use of sedatives or tranquilizers.

A minimal level of aerobic fitness appears necessary for independent living. For older adults without functional impairments, regular physical activity may improve cerebral function and sleep patterns, provide opportunities for social contact, and increase energy intake and expenditure.

Economic

The overall well-being of older individuals is inextricably linked to their economic well-being. It is a determinant of lifestyle, including standards of housing, levels of health care, availability of economic assistance programs, and dietary adequacy.

In 1993, 20% (6.1 million) of elderly persons were classified as poor (income below the poverty level) or near poor (income between the poverty level and 125% of this level) (Bureau of the Census, 1994). Approximately 11% of elderly whites, compared to 28% of elderly blacks and 21% of elderly Hispanics, were poor or near poor. Women were more likely than men to be poor, as were older adults living alone or with non-relatives.

Older persons may have to depend on family members, friends, or public transportation to shop, seek health care, and socialize.

An individual's ability to perform the customary activities of daily living is often referred to as her functional status. Functional status is measured by the degree of assistance required with basic self-management activities called activities of daily living (ADLs) or with home management activities referred to as instrumental activities of daily living (IADLs). Table 12–6 outlines the components of these two groups of activities. In 1986 about 23% of older people living in the community had difficulty with one or more ADLs (self management) and 28% had difficulty with one or more instrumental activities of daily living (home management) (Dawson et al, 1987). The per-

TABLE 12–6 Functional Activities Associated with Mobility and Independence in Older Adults

Activities of Daily Living (ADL)	Instrumental Activities of Daily Living (IADL)
Bathing	Food preparation
Continence	Use of the telephone
Dressing	Housekeeping
Eating	Laundry
Toileting	Use of transportation
Transferring from bed or chair	Responsibility for medication
Walking	Managing money
Getting outside	Shopping

Low-income elderly often have limited access to food and fewer food choices, particularly when needs perceived as more pressing take precedence. Housing costs may consume as much as one-third of their incomes, and for many, medical care (even with Medicare) may consume a large portion of the budget, thus limiting the availability of dollars to purchase adequate food.

Psychosocial

With aging, mental processes slow, but the individual remains in touch with reality and is well oriented (Council on Scientific Affairs, 1990). Important contributors to poor food intake include psychological factors such as bereavement, confusion, and depression and dementia. Several million people over 65 suffer from some type of **dementia**, with the prevalence increasing to approximately 20% or more by age 80 (Woolf et al, 1990). Manifestations of dementias are memory loss, disorientation, indifference, impaired judgment, and coexistent anxiety and restlessness. These often lead to reduced food intake and alteration in physical activity. Dehydration, often unrecognized in older adults, may exacerbate the dementia.

Depression is more common with increasing age. Depression disorders have a significant impact on level of function, productivity, and perceived physical and mental health. Frequent components of depression are loss of enthusiasm and appetite and declining body weight and nutrition status. Distorted attitudes toward food and body image may occur in some older adults, but the pattern of abnormalities may not be that of classical anorexia nervosa (Morley and Solomon, 1994).

The longer individuals live, the more they become the survivors of their generation. Over time they lose spouse, family, neighbors, and vital social and occupational roles in the community. The older individual lives in an increasingly isolated world. Because eating is generally a social activity, social isolation may result in reduced food intake and compromised nutrition status. Older adults who live alone and who, for whatever reason, are unable to go out regularly and have few friends or relatives to visit them may lose the incentive to prepare and consume regular nutritious meals.

Health Status

Degenerative diseases that first appear in middle life persist and become more severe in old age. Most older persons have at least one chronic condition, and many have multiple conditions (Table 12–7). Treatment of chronic health problems increases the demand for economic and social services as well as healthcare resources.

In 1992, older people accounted for 46% of all days of care in hospitals (Bureau of the Census, 1994). Compared

TABLE 12–7 Ten Most Common Chronic Conditions in Non-Institutionalized Older Persons	
Condition	**Adults over 65 years Affected (%)**
Arthritis	48
Hypertension	36
Hearing impairment	32
Heart disease	32
Deformity or orthopedic impairment	19
Cataracts	17
Chronic sinusitis	16
Diabetes	11
Visual impairment	9
Tinnitus	9

From U.S. Department of Health and Human Services Vital and Health Statistics: Current Estimates from the National Health Interview Survey: United States, 1992. Washington, DC: National Center for Health Statistics, 1994.

to younger adults, they had longer stays (an average of 8.2 days compared to only 5.1 days), and twice as many contacts with physicians. Older Americans use approximately 25% of the prescription drugs dispensed each year, and two-thirds take more than one prescription drug (Council on Scientific Affairs, 1990). The most frequently prescribed drugs are antibiotics, diuretics–antihypertensive agents, nonsteroidal antiinflammatory agents, cardiotonics, antiarrhythmics, steroids, tranquilizers, antidepressants, lipid-lowering drugs, and anticoagulants.

Because of multiple chronic health problems, polypharmacy is a real concern in older adults. They are likely to take multiple prescription medications, perhaps from more than one health care provider, and may also use several over-the-counter products. This is a concern because drugs are likely to have greater potency in an older person. This is due to increased brain and organ sensitivity, lower water and blood volume, changes in body composition,

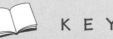 **K E Y   T E R M S**

dementia: organic loss of intellectual function
depression: psychiatric syndrome consisting of dejected mood, psychomotor retardation, insomnia, and weight loss

RESEARCH UPDATE
Alzheimer's Disease

Alzheimer's disease is the epitome of the fears expressed by older people when they say they don't want to become a burden to their families. Over a span of 5 to 7 years, until death from complications such as pneumonia, the disease robs victims of their memory, thinking ability, normal behavior, and often their life savings as they become unable to care for themselves.

Four million Americans suffer from Alzheimer's (Wolf-Klein and Silverstone, 1994). Nearly 10% of persons aged 65 years or over suffer from it; 50% of those over 85 are affected. It is the most common form of dementia, responsible for half of nursing home admissions. The annual cost to American society, estimated at $100 billion, is likely to increase as more adults live longer.

Alzheimer's is an abnormal progressive deterioration of the brain. Unfortunately, the cause is mysterious and there are no signs of the disease's progression until substantial brain damage has occurred. Diagnosis is difficult, but characteristic symptoms are gradual loss of memory and reasoning, loss of the ability to communicate, loss of physical capabilities, and, eventually, loss of life. The only conclusive diagnosis is examination of brain tissue at autopsy.

The brain of a person with Alzheimer's disease contains a large number of abnormal structures called "senile plaques." These plaques consist of a **beta amyloid** surrounded by nerve cells with abnormally twisted protein fibers. The significance of beta amyloid has been the source of much debate. Some researchers argue that the deposition of beta amyloid in plaques is the result of neuron (brain cell) breakdown from an unknown cause. The opposing view contends that the protein causes a pathologic cascade of events in which beta amyloid is produced, escapes from neurons, forms plaques, and kills off other neurons, with dementia as the result.

It appears that normal neurons release beta amyloid and that overproduction of beta amyloid results in the accumulation of insoluble paired helical filaments. Beta-amyloid protein has been demonstrated to be neurotoxic to rodent brain cell cultures, resulting in memory loss for recently acquired events but not for previously learned events in senescence-accelerated mice. Continuing studies have indicated that a number of small peptides may inhibit the **amnestic** effect of the beta-amyloid protein. If proven true, drug intervention to block beta amyloid production may be possible.

Nutrition status and specific nutrient deficiencies affect the brain in several ways, but Alzheimer's is an identifiable disease, the course of which is probably not influenced by nutrition. However, a number of studies of the nutrition status of individuals with Alzheimer's disease have reported weight loss that cannot be explained by food intake or physical activity (Wolf-Klein and Silverstone, 1994; Renvall et al, 1993). It is not clear whether this weight loss is a component of or a consequence of the disease, but such observations suggest systemic and metabolic alternations in Alzheimer's disease.

---

and declining kidney and liver function, which decrease metabolism and excretion. Drug problems may be dismissed as signs of aging. Often no one person providing health care knows the full scope of the drug usage, making side effects almost impossible to identify and correct.

Foods or specific nutrients can affect drug action by altering digestion, absorption, distribution, metabolism, and/or excretion. Drugs, self-administered or prescribed, may influence the nutrition status of an individual in several ways, including changing energy and nutrient needs, reducing food ingestion, or altering nutrient absorption, metabolism, and excretion. The risk of adverse side effects increases with the number of drugs taken and the duration of exposure to drugs.

Alcohol

Although age does not affect the rate of absorption or elimination of alcohol, the decline in lean body mass and corresponding decrease in the volume of total body water mean that alcohol is distributed over less area. Therefore, an identical amount of alcohol will result in a higher blood alcohol concentration in an older adult than in a younger individual of the same size and gender (Dufor and Fuller, 1995).

There is limited information regarding the prevalence of alcohol use among older adults or specific characteristics of elderly drinkers and nondrinkers. In a USDA interim study of almost 600 adults between the ages of 60 and 95 years, 53% of men and 44% of women reported drinking at least two drinks per week (Sulsky et al, 1990). The level of alcohol consumption decreased with age and was positively associated with education and smoking.

Moderate alcohol consumption (1 to 2 drinks per day) may increase feelings of freedom from care while lessening inhibitions, stress, and depression, and may actually enhance appetite for some individuals. However, with reduced energy intake, calories from alcoholic beverages have the potential to displace more nutrient-dense sources of energy. The relationship of moderate alcohol consumption with reduced total and cardiovascular mortality that has been well documented in middle-aged populations appears to occur in older populations as well. A study of more than 6000 men and women aged 65 and older found that low to moderate alcohol consumption was associated with statistically significant lowering of total and cardiovascular mortality (Scherr et al, 1992). However, a 15-year follow-up of Japanese American men in the Honolulu Health Program found that, as alcohol consumption increased, so did the risk of stroke and cancer (Goldberg et al, 1994).

An important concern about alcohol use by older adults is the potential for interactions with both prescription and over-the-counter medications. In a random sample of community-dwelling older adults, the majority (57%) reported using alcohol. In addition, 25% of drinkers took one or more other drugs, most commonly over-the-counter pain medications, for many of which alcohol could exaggerate or negate the effect. This placed them at potential risk for drug-related interactions (Forster et al, 1993). In addition, consumption of alcoholic beverages may exacerbate cognitive impairment and dementias of other etiology.

Cigarette Smoking

Cigarette smoking is the #1 avoidable cause of mortality in the United States. In addition to the well-known health risks associated with smoking, older smokers were found to be weaker and had poorer balance and poorer performance on measures of integrated physical function than nonsmokers (Nelson et al, 1994). The decrease in function (muscle strength, agility, coordination, gait) was 50% to 100% as great as that associated with a 5-year increase in age, and most measures worsened with increasing number of pack-years.

ENERGY AND NUTRIENT NEEDS

■ How have nutrient needs been established for older adults?

■ What happens to nutrient needs with aging?

■ Is there evidence that the RDA for some nutrients should be revised?

Over several decades the changes of aging can influence energy and nutrient needs, patterns of food intake, and physical activity. Most of the nutrient recommendations for older persons have been derived by extrapolation of data from younger adults. Because of limited data on the effects of age on nutrient needs, the 10th edition of the Recommended Dietary Allowances (RDA) makes one set of recommendations for adults 51 years and older (Table 12–8). The very heterogeneous nature and wide age range of older population make it difficult to generalize. The physiologic and health status of persons who are 60 years old is very different from that of persons who are 80 or 90. For these reasons, it has been recommended that future editions of the RDA include a category for adults over age 70 years.

Current evidence suggests that the current RDA for older adults may be too low for protein, calcium, vitamin D, vitamin E, vitamin B_6, vitamin B_{12}, and folate, and too high for vitamin A (Blumberg, 1994). Only energy and those nutrients for which changes in recommendations seem appropriate are discussed here.

Energy Needs

Energy is required for metabolic processes at the cellular level, for maintaining homeostasis of turnover processes (mainly protein turnover), and for muscular work. Energy needs decline with age in association with decreased body size, a loss of lean body mass, and a diminution of physical activity. The 1989 RDA for energy intakes are 2300 kcal for the reference 77 kg older male and 1900 for the 65 kg older female (Food and Nutrition Board, 1989). These levels are approximately 30 kcal/kg/day, representing a reduction from the 33 to 34 kcal/kg/day that are the bases for younger adults.

While energy needs decline, requirements for many nutrients may increase. That means older adults require a careful selection of nutrient-dense foods to meet their nutritional needs in fewer kilocalories. Physical activity is important compensation for decreased energy intake, because it increases energy expenditure and food intake and delays lean body mass decline and improves independence.

 KEY TERMS

beta amyloid: a fragment from a large, normally-occurring protein called beta amyloid precursor protein
amnestic: causing loss of memory

TABLE 12–8 Recommended Dietary Allowances for Adults over 51 Years of Age

	Males	Females
Energy (kcal)	2300	1900
Protein (g)	63	50
FAT-SOLUBLE VITAMINS		
Vitamin A (μg RE)*	1000	800
Vitamin D (μg)†	5	5
Vitamin E (mg α-TE)‡	10	8
Vitamin K (μg)	80	65
WATER-SOLUBLE VITAMINS		
Vitamin C (mg)	60	60
Thiamin (mg)	1.2	1.0
Riboflavin (mg)	1.4	1.2
Niacin (mg NE)§	15	13
Vitamin B_6 (mg)	2.0	1.6
Folate (μg)	200	180
Vitamin B_{12} (μg)	2.0	2.0
MINERALS		
Calcium (mg)	800	800
Phosphorus (mg)	800	800
Magnesium (mg)	350	280
Iron (mg)	10	10
Zinc (mg)	15	12
Iodine (μg)	150	150
Selenium (μg)	70	55

* I RE (retinol equivalent) = I μg or 6 μg β-carotene.
† As cholecalciferol. 10 μg cholecalciferol = 400 IU vitamin D.
‡ α-Tocopherol equivalents. I mg d-α = I α-TE.
§ I NE (niacin equivalent) = I mg of niacin or 60 mg dietary tryptophan.

Protein

The RDA for protein, 0.8 g/kg body weight per day, has been assumed to be adequate for older adults when energy intakes exceed 30 kcal/kg/day. However, at usual energy intakes for older individuals, that level may not be sufficient to attain nitrogen balance. Studies have documented a requirement of approximately 1 g or more of protein per kg per day to establish nitrogen **equilibrium**. Lower intakes have been shown to compromise lean tissue, immune response, and muscle function (Castaneda et al, 1995). A safe protein intake for older adults would be 1.0 to 1.25 g/kg/day of high-quality protein (Campbell et al, 1994).

Fat-Soluble Vitamins

Vitamin A

The 1989 RDAs for vitamin A for adults 51 years of age and older are 1000 μg retinol equivalents for males and 800 for females. Current evidence supports a decreased requirement for preformed vitamin A in this age group (Russell and Suter, 1993). This is associated with age-related increases in absorption, as well as delays in the clearance of dietary vitamin A by the liver and other peripheral tissues. Accumulation of vitamin A increases the risk of toxicity. On the other hand, beta carotene and other carotenoids, due to their antioxidant properties, may have health benefits related to cardiovascular disease, cataracts, and cancer (Gerster, 1993). Therefore, it is important that a large fraction of the vitamin A intake come from the carotene-containing fruits and vegetables.

Vitamin D

Blood levels of 25-hydroxyvitamin D are reduced with age. In addition to decreased exposure to sunlight and use of sunscreens, older persons have a decreased capability to synthesize vitamin D_3 in the skin. Vitamin D_3 is hydroxylated to 25-cholecalciferol in the liver and to its active form, 1,25-hydroxyl cholecalciferol, in the kidney. With age there is a decline in the hydroxylation in the kidney and vitamin D receptors in the gastrointestinal tract (Russell and Suter, 1993), all of which may contribute to deficiency.

The RDA for vitamin D for adults 51 years and older is 5 μg. In some populations of older adults with limited exposure to sunlight, vitamin D intakes of 10 to 20 μg were necessary to maintain adequate vitamin D status (O'Dowd et al, 1993). This has resulted in recommendations for 10 μg (400 IU per day), or twice the RDA, for the homebound elderly, those in nursing homes, and others who may have limited exposure to sunlight.

Food sources include vitamin D–enriched milk, fish oils, and liver. In the United States and Canada, the principal food source for vitamin D is fortified milk. However, the amount of vitamin D in milk is variable, and some skim milks contain no vitamin D at all (Hollick, 1994).

Vitamin E

There is considerable interest in the antioxidant role that vitamin E (tocopherol) may play in aging or prevention of chronic disease. No deficiency of vitamin E has been reported in healthy older adults. However, vitamin E supplements have been shown to improve immune responses (Meydani et al, 1995) and decrease the risk of cardiovascular disease in older adults (Hodis et al, 1995).

Water-Soluble Vitamins

Although there are insufficient data to justify a change in the current recommendations for most water-soluble vitamins for older adults, there has been increased evidence for age-related changes in recommendations for vitamins B_6, B_{12}, and folate.

Older adults tend to be at greater risk of vitamin B_6 deficiency. Data from NHANES III showed that mean intakes of vitamin B_6 of adults over 50 years were below the RDA. Serum B_6 levels decrease with age, suggesting that metabolic utilization is less efficient and that the requirement for vitamin B_6 may be higher for older individuals (Pannemans et al, 1994). Impaired cell-mediated immune responses have been associated with vitamin B_6 deficiency.

Low serum or plasma vitamin B_{12} levels are twice as common in older adults as in young adults (Lindenbaum et al, 1994). A low intake, especially among the poor elderly, and impaired absorption due to atrophic gastritis may be important factors. In addition, bacterial overgrowth in the small bowel may lead to competition for vitamin B_{12}. Anemia occurs in the most severely vitamin B_{12}–depleted individuals, and neuropsychiatric manifestations and metabolic abnormalities often occur before low serum concentrations are observed (Allen and Casterline, 1994). The decrease in hydrochloric acid secretion may reduce absorption of dietary folate.

These three vitamins have been associated with epidemiologic observations that an elevated blood level of homocysteine is an independent risk factor for cardiovascular (Pancharuniti et al, 1994) and cerebrovascular disease (Selhub et al, 1995) (see page 288). It has been suggested that increased dietary intakes of these vitamins will normalize homocysteine levels and may reduce risk of atherosclerotic disease.

Minerals

Calcium

Bone mass continues to increase up to the third decade of life and then plateaus. Inadequate calcium during the growth period may result in failure to reach peak bone mass, contributing to decreased skeletal integrity and fracture in older adulthood. In later decades, adequate calcium intake is needed to maintain or minimize bone loss.

Surveys of food habits of older Americans reveal that most women and many men do not ingest sufficient quantities of calcium to meet the RDA of 800 mg. Accumulating scientific evidence indicates that the RDA for calcium is inadequate to meet the needs of the aging populations (National Institutes of Health Consensus Development Panel, 1994). In particular, intestinal calcium absorption is often reduced because of the effects of estrogen deficiency in women and the age-related reduction in renal 1,25-dihydroxyvitamin D of production in the kidney. A 1994 National Institutes of Health (NIH) Consensus Statement, "Optimal Calcium Intake," recommended a daily intake of 1500 mg of calcium for men and women over 65 (1000 mg for women on estrogen).

Iron

Iron absorption per se does not appear to decline significantly with age, and iron stores appear to increase. However, iron deficiency still occurs in the elderly due to inadequate iron intake or reduced nonheme iron absorption secondary to the hypochlorhydria of atrophic gastritis. In the NHANES I and II studies, the prevalence of iron deficiency anemia in older adults was low and was most often attributable to chronic conditions such as infection, rheumatoid arthritis, cancer, and renal failure than to iron deficiency, indicating that the RDA for the elderly is adequate.

Water

For adults, daily water intake should approximate 30 mL/kg body weight (or about 1.9 liters for the reference female and 2.3 liters for the male) to compensate for usual losses through skin, lungs, kidneys, and bowel. Additional amounts may be necessary to compensate for unusual losses due to excessive perspiration, fever, diarrhea, vomiting, or hemorrhage.

Fluid balance deserves particular attention in older adults because dehydration often goes unrecognized in this group. In part, dehydration may be the result of decreased thirst sensitivity, and older adults need to be encouraged to consume about 1.5 to 2.0 liters of fluid each day. Inadequate water intake can lead to dehydration, hypertension, elevated body temperature, constipation, nausea and vomiting, dryness of the mucosa, decreased urinary excretion, and mental confusion.

In summary, to meet their energy and nutrient needs, the healthy aging population needs to consume a balanced, nutrient-dense diet containing a variety of foods of moderate to low fat content. In addition, an adequate intake of fluids and regular moderate physical activity (strength training and aerobic exercise) are recommended to maintain a healthy vigorous life for as long as possible.

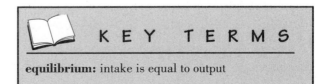

KEY TERMS

equilibrium: intake is equal to output

DIETARY INTAKES OF OLDER ADULTS

Major national surveys assessing the dietary intakes of older persons include NHANES I and II Surveys (National Center for Health Statistics, 1979; National Center for Health Statistics, 1983) and the Ross Laboratory Elderly Dietary Survey (Ryan et al, 1992). The NHANES I and II data were limited to individuals up to age 74 years. There has been limited information regarding intakes of adults 75 years and older, but NHANES III has no upper age limit and will provide data on the very old.

Several studies have documented a progressive decline in energy intakes with advancing age. Males and females aged 65 to 74 followed in NHANES II consumed an average of 1800 and 1400 kcal per day, respectively. A reported downward trend in energy and nutrient intakes with increasing age (Popkin et al, 1992) is shown in preliminary data from NHANES III (Table 12–9). The 31% to 34% of energy from dietary fat represents a decrease from previous surveys but is still above levels recommended in the Dietary Guidelines.

Studies that have measured dietary intakes of healthy community-dwelling older adults show that mean intakes for most nutrients approach the level of the 1989 RDA. Older persons may consume less than the RDA for calcium, magnesium, zinc, folate, vitamin E, and vitamin B_6. Loss of autonomy in such individuals is associated with increased risk of nutritional problems (Payette et al, 1995), and older adults who are homebound are at high risk of in-

adequate intake of protein and energy (Gray-Donald et al, 1995).

Use of Supplements

Americans are users of supplements. Nowhere is this more apparent than in older adults. Studies indicate that 35% to 70% of older Americans use nutritional supplements on a regular basis (Sheehan et al, 1989; Payette and Gray-Donald, 1991). In addition, many older adults are taking more than one supplement each day; some take as many as 20 or 30 tablets, pills, capsules, or drinks each day. Women tend to take supplements more than men. As with other age groups, the older adults who take supplements are often the ones who have the best diets and the least need for supplements to meet nutritional needs. Many older people are motivated to use a myriad of dietary supplements promoted for their purported ability to slow aging, improve health, increase energy levels, or prevent chronic diseases.

Although a single multivitamin supplement may be appropriate for older individuals, the cost-benefit ratio of using multiple supplements must be questioned. Excess intake of vitamins and minerals can occur in elderly adults who regularly use single or small groups of vitamins or minerals as supplements (Mares-Perlman, 1993).

Exercise

In the last few years there has been increased interest in the role that physical activity or exercise can play in the health and overall well-being of older adults. Several studies have demonstrated that weight training and aerobic exercise can enhance lean body mass and reduce fat mass even in the very old (Fiatarone et al, 1994). Exercise has been shown to increase endurance, flexibility, agility, and mobility and reduce falls and injuries in older adults who are ambulatory and cognitively intact (Province et al, 1995). Other health advantages of exercise in the elderly include decreased blood pressure and increased high-density-lipoprotein cholesterol levels (Rauramaa et al, 1995). In addition, expending increased amounts of energy allows a greater caloric intake, which can enhance the nutrient content of the diet.

TABLE 12–9 Mean Daily Total Food-Energy Intake (TFEI), Percentages from Dietary Fat, and Saturated Fat

Age Group (years)	Sample Size	TFEI	TFEI from Dietary Fat (%)	TFEI from Saturated Fat (%)
MALES				
60–69	546	2110	33.3	11.3
70–79	444	1887	33.8	11.6
≥80	296	1776	33.3	11.4
FEMALES				
60–69	560	1578	32.8	11.0
70–79	407	1435	32.3	10.8
≥80	313	1329	31.3	10.8

From Third National Health and Nutrition Examination Survey, Phase I, 1988–91. MMWR 1994;43:117.

ASSESSMENT OF NUTRITION STATUS

■ How well nourished are older adults?

■ Why is nutrition an essential component of geriatric assessment?

■ How and by whom can nutrition screening be initiated?

■ How does nutrition assessment of older adults differ from that for younger individuals?

Undernutrition

Undernutrition in older adults is conventionally defined as an unintentional weight loss of 1% to 2% per week, 5% per month, or 10% over a period of 6 months. Clinical features of early protein-energy malnutrition include confusion and low levels of serum albumin, total lymphocytes, and hemoglobin.

Undernutrition has been reported in 17% to 65% of older persons in hospitals and in 26% to 59% of those in long-term care institutions (Morley, 1993). The incidence of undernutrition in free-living adults is lower but less well defined. A 1992 study in New England that screened a random sample of Medicare beneficiaries aged 70 years and older identified 24% as being at high nutritional risk, and 38% had intakes of less than 75% of the RDA for three or more nutrients (Posner et al, 1994). The Administration on Aging (1994) estimates that 2.5 million community-dwelling older adults are likely to suffer from food insecurity in any 6-month period. In addition, it has been estimated that 85% of older Americans have chronic diseases and conditions that may benefit from nutrition intervention.

Nutrition Screening

Because of skyrocketing health care costs and because the average personal health care expenditure for those over 65 years of age is four times that for younger individuals, geriatric assessment has become an integral component of health care services for older adults. In general, geriatric assessment has concentrated on issues relating to polypharmacy, functional status, cognitive problems, depression, and incontinence (Reuben et al, 1995). There is substantial evidence that geriatric assessment and rehabilitation improves functional status in some older persons and reduces mortality rates (Stuck et al, 1993).

Recently some geriatric assessment programs have focused on nutrition assessment as a major component. It is an important and logical part because of the integral relationship between nutrition and health status in aging. Undernutrition develops in a fairly predictable fashion, and evidence of marginal or poor nutrition status exists long before clinical signs and symptoms occur. Screening for risk factors allows implementation of preventive measures before the overt manifestations of nutritional problems occur.

Nutrition screening and early intervention are primary steps in the development of a system of health care that is affordable or accessible to all older adults (White, 1994).

The Nutrition Screening Initiative (NSI) is an intensified effort to promote screening, identification and aggressive nutrition support. The NSI, a collaborative effort of numerous health professional organizations, began in 1990 with identification of potential risk factors and major indicators of poor nutrition status and development and validation of tools for screening.

An initial tool for identifying nutritional risk is the checklist "To Determine Your Nutrition Health" (Fig. 12–4). It is designed as a public awareness tool for self-assessment by older adults or for assessment by friends, loved ones, and care givers. Level I screen tools, to be completed by a social service or healthcare professional, are designed to identify warning signs of nutritional risk (Fig. 12–5). Individuals identified as at risk using the Level I screen would be further assessed using the Level II screen, which includes more specific diagnostic information. Level II screening is a nutrition assessment to be completed in a healthcare setting such as physician's office, a hospital, or a nursing home. A tool for Level II screen is found in Appendix 9.

The inclusion of nutrition screening in an overall geriatric assessment identifies individuals at risk so that intervention can be initiated early. Such intervention can alleviate remediable problems or control or ameliorate those problems that cannot be prevented. Six areas or priorities for nutrition intervention concentrations are social services, oral health, mental health, medication use, nutrition education and counseling, and nutrition support (Nutrition Screening Initiative, 1991).

Assessment of Nutrition Status

In aging uncomplicated by disease, older individuals have nutritional reserves and nutrition status is similar to that of younger adults. However, with aging an increasing proportion of older persons deplete their reserve capacity and become at nutrition risk. Assessment of older adults is based on anthropometric, laboratory, clinical, and dietary indicators, as discussed in Chapter 2. Table 12–10 outlines major indicators of poor nutritional status identified in the Nutrition Screening Initiative. Most often undernutrition is secondary to physical, economic, and psychosocial factors, which are compounded by the numerous physiologic changes that occur at different rates as individuals age. This is further complicated by the stresses of disease, multiple medications, and trauma.

Compared to that for younger adults, the amount of reference data for nutrition assessment for older adults is limited, particularly for those over 75 years of age. However, population data of adults over 74 years of age will be available soon from the third National Health and Nutrition Examination Survey (NHANES III), a 6-year survey completed in 1994.

The Warning Signs of poor nutritional health are often overlooked. Use this checklist to find out if you or someone you know is at nutritional risk.

Read the statements below. Circle the number in the yes column for those that apply to you or someone you know. For each yes answer, score the number in the box. Total your nutritional score.

DETERMINE YOUR NUTRITIONAL HEALTH

	YES
I have an illness or condition that made me change the kind and/or amount of food I eat.	2
I eat fewer than 2 meals per day.	3
I eat few fruits or vegetables, or milk products.	2
I have 3 or more drinks of beer, liquor or wine almost every day.	2
I have tooth or mouth problems that make it hard for me to eat.	2
I don't always have enough money to buy the food I need.	4
I eat alone most of the time.	1
I take 3 or more different prescribed or over-the-counter drugs a day.	1
Without wanting to, I have lost or gained 10 pounds in the last 6 months.	2
I am not always physically able to shop, cook and/or feed myself.	2
TOTAL	

Total Your Nutritional Score. If it's ---

0-2 **Good!** Recheck your nutritional score in 6 months.

3-5 **You are at moderate nutritional risk.** See what can be done to improve your eating habits and lifestyle. Your office on aging, senior nutrition program, senior citizens center or health department can help. Recheck your nutritional score in 3 months.

6 or more **You are at high nutritional risk.** Bring this checklist the next time you see your doctor, dietitian or other qualified health or social service professional. Talk with them about any problems you may have. Ask for help to improve your nutritional health.

 The Nutrition Screening Initiative
2626 Pennsylvania Avenue, NW, Suite 301
Washington, DC 20037

The Nutrition Screening Initiative is funded in part by a grant from Ross Laboratories, a division of Abbott Laboratories.

These materials developed and distributed by the Nutrition Screening Initiative, a project of:

 AMERICAN ACADEMY OF FAMILY PHYSICIANS

 THE AMERICAN DIETETIC ASSOCIATION

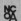 NATIONAL COUNCIL ON THE AGING

Remember that warning signs suggest risk, but do not represent diagnosis of any condition. Turn the page to learn more about the Warning Signs of poor nutritional health.

 46

FIGURE 12–4. Checklist to determine nutritional health. (From Report of Nutrition Screening I: Toward a common view. The Nutrition Screening Initiative. Washington, DC, 1991. Reprinted with permission by the Nutrition Screening Initiative, a project of the American Academy of Family Physicians, the American Dietetic Association and the National Council on the Aging, Inc., and funded in part by a grant from Ross Products Division, Abbott Laboratories.)

MARYLAND NUTRITION SCREENING

LEVEL I SCREEN

SSN#: _____

Race:
- ☐ 001 American Indian/Alaskan
- ☐ 002 Asian/Pacific Islander
- ☐ 003 African American
- ☐ 004 Hispanic
- ☐ 005 White, Not Hispanic

Address: _____

Name: _____
        Last   First

Age: _____   Sex: _____ (M/F)

County: _____   Telephone #: (__) _____

Site: _____   Date: _____

Health Indices

- 006   Height (in): _____
- 007   Weight (lbs): _____
- 008   Body Mass Index: _____
- 009   Blood Pressure: _____
- 010   Blood Cholesterol: _____
- 011   Blood Glucose: _____

Check any boxes that are true for the individual:

Weight Status

- ☐ 100   Has lost/gained 10 lbs. or more in the past 6 months
- ☐ 101   Body mass index < 22
- ☐ 102   Body mass index > 30

Eating Habits

- ☐ 200   Eats vegetables ≤ two daily
- ☐ 201   Eats milk/milk products < one daily
- ☐ 202   Eats fruit/drinks fruit juice ≤ one daily
- ☐ 203   Eats breads, cereal, pasta, rice or other grains ≤ five daily
- ☐ 204   Has more than one alcoholic drink per day (if woman); more than two drinks per day (if man)
- ☐ 205   Is on a special diet _____
- ☐ 206   Has chronic illness _____
- ☐ 207   Is taking 3 or more different prescribed or over-the-counter medications per day
- ☐ 208   Usually eats alone
- ☐ 209   Has difficulty chewing or swallowing
- ☐ 210   Has pain in mouth, teeth or gums
- ☐ 211   Has poor appetite
- ☐ 212   Does not have enough food to eat each day
- ☐ 213   Does not eat anything on one or more days each month
- ☐ 214   Participates in "Eating Together Program"
- ☐ 215   Participates in HDM Program

Functional Status

Usually or always needs assistance—check all that apply

- ☐ 300   Bathing
- ☐ 301   Dressing
- ☐ 302   Grooming
- ☐ 303   Toileting
- ☐ 304   Eating
- ☐ 305   Walking or moving about
- ☐ 306   Traveling outside the home
- ☐ 307   Preparing food
- ☐ 308   Shopping for food or other necessities

Living Environment

- ☐ 400   Lives on an income of less than $6,000 per year (per individual in the household)
- ☐ 401   Lives alone
- ☐ 402   Is housebound
- ☐ 403   Is concerned about home security
- ☐ 404   Lives in a home with inadequate heating or cooling
- ☐ 405   Does not have a stove and/or refrigerator
- ☐ 406   Is unable or prefers not to spend money on food (< $25-$30 per person spent on food each week)
- ☐ 407   Participates in Senior Center Programs
- ☐ 408   Participates in Senior Care

Mental/Cognitive Status

- 500   Folstein: _____
- 501   GDS: _____
- 502   Beck Inventory: _____
- ☐ 503   Clinical Impairment—Folstein < 26
- ☐ 504   Depressive Illness—GDS > 10; Beck > 15

Interest Profile

- ☐ 601   Extension Service Programs
- ☐ 602   Nutrition Topics
- ☐ 603   Shopping/Budgeting
- ☐ 604   Physical Fitness

Comments/Referral: _____

FIGURE 12–5. Example of a nutrition screening initiative. Level I Screen. (From Protocol for implementing nutrition screening at health promotion events. Maryland Nutrition Screening Initiative. Baltimore, MD: Maryland Office on Aging.)

TABLE 12–10 Major Indicators of Poor Nutrition Status

Significant loss of weight over time
  5% of body weight in 1 month
  7.5% or more in 3 months
  10% or more in 6 months
  Unintended weight loss of more than 10 pounds

Significantly low weight for height
  MRW <80%

Significant change in functional status
  Change from independence to dependence in two of the self-care skills (activities of daily living)
  Change from independence to dependence in nutrition-related skills

Significant reduction in serum protein measures
  serum albumin <3.5 g/dL

Significant and sustained reduction of nutritional intake below RDA
  3 months or more when intake is below the minimum from one or more of the five food groups

Significant reduction in midarm circumference
  <10th percentile

Significant increase or decrease in the triceps skinfold measurement <10th or >95th percentile

Significant obesity
  MRW >120%
  BMI ≥27

Nutrition-related disorders
  Osteoporosis
  Osteomalacia
  Folate deficiency
  Vitamin B$_{12}$ deficiency

From The Nutrition Screening Initiative. Report of Nutrition Screening I: Toward a common view. Washington, DC: 1991. Reprinted with permission by the Nutrition Screening Initiative, a project of the American Academy of Family Physicians, the American Dietetic Association and the National Council on the Aging, Inc., and funded in part by a grant from Ross Products Division, Abbott Laboratories.

Anthropometry

Generally, height declines by approximately 0.5 to 1.5 cm per decade with aging due to vertebral collapse or compaction. It may be difficult to accurately measure someone who is ambulatory because of **kyphosis**, bowing of the legs, or other loss of the ability to stand erect. Stature cannot be measured accurately in non-ambulatory older individuals, but height can be estimated from recumbent length, knee height, or arm length (Appendix 10). A recorded height that is 2 to 3 inches less than that recalled by the individual may precede the development of osteoporosis by several years.

The limitations of the Metropolitan Height Weight tables were discussed in Chapter 2. These tables may be less appropriate for older adults because they are based on weight data for individuals between 20 and 59 years of age. A more important predictor of risk is involuntary weight loss (Wallace et al, 1995). Extremes of high and low body mass index (BMIs) confer increased risk of mortality, but there is a broad range for body mass index (BMI) over which mortality does not vary.

Midarm circumference and fatfold measurements are less reliable in those over 65 years than in younger adults because of difficulty in accurately locating anatomic landmarks, increased compressibility of subcutaneous adipose tissue, age-related loss of skin elasticity, and changes in hydration status. As people age, the thickness of adipose tissues decreases on the arm and leg and increases on the trunk. Therefore, if general standards are applied, midarm muscle circumference (MAMC) and midarm muscle area (MAMA) will overestimate somatic protein status whereas the triceps fatfold will underestimate body fatness.

Biochemical

The most commonly used biochemical indicators of protein status are serum proteins that are synthesized in the liver. Serum albumin has prognostic value for subsequent mortality and morbidity in older adults (Ferguson et al, 1993). Proteins with shorter half-lives and smaller body pools, such as transferrin, retinol-binding protein, and prealbumin may be better suited to monitor status during acute illness and convalescence. Although total lymphocyte count (TLC) values for older adults are somewhat below the base for younger individuals, a TLC less than 1500/cm^3 indicates deficit and the need for further assessment. In older adults, the creatinine height index (CHI) may be less accurate in assessing muscle mass or somatic protein because of age-related declines in kidney function, which result in decreased clearance of creatinine. In addition, age-related standards have not been developed.

Because vitamin B$_{12}$ deficiency is more common among older adults, especially those with atrophic gastritis, periodic screening of serum levels for vitamin B$_{12}$ status is recommended after age 55 to 60 years (Allen and Casterline, 1994). Recently it has been demonstrated that older adults with normal serum vitamin concentrations of folate, vitamin B$_6$, and vitamin B$_{12}$ may have increased levels of metabolites that suggest vitamin inadequacies (Joosten et al, 1993; Lindenbaum et al, 1994). Measurement of metabolites of these vitamins in blood or urine may be more appropriate indicators of status for these vitamins.

Clinical Signs

Physical signs that suggest possible nutritional deficiency were outlined in Table 2–7. Clinical signs of malnutrition may be "softer" in older adults in that they are more difficult to identify because of age-related changes in hair, skin, nails, and body fat distribution. They may not correlate well with dietary intakes or even serum levels in older adults.

Dietary Assessment

In some ways, collecting dietary information from older adults can be easier than for other age groups because their dietary patterns tend to be less variable than those of younger adults. Also, many older adults, concerned about nutrition and health, are eager to share information about their dietary intakes and can be very conscientious about maintaining dietary records. Age-associated decline in short-term memory may make self-reported intakes, especially the 24-hour dietary recall, unreliable, however. A dietary history method, although time-consuming, may be an effective means to estimate usual or typical dietary patterns (van Staveren et al, 1994). In some instances it may be necessary to gather dietary information from caregivers and family members. Accurate assessment includes information about appetite, eating or chewing problems, problems with swallowing or bowel function, food avoidances, and alcohol and tobacco use, as well as health problems and use of drugs that may influence appetite or nutrient utilization. Because older adults tend to use more dietary supplements with greater frequency than other population groups, it is important to include this information in dietary assessment.

PROMOTING NUTRITION FOR OLDER ADULTS

■ What are the health and nutrition guidelines for optimum health for older adults?

■ What community resources are available for older adults at nutritional risk?

Consuming a nutritionally adequate diet and maintaining physical activity contribute significantly to the maintenance of health and well-being among older adults and may delay the decline of functional capacity that accompanies the normal process of aging. In addition, diet is an important factor in the treatment of chronic disease. Recommended intakes for older adults follow the Food Guide Pyramid (see Chapter 1). Because caloric intakes diminish with age, particular attention must be given to the nutrient density of the diet.

The Interventions Roundtable convened by the Nutrition Screening Initiative identified nutrition interventions that are appropriate for the nutrition concerns identified with the Checklist to DETERMINE Nutritional Health (Fig. 12–4) and the Level I (Fig. 12–5) and II Screens (Appendix 10). They can be classified into six areas:

• Obtain, prepare, and eat appropriate diets.
• Maintain adequate oral health.

• Maintain mental health.
• Use medications appropriately.
• Be aware of changing eating habits.
• Provide nutrition support for those individuals who cannot eat an adequate diet.

Identification of nutrition risk in older adults is significant only if steps are taken to improve status. Intervention must be individualized to use specific resources available to meet the unique needs of the older individual. Access to adequate quantity and quality of food is essential. Community-based resources can provide assistance with shopping for food and access to food assistance programs, including home-delivered meals. These services may be accessed through health maintenance organizations, health care agencies, and a series of community volunteer organizations. Nutrition services for older adults at the community level are available from a variety of resources but particularly from programs supported by Title III of the Older Americans Act (see Application at the end of this chapter).

CHRONIC HEALTH CONCERNS

Many chronic diseases first assert themselves in middle life and persist into old age. Food habits are prime factors in the development of some of these diseases. In addition, nutrition may be of prime importance in the treatment of chronic diseases of aging. Nutrition therapy is particularly appealing for those over 65 years of age because it is relatively inexpensive compared to medications and has no side effects.

Of the 2.2 million Americans who died in 1991, 1.6 million, or 7 of 10, were elderly (Bureau of the Census, 1995). Seventy percent of the deaths among older adults could be attributed to cardiovascular disease, cancer, or stroke. These diseases are also the principal causes of morbidity, impaired mobility, and decreased cognitive function.

Cardiovascular Disease

Excess body weight is associated with an increased risk of developing diabetes and cardiovascular disease. Avoidance of obesity and moderate increases in physical activity have been associated with longevity in middle-aged

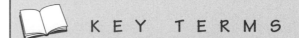

K E Y   T E R M S

kyphosis: abnormally increased convexity in the curvature of the spine; hunchback

men (Paffenbarger et al, 1993) and have positive health benefits for older adults. The relationship between mortality and body weight is a J-shaped curve, with the greatest risk at the extremes of leanness and obesity.

Coronary Heart Disease

Recognizing that cardiovascular disease is the leading cause of death among older people and that more than half of all coronary mortality occurs in those over 65 years of age, the National Cholesterol Education Program (NCEP) panel has recommended application of its lipid screening and management guidelines to management of older individuals (see page 293). However, application of the NCEP guidelines to elderly persons in particular has been criticized.

Hypercholesterolemia, especially elevated levels of low-density-lipoprotein cholesterol (LDL-C), is a recognized risk factor for coronary heart disease (CHD). Major prospective studies have demonstrated the importance of high serum TC and LDL-C and a high ratio of LDL-C to high-density-lipoprotein cholesterol (HDL-C) in CHD incidence and mortality (Anderson et al, 1989; Multiple Risk Factor Intervention Trial, 1990; Lipid Research Clinics Programs, 1984). However, the clinical evidence indicating that a reduction in blood TC or LDL-C levels reduces risk for CHD was obtained from major studies in middle-aged hypercholesterolemic adults.

Several recent analyses have found a positive association between serum cholesterol and coronary disease risk among older adults, but the observed risk was smaller than that among younger individuals (Manolio et al, 1992). Others have found that elevated serum TC or low HDL-C levels were not significant risk factors for all-cause mortality, coronary heart disease mortality, or hospitalization for myocardial infarction in persons older than 70 years (Krumholz et al, 1994; Ostlund et al, 1990). A recent analysis of data collected from 5209 men and women who were enrolled in the Framingham Heart Study from 1948 through 1980 found that the relationship between TC level and all-cause mortality was positive at age 40 years, negligible at ages 50 to 70 years, and negative at age 80 years (Krommal et al, 1993). The relationship of TC to CHD mortality was positive at ages 40, 50, and 60 years, but attenuated with age until the relationship was not significant at ages 70 and 80 years. For non–CHD mortality, cholesterol was negatively related for ages 50 and above. Thus, it appears that for older adults, serum TC and LDL-C concentrations should be interpreted with caution and initiation of cholesterol-lowering treatment in men and women above 65 to 70 years of age reconsidered.

In epidemiologic studies, hypocholesterolemia has been associated with increased mortality from noncardiovascular causes (Goichot et al, 1995). It may be that low cholesterol concentration is a nonspecific feature of poor health status that is independent of nutrient or energy intake.

Hypertension

Normal blood pressure is usually defined as systolic pressure < 85 mm Hg and diastolic pressure < 130 mm Hg (Joint National Committee, 1993). There is a J-shaped curve between blood pressure and mortality in older persons, with both low blood pressure and high blood pressure associated with increased risk of death. In older adults, low blood pressure is often associated with overmedication, protein energy undernutrition, inadequate sodium intake, anemia, dehydration, or an adrenal disturbance. All are potentially treatable conditions that should be considered when an older person has low blood pressure.

Blood pressure tends to rise with increasing age. The increase in blood pressure is related to many factors, including genetics, body weight, physical exercise, alcohol consumption, and cigarette smoking. **Hypertension**, a common problem in older persons, is present in approximately 60% of Hispanics and non-Hispanic whites and 71% of non-Hispanic African-Americans aged 60 years or older (Joint National Committee, 1993).

Hypertension, while without symptoms, is an established risk factor for coronary artery disease, congestive heart failure, transient ischemic attacks, kidney failure, and **retinopathy** (Joint National Committee, 1993). Treatment of hypertension in men and women over 60 years of age reduces the incidence of stroke by about 40%, and some trials have also shown reductions in coronary events (Fletcher and Bullpit, 1994).

The initial treatment is likely to be lifestyle changes, which include weight loss, increased physical activity, and moderation of alcohol and sodium intake. Since the early 1990s, a number of major studies of treatment of hypertension in older persons have been completed. Overall, treatment of hypertensive older adults with **diuretics** and **beta-blockers** produces a significant benefit. A meta-analysis of nine major clinical trials involving more than 15,000 individuals older than 59 years found that overall, treatment reduced all-cause mortality by approximately 12%, stroke mortality by 36%, and coronary heart disease mortality by 25% (Insua et al, 1994).

Antihypertensive drug therapy is carried out with caution because older persons may be more sensitive to decreases in fluid volume and sympathetic nervous system inhibition than younger individuals. Treatment is usually initiated with smaller doses and smaller increases in dosage spaced at longer intervals.

Although there has been extensive research regarding the impact of various dietary components (fatty acids, calcium, sodium, potassium, chloride, and magnesium) on blood pressure, the data currently available do not offer definitive conclusions or evidence for dietary intervention, except for weight loss and moderation of alcohol consumption (Reusser and McCarron, 1994). Some, but not all, individuals respond to a decrease in dietary sodium and an increase in potassium.

Osteoporosis

Most bone is made up of an outer layer of **compact bone** surrounding trabecular or **cancellous** bone structure. Bone loss occurs with age. The rate of loss is greatest in areas of cancellous bone—the vertebrae (the 33 bones of the spinal column), the proximal **femur**, and the distal **radius**.

Osteoporosis is a disorder of the skeleton resulting from an alteration in bone remodeling, the process in which bone is broken down or resorbed and replaced with new bone. It is characterized by increased osteoclastic activity and accelerated reduction in bone mass (Fig. 12–6) and a consequent deterioration in the microarchitecture of bone leading to enhanced bone fragility and an increased risk of fracture. Osteoporosis is a major public health problem in the United States. It affects more than 25 million people (mostly women) and contributes to some 1.3 million fractures each year at a cost of $10 billion (National Institutes of Health, 1993).

Osteoporotic fractures occur most frequently in the hips, vertebrae, and wrists. Hip fracture, usually the result of a fall, is a major cause of mortality and morbidity in older women. The incidence increases with age, and between 12% and 20% of all individuals with hip fracture die in the hospital of complications (Riggs and Melton, 1992). Approximately one-third of survivors are left with some disability, which limits their independence. Wrist fractures, which are also usually incurred during a fall, generally heal completely with few lasting effects.

Vertebral fractures are often called "crush fractures" because they can lead to vertebral compression and a loss of height. When several vertebrae are involved, compression

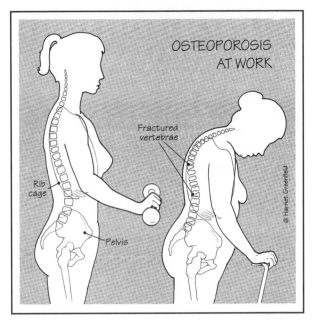

FIGURE 12–7. Compression fractures of the vertebrae lead to loss of height and forward bending of the upper spine. (Reprinted with permission. Copyright Harriet R. Greenfield, 1993.)

can distort the spinal column, leading to "dowager's hump" (Fig. 12–7). As spinal curvature increases, the rib cage sinks toward the pelvis, causing internal organs to become cramped and consequently creating difficulties with breathing and gastrointestinal discomfort.

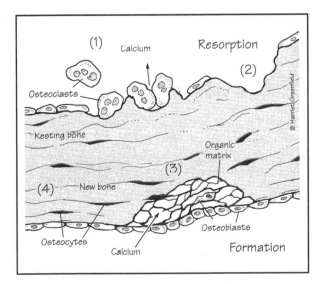

FIGURE 12–6. Bone is constantly remolded during osteoblastic and osteoclastic activity. (Reprinted with permission. Copyright Harriet R. Greenfield, 1993.)

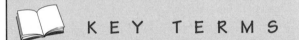

KEY TERMS

hypertension: systolic blood pressure $\geq$140 mm Hg; diastolic blood pressure $\geq$90 mm Hg

retinopathy: a condition of the retina that can lead to blindness

diuretic: a drug that decreases blood pressure by increasing sodium and water loss via the kidney

beta-blockers: drugs that block responses of the sympathetic nervous system

compact bone/cortical bone: dense bone with slow turnover

cancellous: the spongy or lattice-like internal network of bone, which has a higher rate of turnover

femur: the bone that extends from the pelvis to the knee

radius: the bone along the forearm on the outer side when the hand is palm up

RISK FACTORS Bone mass in old age depends on peak bone mass achieved in early adulthood and the rate of bone loss. Bone loss, while primarily due to a reduction in the supply of estrogen, is influenced by many characteristics and behaviors that can predict the potential for osteoporotic fractures (Bauer et al, 1993). Risk factors among osteoporotic women over age 65 years are summarized in Table 12–11.

DETECTION There are several techniques for estimating bone density. Single photon absorptiometry (SPA) and single x-ray absorptiometry (SXA) are used to assess mineral content of the forearm. They measure primarily cortical bone in which tissue loss is not apparent until late in the course of the disease. Dual x-ray absorptiometry (DXA) gives a more accurate estimate of risk, measuring the mineral content of the total cortical and trabecular bones of the hip and spine and total bone mass. Radiation exposure for this procedure is less than that of a standard spine x-ray.

TABLE 12–11 Risk Factors Linked to Osteoporosis

Gender: Women are at greater risk.

Age: Risk increases as bone loss increases with time.

Frame size: Women who are thin and have small frames are at greater risk.

Weight loss: Weight loss after age 50 is associated with lower bone mass.

Heredity: Women whose mothers had vertebral fractures seem to have less bone mass.

Race: Caucasians and Asians are at greater risk than Africans and African Americans.

Decreased estrogen: Postmenopausal women, women whose ovaries have been surgically removed, and young women with low body fat who have little estrogen and irregular menses are at greater risk.

Low dietary calcium can increase bone resorption and lead to bone loss.

Inactivity: Lack of physical activity increases bone resorption.

Smoking: Cigarette smoking increases bone resorption.

Caffeine: Women who consume large amounts of caffeine regularly (3 or more cups of coffee per day) have lower bone density and more fractures.

Alcohol: Two or more drinks per day can accelerate bone loss.

Some drugs: Glucocorticoids such as prednisone (used to treat inflammatory diseases) and antiseizure drugs such as Dilantin can lead to bone loss.

PREVENTION Prevention of osteoporosis is of the utmost importance because, although preliminary research on fluoride looks promising, there are currently no effective, safe methods for restoring high-quality bone to the osteoporotic skeleton (National Institutes of Health, 1993). Approaches to prevention include maximizing peak bone mass in early life and reducing postmenopausal and age-associated bone loss.

Hormone Replacement Therapy

Many studies have shown that estrogen intervention, or hormone replacement therapy (HRT), reduces the rate of bone loss (see page 279). The effects of estrogen in preventing bone loss can be seen immediately after menopause, in women over 70 years old, and in those with established osteoporosis (Priestwood et al, 1994). Long-term estrogen use (more than 5 years), is associated with a reduction in the risk of fractures of the hip and distal radius as well as of vertebral crush fracture (Kanis et al, 1992).

The mode of action of estrogen on bone is unclear. Recently estrogen receptors have been found in osteoblastic cells, suggesting a stimulation of bone synthesis. Estrogens may also influence calcium homeostasis in the body by increasing the hydroxylation of 25-hydroxyvitamin D to its active 1,25 form.

CALCITONIN Calcitonin is a thyroid hormone that, with the parathyroid hormone, regulates calcium metabolism. Several studies have demonstrated that injections or intranasal spray of this hormone inhibit trabecular bone loss and may reduce the incidence of osteoporotic fracture (Kanis et al, 1992). In 1995, FDA approved the intranasal spray of calcitonin for treatment of osteoporosis.

AMINOBISPHOSPHONATE Aminobisphosphonates are a class of new drugs that are potent inhibitors of bone resorption that do not retard bone formation. They are being tested in women with osteoporosis and appear to increase trabecular bone mass significantly without impairment of cortical bone. A recent 3-year study with this drug and 500-mg supplements of calcium found a lower rate of fracture in treated versus placebo-controlled subjects (Reginster, 1995). Application has been made to the Food and Drug Administration for approval in treatment for osteoporosis.

CALCIUM Osteoporosis is not a disease resulting from obvious deficiencies in vitamin D, calcium, and phosphate, but subtle deficiencies may account for the ability of calcium and vitamin D supplements to have a beneficial effect on bone (Bikle, 1994). Reduced calcium intake clearly can cause bone loss by necessitating the use of skeletal calcium to maintain a constant serum calcium level. Although less effective than HRT, daily intakes of 1500 to 1700 mg of calcium with 5 to 10 mg (400 to 800 IU) of vitamin D in the early postmenopausal period have been shown to significantly retard bone loss from the lumbar spine (Reid et al, 1993) and proximal femur (Aloia et al, 1994) and to reduce the risk of hip and other nonvertebral fractures (Chapuy et al, 1992).

VITAMIN D Recently, Dawson-Hughes and coworkers (1995) found that although intakes of 5.0 μg of vitamin D are sufficient to limit bone loss from the spine and the whole body, amounts as high as 20 μg were needed to reduce bone loss from the hip (femoral neck). Recommendations from the Consensus Development Conference (1993) are for 5 to 10 μg of vitamin D intake.

A synthetic form of calcitrol (1,25-dihydroxyvitamin D_3), the most physiologically active metabolite of vitamin D, has been used pharmacologically in treatment of postmenopausal osteoporosis with conflicting results. One clinical trial of 622 women with mild to moderate disease

reported a significantly lower rate of new vertebral fractures after 3 years of treatment (Dechanti and Goa, 1994).

FLUORIDE Fluoride stimulates bone formation by promotion of osteoblast proliferation (see Fig. 12–6), resulting in increases in trabecular bone compared to cortical bone and increases in spinal bone density (Phipps, 1995). Recent research makes fluoride treatment look promising, but optimal dose and regimens remain to be established (Reginster, 1995).

The NIH Consensus Development Conference (1993) concluded that fluoride did not appear to lower the rate of vertebral fracture and may increase cortical fracture. However, preliminary studies of a 2.5-year treatment regimen of slow-release sodium fluoride and 400 mg of calcium citrate twice daily reported improved lumbar bone mass, improved cancellous bone quality, and a significant reduction in vertebral fracture rates (Pak et al, 1994). However, other trials, which administered sodium fluoride and calcium carbonate to women with postmenopausal osteoporosis for 4 years, found no significant decrease in

RESEARCH UPDATE
Are Calcium Supplements Safe?

The recent NIH Consensus Development Panel on Optimal Calcium Intake (1994) recommended a daily intake of 1500 mg per day for men and women over 65 years of age. That is almost twice the RDA, an amount difficult to get from food alone. Although it is preferable for calcium needs to be met using food sources, many older adults may be unable to attain this level without supplements.

There are more than a dozen commonly prescribed calcium supplements and hundreds of different formulations commercially available (Table 12–12). The cost varies widely among different types of calcium preparations and among different brands of similar preparations. The most common and economical supplement, calcium carbonate, has the highest content of calcium—40% by weight. However, carbonate is a relatively insoluble form of calcium, especially at neutral pH, which may occur in the intestines of many older adults with atrophic gastritis and achlorhydria. Most other commercial calcium preparations contain 28% to 31% calcium by weight.

Calcium supplements should be taken throughout the day on an empty stomach to enhance absorption. Although calcium supplements in the range of 1 to 2 g per day are usually very well tolerated, some side effects are seen. Constipation, intestinal bloating, and excess gas are often reported. Supplemental calcium can suppress the absorption of other nutrients, especially iron and zinc, and may impede the absorption of concurrently administered drugs such as tetracyclines. Conversely, calcium absorption is impaired by concurrent ingestion of aluminum-containing antacids, cholestyramine, and phosphate.

It has been known for more than a decade that calcium supplements that contain bone meal and dolomite have biologically significant concentrations of lead. Recently this has been recognized to be true of fossil shell calcium carbonate brands labeled "oyster shell" or "natural source" as well (Bourgoin, 1993). Other contaminants include aluminum, arsenic, mercury, and cadmium. The issue of contamination in calcium supplements illustrates that the safety of a nutrient supplement is not limited to concerns about excess intake of the nutrient itself.

TABLE 12–12 **Characteristics of Calcium Preparations**

Form of Calcium	Elemental Calcium (%)	Average Absorption (%)	Characteristics	Considerations
Calcium carbonate	40	26	Relatively insoluble, especially at neutral pH. Do not take with food or milk	Absorption is very poor with achlorhydial constipation, gastric distention, flatulence
Calcium lactate	13	32–34	Contains lactose—milk yogurt	Less constipating than calcium carbonate
Calcium phosphate	38	28	Tend to be insoluble; contain substantial amounts of phosphate	
Dicalcium phosphate	31	28		
Calcium gluconate	8	26–34	More soluble than calcium carbonate—low calcium content	Less constipating than calcium carbonate
Calcium citrate	21	22	More soluble than calcium carbonate	
Calcium malate-citrate	21	34	More soluble than calcium carbonate	
Oyster shell	28–31	?	Relatively insoluble calcium carbonate	May contain many noncalcium compounds: lead, mercury, aluminum, cadmium
Bone meal	31	?	Less constipating than calcium carbonate	May contain noncalcium compounds: lead, mercury, aluminum, cadmium
Dolomite	22	?	Less constipating than calcium carbonate	May contain noncalcium compounds: lead, mercury, aluminum, cadmium

vertebral fracture rate with the fluoride treatment (Riggs et al, 1994).

EXERCISE The skeleton is subjected to weight-bearing stress of gravity and forces from muscle contraction. These forces change the shape of the bone. Bone mass increases in response to mechanical stress. Physical exercise enhances bone development, and vigorous exercise augments bone mineral density. Physically active people appear to have higher bone density than those who are sedentary, and some studies have reported a positive association between muscle strength and bone mass, especially in premenopausal women (Snow-Harter et al, 1993). In addition, there is evidence that a variety of exercise programs have been associated with reduced risk of falls in older adults (Province et al, 1995).

RECOMMENDATIONS It is never too early or too late to initiate lifestyle changes to reduce loss of bone mass. Adolescents and young adults can build maximal peak bone mass with exercise and a balanced diet containing 1200 mg of calcium and 5 μg of vitamin D. For older women, HRT can minimize bone loss and, in some instances, promote osteogenic activity. Weight-bearing physical activity has the potential not only to protect from further bone loss but also to improve strength, mobility, flexibility, agility, and muscle strength, which may indirectly decrease the incidence of osteoporotic fractures by lessening the likelihood of falling (American College of Sports Medicine, 1995). Calcium and vitamin D are key dietary ingredients. Current recommendations (1500 mg calcium, 10 to 20 μg vitamin D) for these nutrient amounts exceed the RDA and may be difficult to obtain through food alone. Supplements should be used with caution, though, because excess vitamin D can cause bone loss and neurologic problems. Other therapies, including fluoride, vitamin D analogs, and calcitonin, will undoubtedly have greater potential in the future.

CONCEPTS TO REMEMBER

▶ Aging is a process that is associated with functional decline, diminished physiologic reserves, and increased vulnerability to disease.

▶ Adults over the age of 65 years make up more than 12% of the American population, and the number increases daily.

▶ Older adults are a heterogeneous group of individuals who age at vastly different rates.

▶ Being old is less a chronologic age than a state of mind and physical status.

▶ The aging process is influenced by genetic and environmental factors.

▶ Aging is accompanied by numerous changes in physiologic status and body composition.

▶ The physiologic, social, economic, and health changes associated with aging are important determinants of an individual's ability to function independently and determine his or her quality of life.

▶ Although energy needs decline, requirements for most nutrients, except vitamin A, are equal to or greater than those of younger adults.

▶ Nutrition screening and assessment are essential components of geriatric assessment.

▶ Nutrition screening is important for identifying risk for poor nutrition and serves as a basis for intervention.

▶ Nutrition intervention is an important component of health care that allows older adults to maintain quality of life and independence.

▶ Older adults are more likely to have health problems and suffer from chronic diseases than younger persons.

▶ Nutrition is important in the prevention and treatment of chronic diseases including osteoporosis, coronary heart disease, and hypertension.

▶ Multiple medications required by older adults may interfere with nutrition status and increase overall health risks.

References

Administration on Aging. A profile of older Americans. Washington, DC: U.S. Department of Health and Human Services, American Association of Retired Persons, 1994.

Allen LH, Casterline J. Vitamin B_{12} deficiency in elderly individuals: diagnosis and requirements. Am J Clin Nutr 1994;60:12.

Aloia JF, et al. Calcium supplementation with and without hormone replacement therapy to prevent postmenopausal bone loss. Ann Intern Med 1994;120:97.

American College of Sports Medicine. ACSM position stand on osteoporosis and exercise. Med Sci Sports Exerc 1995;227:i.

Anderson KM, et al. Cholesterol and mortality: 30 years of follow-up from the Framingham Study. JAMA 1989;257:2176.

Bauer DC, et al. Factors associated with appendicular bone mass in older women. Ann Intern Med 1993;118:657.

Bikle DD. Role of vitamin D, its metabolites, and analogs in the management of osteoporosis. Rheum Dis Clin N Am 1994;20:759.

Blumberg J. Nutrient requirements of the healthy elderly—should there be specific RDAs? Nutr Rev 1994;52:S15.

Bogden JD, et al. Daily micronutrient supplements enhance delayed-hyposensitivity skin test responses in older people. Am J Clin Nutr 1994;60:437.

Bourgoin BP, et al. Lead content in 70 brands of dietary calcium supplements. Am J Public Health 1993;83:1155.

Bureau of the Census. Statistical Brief 94. Washington, DC: U.S. Department of Commerce, 1994.

Bureau of the Census. Statistical Brief 95–8. Sixty five plus in the United States. Washington, DC: U.S. Department of Commerce, 1995.

Campbell WW, et al. Increased energy requirements and changes in body composition with resistance training in older adults. Am J Clin Nutr 1994;60:167.

Carmeli E, Reznich AX. The physiology and biochemistry of skeletal muscle atrophy as a function of age. Proc Soc Exp Biol Med 1994;206:103.

Castaneda C, et al. Elderly women accommodate a low-protein diet with losses of body cell mass, muscle function, and immune response. Am J Clin Nutr 1995;62:30.

Chandra R. Nutrition and immunity in the elderly: clinical significance. Nutr Rev 1995;53(Suppl):S80.

Chapuy MC, et al. Vitamin D_3 and calcium to prevent hip fractures in elderly women. N Engl J Med 327;23:1637.

Committee on Diet and Health. Diet and health: implications for reducing chronic disease risk. Washington, DC: National Academy Press, 1989.

Council on Scientific Affairs. American Medical Association White Paper on Elderly Health. Ann Intern Med 1990;150:2459.

Dawson D, et al. Aging in the eighties: functional limitations of individuals age 65 years and over. Advanced data from Vital Health Statistics of the National Center for Health Statistics, No. 133. Rockville, MD: U.S. Department of Health and Human Services, Public Health Service. June 10, 1987.

Dawson-Hughes B, et al. Rates of bone loss in postmenopausal women randomly assigned to one of two dosages of vitamin D. Am J Clin Nutr 1995;61:1140.

Dechanti KL, Goa KL. Calcitrol, a review of its use in the treatment of postmenopausal osteoporosis and its potential in corticosteroid-induced osteoporosis. Drugs and Aging 1994;5:300.

Dufor M, Fuller RK. Alcohol in the elderly. Ann Rev Med 1995;46:123.

Evans DA, et al. Prevalence of Alzheimer's disease in community populations of older persons. JAMA 1989;262:2551.

Ferguson RP, et al. Serum albumin and prealbumin as predictors of clinical outcomes of hospitalized elderly nursing home residents. JAGS 1993;41:545.

Fiatarone M, et al. Exercise training and nutritional supplementation for physical frailty in very elderly people. N Engl J Med 1994;330:1769.

Fletcher A, Bulpitt C. Epidemiology of hypertension in the elderly. J Hypertension 1994;12:S3.

Flynn MA, et al. Aging in humans: a continuous 20-year study of physiologic and dietary parameters. J Am Coll Nutr 1992;11:660.

Fontera WR, et al. A cross-sectional study of muscle strength and mass in 45- to 78-year-old men and women. J Appl Physiol 1991;71:644.

Food and Nutrition Board. Recommended dietary allowances. 10th ed. Washington, DC: National Academy Press, 1989.

Forster LE, et al. Alcohol use and potential risk for alcohol-related reactions among community-based elderly. J Comm Health 1993;18:225.

Galanos AN, et al. Nutrition and function: is there a relationship between body mass index and the functional capabilities of community dwelling elderly? J Am Geriatr Soc 1994;42:368.

Gerster H. Anticarcinogenic effect of common carotenoids. Inter J Vit Nutr Res 1993;63:93.

Goichot B, et al. Low cholesterol concentrations in free-living elderly subjects: relations with dietary intake and nutritional status. Am J Clin Nutr 1995;62:547.

Goldberg RJ, et al. A prospective study of the health effects of alcohol consumption in middle-aged and elderly men. The Honolulu Heart Program. Circulation 1994;89:651.

Gray-Donald K. The frail elderly: meeting the nutritional challenge. J Am Diet Assoc 1995;95:538.

Hodis HN. Serial coronary angiographic evidence that antioxidant vitamin intake reduces progression of coronary artery atherosclerosis. JAMA 1995;273:1849.

Hollick MF. Vitamin D—new horizons for the 21st century. Am J Clin Nutr 1994;60:619.

Holt PR, Balint JA. Effects of aging on intestinal lipid absorption. Am J Physiol 1993;264:1.

Insua JI, et al. Drug treatment of hypertension in the elderly: a meta-analysis. Ann Intern Med 1994;121:355.

Joint National Committee on Detection, Evaluation, and Treatment of High Blood Pressure. The fifth report of the Joint National Committee on Detection, Evaluation, and Treatment of High Blood Pressure (JNC V). Arch Intern Med 1993;153:154.

Joosten E, et al. Metabolic evidence that deficiencies of vitamin B_{12} (cobalamin), folate and vitamin B_6 occur commonly in elderly people. Am J Clin Nutr 1993;58:468.

Kanis JA, et al. Evidence for efficacy of drugs affecting bone metabolism in preventing hip fracture. BMJ 1992;305:1124.

Krommal RA, et al. Total serum cholesterol levels and mortality risk as a function of age. A report based on the Framingham data. Arch Intern Med 1993;153:1065.

Krumholz HM, et al. Lack of association between cholesterol and coronary heart disease mortality and morbidity and all-cause mortality in persons older than 70 years. JAMA 1994;272:1335.

Lee AT, Cerami A. Role of glycation in aging. Ann NY Acad Sci 1992;663:63.

Lindenbaum J, et al. Prevalence of cobalamin deficiency in the Framingham elderly population. Am J Clin Nutr 1994;60:2.

Lipid Research Clinics Program. The Lipid Research Clinics Coronary Primary Prevention Trial results. I: reduction in incidence of coronary heart diease JAMA 1984;251:351.

Makinodan T. Patterns of age-related immunologic changes. Nutr Rev 1995;53:S27.

Manolio TA, et al. Cholesterol and heart disease in older persons and women. Review of NLIBI workshop. Ann Epidemiol 1992;2:161.

Mares-Perlman JA, et al. Nutrient supplements contribute to the dietary intake of middle- and older-aged adult residents of Beaver Dam, Wisconsin. J Nutr 1993;123:176.

Meydani SN, et al. Vitamin E enhancement of T cell-mediated function in healthy elderly: mechanism of action. Nutr Rev 1995;53:S52.

Miller RA. The biology of aging and longevity. In: Hazzard WR, et al (eds). Principles of geriatric medicine and gerontology. New York: McGraw-Hill, 1994.

Morley JE. Why do physicians fail to recognize and treat malnutrition in older persons? J Am Geriatr Soc 1993;39:1139.

Morley JE, Solomon DH. Major issues in geriatrics over the last five years. J Am Geriatr Soc 1994;42:218.

Multiple Risk Factor Intervention Trial Reseach Group. Mortality rates after 10.5 years for participants in the Multiple Risk Factor Intervention Trial. JAMA 1990;263:1795.

National Center for Health Statistics. Dietary Intake Source Data, United States 1971–1974. PHS 79–1221. U.S. Department of Health, Education and Welfare. Hyattsville, MD: Public Health Service, 1979.

National Center for Health Statistics, Carroll MD. Dietary Intake Source Data, United States 1976–1980. PHS 83–1681. U.S. Department of Health and Human Services. Hyattsville, MD: Public Health Service, 1983.

National Institutes of Health. Consensus Development Conference. Diagnosis, prophylaxis, and treatment of osteoporosis. Am J Med 1993;94:646.

National Institutes of Health Consensus Development Panel on Optimal Calcium Intake. Optimal calcium intake. JAMA 1994;272:1942.

Nelson HD, et al. Smoking, alcohol, and neuromuscular and physical function of older women. JAMA 1994;272:1825.

Nutrition Screening Initiative. Report of Nutrition Screening I: toward a common view. Consensus Conference, Washington, DC:1991.

O'Dowd KJ, et al. Exogenous calciferol (vitamin D) and vitamin D endocrine status among elderly nursing home residents in the New York City area. J Am Geriatr Soc 1993;41:414.

Ostlund RE, et al. The ratio of waist-to-hip circumference, plasma insulin level and glucose intolerance as independent predictors of the HDL2 cholesterol level in older adults. N Engl J Med 1990;322:229.

Paffenbarger RS, et al. The association of changes of physical activity level and other lifestyle characteristics with mortality among men. N Engl J Med 1993;328:538.

Pak CY, et al. Slow-release sodium fluoride in the management of postmenopausal osteoporosis. A randomized controlled trial. Ann Intern Med 1994;120:625.

Panchararuniti N, et al. Plasma homocysteine, folcite and vitamin B_{12} concentrations and risk for early-onset coronary artery disease. Am J Clin Nutr 1994;59:940.

Pannemans DL, et al. The influence of protein intake on vitamin B_{12} metabolism differs in young and elderly humans. J Nutr 1994;124:1207.

Parker DR, et al. Relationship of dietary saturated fatty acids and body habitus to serum insulin concentrations: the Normative Aging Study. Am J Clin Nutr 1993;58:129.

Payette H, et al. Predictors of dietary intake in a functionally dependent elderly population in the community. Am J Public Health 1995;85:77.

Phipps K. Fluoride and bone health. J Public Health Dent 1995;55:53.

Popkin BM, et al. Dietary changes in older Americans. Am J Clin Nutr 1992;55:823.

Posner B, et al. Nutritional risk in New England elders. J Gerontol 1994;49:M123.

Priestwood KM, et al. The short term effects of conjugated estrogen on bone turnover in older women. J Clin Endocrinol Metab 1994;79:366.

Province MA, et al. The effects of falls on elderly patients. A preplanned meta-analysis of the FICSIT Trials. Frailty and injuries: cooperative studies of intervention techniques. JAMA 1995;273:1341.

Rauramaa R, et al. Inverse relation of physical activity and apolipoprotein AI to blood pressure in elderly women. Med Sci Sports Exercise 1995;27:164.

Reginster JY. Treatment of bone in elderly subjects: calcium, vitamin D_2, fluoride, bisphosphates, calictonin. Hormone Res 1995;43:83.

Reid IR, et al. Effect of calcium on bone loss in postmenopausal women. N Engl J Med 1993;328:460.

Renvall MJ, et al. Body composition of patients with Alzheimer's disease. J Am Diet Assoc 1993;93:47.

Reuben DB, et al. Nutrition screening in older persons. J Am Geriatr Soc 1995;43:415.

Reusser ME, McCarron DA. Micronutrient effects on blood pressure regulation. Nutr Rev 1994;52:367.

Rhodus NL, Brown J. The association of xerostemia and inadequate intake in older adults. J Am Diet Assoc 1990;90:1688.

Riggs BL, Melton LJ. The prevention and treatment of osteoporosis. N Engl J Med 1992;327:620.

Riggs BL, et al. Clinical trial of fluoride therapy in postmenopausal osteoporotic women: extended observations and additional analysis. J Bone Miner Res 1994;9:265.

Rosenberg IH, Miller JW. Nutritional factors in physical and cognitive functions of elderly people. Am J Clin Nutr 1992;55:1237S.

Russell RM, Suter PM. Vitamin requirements of elderly people: an update. Am J Clin Nutr 1993;58:4.

Ryan A, et al. Nutrient intakes and dietary patterns of older Americans: a national study. J Gerontol 1992;47:M145.

Scherr PA, et al. Light to moderate alcohol consumption and mortality in the elderly. J Am Geriatr Soc 1992;40:651.

Seddon JM, et al. Dietary carotenoids, vitamins A, C, and E, and advanced age-related macular degeneration. Eye Disease Case-Control Study Group. JAMA 1994;272:1413.

Selhub J, et al. Association between plasma homocysteine concentrations and extracranial carotid-artery stenosis. N Engl J Med 1995;332:286.

Sheehan E, et al. Vitamin and food supplement practices and nutrition beliefs of the elderly in seven western states. Nutr Res 1989;9:251.

Snow-Harter C, et al. Determinants of femoral neck BMD in pre- and post-menopausal women. Med Sci Sports Exerc 1993;25:5856.

Stuck AE, et al. Comprehensive geriatric assessment: a meta-analysis of controlled trials. Lancet 1993;342:1032.

Taylor A. Role of nutrients in delaying cataracts. Ann NY Acad Sci 1992;669:111.

van Staveren WA, et al. Assessing diets of elderly people: problems and approaches. Am J Clin Nutr 1994;59:221S.

Vellas BJ, et al. Diseases and aging: patterns of morbidity with age: relationship between aging and age-associated diseases. Am J Clin Nutr 1992;55:1225S.

Vitale S, et al. Plasma antioxidants and risk of cortical and nuclear cataract. Epidemiology 1993;4:195.

Wallace JI, et al. Involuntary weight loss in outpatients: incidence and clinical significance. J Am Geriatr Soc 1995;43:329.

White JV. Risk factors for poor nutritional status. Prim Care: Clinics in office practice 1994;21:19.

Wilson PWF, et al. Determinants of change in total cholesterol and HDL-C with age: The Framingham Study. J Gerontol 1994;49:M52.

Wolf-Klein GP, Silverstone FA. Weight loss in Alzheimer's disease: an international review of the literature. Int Psychogeriatr 1994;6:135.

APPLICATION: Programs for Older Adults

George was 67 years old when he joined the Senior Center of the local Recreation Department. He and his wife participated in many activities together until her death 4 years later. After that, George still came to play pool and learned to play bridge. Sometimes he would go on sight-seeing trips for seniors.

In his early seventies George developed hypertension, and his physician prescribed a diuretic medication and recommended that he lose weight. George would take the medicine "when he remembered" but made no attempt to lose weight. A couple of years later, George began to feel tired and had frequent headaches. His physician adjusted his medication but insisted that he must get his weight down and referred him to the dietitian at the Community Senior Health Clinic where he could receive nutrition counseling for a sliding scale fee based on his income. When George appeared at the health clinic he was 74 years old. Five years ago George weighed 85 kg (188 lb), but his current weight, 96 kg (212 lb), has been stable for about a year. For his height, 180 cm (5'11"), his BMI was 30.

In the session with the dietitian, George reported he took a number of food supplements, including garlic capsules, which he sometimes used in place of his antihypertensive medication to save money. The dietitian tried to convince him to stick to his prescribed medication and stop experimenting with supplements and panaceas. A 24-hour dietary recall revealed that George's diet consisted primarily of fast and convenience foods, since, by his own admission, he did not like to cook. Consumption of fruits and vegetables was low. In fact, for the previous day his only vegetable had been french fries. He considered the potatoes interchangeable with a cooked vegetable or a small green salad.

The dietitian suggested he eat foods of low caloric density for breakfast, such as cereal, skim milk, and fruit, which would require little preparation. Suggestions for low-fat snacks to be eaten with his beer, and substitutes for sweet snacks and desserts were given. George was resistant to changes in his eating habits, but when the dietitian reinforced the physician's claim that he would feel better, he agreed to try. George made an appointment to see the dietitian the following week to review his progress. Because of the sliding payment schedule he was able to see her regularly. After about three visits, George reported that the changes were not as bad as he expected. Breakfast was simple, and he had begun to eat lunch at the local congregate meals site. The dietitian helped him plan simple evening meals and snacks. Gradually George began to lose weight. At the suggestion of the recreation leader at the senior center he joined some other older adults in walking in the early morning at a local shopping mall.

With the assistance of the dietitian and the nurse at the senior health clinic George learned to monitor his blood pressure and regulate his food intake, continuing to lose weight. As he began to feel better, he found he could do more. He even started going to dances at the senior center, something he loved to do when he was younger.

The following year, George developed a urinary tract infection. He didn't want to go all the way to his physician's office, so he went to the walk-in clinic near his house. The physician on duty prescribed a sulfa antibiotic without discovering that George is allergic to sulfa drugs. Two days later George developed hives. He was so miserable that, at the suggestion of his neighbor, he went to her dermatologist, who prescribed an anti-itch medication for allergies of unknown origin. That drug controlled the hives but actually caused central nervous system depression and lethargy. George became absent-minded and withdrawn, and lost interest in his usual activities, even declining to visit his grandchildren. George's family became concerned because his mind appeared to be "slipping" and wanted him to move in with one of them. George resisted because he did not want to leave his home. His daughter, who visited regularly to help him with some things around the house, continued to have the prescription for the anti-itch medication filled long after he had completed the course of sulfa because no one made the connections between the sulfa and hives or between the anti-itch drug and depression. George ap-

congregate meals—a federally funded meals program for older adults

Older adults often obtain medication from more than one source without the provider knowing the total of medications taken.

Side effects of drugs are often unrecognized or misinterpreted.

peared to become more depressed, had no appetite, and was losing weight. His daughter became increasingly concerned and took him to the clinic at a local hospital. A third physician put him on medication for "depression," promising he would feel better soon. Although he improved somewhat with this medication, George still didn't "perk up" and his family had him evaluated for home health care. A nurse from the senior community health program visited George at home to assess his case for home assistance. She discovered that he was taking multiple medications and suggested an appointment with a physician who specializes in geriatrics. This physician took him off all medication. The depression lifted as his mind cleared, and he improved dramatically. Eventually the only medications George was taking were a diuretic for hypertension and aspirin for arthritis.

Almost 5 years later, George, usually happy and active, began to lose weight and came to the senior center less often. He became fatigued just getting to the center or doing a small amount of grocery shopping. He complained of chest pain and shortness of breath. The diagnosis of advanced atherosclerotic disease resulted in a prescription for a lipid-lowering drug, cholestyramine, and medication to reduce chest pain, in addition to a stronger diuretic and an anti-inflammatory agent for arthritis. A walker allowed him to get around more comfortably.

While George's family encouraged him to move in with one of them, he valued his independence and wanted to stay in his apartment. The physician's office referred them to a community services agency of the County Health Department. Over a period of several weeks, arrangements were made for home nursing visits, assistance with shopping and housekeeping, and a home-delivered meals program on weekdays. Someone from the family arranged to visit several times a week and to make sure George had suitable foods on hand for breakfast and dinner. A community services van takes George to medical and dental appointments.

George loves the meals program deliveries and looks forward to lunch and chatting with the driver who delivers his meals. He is much happier at home than anywhere else, and the community-based services, including the meals program, allow him an acceptable quality of life while permitting him to maintain some level of independence.

For many older adults like George, the alternative to community-based long-term care is admission to a nursing home care or extended care facility. The high cost of nursing home care depletes the life savings of thousands of older persons every year. In addition, the cost of extended health care has consumed an ever-growing portion of federal and state government budgets. There will be substantial increases in the need for long-term health care as the number of persons aged 85 and over (the most frail) increases. Due to these growing expenditures, nursing homes can no longer be considered the best solution to meet the needs for services of a functionally compromised older population (Torres-Gil et al, 1995).

Programs for Older Americans

Numerous food and nutrition programs and resources are available to support community-based long-term care for older persons. If they meet the income guidelines, they are eligible for the regular federal food assistance available to all low-income individuals and families (see Table A9–1, page 245). These include the Food Stamp Program, which improves quality of the diet by increasing food-buying power, and the Surplus Agricultural Commodities Distribution Program, which provides direct food supplements and nutrition education. This program can provide monthly food packages of staple food items, but it is not available in all areas.

Social Security celebrated its 60th anniversary in 1995, and Medicare, Medicaid, and the Older Americans Act were 30 years old. These programs are important in providing services that improve the quality of life of older adults. Optimal nutrition status is essential to the well-being, health, independence, and quality of life for all older adults ranging from the healthy to the frail, vulnerable, and functionally impaired (American Dietetic Association, 1994). Nutrition programs and services do not function in isola-

Depression is often associated with decreased appetite and weight loss.

Older adults value independence. Community-based health care allows many to remain at home.

Home-delivered meals are essential to allow older adults to live independently.

tion, however. They are an integral part of health and medical services as well as a broad, comprehensive system that encompasses social and supportive services that allow older adults to remain in their homes and communities.

The Nutrition Program for Older Americans (Title VII) of the Older Americans Act was authorized by Congress in 1972 to provide services such as outreach, escort and transportation, health, information, and referral, as well as health and welfare counseling and nutrition and consumer education. The 1978 amendments to the Older Americans Act included Title III, which provided funding from the USDA for congregate and home-delivered meals operated through local area agencies on aging.

The Congregate Meals or Dining Program, created in 1965, was the first federal nutrition program specifically designed to improve the diets of older adults. It provides some food security to older Americans with nutritionally balanced meals at little or no cost. These meals are prepared at or delivered to a variety of centrally located public or private community facilities that are accessible to older people. Older persons gather for a nutritious noon meal as well as social interaction and nutrition education. Meals are usually available 5 days a week in urban settings and 2 to 3 days a week in rural communities. Depending on location, congregate meals participants have access to a variety of support services such as shopping assistance, medical assistance and referral, transportation, weatherization, and fuel assistance. Meals programs are often located in community facilities, which may provide access to other programs such as recreation, fitness, or even legal assistance.

For decades there have been home-delivered meals programs throughout the United States. Often referred to as "Meals on Wheels," such programs frequently were operated by nonprofit community organizations who delivered hot meals to those unable to get out or to prepare meals for themselves. Usually the meals, delivered by volunteers, were prepared by the food service of local hospitals, nursing homes, schools, or churches. The Home Delivered Meals Program funded by Title III, is designed to provide nutritious meals for homebound persons. Meals are delivered to the individual's home by couriers or volunteers. In addition to supporting nutritional needs for the older adult, the program provides regular human contact. The courier may be the only person the housebound individual sees during the day. In some locations, a cold meal for supper or food for breakfast the next morning is delivered with the noon meal. For many older adults this program is essential to their ability to get an adequate diet and to continue to live independently.

Because resources are limited, the Meals programs strive to target higher risk older persons. This is usually defined as advanced age (usually over 80), low income, social isolation, minority status, mobility impairment, or limited ability to speak English. Many participants have a high level of risk for nutritional deficiency. A study that assessed the nutrition status of home-delivered meals participants revealed that there was a high prevalence of low nutrient intake levels and that more than one-third of the participants were at risk of protein energy malnutrition (Lipschitz et al, 1985). In 1994 the Federal Administration on Aging distributed almost $500 million to 57 states and territories and an additional $16 million to Indian tribes earmarked for both congregate and home-delivered nutrition services (Administration on Aging, 1994). Funds from the United States Department of Agriculture Cash and Commodity Program, participant donations, and state and local sources added to OAA funding brought the total to over $1 billion a year for nutrition programs.

Over 230 million meals were served in 1995 through a network of more than 2200 Title III Elderly Nutrition Projects (Title III Elderly Nutrition Program Data, 1994). Of those meals, 45% were provided in the homes of the elderly. There were almost 16,000 meal sites in operation every day.

The ideal systems of long-term care are a continuum of home and community-based services as well as institutional care, housing alternatives such as assisted living, transportation, nutrition, and other social services (Torres-Gil et al, 1995). Nutrition services, specifically meals delivered to those living at home, are a fundamental core service necessary for keeping functionally limited older people in their homes and in the community.

Congregate Meals or Dining Programs:

- Provide balance meals
- Require little or no expense to participant
- Are served at centrally located sites
- Promote social interaction
- Often allow access to a variety of support services

REFERENCES

Administration on Aging may get $5 million more; Up from $872 million in FY '95. Older Americans Report, p. 315. Sept. 23, 1994.

American Dietetic Association. Position of the American Dietetic Association: nutrition, aging and the continuum of health care. J Am Diet Assoc 1993;93:80.

Lipschitz DA, et al. Nutritional evaluation and supplementation of elderly subjects participating in a "Meals on Wheels" program. JPEN 1985;9:343.

Title III Elderly Nutrition Program Data. US Administration on Aging, Washington, DC:OFO (OPCA) 94–63, July 13, 1994.

Torres-Gil FM, et al. Role of elderly nutrition in home and community-based care. Persp Appl Nutr 1995;2:9.

PART V

SPECIAL CONCERNS ACROSS THE LIFE SPAN

CHAPTER 13

EATING DISTURBANCES: DIETARY RESTRAINT, BINGING, PURGING, AND EXCESSIVE CONSUMPTION

Eating Disorders
Anorexia Nervosa
Bulimia Nervosa
Binge Eating Disorder

Overweight/Obesity
Excess Weight Across the Life Span
Concepts to Remember

Emily is a 35-year-old housewife who is 173 cm (68 in) tall, weighs 48 kg (106 lb; reference weight : 140 lb). She weighed 127 kg (280 lb) or more for most of her adult life, but she began to lose weight after her father died a year ago. Now she refuses to stop her weight-loss routine. Emily has numerous rituals that interfere with her life and that of her family. She has many cleaning compulsions. She does not allow guests in her home, and, if someone visits unexpectedly, she spends hours cleaning after they leave. She insists on eating the same thing every day, at the same time and place. Her husband tolerates her peculiarities but is concerned that she eats so little and has lost so much weight. Emily's last menstrual period was 8 months ago. She frequently complains of being cold, sleeps poorly at night, and thinks her hair is thinner. She spends at least 2 hours each day exercising using two different aerobic tapes. If she feels fatter than usual, she exercises for an additional hour.

A typical dietary pattern for Emily is breakfast at 7:00 a.m., consisting of one piece of dry whole wheat toast and one cup of regular coffee. Lunch at noon is one piece of fruit (usually an apple or orange), 6 ounces of lowfat yogurt, and two glasses of diet cola. Emily is a good cook. She always prepares a balanced meal for her family, and dinner is always at 6:00 p.m. However, Emily eats only a slice of whole wheat toast, one-half cup of cottage cheese, and a glass of water. At bedtime she allows herself two crackers and another piece of fresh fruit. Originally Emily planned to stop dieting when she reached 50 kg (110 lbs), but when she reached that point she refused to change her routine and rebuffed suggestions that she add more foods to her diet. She continued to lose weight. After several weeks it was apparent that her dieting was out of control. At the insistence of her physician, Emily began to see a counselor who attempted to involve her in psychotherapy to motivate her to eat. By that time, Emily was so cognitively impaired by starvation that she was unable to respond to the proposed therapy. When Emily reached 41 kg (90 lb) about 2 months later, she was hospitalized near death.

In affluent countries cultural perpetuation of slimness has created an unrealistic standard for **body image** of women and, to a lesser extent, for men (Abrams et al, 1994). Preoccupation with body weight and appearance contribute to food-related behaviors that range from dietary restraint to unhealthy dietary practices to excessive food consumption and binging.

Eating disturbances occur across a continuum from severe underweight (anorexia nervosa) through unusual dietary practices to maintain body weight (bulimia nervosa)

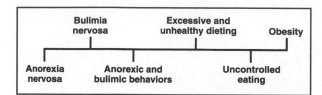

FIGURE 13–1. The spectrum of eating disturbances: bulimia (excessive and nervosa), unhealthy dieting, and obesity; [anorexia and uncontrolled nervosa; bulimic behaviors; eating.] (From Neumark-Sztainer D. Excessive weight preoccupation. Nutr Today 1995;30:68. Reprinted by permission of Williams & Wilkins.)

to binge eating and obesity (Fig. 13–1). All are associated with negative physiologic and psychological health consequences.

EATING DISORDERS

The American Psychiatric Association (1994) has established diagnostic criteria for eating disorders. The most recent edition of the *Diagnostic and Statistical Manual for Mental Disorders* (DSM-IV) includes Anorexia Nervosa and Bulimia Nervosa and subtypes within each group. A new provisional category, Eating Disorders Not Yet Specified, is reserved for disorders of eating that do not meet the criteria for anorexia nervosa or bulimia nervosa. Within this category, research criteria have been specified for Binge Eating Disorder (BED). Another related behavior pattern, excessive exercise, is also discussed in this section.

Although various forms of **disordered eating** have been described, an individual is likely to manifest symptoms or characteristics of more than one disorder (Gralen et al, 1990). For example, 30% to 80% of those who meet diagnostic criteria for bulimia nervosa have a history of anorexia nervosa (Haller, 1992), and individuals with anorexia nervosa and bulimia nervosa often use excessive exercise as another method to control body weight.

ANOREXIA NERVOSA

■ What is anorexia nervosa?

■ Do eating disorders serve a purpose for the individual?

■ What factors predispose an individual to anorexia nervosa?

■ What are the signs, symptoms, and complications of anorexia nervosa?

■ How is anorexia nervosa treated? How successful is treatment?

Definition and Incidence

Anorexia nervosa is characterized by self-imposed starvation resulting in excessive weight loss. The affected individual has a distorted body image and an intense fear of becoming fat even when underweight. The diagnostic criteria for anorexia nervosa established by the American Psychiatric Association are listed in Table 13–1. The prevalence of anorexia nervosa in affluent societies is approximately 1% of young women and 0.5% in adolescent girls (Lucas et al, 1991). Although it occurs primarily in females, 5% to 10% of the cases are in males (Touyz et al, 1993). Traditionally, the typical individual with anorexia nervosa has been described as a young, achievement-oriented, perfectionist female from a successful Caucasian middle or upper class family with high expectations of achievement for its offspring. Over the past decade, however, anorexia nervosa has been noted in males and in all ethnic and socioeconomic groups (Rastam and Gillberg, 1991).

TABLE 13–1 DSM-IV Diagnostic Criteria: Anorexia Nervosa

A. Refusal to maintain body weight at or above a minimally normal weight for age and height (e.g., weight loss leading to maintenance of body weight less than 85% of that expected; or failure to make expected weight gain during period of growth, leading to body weight less than 85% of that expected)

B. Intense fear of gaining weight or becoming fat, even though underweight

C. Disturbance in the way in which one's body weight or shape is experienced; undue influence of body weight or shape on self-evaluation, or denial of the seriousness of the current body weight

D. In postmenarchal females, amenorrhea (i.e., the absence of at least three consecutive menstrual cycles). (A woman is considered to have amenorrhea if her periods occur only following hormone, e.g., estrogen, administration.)

SPECIFY TYPE:
Restricting type: During the episode of anorexia nervosa the person does not regularly engage in binge eating or purging behavior (i.e., self-induced vomiting or the misuse of laxatives or diuretics).

Binge eating/purging type: During the episode of anorexia nervosa, the person regularly engages in binge-eating or purging behavior (i.e., self-induced vomiting or the misuse of laxatives or diuretics).

Reprinted with permission from the Diagnostic and Statistical Manual of Mental Disorders, Fourth Edition. Copyright 1994 American Psychiatric Association.

Etiology

The etiology of anorexia nervosa is multifactorial, encompassing societal, biologic, psychological, and familial factors. The role of society is the cultural focus on being slender, which drives a youngster to the "pursuit of thinness." Anecdotal records of cases of anorexia nervosa indicate that restrictive food behavior can be triggered by something as small as a passing comment by a parent or peer suggesting the individual is heavy or overweight.

More than three decades ago it was observed that persons with eating disorders had disturbances in perception and interpretation of visceral and emotional stimuli and a sense of ineffectiveness (Bruch, 1973). Recent studies have found that, unlike their normal peers, adolescents with anorexia nervosa have low scores on measures of body and self-image, social relationships, and sexual attitudes (Grant and Fodor, 1986), and less self-acceptance and self-protection (Swift et al, 1986).

Many studies have shown relationships among anxiety, depression, and life stress and eating disorders (Fisher et al, 1995). Adolescents with eating disorders have more first- and second-degree relatives with eating disorders (Herzog et al, 1991) and more first-degree relatives with depression and alcoholism (Strober et al, 1984).

Family dysfunction often exists for a long time before the onset of illness. Typical family characteristics are success orientation, rigidity, overprotectiveness, enmeshment, and avoidance of conflict (Rastam and Gillberg, 1991). There is generally poor communication within the family, unrealistic expectations for achievement, and belittling, rejection, or neglect (Garfinkel et al, 1983). An individual with anorexia nervosa often struggles for autonomy, identity, self respect, and self control. She feels out of control, insecure, and ineffective. Control of her diet and body weight may give her a sense of control, confidence, and autonomy.

Characteristics

Emily is older than the "typical" anorexic, but the pattern of her behavior is representive of a sequence of events that might occur. The term "anorexia" is a misnomer. In actuality, anorexics are preoccupied with thoughts of food and may be intensely hungry, but they are even more concerned with a "terror of fat" that causes high degrees of dietary restraint.

Psychological Characteristics

The person with anorexia nervosa has a distorted image of her body. While she can accurately perceive the relative body fatness of other individuals, she is unable to perceive herself as anything but fat. Even an individual who is 170 cm (67 in) tall and weighs 39 kg (85 lb) will maintain that she is too fat.

In addition to morbid fear of gaining weight and denial of the degree of emaciation, anorexia nervosa is characterized by obsessive-compulsive behaviors, some of which may relate to dietary intake, such as detailed calorie counting, ritualistic eating mannerisms, recipe collection, and food hoarding (Thiel et al, 1995; Vitousek and Manke, 1994). Persons with anorexia nervosa tend to be perfectionists who struggle to live up to performance standards, often self-imposed. Furthermore, the anorexic is plagued by a pervasive sense of personal ineffectiveness. Distorted perceptions of stimuli arising in the body allow the individual to deny feelings of hunger and fatigue, resulting in semi-starvation or exercising beyond the point of exhaustion for most individuals. Another characteristic, increasing social isolation, can be an early clue for parents and teachers of potential problems.

Physical Characteristics

Many characteristics distinguish anorexia nervosa from other eating disorders. The most significant characteristic is intentional, severe loss of body weight. The anorexic will refuse to eat and refuse to maintain a body weight that is within 15% of the expected weight for height.

Unchecked anorexia nervosa can result in a multitude of health problems and even death (Table 13–2). Anorexia nervosa has the highest mortality rate of any psychiatric disorder, ranging from 6% to 20% (Schwartz and Thompson, 1981; Yates, 1990). Most of the complications of anorexia nervosa are the result of severe weight loss caused by inadequate food intake and, in some cases, purging. Starvation itself causes sleep disturbances, impaired concentration, irritability, anxiety, depression, and preoccupation with food (Garfinkel and Kaplan, 1985; Turner and Shapiro, 1992). In early stages, the complications of malnutrition are reversible with increased food intake and weight gain. The catabolic state of anorexia results in decreased body weight, decreased muscle mass, and declines in stores of body fat as well as depletion of liver and mus-

 K E Y   T E R M S

body image: a person's perception of the physical size and appearance of the body. It includes the attitudes, feelings, and behavioral reactions of the individual regarding his or her body. Body image is central to how individuals feels about themselves.

disordered eating: restrained eating, binge eating, fear of fatness, purging, and distorted body image

TABLE 13–2 Complications of Eating Disorders

ANOREXIA NERVOSA
Dizziness, confusion

Dry skin

Dry, brittle hair

Lanugo-type hair

↓ Blood pressure, pulse, bradycardia

Weight loss

↓ Metabolic rate and malnutrition

Muscle wasting, ↓ body fat, hypothermia

Growth failure; delayed sexual maturation

↓ Estrogen secretion

Amenorrhea

Decreased bone mass

↓ Follicle-stimulating hormone secretion

↓ Kidney function (↓ glomerular filtration rate)

Dehydration

Delayed gastric emptying

Constipation; fecal impaction

BULIMIA NERVOSA
Frequent weight fluctuations

Irregular menses

WITH VOMITING
Parotid (salivary) gland enlargement

Erosion of dental enamel, dental caries

Esophageal dysmotility, esophagitis, impaired gastric emptying

Calluses on knuckles

WITH LAXATIVE ABUSE
Alternating diarrhea, constipation

WITH VOMITING AND LAXATIVE/DIURETIC ABUSE
Hypokalemia

Hypocholoridemia

Metabolic alkalosis

Dehydration

Arrhythmia

usually, but not always, return. A long-term complication of estrogen deficiency is **osteopenia**. Adolescents with anorexia nervosa accompanied by amenorrhea have deficits in bone mass of 10% to 30% compared to age- and gender-matched control subjects (Bachrach et al, 1990; Davies et al, 1990). Unfortunately, the age at which anorexia most frequently occurs is a critical stage of development of maximum bone mass, which is related to long-term bone health (Matkovic, 1992).

Severe weight loss can have an effect on many body functions, including those of the heart, kidneys, and gastrointestinal tract. Cardiac manifestations include decreased cardiac output, **bradycardia**, tachycardia, arrhythmias, and hypotension. As kidney function decreases, the **glomerular filtration rate (GFR)** declines, resulting in increased levels of solutes in the blood and associated dehydration.

Chronic restriction of food intake can result in delays in gastric emptying and intestinal motility. In the absence of the stimulus of food, function of the colon may decline, resulting in chronic constipation and increasing the risk of **fecal impaction**. Some anorexics may induce vomiting or abuse laxatives or diuretics, which further complicates their medical condition (such abuse is discussed in the section Bulimia Nervosa). Induction of vomiting, in addition to lowering body weight, can lead to fluid and electrolyte depletion and potentially to **alkalosis**, hypochloremia (low blood chloride), and hypokalemia (low blood potassium).

Treatment

Treatment of anorexia nervosa is complex and requires an ongoing, comprehensive plan to deal with multiple problems. Many individuals have lived with their illness for years, and treatment involves a long-term commitment from both the patient and the treatment provider. Success of treatment can be predicted by certain prognostic signs (Table 13–3). Individuals with good prognostic signs may respond to outpatient treatment—usually a combination of individual and family psychotherapy and nutrition counseling. Those with poor prognostic signs are likely to require long-term treatment and possibly hospitalization if weight loss has been so prolonged or so rapid that life-threatening complications must be averted.

As eating disorders become more entrenched, the behaviors and their consequences become less reversible. It is hoped that the sooner the weight loss is stopped, the greater the chances are for a more complete recovery (Fisher et al, 1995).

The aims of treatment are to restore normal eating patterns, establish normal body weight, and resolve underlying psychological conflicts. It is often easier to change eating behaviors than to correct psychological problems, but long-term recovery depends on the resolution of the un-

cle glycogen. The decline in the basal metabolic rate is one of the body's mechanisms to maintain itself during the shortage of energy intake. A loss of the ability to regulate body temperature causes the individual to complain of feeling cold, especially in the extremities.

Severe weight loss results in decreased secretion of estrogen from the ovary and of the follicle-stimulating hormone (FSH) from the pituitary gland, which causes amenorrhea (Stewart, 1992). With weight gain, normal cycles

TABLE 13–3 Prognostic Signs for Recovery from Anorexia Nervosa

GOOD PROGNOSTIC SIGNS FOR RECOVERY

Young age of onset, recent onset

Normal premorbid weight

No bulimic symptomatology

Insignificant family pathology

POOR PROGNOSTIC SIGNS FOR RECOVERY

Late onset, long duration

Low body weight

Weight has decreased by 25%

Presence of bulimic symptoms

Disturbed relationships with family

Concomitant psychiatric illness

Severe metabolic disorders

Failed previous treatment

Greater social difficulties

Increased somatic or obsessional disorders

derlying conflicts. Currently, the most successful early therapies are multidisciplinary approaches that incorporate weight restoration accompanied by individual and family psychotherapy (American Psychiatric Association, 1993).

Nutrition Intervention

Intervention involves nutrition education, counseling and management (American Dietetic Association, 1994). The highest priority for treatment of anorexia nervosa is to reverse the individual's poor nutrition status. The first goal is cessation of weight loss. It is important to improve nutrition status even while the individual maintains a low weight and then to encourage gradual weight gain through self-feeding. It is important to recognize that an anorexic in a state of starvation is cognitively impaired and a poor candidate for psychotherapy. Thus, weight resolution is a prerequisite to other treatment modalities (Brown, 1993).

For the most severe cases, hospitalization and nutrition replacement via parenteral or nasogastric tube feeding may be appropriate to reverse potentially fatal self-starvation. Such feeding may increase medical and psychological risks, and refeeding must be monitored carefully. Medical risks include fluid retention and changes in electrolyte and mineral status (Wilfley et al, 1993). Significant psychological risks of rapid refeeding are associated with the patient's perceived loss of control, loss of identity, increased body distortion, and mistrust of the treatment team (American Dietetic Association, 1994).

Treatment involves a careful nutrition assessment, determination of caloric need, and design of an appropriate diet plan for weight maintenance, followed by the gradual progression to meet weight gain expectations and, finally, design of a diet plan for maintenance of an acceptable weight. Guidelines for Nutrition Therapy appear in Table 13–4. Nutrition rehabilitation must be performed slowly. Treatment usually begins with a caloric level that is 130% of the resting energy expenditure (REE). When available, **indirect calorimetry** measurements of resting energy expenditure serve as the basis for energy intake calculations. If indirect calorimetry is not available, the Harris-Benedict equations for the prediction of resting energy expenditure, with an adjustment for the hypometabolic state, have been utilized with the following formulas:

RESTING ENERGY EXPENDITURE:

Females:
$$\text{REE (kcal)} = 655 + (9.56 \times \text{wt [kg]}) + (1.85 \times \text{ht [cm]}) - (4.68 \times \text{age [yr]})$$

Males:
$$\text{REE (kcal)} = 66.5 + (13.75 \times \text{wt [kg]}) + (5.0 \times \text{ht [cm]}) - (6.78 \times \text{age [yr]})$$

Using this formula for Emily at the point at which she was admitted to the hospital, it would yield:

$$\text{REE} = 655 + (9.56 \times 41) + (1.85 \times 173) - (4.68 \times 35)$$

$$\text{REE} = 655 + 392 + 320 - 164$$

$$\text{REE} = 1203 \text{ kcal}$$

KEY TERMS

osteopenia: reduced bone mass due to a decreased rate of synthesis to a level insufficient to compensate for breakdown

bradycardia: abnormally slow heart rate

glomerular filtration rate: rate at which the kidney filters blood. When the rate is decreased, the blood may contain substances ordinarily filtered out by the normal kidney.

fecal impaction: a collection of hardened feces in the rectum or sigmoid colon

alkalosis: a condition resulting from accumulation of base or a decrease of acid (hydrogen ion) in body fluids characterized by an increase in pH

indirect calorimetry: measurement of oxygen used or carbon dioxide exhaled to estimate energy expenditure

---

TABLE 13–4 Guidelines for Nutrition Therapy in Anorexia Nervosa and Bulimia Nervosa

Anorexia Nervosa	Bulimia Nervosa
ENERGY	**ENERGY**
1.3 × REE* for weight gain	Weight maintenance
Initial caloric prescriptions: generally in the range of 1000 to 1400 kcal/day	1.2 × REE for sedentary activity
	1.3 × REE for moderate activity
Additional kcal for physical activity	Monitor anthropometric status and adjust caloric prescription for weight maintenance.
Increase daily caloric prescription to promote steady weight gain: 100 kcal increments in early treatment; 200 kcal increments in late treatment	Avoid weight reduction diets until eating patterns and body weight have stabilized.
MACRONUTRIENTS	**MACRONUTRIENTS**
Protein: minimum 0.8 g/kg target body weight	Protein: minimum 0.8 g/kg target body weight
Carbohydrate: 50–55% kcal	Carbohydrate: 50–55% kcal
Encourage water-soluble fiber to reduce constipation	Encourage water-soluble fiber to reduce constipation
Fat: 25–30% kcal	Fat: 25–30% kcal
MICRONUTRIENTS	**MICRONUTRIENTS**
100% RDA	100% RDA
Multivitamin supplement may be necessary	Multivitamin supplement may be necessary

* REE, resting energy expenditure. Can be measured by indirect calorimetry or calculated using the Harris-Benedict equation (see text).

From Luder E, Schebendach J. Nutrition management of eating disorders. Top Clin Nutr 1993;8:48. © 1993. Aspen Publishers, Inc.

The calculation is then adjusted for the hypometabolic rate (Schebendach et al, 1995) as follows:

$$1.84 - \text{calculated REE } (1193) - 1435$$
$$2195 - 1435 = 760 \text{ kcal}$$
(adjusted REE for anorexia nervosa)

As the anorexic improves with refeeding, the resting metabolic rate increases beyond that which can be explained by the increased body mass alone (Obarzanek et al, 1994; Salisbury et al, 1995). Therefore, caloric requirements for weight restoration may be greater than anticipated, and monitoring of the response of the individual will be necessary to plan increases in dietary intake. The expected rate of weight gain varies among treatment programs, but a rate of 0.36 lb/day has been shown to be safe in adolescents with anorexia nervosa (Solanto et al, 1994).

Dietary education, counseling, and management are important components of overall treatment for anorexia nervosa. Nutrition therapy for eating disorders is usually a lengthy process (American Dietetic Association, 1994). It can be divided into an education phase and an experimental phase (Table 13–5). The primary focus of the education phase is to provide nutrition information, and patient interaction is limited. The experimental phase is based on a long-term counseling relationship between the client and the registered dietitian, who is part of the multidisciplinary treatment team. The experimental phase requires a dietitian with training and experience in the area of eating disorders.

Initial use of small quantities of food may meet the psychological need of a person with anorexia nervosa who is fearful of gaining weight rapidly and becoming fat. Dietary patterns usually consist of three meals a day plus snacks. Oral liquid supplements may be of value in meeting caloric needs, because the person suffering from anorexia nervosa typically has problems consuming the increased amounts of food required for weight gain.

Behavior Modification

The behavioral component of treatment provides the structure needed for the anorexic to interfere with his or her self-destructive behaviors. It usually begins with strict monitoring of behavior. As the individual is better able to contain the deleterious behavior, the amount of autonomy and responsibility received increases. In this system the client agrees to a contract with a predetermined target weight to be rewarded with a variety of privileges. Initially physical exercise is kept to a minimum to avoid increases in energy expenditure.

TABLE 13–5 Phases of Nutrition Therapy for Eating Disorders

EDUCATION PHASE

The dietitian educates the client about her eating disorder. The dietitian:

Collects relevant information.

Establishes a collaborative relationship with the client.

Defines and discusses relevant principles and concepts of food, nutrition, and weight regulation.

Presents examples of typical hunger patterns, food intake patterns, and caloric intakes of someone who has recovered.

Works to educate the family.

EXPERIMENTAL PHASE

The dietitian helps the client make changes in food- and weight-related behaviors in a safe environment. The client:

Separates food- and weight-related behaviors from feelings and psychological issues.

Makes gradual, incremental changes in food behaviors until food intake patterns are normalized.

Slows increase or decrease in weight.

Learns to maintain a weight that is healthful for the individual without using abnormal food- and weight-related behaviors.

Learns to be comfortable in social eating situations.

From The American Dietetic Association. Position of the American Dietetic Association: Nutrition intervention in the treatment of anorexia nervosa, bulimia nervosa and binge eating. J Am Diet Assoc 1994;94:900. Copyright The American Dietetic Association. Reprinted by permission from Journal of the American Dietetic Association.

PSYCHOTHERAPY For the individual with anorexia nervosa to develop autonomy, he or she must identify feelings and their relationship to behavior. Individual psychotherapy facilitates personal growth, helping individuals to take responsibility for themselves. Counseling is likely to be required for several years. Issues specific to adolescents involve assertiveness, educational achievement, social skills, family interaction, substance use, and sexual behavior.

Family Therapy

It is important for adolescents to identify the underlying dysfunctional family patterns that have prohibited development of independence. Involving parents is essential in building an alliance between the treatment team and the family and client because young adolescents are not emotionally or situationally autonomous (Crisp et al, 1991; Russell et al, 1987). Later in the course of treatment, family therapy should center on separation and autonomy, family expression of feelings, and conflict resolution.

Pharmacotherapy

No single medication has proven to be especially effective for treating anorexia nervosa (Schwartz and Thompson, 1981; Fisher et al, 1995) and routine use of medications is not recommended (American Psychiatric Association, 1993). The medications most often used are antidepressants for individuals with depression, but they are not given until after weight gain when the psychological effects of malnutrition are resolving. Malnourished patients may be less responsive to medications and are more prone to side effects.

Prognosis

Anorexia nervosa is a chronic condition that requires long-term treatment programs to prevent **relapse**. For treatment to be successful, the chronic nature of the disorder must be considered. Follow-up studies of seriously ill anorexics show that 40% to 50% recovered (Hsu, 1990). Another 25% show some improvement, but approximately 30% had a poor outcome and mortality was zero to 18% (Fisher et al, 1995). Criteria of recovery were normal stable body weight (within 15% of recommended levels) and establishment of regular menses. Studies of milder cases of anorexia nervosa indicate as many as two-thirds of recovering anorexics still worried about body shape and had persistent abnormal eating behavior (Halmi et al, 1991).

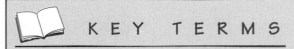

KEY TERMS

relapse: return of symptoms at least weekly for a minimum of 2 months

Sue is 163 cm (64 in) tall and weighs 50 kg (109 lb). Her reference weight range is 51 to 58 kg (113 to 128 lb). Sue weighed about 55 kg (120 lb) when she was 15 years old. She started dieting when her best friend suggested she would look really great if she were thinner. During her senior year in high school, Sue discovered that if she ate and immediately vomited, she could achieve almost the same effect as her restrictive diet. Her daily intake pattern is to skip breakfast. If her mother insists that she eat before going to school, she vomits before she leaves. Lunch is a diet cola or a piece of fruit. Sue has cheese and crackers or a candy bar before tennis practice, and she eats a large evening meal. She snacks most of the evening while studying or watching television. She usually vomits before going to bed. In addition, she takes laxatives, usually 3 to 4 every night, unless she really feels fat, in which case she may take up to 30. Sue really likes the new freedom to eat she has found, but she doesn't like the fact that she feels bad most of the time. She is chronically depressed and spends less time with friends because her binging rituals take up a great deal of time. Frequently she feels faint after long spells of vomiting or during her nightly diarrhea. Although Sue wants to stop the binging/purging pattern, she desperately wants to keep her weight under control and is not sure she can stop. She feels miserable most of the time.

BULIMIA NERVOSA

■ What are the signs and symptoms of bulimia nervosa? Who is at greatest risk?

■ Describe binging and purging.

■ What are the biologic, social, and emotional factors that predispose an individual to bulimia nervosa?

■ What are the health risks of bulimia nervosa?

■ How is bulimia nervosa treated?

Definition and Incidence

In contrast to anorexia nervosa, those with bulimia nervosa have recurrent episodes in which they **binge** on copious amounts of food. Because of guilt over that extreme consumption, they tend to **purge** to get rid of the excess food they have consumed. Current diagnostic criteria for bulimia nervosa established by the American Psychiatric Association (1994) appear in Table 13–6. This disorder is estimated to affect between 4% and 20% of adolescent and college females (Drewnowski et al, 1988; Fukagawa, 1992). Bulimia nervosa occurs much less frequently in males (<5%) and is often associated with a history of sexual identity concerns, obesity, defensive dieting or dieting in relation to sports participation (Carlat and Carmago, 1991).

Etiology

Although the causes of bulimia nervosa have been elusive and uncertain, it has been proposed that bulimic be-

---

TABLE 13–6 DSM-IV Diagnostic Criteria: Bulimia Nervosa

A. Recurrent episodes of binge eating. An episode of binge eating is characterized by both of the following:
   1. Eating, in a discrete period of time (e.g., within any 2-hr period), an amount of food that is definitely larger than most people would eat during a similar period of time and under similar circumstances.
   2. A sense of lack of control over eating during the episode (e.g., a feeling that one cannot stop eating or control what or how much one is eating).

B. Recurrent inappropriate compensatory behavior to prevent weight gain, such as self-induced vomiting; misuse of laxatives, diuretics, or other medications; fasting; or excessive exercise.

C. The binge eating and inappropriate compensatory behaviors both occur, on average, at least twice a week for 3 months.

D. Self-evaluation is unduly influenced by body shape and weight.

E. The disturbance does not occur exclusively during episodes of Anorexia Nervosa.

SPECIFY TYPE:
Purging type: During the current episode of bulimia nervosa, the person has regularly engaged in self-induced vomiting or the misuse of laxatives, diuretics or enemas.

Nonpurging type: During the current episode of bulimia nervosa, the person uses other inappropriate compensatory behaviors, such as fasting or excessive exercise, but does not regularly engage in self-induced vomiting or the misuse of laxatives, diuretics, or enemas.

Reprinted with permission from the Diagnostic and Statistical Manual of Mental Disorders, Fourth Edition. Copyright 1994 American Psychiatric Association.

havior may serve to reduce tension, help regulate the self, and provide stimulation needed to dampen feelings of emptiness (Goodsitt, 1983). Biologic, psychological and environmental factors appear to be related to the development of bulimic behavior. Underlying issues are societal pressures, lack of **self esteem**, and perceptions of body image and appearance.

Restrictive dieting produces abnormal eating behaviors, which may disturb intake/satiety regulation mechanisms. Part of the biologic component may be related to dieting and its associated hunger and emotional precipitants, which lead to binging and then, eventually, to purging. The cycle perpetuates a caloric deficit, and biology drives overeating. Several theories have been postulated to explain the biologic mechanism of disordered satiety associated with bulimic behaviors. One study reported a decrease in the secretion of **cholecystokinin** in individuals with bulimia nervosa and suggested that this leads to decreased satiety and the consequent binging behavior (Geracioti and Liddle, 1988).

Other contributors to disordered satiety involve neurotransmitters (serotonin, catacholamines, opiates) of the central nervous system. Most research has focused on serotonin and its dietary precursor, the amino acid tryptophan. Individuals with bulimic symptomatology tend to have lower levels of 5-hydroxyindoleacetic acid, a metabolite of serotonin. It has been suggested that diminished activity of satiety-related pathways regulated by serotonin may cause bulimic symptoms (Brewerton et al, 1992). Additional evidence for such an effect is that antidepressant medications that increase available serotonin have met with success in the treatment of bulimia nervosa.

In bulimia nervosa, self-concept and self-esteem play critical causal roles. Adolescents particularly experience significantly lower self-esteem, more self-regulating difficulties, frustration intolerance, and impaired ability to express feelings than those without eating disorders (Gross and Rosen, 1988). The psychological component may also be associated with food restriction, which leads to a decreased frustration tolerance and a decreased sense of well-being. For dieters, eating may renew frustration tolerance, becoming an emotional reflex, and over time eating may become a regulator of tension. They may use food to deflect emotions and avoid confrontation.

Symptoms of anxiety and depression are more common among those with clinical and subclinical bulimia nervosa (Lancelot et al, 1991; Gross and Rosen, 1988; Killen et al, 1987). It is not known whether the anxiety and depression are primary or secondary to the eating disorder. A number of studies have demonstrated a relationship between the occurrence of stressful or traumatic life events and eating disorders (Yaeger et al, 1993; Strober, 1984). Persons with bulimia nervosa often have other impulsive behaviors such as drug abuse, shoplifting, and alcohol abuse (Timmerman et al, 1990). They share characteristics with other substance abusers, especially self-perpetuating lifestyle— i.e., they develop a lifestyle to accommodate times, places, and money to support the binge/purge pattern.

Characteristics

Bulimia nervosa is characterized by alternating episodes of binging and purging. Figure 13–2 illustrates a cycle of events that is characteristic of bulimia: anxiety, binge eating, guilt, purging, semi-starvation, obsession, hunger, and binging.

The individual has a sense of being unable to control eating once a binge begins. A binge is terminated only by abdominal pain, sleep, social interruption, or vomiting. The loss of control results in shame and guilt, which in turn are usually followed by purging (self-induced vomiting, abuse of laxatives or diuretics, or excessive exercise). In many instances, guilt for having lost control results in severe dietary restraint until stress and/or hunger again precipitates a binge/purge episode. These behaviors have many medical consequences (see Table 13–2).

The individual is aware that his or her eating pattern is abnormal, but for most bulimics binging episodes are secret and they deny the presence of the problem to other people. There are two major differences between bulimia nervosa and anorexia nervosa: the individual with bulimia (1) does not feel as personally ineffective as the one with anorexia nervosa and (2) is more aware of his or her emotions, even if unable to control them.

Purging

A variety of behaviors may be used to "purge" excess calories to control body weight, including vigorous exercise, diuretics, inducing vomiting, laxatives, and taking **sorbitol** to cause diarrhea. Purging behaviors have major health consequences (see Fig. 13–2).

Vomiting

About 60% to 80% of bulimics vomit repeatedly to rid themselves of huge quantities of food. Some use the **emetic ipecac**, which can cause dry heaves for several

K E Y   T E R M S

binge: rapid consumption of large quantities of food
purge: overuse of laxatives, self-induced vomiting, rigorous dieting, and fasting to counteract effects of binge eating
self esteem: confidence and satisfaction in one's self
cholecystokinin: a hormone that stimulates release of bile and produces satiety in humans
sorbitol: alcohol from sugar that is used as a sweetener in some food products
emetic: something that causes vomiting
ipecac: dried roots of the plant *Cephaelis ipecacuanha* or *acuminata* used as an emetic

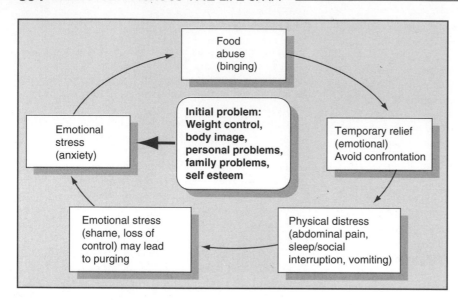

FIGURE 13–2. The dynamics of the food abuse process.

hours, to induce vomiting. Because ipecac has a long half-life, it may accumulate in the body with use on a regular basis and may become cardiotoxic. Repeated vomiting may lead to dental disease, perimolysis, in which the teeth are progressively decalcified and dissolved due to contact with hydrochloric acid during regurgitation (Zachariasen, 1995). The enamel layer of teeth gets thinner, causing sensitivity to hot, cold, and acid substances. In some instances, fillings become loose as the tooth structure to support them diminishes.

Perioral trauma may be associated with vomiting. The **parotid gland** may enlarge, giving a puffy chipmunk facial appearance. The cause is unknown, but it is associated with malnutrition and chronic stimulation by the repeated ingestion of very large amounts of carbohydrate.

Esophageal disorders induced by repeated retching and vomiting include a painful sore throat, esophagitis, esophageal ulcers, and esophageal bleeding and rupture. **Aspiration** is always a danger with regurgitation. Acute dilation and rupture of the stomach after binge eating episodes have been reported (Mitchell et al, 1987). Many individuals develop calluses on their knuckles from using their fingers to induce vomiting. Severe metabolic complications of vomiting include hypokalemia and hypochloremia, which may lead to **metabolic acidosis** and, if severe, arrhythmias and sudden death.

Laxative Abuse

As many as 40% to 60% of those with bulimia nervosa use laxatives and diuretics on a regular basis. The laxative abuse syndrome is associated with excess use of one or several of the stimulant type **cathartics**. Laxative abuse leads to watery diarrhea, which can cause dehydration and may exaggerate electrolyte depletion. Acute episodes of laxative abuse may be associated with nonspecific symptoms such as pain and vomiting. However, chronic use can

lead to more severe problems such as **cathartic colon**. Symptoms characteristic of cathartic colon are alternating diarrhea and constipation, but the individual may also experience nausea, vomiting, and weight loss.

Diuretic Abuse

Diuretics are substances that increase kidney output. They vary from caffeine to alcohol to prescription drugs. However, many diuretics increase the excretion of other nutrients, especially potassium and magnesium. Diuretic abuse results in major losses of electrolytes, which may lead to severe metabolic imbalances, including hypokalemia and hypocalcemia. The combination of the abuse of laxatives and abuse of diuretics is particularly dangerous.

Treatment

People with bulimia nervosa can become so obsessive that the victims literally cannot stop their self-destructive behavior without professional help. Treatment is often difficult because of denial and the need for the individual to acknowledge the problem before treatment can begin. The biopsychosocial nature of bulimia nervosa indicates a need for interdisciplinary approaches. Intervention strategies include cognitive, behavioral, psychodynamic, and pharmacologic approaches in individual and/or group settings (Brambilla et al, 1995).

The goals of treatment of bulimia nervosa are to restructure and normalize eating patterns, to eliminate the binge/purge cycle, and to normalize perceptions of body build and shape. Treatment early in the course of the disorder provides the most likelihood of recovery (Woodside, 1995). Hospitalization is seldom necessary except for those who do not make progress or who have concurrent drug or alcohol abuse problems or other severe medical problems (American Psychiatric Association, 1993).

Nutritional Intervention

Appropriate nutrition therapy for the treatment of bulimia nervosa (see Table 13–4) will be implemented using the education and behavioral strategies outlined in Table 13–5. The primary goal is to structure eating patterns. The individual cannot diet or lose weight while learning to normalize eating habits. Dietary modifications include spreading kilocalories throughout the day and avoiding fasting. Techniques are learned to develop alternatives to eating to get past boredom, anxiety, and restlessness and to isolate and manage foods that "trigger" binging episodes. Therapy encourages strategizing, substituting, and sublimating to increase "free days" (those free of binging or purging) and broaden coping strategies.

Psychosocial Treatment

Most treatment for bulimia nervosa is based on the cognitive–behavioral approach in which habits and attitudes are the key targets (Fairburn et al, 1991). The goal is to change the bulimic's attitude in order to change behavior. This treatment is similar to that of other indulgent behaviors such as alcohol, nicotine, and cocaine, which are associated with short-term gratification and long-term punishment.

Bulimics have a high rate of **comorbid** mood, anxiety, and personality disturbances and unresolved conflicts. Many recovering bulimics may require extended psychotherapy or psychoanalysis that addresses these intrapsychic and intrapersonal issues, which come into focus as binge/purge associated systems abate (Crow and Mitchell, 1994).

Pharmacology

Antidepressant medications may reduce symptoms of binging and purging in some bulimics (Pope and Hudson, 1986), but antidepressants are just one component of a treatment program. They may be especially helpful for individuals with significant symptoms of depression, anxiety, obsession, or impulse disorder symptoms or for individuals who have failed previous attempts at appropriate psychosocial therapy. Over the past several years, selective serotonin uptake inhibitors have become the most commonly used class of drugs (Crow and Mitchell, 1994). Studies in adults (Fluoxetine Bulimia Nervosa Collaborative Group, 1992; Ayuso-Guitierrez et al, 1994) have demonstrated the usefulness of serotonin-uptake inhibitors for the treatment of bulimia nervosa. Agras et al (1994) found that, after 1 year, the greatest success occurred when the drug was used in combination with cognitive-behavioral therapy.

Prognosis

Although limited data are available on the success of treatment of bulimia nervosa, several studies have reported relapse rates ranging from 30% to 40% at 6 to 8 months to 63% at 18 months after **recovery** (Olmsted et al, 1994). This suggests that relapse is a serious problem. Frequency of continued vomiting appears to be an important prognostic indicator of relapse (Olmsted et al, 1994).

Reiss and co-workers (1995) reported that a stable satisfactory relationship was associated with a good outcome. One 10-year follow-up of persons treated for bulimia nervosa found that more than half had full recovery (Collings and King, 1994). While the remainder continued to experience some symptoms, only 9% continued to suffer the full syndrome.

Prognosis is much better for adolescents with bulimia nervosa than for adults (Fisher et al, 1995). This supports the value of early aggressive treatment in adolescents with eating disorders. To date, there are no studies that have evaluated the outcome of adolescent patients with bulimia nervosa.

BINGE EATING DISORDER

■ What are the characteristics of individuals with binge eating disorder?

■ Why has binge eating been given a provisional category as an eating disorder?

■ What are the health implications of binge eating disorder? How is it treated?

Binge eating, first described in 1959, has long been recognized as a serious clinical problem in obesity (Stunkard,

K E Y   T E R M S

parotid gland: a gland located near the ear
aspiration: breathing vomitus or mucus into the respiratory tract
metabolic acidosis: a condition resulting from a depletion of the alkaline resins (bicarbonate) in body fluids characterized by a decrease in pH
cathartic: an agent that causes evacuation of the bowels by increasing motor activity of the intestine
cathartic colon: thinning of the colon wall and structural defects associated with changes in motility
comorbid: disorders or diseases that occur concurrently
recovery: abstinence from or substantial decrease in binge eating or purging

■ What are the health implications of binge eating disorder? How is it treated?

Binge eating, first described in 1959, has long been recognized as a serious clinical problem in obesity (Stunkard, 1959; Loro and Orleans, 1981). Often referred to as compulsive overeating, binging occurs without the regular use of inappropriate compensatory purging behaviors (Walsh 1990; Spitzer et al, 1993). Binge eating disorder (BED) is included in the fourth edition of the *Diagnostic and Statistical Manual of Mental Disorders* (DSM-IV) as a provisional category warranting further study (American Psychiatric Association, 1994). Research criteria for this disorder appear in Table 13–7.

Definition and Incidence

TABLE 13–7 Research Criteria for Binge Eating Disorder

Recurrent episodes of binge eating. An episode of binge eating is characterized by both of the following:
1. Eating in a discrete period of time (e.g., within any 2-hour period), an amount of food that is definitely larger than most people would eat in a similar period of time under similar circumstances
2. A sense of lack of control over eating during the episodes (e.g., a feeling that one cannot stop eating or control what or how much one is eating)

The binge-eating episodes are associated with three (or more) of the following:
1. Eating much more rapidly than normal
2. Eating until feeling uncomfortably full
3. Eating large amounts of food when not feeling physically hungry
4. Eating alone because of being embarrassed by how much one is eating
5. Feeling disgusted with oneself, depressed, or very guilty after overeating

Marked stress regarding binge eating is present.

The binge eating occurs, on average, at least 2 days a week for 6 months.

Note: The method of determining frequency differs from that used for Bulimia Nervosa; future research should address whether the preferred method of setting a frequency threshold is counting the number of days on which binges occur or counting the number of episodes of binge eating.

The binge eating is not associated with the regular use of inappropriate compensatory behaviors (e.g., purging, fasting, excessive exercise) and does not occur exclusively during the course of Anorexia Nervoxsa or Bulimia Nervosa.

Reprinted with permission from the Diagnostic and Statistical Manual of Mental Disorders, Fourth Edition. Copyright 1994 American Psychiatric Association.

Although it has only recently been recognized as a distinct condition, binge eating disorder is probably the most common eating disorder. Most people with binge eating disorder are obese, but people of normal weight can be affected. The disorder affects approximately 2% of all adults, or 1 million to 2 million Americans (U.S. Public Health Service, 1993). Binge eating disorder occurs in approximately 10% to 15% of mildly obese people in self-help or commercial weight loss programs and in 20% to 50% of those enrolled in medically supervised weight loss programs (Marcus, 1993; Yanovski et al, 1993). In general, binge eating disorder affects three women for every two men (U.S. Public Health Service, 1993).

Characteristics

Compulsive overeating of sweet and high-fat foods and heightened cravings for these foods are typical of the binge eating disorder. Binge eating has been likened to drug abuse because both behavioral syndromes involve intense cravings and loss of control (Drewnowski et al, 1992). Drewnowski and co-workers (1995) have suggested that food preferences and binge episodes may be influenced by endogenous **opiate** peptides. They observed that a drug that blocked opiate function reduced the consumption of sweet and high-fat foods among women who had a history of binge eating but did not have that affect in nonbinging women.

Individuals with binge eating disorder share many characteristics with those who suffer from anorexia nervosa and bulimia nervosa. They have impaired social functioning and undue concerns about body weight (Spitzer et al, 1993). Obese binge eaters have been shown to have more psychopathology (e.g., major depression, panic disorder, and borderline personality disorders) than normal-weight or obese individuals who do not binge (Antony et al, 1994) but less psychiatric disturbance than normal-weight women with bulimia nervosa (Brody et al, 1994; McCann et al, 1991).

Treatment

Many obese individuals with binge eating disorder are able to lose weight with traditional diet, exercise, and behavioral self-management methods, but the effects are short-term and most regain virtually all the weight within a few years.

Researchers are still trying to determine which method or combination of methods is most effective in controlling binge eating disorder (Walsh, 1990; Spitzer et al, 1993). Options currently being used center on cognitive-behavioral therapy, which teaches clients techniques for monitoring and changing eating habits and interpersonal psychotherapy, which assists them in developing skills to

nature of the problem and are individualized for his or her special needs. Structured approaches similar to those used for treatment of anorexia nervosa and bulimia nervosa appear to be most effective (Bruce and Wilfley, 1996).

Prevention of Eating Disorders

Disordered eating is a society-wide concern that has major health consequences (Neumark-Sztainer, 1995). Preoccupation with body weight and concern about dieting begin early. In one study, the weight-related concerns of 457 boys and girls between 9 and 11 years revealed that children are concerned about body image and with food and weight control (Gustafson-Larson and Terry, 1992). Almost two-thirds of the children reported they desired to be thinner, and 80% reported that they avoided foods they felt would make them fat. A similar study of adolescent girls and young women found that 67% were dissatisfied with their weight and 54% were dissatisfied with their body image. Binging, dieting, and fasting to control body weight were reported by more than one-third of these subjects (Moore, 1988).

The large numbers of children and adolescents with abnormal attitudes toward body image and eating make the issue of early prevention and intervention particularly pertinent (Fisher et al, 1995). It is essential for healthcare professionals to encourage parents and their children to develop healthy attitudes about their weight, body image, and self esteem and to ameliorate the sociocultural influences that promote eating disorders.

OVERWEIGHT AND OBESITY

■ How are overweight and obesity assessed? What is the prevalence?

■ What are the risks of excess body weight and fat?

■ Describe the genetic, physiologic, social, cultural, and psychological factors that contribute to excess body weight.

■ What are appropriate treatment modalities and programs for overweight and obesity?

■ Discuss the advantages and disadvantages of weight reduction.

■ How can the onset or progression of obesity be prevented or delayed?

In affluent societies, excess body weight is the most common nutrition-related health problem. Obesity is a complicated disordered condition or group of conditions that has physiologic, psychological, and social consequences. Unfortunately, the precise etiologies of obesity are poorly understood, and treatment programs are characterized by high rates of **recidivism**.

Assessment

Overweight is a condition in which an individual's weight exceeds a reference weight based on height. It is characterized by an excess accumulation of body fat. Assessment of body weight and body fat is discussed in Chapter 2 (see page 32). Overweight and obesity have traditionally been defined in terms of excess body weight and reported as a percentage of the reference weight, usually the Metropolitan Height–Weight Tables (see the inside back cover). A preferred method to assess obesity is the body mass index (BMI). BMI is based on weight and height, but has minimal correlation with height, making it a better indicator of relative fatness for both children and adults (Manson et al, 1987; Gasser et al, 1994). Table 13–8 gives the Metropolitan Relative Weights and BMIs used to define overweight and obesity.

Because obesity is defined in terms of fatness, fatfolds (skinfolds) may be useful for assessment. The thickness of the fatfold measurement increases and decreases when an individual gains or loses body fat. A fatfold value that exceeds the 85th percentile of the NHANES date (Appendices 3A and 3B) is generally considered indicative of obesity; a value greater than the 95th percentile indicates extreme obesity.

The distribution of body fat is an important determinant of health risks. An excessive amount of fat on the trunk and abdominal area (android) compared to gluteo-femoral fat (gynoid) is associated with increased risk for a variety of illnesses and overall mortality (Larsson et al, 1992). The **waist-to-hip ratio** (WHR) is currently the practical surrogate measure of abdominal or visceral fat. A WHR that exceeds 0.80 for women and 1.0 for men suggests a weight distribution that poses increased risks to health compared to excess weight alone (Institute of Medicine, 1995).

Prevalence

Healthy People 2000 Objective 2.3 for health promotion is to reduce the prevalence of overweight to no more than 20% among people aged 20 and older and to no more than 15% among adolescents 12 through 19 years of age. The

K E Y   T E R M S

opiate: any compound that induces sleep
recidivism: tendency to relapse into a previous condition or mode of behavior
waist-to-hip ratio: waist circumference divided by hip circumference

RESEARCH UPDATE
Can You Exercise Too Much?

About 2 years ago, Judy, a 32-year-old healthcare professional, was exercising at least 4 hours a day. She didn't have a VCR, so she listened to exercise tapes. She'd play them again and again. Then, when others might be ready to relax, she went to the health spa, convinced that if she went one day without doing this, she would gain weight. Exercise became as much an addiction for her as food is for the binge eater. The more involved she became, the more rituals she developed. She was at the spa at 9 a.m. every day, even when she had a cold or developed the flu.

Gradually Judy developed a pattern. At first, she was getting the exercise out of the way so she could enjoy something, such as meals. Then she cut herself to two meals, then one, then a carton of yogurt. As she cut herself off from food, she also avoided the rest of the world. She stopped seeing her friends. The spa came first, and she was too busy all the time. By this time, the 157 cm (62 in) Judy weighed 35 kg (78 lb). Other problems developed when she had to have intestinal surgery for an unrelated illness. Although she was told not to exercise after the surgery, she felt she had to. She ripped open her incision and had to undergo surgery again. Judy was scared, and she finally realized she had a problem.

Decades of epidemiologic research have established a consensus that regular physical activity provides a number of benefits, reducing both mortality and morbidity of coronary heart disease, hypertension, and osteoporosis (Bouchard et al, 1990). However, that "healthful" practice can get out of control. For some individuals, excessive or compulsive exercise becomes a means to control body weight and emotional frustrations. Often such exercise is expressed by intensive and highly ritualized daily activities such as performing a specified number of sit-ups, swimming a set of number laps, or running set distances (Yates et al, 1994). Rituals become more pronounced and in-

volved as the individual becomes "exercise dependent" (Pierce, 1994). "Excessive" has not been defined for exercise, but some researchers suggest that criteria include: exercise 2 to 3 hours a day, exercising despite injury or pain, and withdrawal without activity after 24 to 36 hours (Hauck, 1992; Pierce, 1994).

Clearly, there is harm in too much exercise. Body fat stores become depleted, and continuing to exercise will cause degradation of muscle to meet energy needs. Low body weight may contribute to decreased bone mass and eventually to osteoporosis. Those who overexercise may experience more stress fractures, and when they exercise despite injuries, they develop more serious injuries.

There is considerable overlap between compulsive athleticism and eating disorders. Both are associated with patterns of distorted self esteem, distorted body image (Sundgot-Borgen, 1993; Beumont et al, 1994), depression (Specker et al, 1994), and obsessive-compulsive behavior personality disorders such as perfectionism (Yates, 1994). One study of 88 men and 97 women found a strong relationship between exercise and weight preoccupation among men and women and between exercise and obsessive-compulsiveness among men (Davis et al, 1993).

The overexerciser may need assistance in recognizing and acknowledging the problem before it can be confronted or treatment can be initiated. Treatment may be especially difficult because controlling the exercise may be only part of the problem. Former overexercisers often turn to other weight control methods, and they may become bulimic. Treatment approaches are similar to those used for eating disorders. Beumont and co-workers (1994) have developed an exercise program to be incorporated into the treatment of eating disordered individuals that includes behavior modification, education, and shared responsibility.

Prevalence

Healthy People 2000 Objective 2.3 for health promotion is to reduce the prevalence of overweight to no more than 20% among people aged 20 and older and to no more than 15% among adolescents 12 through 19 years of age. The

baseline for this objective was a prevalence of 26% from the NHANES II (1976–1980) data. Rather than decreasing, however, the prevalence of overweight in adults in the United States has increased by approximtely 8%. According to data from NHANES III (1988–1991), Phase I, one-third of all American adults are overweight (Kuczmarski et

TABLE 13–8 Definition of Overweight and Obesity by Metropolitan Relative Weight (MRW) and Body Mass Index (BMI)

Degree of Excess Weight	MRW	BMI
Overweight	<120	20–24
Mild obesity	120–140	25–29
Moderate obesity	140–200	30–39
Severe obesity	>200	>40

Metropolitan Relative Weight = 100 × actual weight/reference weight from the height and frame size on Metropolitan Height–Weight Tables.
BMI = wt (kg)/ht (cm²)

al, 1994). Overweight is more frequent in women (35%) than men (31%) (Fig. 13–3). Minority populations, especially women, are affected disproportionately; nearly 50% of African American women, Mexican American women, and Native American women are overweight (National Task Force, 1994). Poverty and lower educational attainment increase the susceptibility to obesity and its progression (Kumanyika, 1994; Gortmaker et al, 1993).

Health Risks

The Consensus Development Conference on Obesity concluded that a BMI greater than 27.8 for males or greater than 27.2 for females has adverse affects on health and longevity (National Institutes of Health, 1985). Table 13–9 lists the most common risks of excess body weight. Optimum body weight for health is a subject of debate (Blackburn et al, 1994), but morbidity and mortality increase as weight increases (Van Itallie, 1985).

Mortality

The relationship between body weight and mortality from three major national studies is illustrated in Table 13–10. An excess body weight of 30% is associated with an increase of 25% to 42% in mortality, and mortality increases with increasing body weight (Kushner, 1993). For those instances in which increased risk occurred with underweight, it is uncertain if that risk is related to leanness or unhealthy lifestyle habits, preclinical disease processes, or other unidentified factors.

Lee and co-workers (1993) at Harvard University conducted a follow-up of 17,297 healthy men who completed health questionnaires in 1962 and 1966. After 27 years, the lowest mortality occurred among those who weighed

approximately 20% below the United States average for men of comparable age and height. A similar observation from the longitudinal Nurses Health Study was that for middle-aged women, mortality was lowest when they weighed at least 15% less than the average weight for women in the U.S. (Manson et al, 1995).

Morbidity

Much of the morbidity associated with obesity is due to an increase in the occurrence of hypertension, hyperlipidemia, and non–insulin-dependent diabetes mellitus (NIDDM), all of which contribute to an increased risk of cardiovascular disease (Sjostrom, 1992; Denke et al, 1993). Moreover, the health risks from these comorbidities increase with the duration and severity of the obesity. Although the morbidity of obesity is not as prominent in women as in men, the association of obesity with cardiovascular disease is as strong in women as men, particularly with weight gains of more than 20 lbs (Manson et al, 1987). Excessive weight also increases the risk for gallbladder disease, **gout**, pulmonary and orthopedic problems, particularly osteoarthritis, and some types of cancer (Sjostrom, 1992).

The pattern of adipose tissue distribution can alter the health risks of obesity independent of total body fat. Excessive accumulation of intra-abdominal fat is linked to other metabolic complications such as hyperinsulinemia/**insulin resistance** and hypertension, which are known risk factors for cardiovascular disease (Bjorntorp, 1987; Van Itallie, 1985). The clustering of these abnormalities has been referred to as syndrome X (Reaven et al, 1993). In fact, abdominal obesity is as strong a predictor of **myocardial infarction** as the leading risk factors, hypercholesterolemia, hypertension, and smoking (Bouchard et al, 1990).

Excess body weight has substantial socioeconomic and psychological ramifications that can impair the day-to-day functioning of an obese person (Kral et al, 1992). For ex-

KEY TERMS

gout: a form of arthritis characterized by excess uric acid in the blood and recurrent attacks of acute arthritis involving a peripheral joint followed by complete remission

insulin resistance: a condition in which insulin is present in the blood and does facilitate glucose uptake by cells, but very slowly

myocardial infarction: blockage of artery to the heart resulting in tissue damage

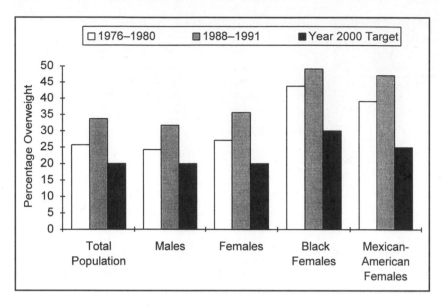

FIGURE 13–3. Prevalence of overweight among U.S. adults aged 20–74. Data are from the National Health and Nutrition Examination Surveys (NHANES) II (1976–1980) and III (Phase 1, 1988–1991), conducted by the National Center for Health Statistics. Target goals are from Healthy People 2000 (DHHS, 1991). (From Committee to Develop Criteria for Evaluating the Outcomes of Approaches to Prevent and Treat Obesity. Food and Nutrition Board. Washington, DC: National Academy Press, 1995.)

dividuals in a negative fashion. This is often reflected in discrimination toward those with excess body weight (Stunkard, 1993).

Etiology

The fundamental basis of obesity is imbalance between energy intake and expenditure, but underlying origins are multifactorial, reflecting genetic, environmental, metabolic, cultural, socioeconomic, and psychological factors.

Genetics

The observation that the adult weight of twins who have been raised in separate homes is very similar (Stunkard et al, 1990; Sorenson et al, 1992) suggests heredity is a strong determinant of body weight. Specific genes responsible for excessive fatness have been identified in animals. Researchers at Rockefeller University identified a gene, called the ob gene, that regulates energy balance in the mouse. Mutation of the ob gene results in profound obesity and type II diabetes as part of a syndrome that resembles morbid obesity in humans (Zhang et al, 1994). The ob gene is believed to regulate the size of the body fat depot by causing the formation of a signaling pattern or product that sends the satiety message to the brain. Recently scientists have isolated such a substance, called leptin, in the blood of human beings and have observed that obese individuals have elevated levels. It would appear that at least some obese persons lack receptors (probably controlled by another gene or genes) for leptin or have a problem with its transport to the brain (Rink, 1994).

Researchers are identifying an increasing number of obesity genes in animal models. Of particular relevance to human obesity are studies attempting to identify genes that increase the susceptibility of animals to gaining weight when fed high-fat diets. Diet-induced models of animal obesity may more closely mimic human obesity than the genetic model.

Regulation of Food Intake

Each day we make many choices about when, what, and how much we eat. While these decisions illustrate the voluntary nature of eating, there is a complex relationship between eating behavior and its molecular determinants (Hirsch, 1994). Most adults maintain a relatively constant body weight, and gains or losses are usually temporary as adipose tissue expands and contracts to accommodate variations in energy balance. Mechanisms that balance food intake and energy expenditure determine who will be obese and who will be lean.

Food intake appears to have both internal and external controls, which act cojointly to control hunger, satiety, and eating behavior (Fig. 13–4). These are integrated by the **cortex** of the brain. Internal controls are concerned with physiologic changes that signal depletion and need to ingest food or satiation and cessation of eating. External controls reflect a learned association between external stimuli and food intake that may modify the externally regulated eating behavior (Van Itallie et al, 1988). Internal control of body fat appears to be a relationship between long-term feeding regulation, which maintains the nutrient stores of the body, and short-term feeding regulation concerned with hunger and satiety.

TABLE 13-9 Health Risk Factors Associated with Obesity

Increased mortality
> >30% of weight for height, especially in younger age groups

Respiratory difficulties
> Pickwickian syndrome

Cardiovascular
> Coronary artery disease
>> Hypercholesterolemia
>> Myocardial infarction
> Hypertension

Cerebrovascular

Endocrine
> Non–insulin-dependent diabetes
> Irregular menstrual cycles
> Infertility

Increased obstetric risk
> Macrosomic infants
> Prolonged labor, delivery complications
> More gestational diabetes

Higher risk with surgery
> Fat layer must be dissected first
> Anesthesia needed longer
> Difficult to find blood vessel for intravenous infusion
> Increased sepsis and wound rupture

Gallbladder disease

Musculoskeletal problems
> Gout
> Osteoarthritis

Some skin disorders

Some forms of cancer
> Males: colon, rectum, prostate
> Females: gallbladder, breast, cervix, uterus, ovaries, endometrium

Psychological problems

---

gest food or satiation and cessation of eating. External controls reflect a learned association between external stimuli and food intake that may modify the externally regulated eating behavior (Van Itallie et al, 1988). Internal control of body fat appears to be a relationship between long-term feeding regulation, which maintains the nutrient stores of the body, and short-term feeding regulation concerned with hunger and satiety.

SHORT-TERM CONTROL   The **hypothalamus** is believed to be the internal physiologic regulator for hunger and satiety (Weingarten, 1985). The ventromedial nucleus appears to be the satiety center, whereas the lateral hypothalamic area acts as the feeding center. Signals from the body reach the hypothalamus via various neuro-

transmitters and **brain peptides**, which may stimulate, inhibit, or modulate feeding. The hypothalamus regulates the release of certain pituitary hormones that influence food intake via stimulation of the **autonomic nervous system**.

Within the biologic system, the control of hunger and satiety involves post-digestive signals from the gastrointestinal tract and the release of hormones when food is processed. Postprandial sensations of satiety appear to respond to the activity of intestinal nutrient receptors. Cholecystokinin (CCK), released by the duodenum in response to dietary lipids and peptides, causes satiety by desensitizing gastric nerves (Read et al, 1994).

LONG-TERM CONTROL   Depot fat appears to be primary in the long-term control of food intake, but the mechanisms by which this occurs are not clear. Recent research indicates that the activity level of adipose tissue **lipoprotein lipase** (LPL) is a regulator of body fat cell mass (Eckel, 1989). LPL facilitates fat storage. Lipoprotein lipase levels are elevated in obesity, which may be a primary defect that promotes the development of obesity or a defect secondary to the enlarged fat cells that develop as the result of obesity. The activity of LPL rises with weight loss and returns to lower values when weight is regained. This elevation of LPL with weight loss acts to enhance triglyceride storage. The net effect may be rapid regain of lost weight and greater difficulty with succeeding

KEY TERMS

cortex: a thin layer of gray matter on the surface of the cerebral hemisphere. It is responsible for higher mental functions, general movement, visceral functions, perception, and behavioral reactions and for the association and integration of these functions.
hypothalamus: a small gland in the midbasal brain area that controls and integrates peripheral autonomic mechanisms, endocrine activity, and many somatic functions, e.g., regulation of food intake, water balance, body temperature, and sleep
brain peptides: a chain of amino acids that can influence feeding functions, such as opioids, calcitonin, gastrin-releasing peptide, bombesin, cholecystokinin, thyrotropin-releasing hormone, and neurotensin
autonomic nervous system: autonomic, self-controlling, functionally independent; the portion of the nervous system concerned with regulation of the activity of cardiac muscles, smooth muscle, and glands
lipoprotein lipase: an enzyme located at the lining of the capillaries that promotes breakdown of circulating triglycerides and cell uptake of fatty acids.

TABLE 13–10 Mortality Ratios According to Variations in Weight*

Weight Group	Build and Blood Pressure Study 1959		American Cancer Society Study		Build and Blood Pressure Study 1979	
	Male	Female	Male	Female	Male	Female
20% Underweight	95	87	110	110	105	110
10% Underweight	90	89	100	95	94	97
10% Overweight	113	109	107	108	111	107
20% Overweight	125	121	121	123	120	110
30% Overweight	142	130	137	138	135	125
40% Overweight	167	—	162	163	153	136
50% Overweight	200	—	210	—	177	149
60% Overweight	250	—	—	—	210	167

* Mortality compared to body weights for which the mortality would be 100 as defined in each study.
From Van Itallie TB. Obesity: adverse effects on health and longevity. Am J Clin Nutr 1979;32:2723. © Am J Clin Nutr. American Society for Clinical Nutrition.

is approximately a fivefold increase in fat cell number from infancy to adulthood. It appears that in severely obese people (those with a BMI greater than 40) hyperplasia of adipocytes may continue as long as positive energy balance continues. Weight loss will diminish the size of adipocytes but not the number. Refeeding of animals that have lost weight seems to continue until fat cells return to their original size. Thus, adipose tissue appears to exert a regulatory function in energy intake. It has been speculated that leptin originates in adipose tissue and may

act as a long-term satiety hormone that defends the level of depot fat (Rink, 1994).

INSULIN RESISTANCE Excess body weight, especially abdominal fat, is associated with the development of non–insulin-dependent diabetes mellitus (NIDDM). Obesity may be an important environmental determinant of the manifestation of diabetes in genetically susceptible individuals. This condition is characterized by insulin resistance. When fat cells enlarge, their response to insulin is

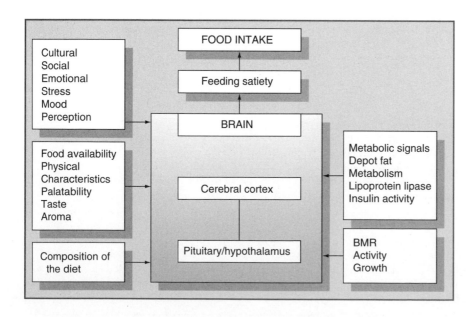

FIGURE 13–4. An overview of factors that regulate food intake.

diminished, even when insulin concentrations are high. Excess body fat is related to low levels of insulin receptors on the outer cell membrane and intracellular defects in glucose metabolism (Lillioja et al, 1988).

Energy Expenditure

The resting energy expenditure (REE) of obese persons expressed per kilogram of body weight generally is lower than that of lean individuals. Although differences in REE among individuals may seem to be small, a low REE and total 24-hour energy expenditure are significant predictors of gains in body weight, especially of regain of lost weight (Ravussin et al, 1992).

The most variable component of energy expenditure is that spent on physical activity. Data from the Health Professionals Follow-Up Study found that among 222,076 males, low levels of physical activity were related to the development of obesity (Ching et al, 1996). Nearly 60% of the adult population of the United States reports engaging in little or no leisure-time physical activity (Siegel et al, 1991).

Composition of the Diet

For years it has been assumed that all calories, regardless of their source, contribute equally to body energy needs and, if in excess, to obesity. Recent evidence indicates that body weight or BMI increases as the percentage of energy from fat increases (Alford et al, 1990). In addition, consumption of diets low in fat is associated with reduced body weight or fat and some increase in lean body mass (Prewitt et al, 1991; Rumpler et al, 1991).

Several theories have been proposed to explain this effect. The most popular maintains that a diet high in carbohydrate results in a spontaneous reduction in total energy intake. However, individuals fed **isocaloric** diets of varying fat content tend to gain weight on high fat intakes. Such observations have lead to suggestions that most dietary carbohydrate is oxidized or used to replenish glycogen stores instead of undergoing the metabolic expensive process of lipogenesis. In fact, it is estimated that on mixed diets, as little as 1% of dietary carbohydrate is synthesized as fat (Dattilo et al, 1992). In contrast, fat storage from dietary fat is believed to be metabolically efficient. Rising and co-workers (1996) found that over a period of 7 years (ages 31 to 38 years) there was a decline in fat utilization. They suggest that this contributes to the slow gain in weight and increase in body fat associated with aging.

Although there is substantial evidence of a genetic predisposition and aberrations in metabolic controls for obesity, environmental, and behavioral factors play a significant role in the development of obesity (Bouchard and Perusse, 1993; Roberts and Greenberg, 1996).

Intervention

Obesity is a chronic disorder with substantial comorbidities. Due to current limitations of treatment, increasing prevalence, high rate of recidivism, and significant associations with morbidity and mortality, intervention becomes a challenge (National Institutes of Health Assessment Conference Panel, 1992).

Benefits of Weight Reduction

HEALTH STATUS Obese individuals who lose even small amounts of weight are likely to improve their health by reducing the risk of comorbidities associated with obesity (Goldstein, 1992; Wadden et al, 1992; Institute of Medicine, 1995). Of adults with NIDDM, 80% to 90% are obese. If weight loss is maintained, insulin sensitivity improves and the need for oral hypoglycemic agents or insulin diminishes (Wing et al, 1991). Similarly, overweight hypertensives who lose weight have a significant reduction in both systolic and diastolic blood pressure that is proportional to weight loss (Stevens et al, 1993; Scotte and Stunkard, 1990). Among obese individuals, total serum cholesterol levels decrease in proportion to the amount of weight lost (Osterman et al, 1992). In one study a decrease of 5% to 6% in BMI was associated with reductions of 16% in total cholesterol and 12% in LDL cholesterol, decreasing the risk of cardiovascular disease (Seim and Holtmeier, 1992).

Weight loss results in improved functional status and greater ease in daily activities such as climbing stairs, getting in and out of an automobile, or going on and off a bus. Improved mobility allows the individual to participate in more physical activities, which may improve overall energy expenditure and health.

WEIGHT CYCLING More than 90% of weight loss programs are unsuccessful in the long term, and many individuals lose and gain hundreds of pounds in a succession of failed attempts at weight reduction. Recognition of this cycling of weight has raised concerns regarding the effects of repeatedly losing and gaining weight (Brownell and Rodin, 1994).

It is difficult to differentiate effects of weight cycling from preexisting health problems and individual motiva-

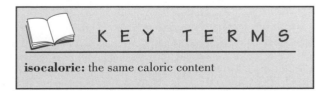

KEY TERMS

isocaloric: the same caloric content

tion (Williamson, 1996). Recently a National Task Force on the Prevention and Treatment of Obesity (1994) reviewed 43 studies (28 human studies) on the effects of weight change or weight cycling on humans or animals. The Task Force concluded that there is no convincing evidence that weight cycling in humans has adverse effects on body composition, energy expenditure, risk factors for cardiovascular disease, or the effectiveness of future efforts at weight loss. They concluded that there was insufficient information to evaluate the psychological impact of weight cycling.

LONG-TERM EFFECTS   Evidence that weight loss reduces mortality risk is meager. In fact, most epidemiologic studies indicate that weight loss is associated with increased mortality, especially for cardiovascular disease (Cutter, 1993). Such an observation is difficult to interpret because none of the current research studies separate intentional from unintentional weight loss or define characteristics associated with it such as diet, exercise, and physical fitness. Individuals who voluntarily lose weight may be those with the most severe disease and greatest motivation.

Weight Reduction Practices

According to the National Health Interview Survey, one-third of Americans consider themselves to be overweight. Fewer than two-thirds of those persons are trying to lose weight, however (Horm and Anderson, 1993). Among 60,681 respondents in the Behavioral Risk Factor Surveillance System telephone survey, 40% of women and 25% of men reported they were trying to lose weight and another 28% of both women and men were trying to maintain their weight (Williamson et al, 1992). A variety of weight reduction regimens have been utilized. Figure 13–5 summarizes the weight loss practices of adults from the FDA's 1992 Weight Loss Practices Survey. Dieting and exercise were the most common weight loss practices for both men and women. Exercise declined with increasing BMI for females but not males. As the BMI increased, participation in organized programs and use of diet supplements tended to increased. Among females, use of over-the-counter products and questionable dietary practices increased with increasing BMI (Levy and Heaton, 1993).

Treatment Approaches

If weight reduction is a primary goal, a plethora of weight loss programs are available. They vary in intensity of treatment, cost, nature of interventions, and degree of involvement of healthcare professionals. An individual may initiate his or her own program, join a commercial program, or enter clinical programs in which services are provided by licensed health professionals. Treatment has been divided into five broad approaches: diet, physical activity, behavior modification, drug therapy, and **gastric surgery** (In-

stitute of Medicine, 1995). Table 13–11 outlines these approaches, their characteristics, and considerations related to nutrition care.

Diets

BALANCED ENERGY DEFICIT DIETS   Balanced energy deficit diets provide 1200 kcal/day or more (22 to 25 kcal/kg of reference weight). These diets can be nutritionally adequate when the minimum number of servings in each group of the Food Guide Pyramid are included. For a 500 kcal/day energy deficit, weight loss would be approximately 0.25 kg/week. By normalizing food patterns, such diets have the potential for promoting permanent changes in eating patterns.

DECREASED DIETARY FAT   As discussed on page 363, when an individual decreases the percentage of energy from fat in the diet, loss of body weight and fat results. In addition, reduction of dietary fat is recommended for prevention of other chronic diseases, especially heart disease and cancer. Dietary changes to reduce fat can be accomplished easily at no risk or additional cost. Dietary patterns are gradually shifted toward lower-fat and lower-energy foods without perceptions of deprivation. This technique, referred to as nonrestrictive dieting, can be particularly important in the maintenance of weight loss.

LOW-CALORIE DIETS   Low-calorie diets provide approximately 800 to 1200 kilocalories per day. Some diets use regular foods while others are based on formulated or fortified products or prepackaged foods designed as meal replacements. For diets using limited amounts of food, a vitamin–mineral supplement may be necessary to meet nutrient recommendations. Weight loss averages 0.5 to 1.5 kg/week, or about 8.5 kg in 20 weeks. Physician approval and supervision from healthcare persons is desirable.

VERY-LOW-CALORIE DIETS (VLCD)   Very-low-calorie diets are modified fasts that provide fewer than 800 kcal/day. Programs utilizing VLCDs are based in hospitals or clinics and include commercial products. They are supervised and administered by a multidisciplinary team of healthcare professionals. Most of the formula products used provide 400 to 700 kcal, most of which is protein (0.8 to 1.5 g/kg reference weight) and up to 100 g of carbohydrate. These programs are usually restricted to individuals who are moderately to severely obese (BMI >30) and who have been unsuccessful in more traditional weight loss approaches or those with BMIs between 27 and 30 when comorbidities are present (National Task Force on the Prevention and Treatment of Obesity, 1993). Average weight loss, 20 kg over 20 weeks, is associated with improved glycemic control, decreased blood pressure, and reductions in total serum cholesterol, LDL cholesterol, and triglyceride levels (Kanders and Blackburn, 1993). In

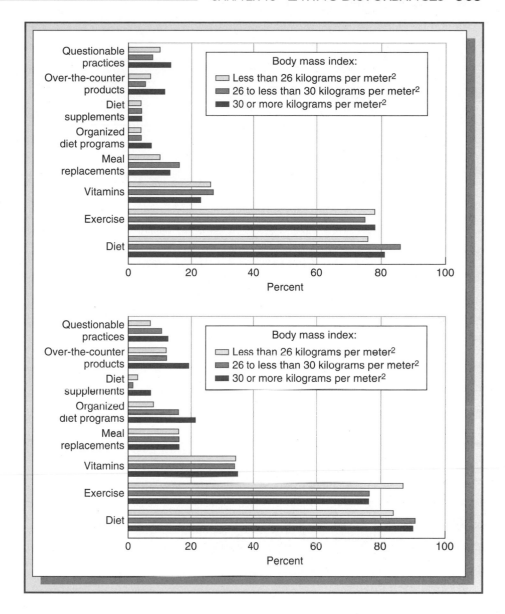

FIGURE 13–5. Weight loss practices by body mass index. (From Food and Drug Administration, Consumer Studies Branch, Weight Loss Practices Survey, 1991.)

the short term, these severely restricted diets generate a rapid weight loss, but long-term maintenance of that loss is limited. The comprehensive VLCD programs can be very expensive compared to other treatment modalities.

Physical Activity

If energy expenditure can be increased by physical activity while energy intake is kept constant, body weight will be reduced. The more vigorous the activity, the more energy stores are utilized. The amount of weight loss depends on the time and intensity of each activity. Success in improving physical fitness depends on selecting activities that appeal to the client and fit into her lifestyle constraints. Exercise has beneficial effects independent of

weight loss, including improved cardiovascular fitness and increased high-density lipoprotein cholesterol levels (Blair, 1995). Inclusion of resistance training can increase lean body mass. Exercise can be an important adjunct to

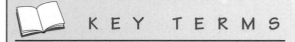

KEY TERMS

gastric surgery: consists of (1) surgical banding or stapling of the stomach to reduce capacity or (2) creation of a small gastric pouch that empties into the jejunum

TABLE 13–11 Approaches for Treating Obesity

Approach	Characteristics	Considerations
Balanced diet, reduced energy level 1200+ kcal/day	Nutritionally adequate Average weight loss 0.25 kg/wk for every 500 kcal/day deficit	Requires little supervision for individuals without underlying medical conditions Group support and monitoring by a healthcare professional have been shown to yield better results
Low energy diet 800–1200 kcal/day	Specially formulated or fortified products and/or prepackaged foods; may require vitamin/mineral supplementation Average weight loss of 0.5 to 1.5 kg/wk (8.5 kg over 20 weeks)	Safe, but need physician approval and supervision by a healthcare provider (especially for clients with comorbid conditions) Most regain weight lost in 5 years
Very-low-calorie diet Modified fast <800 kcal/day	Replace usual foods with supplements; supply 0.8–1.5 g high biologic value protein/ kg; minimum fat for EFA; RDAs for vitamins, minerals and electrolytes Average weight loss 20 kg over 12 wk. Most regain weight lost in 5 years.	Medically supervised and administered by a multidisciplinary team. BMI > 30 (moderate to severe obesity) who have failed at other weight loss therapies May also be appropriate for BMI 27–30 who have comorbid conditions
Physical activity Increased energy output	Ranges in intensity from walking to vigorous activities such as jogging and bicycling Weight loss related to time and intensity of exercise Activities that engage one's interest and lifestyle.	Should have realistic goal before starting Start at low level that feels comfortable and progress to high levels slowly Consult physician before starting.
Behavior modification	Principles include self monitoring, stimulus control, stress management, cognitive behavioral strategy, and social support Weight loss can be 0.5–0.75 kg/wk	All behavioral principles are useful to help individuals adhere to a healthy diet and exercise program and medication therapy. Principles and techniques are tailored to each person's specific problems.
Pharmacotherapy	Drugs currently used: catecholinergic and serotonin antagonists Weight loss 0.23 kg/week compared to placebo in clinical trials Most research based on use < 6 months Some side effects May help maintain lower body weight	If consider obesity chronic disease, need to consider long-term use of drugs. BMI ≥ 30; patients who are medically at risk because of their comorbid conditions Drugs are effective for as long as taken.
Gastric surgery Gastric banding; gastric bypass	Indicated for BMI >40 BMI 35–40 if high risk of comorobidity Substantial weight loss within 12 months Some regain after 2 to 5 years Weight loss improves comorbidity	Risk-benefit ratio must be evaluated for patient Risks—postsurgical complications

Compiled from Institute of Medicine. Weighing the options. Criteria for evaluating weight-management programs. Washington, DC: National Academy Press, 1995.

TABLE 13–12 Behavior Treatment Components

Component	Description	Examples
Self-monitoring	Recording of target behaviors and factors associated with behaviors	Keep food and exercise records; note moods, and environment associated with overeating.
Stimulus control	Restricting environmental factors associated with inappropriate behaviors	Keep away from high-fat foods; eat at specific times and places; set aside time and place for exercise.
Contingency management	Rewarding appropriate behaviors	Give prizes for achieving exercise goals.
Changing behavior parameters	Directly altering target behavior topology	Slow down eating; self-regulate exercise.
Cognitive-behavior modification	Changing thinking patterns related to target behaviors	Counter social pressure to be thin to reduce temptation to diet.

From Foreyt JP, Goodrick GK. Evidence for success of behavior modification in weight loss and control. Ann Intern Med 1993;19:699.

other weight reduction strategies and may diminish the tendency for rapid post-program weight gain (Zelasko, 1995).

Behavior Modification

Behavior treatment of obesity focuses on gradual changes to modify eating behavior and physical activity habits. It can be undertaken alone or through group or individual sessions, under the guidance of professional or lay personnel or in conjunction with other approaches. Principles used are self-monitoring, stimulus control, contingency management, stress management, cognitive behavior strategies and social support (Table 13–12). A typical behavior modification program takes about 16 to 20 weeks and can generate a 0.5 to 0.75 kg/week weight loss. Behavior modification is a method that supports other treatment approaches.

Pharmacotherapy

Recent recognition of obesity as a chronic disease has resulted in increased interest in medication to treat it. The most widely used prescription drugs for weight control are those that act on the neurotransmitters of the central nervous system. Phentermime acts on the nonadrenergic neurotransmitters dopamine and norepinephrine to suppress appetite. The serotonin **reuptake** inhibitors fenfluramine and dexfenfluramine raise brain serotonin levels inducing early satiety, decreased food intake, and increased basal energy expenditure (Bross and Hoffer, 1995).

Recent clinical trials with serotonin uptake inhibitors have demonstrated that these drugs enhance weight loss when used in combination with a diet and exercise program (Darga et al, 1991). In fact, a series of studies have shown that the drug can be used for up to 3.5 years to support weight loss and maintenance without major side effects (Weintraub, 1992). However, drugs should be used as only one component of a comprehensive weight reduction program.

The report of the NIH Workshop on Pharmacologic Treatment of Obesity concluded that pharmacologic agents may be effective in reducing body weight over an extended period of time (Atkinson and Hubbard, 1994). Additional research is needed on long-term efficacy and safety of drugs for obesity and especially for combinations of drugs.

Selecting a Treatment Approach

Healthy People 2000 objective 2.7 is to increase to at least 50% the proportion of overweight people aged 12 years and older who have adopted sound dietary practices combined with regular physical activity to attain an appropriate body weight. Success cannot be measured just by the amount of weight lost during a relatively short period. Appropriate goals are long-term amelioration of med-

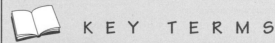

K E Y   T E R M S

reuptake: after a neurotransmitter is released from a neuron and performs its transmitting function, it is removed within seconds by breakdown or reuptake into the cell

Selecting a Treatment Approach

Healthy People 2000 objective 2.7 is to increase to at least 50% the proportion of overweight people aged 12 years and older who have adopted sound dietary practices combined with regular physical activity to attain an appropriate body weight. Success cannot be measured just by the amount of weight lost during a relatively short period. Appropriate goals are long-term amelioration of medical problems and health risks and improved quality of life with or without weight loss (Robinson et al, 1995). Approaches should be health oriented and related to lifestyle changes.

A weight loss treatment for an individual must match treatment approach(es) to the client on the basis of the degree of excess fat, the client's needs, and the kinds of programs available. Brownell and Wadden (1991) have developed a conceptual scheme that outlines these considerations (Fig. 13–6).

The potential benefits to be accrued from weight loss and an individual's potential to maintain such a loss should be considered carefully before a program is initiated. For example, if two women 163 cm (64 in) tall with a reference weight of 57 kg (125 lb) weighed 100 kg (220 lb), they would have a twofold increase in mortality risk. If the first woman is 60 years of age and has osteoarthritis, she will benefit from some weight loss to decrease the physical discomfort of standing and walking. However, because she has a limited ability to exercise, she will have difficulty attaining her reference weight and may not accrue benefits from such weight loss. By contrast, if the second woman were 20 years old with a family history of diabetes and hypertension, reducing to her reference weight could have lifetime benefits, and, because of her age and mobility, she is much more apt to succeed.

EXCESS WEIGHT ACROSS THE LIFE SPAN

Obesity in Childhood and Adolescence

In the United States obesity affects 27% of children and 21% of adolescents (U.S. Public Health Service, 1994). Of even greater concern is evidence that the prevalence of obesity is increasing (Gortmaker et al, 1987). This trend is greater among children in low-income populations (Okamoto et al, 1993) and those subjected to parental neglect (Lissau and Sorenson, 1994). Critical periods for development of obesity appear to occur during infancy, ages 5 to 7 years, and adolescence (Dietz, 1994).

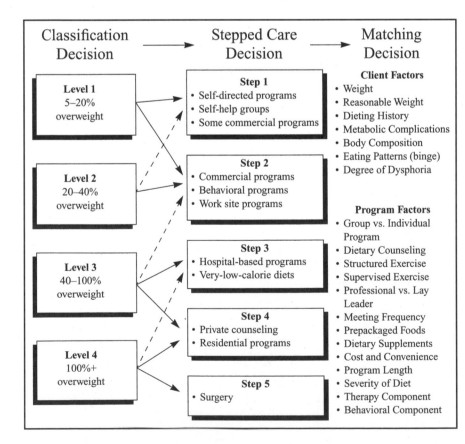

FIGURE 13–6. Conceptual scheme for matching individuals with treatments. (From Brownell KD, Wadden TA. The heterogeneity of obesity: fitting treatments to individuals. Behavior Therapy 1991;228:162. Reprinted with permission from the Association for Advancement of Behavior Therapy.)

TABLE 13–13 90th and 95th Percentile of Body Mass Index for Ages 1 through 19 Years				
Age (y)	**90th Percentile**		**95th Percentile**	
	Females	Males	Females	Males
1	18.6	19.4	19.3	19.9
2	18.0	18.4	18.7	19.0
3	17.6	17.8	18.3	18.4
4	17.5	17.5	18.2	18.1
5	17.5	17.3	18.3	18.0
6	17.7	17.4	18.8	18.1
7	18.5	17.7	19.7	18.9
8	19.4	18.4	21.0	19.7
9	20.8	19.3	22.7	20.9
10	21.8	20.3	24.2	22.2
11	23.0	21.3	25.7	23.5
12	23.7	22.3	26.8	24.8
13	24.7	23.3	27.9	25.8
14	25.3	24.4	28.6	26.8
15	26.0	25.4	29.4	27.7
16	26.5	26.1	30.0	28.4
17	27.1	27.0	30.5	29.0
18	27.4	27.7	31.0	29.7
19	27.7	28.3	31.3	30.1

From National Health and Nutrition Examination Survey (NHANESI), 1971 to 1974.

Assessment

Determination of obesity in childhood and adolescence is compounded by increases in height as well as weight and the changes in body composition associated with growth. BMIs at the 90th and 95th percentiles of BMI distribution at various ages are often used as criteria for obesity and "super" obesity respectively (Table 13–13). A frequently used assessment compares a child's weight for height to the NCHS growth charts (see Figs. 6–5 and 6–6 in Chapter 6). It is important to monitor weight changes over time. Figure 13–7 illustrates growth of a boy who could be considered obese from ages 2 to 8 years. The increase in weight is out of proportion to gains in stature.

A triceps fatfold that exceeds the 85th percentile is a common definition of obesity. A more definitive measurement of childhood obesity would be a combination of triceps and subscapular fat folds that exceed the 80th percentile and a weight greater than the 75th percentile (Rocchini, 1993). Obesity in adolescents is often defined by a weight greater than the 95th percentile and a BMI

greater than 30 (Himes and Dietz, 1994).

Health Risks

RISK OF BECOMING OBESE ADULTS The longer the duration of obesity, the greater is the likelihood that excess body weight will be sustained into adulthood. Although less than 10% of infants who are obese become obese adults, the risk increases to approximately one-third for obese preschool children, 50% for school-age children (Serdula et al, 1993), and 70% to 80% for obese adolescents (Kolata, 1986). In addition, the more severe the disease in childhood, the greater the chance of persistence into adulthood (Serdula et al, 1993; DiPietro et al, 1994, Guo et al, 1994). Risk of obesity in adolescents is associated with early maturation (van Lenthe et al, 1996). There are some gender differences in the effect of childhood weight on adult weight. A 50-year follow-up of individuals who were enrolled in the Harvard Growth Study of 1922–35 at ages 13 to 18 years found that the BMI in childhood and adolescence was a predictor of body size in middle-aged males but not in females (Casey et al, 1992).

IMMEDIATE HEALTH EFFECTS A variety of somatic changes accompany obesity in youth. Height and bone age are increased above the norms expected for children of the same age and gender. Lean body mass (LBM) is increased to support the additional weight and may account for as much as 50% of the excess weight in obese adolescents.

Some of the greatest concerns about obesity in childhood center around increased health risks. As many as 80% of obese adolescents have been found to have elevated systolic or diastolic blood pressure, and 97% already had known risk factors for heart disease, including elevated serum triglyceride and cholesterol levels and decreased high-density lipoprotein (HDL) cholesterol levels (Becque et al, 1988). The relationship of intra-abdominal fat to insulin resistance, hypertension, and hyperlipidemia, observed to increase risk in adults, is present in obese adolescent girls (Caprio et al, 1996).

There is strong prejudice against obese persons regardless of age, gender, race, and socioeconomic status. Such discrimination may be particularly devastating for children, who have little control over their own environments. Obese children experience discrimination by teachers and even parents, but that manifested by peers can be particularly damaging to the child's self esteem (Hill and Silver, 1995). Children as young as 5 years of age, when asked to describe silhouettes of obese youngsters characterized them as lazy, stupid, ugly, cheats, and liars, and consistently rank them as less desirable than children with other handicaps (Staffieri, 1967).

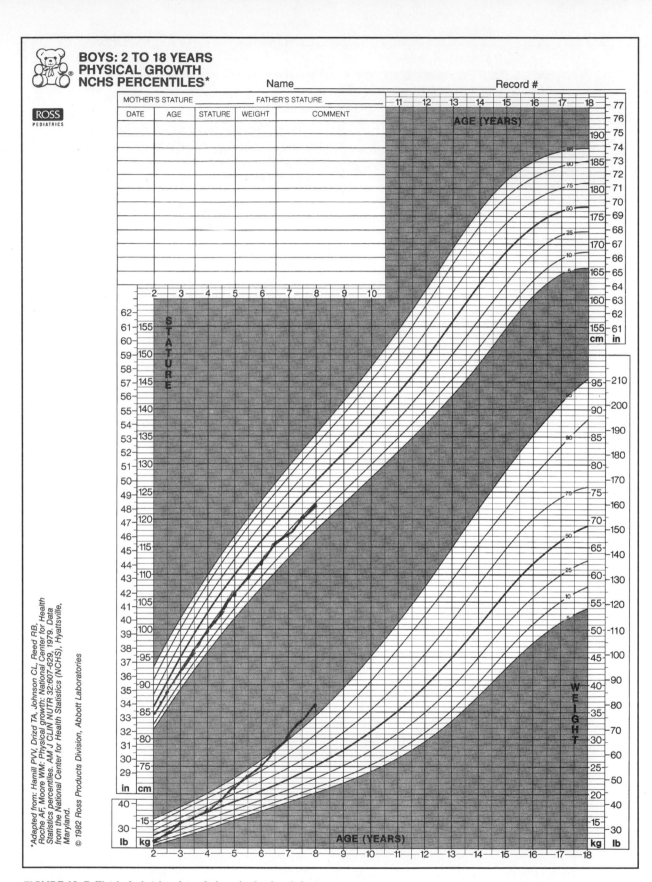

FIGURE 13-7. Weight for height values of a boy who developed obesity

Etiology of Obesity During Growth

Multiple factors contribute to excess of body fat in childhood. In addition to dietary intake and physical activity patterns, the development of obesity in childhood may be influenced by a breakdown in family interactions that precipitates inappropriate food behavior.

Children generally eat best when their parents are neither over-managing nor over-permissive (Burroughs and Terry, 1992). Birch and co-workers (1981) observed that mothers of fatter 4- to 8-year-old children talked less to their children during mealtimes, were less responsive, gave less approval, and made fewer efforts to control inappropriate behavior during mealtime. If the parent is too involved or attempts to manipulate the child's eating, the child may feel too uncomfortable and overeat. A disinterested parent who fails to provide guidance, or who is so enmeshed that he can't say no, may make the child too comfortable. A disengaged family relationship may fail to provide the love and care that a particular child needs for a positive sense of self, leading to emotional overeating and obesity.

ENERGY BALANCE Although the body size of American children has increased over the last several decades, energy intakes have remained relatively stable (Schlicker et al, 1994). For example, a comparison of the intakes of children and adolescents studied in the 1977–1978 and the 1987–1988 National Food Consumption Surveys (NFCS) found that energy and fat intakes were less in 1987–1988 than a decade earlier (Gazzaniga and Burns, 1993). Such observations have led to suggestions that the increase in childhood obesity in the United States is associated with decreased physical activity.

It has been observed that obese youngsters expend more total energy than their leaner peers on a daily basis (Bandini et al, 1990), but expenditure per kilogram of body weight is comparable (Maffels et al, 1993). When energy expenditure was calculated on the basis of lean body mass, there were no differences between obese and nonobese youths. Such observations have led to suggestions that obese children are less physically active than leaner children.

Two large-scale surveys have assessed the behavior of American children and adolescents related to physical activity. The first, using self-reported frequency and duration, determined that most youngsters between the ages of 10 and 17 years had 1 to 2 hours of moderate to vigorous physical activity per day (Pate and Ross, 1987). However, 20% to 30% of the youths reported averaging less than one-half hour of physical activity per day.

In the second study of high school students, half of the males and three-quarters of the females reported participating in moderate or vigorous activity three or fewer times per week (Sallis, 1993). Girls tended to be less physically active than boys, and there was a consistent decline in physical activity over the school years.

A number of studies have shown that physical activity is inversely related to adiposity. An analysis of data from one national study found that 6- to 9-year-old children who were less physically active (based on reports of parents and teachers) tended to have thicker fatfolds (Pate et al, 1990). However, such observations must be interpreted cautiously. It may be that physical inactivity "causes" greater adiposity. It is also possible that higher levels of adiposity predispose youngsters to a less active lifestyle.

Prevention and Treatment

The most practical intervention to prevent obesity in youngsters is to modify the environment in terms of habitual physical activity and food intake. It is vital that tactics be moderate and positive and promote realistic changes while doing no harm. The essential task is to create a structure in which the child's natural ability to regulate food intake is distorted as little as possible by outside influences.

BENEFITS OF TREATMENT There are several benefits to reducing obesity in childhood. In the long term, the most important is the prevention of adult obesity and related hypertension, cardiovascular disease, and diabetes. Short-term benefits include improved fitness, decreased blood pressure and glucose, and a more favorable lipid profile (Sutter and Hawes, 1993). Knip and Nuutinen (1992) reported that weight loss in a group of 32 obese children was associated with decreased levels of serum triglycerides and plasma insulin concentrations and increased high-density-lipoprotein cholesterol levels.

Therapy for or prevention of obesity in childhood or adolescence is complicated and must be sensitive to the child's needs—physical, nutritional, and emotional. A major concern in controlling gains in body weight or fat during growth is that long-term growth might be impaired. A recent study reported that moderate energy restriction in children aged 6 to 12 years did not negatively influence long-term growth after 10 years (Epstein et al, 1993).

DIET AND EXERCISE It is vital that any dietary intervention for obesity provide adequate energy and nutrients to support normal growth patterns, allowing the child to grow into her body. Appropriate goals involve decreasing energy intake and increasing energy output. The results of a number of controlled intervention studies suggest that increased physical activity can modestly decrease or slow the increase in adiposity in obese youth (Sasaki et al, 1987; Epstein et al, 1990). Physical activity as a singular intervention can have a beneficial effect on body composition in obese youngsters, but that intervention is more likely to be effective if dietary changes and behavior modification techniques are used in combination with increased physical activity. Important guidelines for parents are as follows:

- Encourage good eating habits and an exercise routine by being a good role model.
- Take a positive approach. Talk more about making the right food choices rather than about not making poor choices.
- Find out what your child's eating patterns are when he or she is away from home. Then, plan snacks and meals to balance the daily intake of kilocalories, fat, and micronutrients.
- Establish family eating habits that will allow the child to grow and develop normally while keeping his or her body weight under control.
- Make moderate exercise a regular and enjoyable part of your child's life.

FAMILY THERAPY   Parents are very important in determining the behavior of their children. Family therapy assumes that children need parental support and family cohesion to make changes in eating and physical activity habits (Mellin and Frost, 1992). Focus is on the family system and attempts to modify how the family solves problems and resolves conflicts. It involves teaching the child to connect with people rather than food when he is distressed. Support from the entire family promotes long-term changes in behavior such as diet and exercise. In a recent study that involved diet and exercise with and without family therapy, it was observed that adding family therapy to intervention programs improved outcomes as measured by weight, fatfolds, and physical fitness (Floodmark et al, 1993).

Older Adults

The association of excess body weight with mortality and morbidity decreases as aging progresses, and the body weight associated with lowest mortality increases as age advances (Lissner et al, 1991). Data from the NHANES II show that overweight adults aged 45 to 75 years have a lower risk of hypertension and diabetes and higher serum cholesterol levels than those younger than 45 years (Van Itallie, 1985). Although such observations have resulted in higher relative weight standards for older adults (Andres et al, 1985), avoidance of obesity and moderate increases in physical activity are associated with longevity in middle-aged men (Paffenbarger et al, 1993).

Excess body weight in older adults means greater stress on joints that are often arthritic and greater demand on the respiratory and cardiovascular systems. However, it may be exceedingly difficult for older persons to lose weight because of decreased energy expenditure associated with lower basal metabolic rates and reduced activity levels. Women over 65 years are at greater disadvantage than men due to lower energy requirements. When energy needs are as low as 1200 to 1600 kcal/day, most food choices must be restricted to those from the Food Guide Pyramid with relatively little room for calorie-dense foods rich in sugars and fats. Some flexibility may be gained by increasing energy output via a program of exercise.

CONCEPTS TO REMEMBER

▶ Behaviors associated with eating disturbances cover a spectrum from semi-starvation to unhealthy dietary practices to binging and purging to compulsive overeating.

▶ Eating disturbances have potential serious negative psychological and physiologic consequences.

▶ The etiology of eating disorders (anorexia nervosa, bulimia nervosa, and binge eating disorder) is complex and has biologic, social, psychological, and environmental parameters.

▶ Success in treating eating disorders is related to the severity and duration of the disorder and to family circumstances. Therefore, multidisciplinary approaches for prevention, early recognition, and intervention are important.

▶ Obesity, the most common nutrition-related health problem of Americans, has substantial psychological, social, physiologic, and health consequences.

▶ Obesity is a chronic disease for which long-term treatment approaches are needed.

▶ Treatment programs for obesity must be individualized to meet the needs and lifestyles of the individual.

▶ For very obese individuals, pharmacotherapy and gastric surgery may be treatment alternatives.

▶ Obesity is a health concern across all stages of the life span.

References

Abrams KK, et al. Disordered eating attitudes and behaviors, psychological adjustment, and ethnic identity: a comparison of black and white female college students. Int J Eating Dis 1994;14:49.

Agras WS, et al. One year follow-up of psychosocial and pharmacologic treatments for bulimia nervosa. J Clin Psychiatry 1994;55:179.

Alford BB, et al. The effects of variations in carbohydrate, protein and fat content of the diet upon weight loss, blood values, and nutrient intake of adult obese women. J Am Diet Assoc 1990;90:534.

American Dietetic Association. Position of the American Dietetic Association: Nutrition intervention in the treatment of anorexia nervosa, bulimia nervosa and binge eating. J Am Diet Assoc 1994;94:902.

American Psychiatric Association. Practice guidelines for eating disorders. Am J Psychiatry 1993;150:212.

American Psychiatric Association. Diagnostic and statistical manual for mental disorders. 4th ed. (DSM-IV). Washington, DC: American Psychiatric Association Press, 1994.

Andres R, et al. Impact of age on weight goals. Ann Intern Med 1985;103:1030.

Antony MM, et al. Psychopathology correlates of binge eating and binge eating disorder. Compr Psychiatry 1994;35:386.

Atkinson RL, Hubbard VS. Report on the NIH Workshop on Pharmacologic Treatment of Obesity. Am J Clin Nutr 1994;60:153.

Ayuso-Gutierrez JL, et al. Open trial of fluroxamine in the treatment of bulimia nervosa. Int J Eating Dis 1994;15:245.

Bachrach LK, et al. Decreased bone density in adolescent girls with anorexia nervosa. Pediatrics 1990;86:440.

Bandini LG, et al. Energy expenditure in obese and nonobese adolescents. Ped Res 1990;27:198.

Becque MD, et al. Coronary risk incidence of obese adolescents: reductions with exercise plus diet intervention. Pediatrics 1988;81:605.

Beumont PJV, et al. Excessive physical activity in dieting disorder patients: proposals for a supervised exercise program. Int J Eating Dis 1994;15:21.

Birch LL, et al. Mother-child interaction patterns and the degree of fatness in children. J Nutr Educ 1981;13:17.

Bjorntorp P. Classification of obese patients and complications related to distribution of surplus fat. Am J Clin Nutr 1987;45(suppl):1120.

Blackburn GL, et al. Report of the American Institute of Nutrition (AIN) Steering Committee on Healthy Weight. J Nutr 1994;124:2240.

Blair SN. Diet and activity: the synergistic merger. Nutr Today 1995;30:108.

Bouchard C, Perusse L. Genetics of obesity. Ann Rev Nutr 1993;13:337.

Bouchard C, et al, eds. Exercise, fitness and health. Champaign, IL: Human Kinetics, 1990.

Brambilla F, et al. Combined cognitive behavioral, psychopharmacological and nutritional therapy in bulimia nervosa. Neuropsychobiology 1995;32:68.

Brewerton TD, et al. Neuroendocrine response to m-chorophenylpiperazine and L-tryptophan. Arch Gen Psychiatry 1992;49:852.

Brody ML, et al. Binge eating disorder: reliability and validity of a new diagnostic category. J Consult Clin Psychol 1994;62:381.

Bross R, Hoffer LJ. Fluoxetine increases resting energy expenditure and basal body temperature. Am J Clin Nutr 1995;61:1020.

Brown NW. Anorexia nervosa visited and revisited: Weight is the issue. JAMWA 1993;48:23.

Brownell KD, Rodin J. Medical, metabolic and psychological effects on weight cycling. Arch Int Med 1994;154:1325.

Brownell KD, Wadden TA. The heterogeneity of obesity: fitting treatments to individuals. Behavior Therapy 1991;228:162.

Bruce B, Wilfley D. Binge eating among the overweight populations: a serious and prevalent problem. J Am Diet Assoc 1996;96:58.

Bruch H. Eating disorders. New York: Basic Books, 1973.

Burroughs ML, Terry RD. Parents' perspectives toward their children's eating behavior. Top Clin Nutr 1992;8:45.

Caprio S, et al. Fat distribution and cardiovascular risk factors in obese adolescent girls: importance of the intraabdominal fat depot. Am J Clin Nutr 1996;64:12.

Carlat D, Camargo C. Review of bulimia nervosa in males. Am J Psychiatry 1991;148:831.

Casey VA, et al. Body mass index from childhood to middle age: a 50 year follow-up. Am J Clin Nutr 1992;56:14.

Ching PLYH, et al. Activity level and risk of overweight in male health professionals. Am J Publ Health 1996;86:25.

Collings S, King M. Ten-year follow-up of 50 patients with bulimia nervosa. Brit J Psychiatry 1994;164:80.

Crisp AH. A controlled study of the effect of therapies aimed at adolescent and family psychopathology in anorexia nervosa. Br J Psychiatry 1991;159:325.

Crow SJ, Mitchell JE. Rational therapy of eating disorders. Drugs 1994;48:372.

Cutter GR. Obesity and the implications of weight loss (is there death after success?) Perspect Appl Nutr 1993;1:3.

Darga LL, et al. Fluoxetine's effect on weight loss on obese subjects. Am J Clin Nutr 1991;54:321.

Dattilo AM. Dietary fat and its relationship to body weight. Nutr Today 1992;27:13.

Davies MC, et al. Bone mineral loss in young women with amenorrhea. Brit Med J 1990;301:790.

Davis C, et al. Behavioral frequency and psychological commitment: necessary concepts in the study of excessive exercising. J Behav Med 1993;16:611.

Denke MA, et al. Excess body weight. An under-recognized contributor to high blood cholesterol levels in white American men. Arch Int Med 1993;153:93.

Dietz WH. Critical periods in childhood for the development of obesity. Am J Clin Nutr 1994;59:955.

DiPietro L, et al. A 40-year history of overweight children in Stockholm: life-time overweight, morbidity, and mortality. Int J Obesity 1994;18:85.

Drewnowski A, et al. Naloxone, an opiate blocker, reduces the consumption of sweet high-fat foods in obese and lean female binge eaters. Am J Clin Nutr 1995;61:1206.

Drewnowski A, et al. Food preferences in human obesity: carbohydrates versus fats. Appetite 1992;18:207.

Drewnowski A, et al. The prevalence of bulimia nervosa in the U.S. college student population. Am J Public Health 1988;78:1322.

Eckel RH. Lipoprotein lipase: a multifactorial enzyme relevant to common metabolic disease. N Engl J Med 1989;320:1060.

Epstein LH. Growth in obese children treated for obesity. Am J Dis Child 1990;144:1360.

Epstein LH, et al. Effect of weight loss by obese children on long-term growth. Am J Dis Child 1993;147:1076.

Fairburn CG, et al. Three psychosocial treatments for bulimia: a comparative trial. Arch Gen Psychiatry 1991;48:463.

Fisher M, et al. Eating disorders in adolescents: a background paper. J Adolesc Health 1995;16:420.

Floodmark CE, et al. Prevention of progression to severe obesity in a group of obese schoolchildren treated with family therapy. Pediatrics 1993;91:880.

Fluoxetine Bulimia Nervosa Collaborative Study Group. Fluoxetine in the treatment of bulimia nervosa. Arch Gen Psychiatry 1992;49:139.

Fukagawa N. Eating disorders: diagnosis and management. Semin Pediatr Gastroenterol Nutr 1992;3:1.

Garfinkel PE, Kaplan AS. Starvation-based perpetuatory mechanisms in anorexia nervosa and bulimia. Int J Eating Dis 1985;4:651.

Garfinkel PE, et al. A comparison of characteristics in the families of patients with anorexia nervosa and normal controls. Psychol Med 1983;13:821.

Gasser T, et al. Measures of body mass and of obesity from infancy to childhood and their appropriate transformations. Ann Human Biol 1994;21:111.

Gazzaniga JM, Burns TL. Relationship between diet composition and body fatness, with adjustment for resting energy expenditure and physical activity in pre-adolescent children. Am J Clin Nutr 1993;58:21.

Geracioti TD, Liddle RA. Impaired cholecystokinin secretion in bulimia nervosa. N Engl J Med 1988;319:683.

Goldstein DJ. Beneficial health effects of modest weight loss. Int J Obesity 1992;16;397.

Goodsitt A. Self-regulatory disturbances in eating disorders. Int J Eating Dis 1983;2:52.

Gortmaker SL. Increasing pediatric obesity in the United States. Am J Dis Child 1987;141:535.

Gortmaker SL, et al. Social and economic consequences of overweight in adolescence and young adulthood. N Engl J Med 1993;329;1008.

Gralen SJ, et al. Dieting and disordered eating during early and middle adolescence. Do the influences remain the same? Int J Eating Dis 1990;9:501.

Grant CL, Fodor IG. Adolescent attitudes toward body image and anorexic behavior. Adolescence 1986;23:269.

Gross J, Rosen JC. Bulimia in adolescents: Prevalence and psychosocial correlates. Int J Eating Dis 1988;7:51.

Guo S, et al. The predictive value of childhood body mass index values for overweight at age 35 years. Am J Clin Nutr 1994;59:810.

Gustafson-Larson AM, Terry RD. Weight-related behaviors of fourth-grade children. J Am Diet Assoc 1992;92:818.

Haller E. Eating disorders: a review and update. West J Med 1992;157:658.

Halmi KA, et al. Comorbidity of psychiatric diagnoses in anorexia nervosa. Arch Gen Psychiatry 1991;48:712.

Hauck ER, Blumenthal JA. Obsessive and compulsive traits in athletes. Sports Med 1992;14:215.

Herzog DB, et al. Bulimia nervosa in adolescence. J Devel Behav Pediatr 1991;12:191.

Hill AJ, Silver EK. Fat, friendless and unhealthy: 9-year old children's perception of body shape stereotypes. Int J Obesity 1995;19:423.

Himes JH, Dietz WH. Guidelines for overweight in adolescent preventive services: recommendations from an expert committee. Am J Clin Nutr 1994;59:307.

Hirsch J. Herman Award Lecture, 1994: Establishing a biologic basis for human obesity. Am J Clin Nutr 1994;60:615.

Horm J, Anderson K. Who in America is trying to lose weight? Ann Intern Med 1993;119:672.

Hsu LKG. Eating disorders. New York: Guilford Press, 1990.

Institute of Medicine. Weighing the options. Criteria for evaluating weight-management programs. Food and Nutrition Board. Washington, DC: National Academy Press, 1995.

Kanders BS, Blackburn GL. Very low calorie diets for the treatment of obesity. In: Blackburn GL, Ganders BS, eds. Obesity: pathophysiology, psychology and treatment. New York: Guilford Press, 1993.

Killen JD, et al. Depressive symptoms and substance use among adolescent binge eaters and purgers: a defined population study. Am J Public Health 1987;77:1539.

Knip M, Nuutinen O. Long-term effects of weight reduction in serum lipid and plasma insulin in obese children. Am J Clin Nutr 1992;57:490.

Kolata G. Obesity in children: a growing problem. Science 1986;232:20.

Kral J, et al. Assessment of quality of life before and after surgery for severe obesity. Am J Clin Nutr 1992;55(suppl):611S.

Kuczmarski RJ. Prevalence of overweight and weight gain in the United States. Am J Clin Nutr 1992;55:495S.

Kuczmarski RJ, et al. Increasing prevalence of overweight among U.S. adults: The National Health and Nutrition Examination Surveys, 1960 to 1991. JAMA 1994;272:205.

Kumanyika SK. Obesity in minority populations. Obes Res 1994;2:166.

Kushner RF. Body weight and mortality. Nutr Rev 1993;51:127.

Lancelot C, et al. Comparison of DSM-III and DSM-III-R bulimia nervosa classifications for psychopathology and other eating behaviors. Int J Eating Dis 1991;10:57.

Larsson B, et al. Is abdominal body fat distribution a major explanation for the sex difference in the incidence of myocardial infarction? Am J Epidemiol 1992;135:266.

Lee I, et al. Body weight and mortality. A 27-year follow-up of middle aged men. JAMA 1993;270:2823.

Levy AS, Heaton AW. Weight control practices in U.S. adults trying to lose weight. Ann Int Med 1993;119:661.

Lilloja S, et al. Impaired glucose tolerance as a disorder of insulin action. N Engl J Med 1988;318:217.

Lissau L, Sorensen TIA. Parental neglect during childhood and increased risk of obesity in young adulthood. Lancet 1994;343:324.

Lissner L, et al. Variability of body weight and health outcomes on the Framingham population. N Engl J Med 1991;324:1839.

Loro AD, Orleans CS. Binge eating in obesity: preliminary findings and guidelines for behavioral analyses and treatments. Addict Behav 1981;6:155.

Lucas AR, et al. 50-year trends in the incidence of anorexia nervosa in Rochester, MN: a population-based study. Am J Psychiatry 1991;148:917.

Maffels C, et al. Resting metabolic rate in six- to ten-year-old obese and nonobese children. J Pediatr 1993;122:556.

Manson JE, et al. Body weight and mortality among women. N Engl J Med 1995;333:677.

Manson J, et al. A prospective study of obesity and risk of coronary heart disease in women. N Engl J Med 1990; 322:882.

Manson JE, et al. Body weight and longevity: a reassessment. JAMA 1987;257:353.

Marcus MD. Binge eating in obesity. In: Fairburn CG, Wilson GT, eds. Binge eating: nature, assessment and treatment. New York: Guilford Press, 1993.

Matkovic V. Calcium intake and peak bone mass [editorial]. N Engl J Med 1992;327:120.

McCann UD, et al. Nonpurging bulimia: a distinct subtype of bulimia nervosa. Int J Eating Dis 1991;10:679.

Mellin LM, Frost L. Child and adolescent obesity: the nurse practitioner's use of the SHAPEDOWN method. J Ped Health Care 1992;6:187.

Mitchell JE, et al. Medical complications and medical management of bulimia. Am Inter Med 1987;107:71.

Moore DC. Body image and eating behavior in adolescent girls. Am J Dis Child 1988;142:1114.

Must A, et al. Long-term morbidity and mortality of overweight adolescents. N Engl J Med 1992;327:1350.

National Institutes of Health Consensus Development Conference statement. Health implications of obesity. Ann Intern Med 1985;103:147.

National Institutes of Health, Methods for Voluntary Weight Loss and Control. Technology Assessment Conference Statement. Nutr Today 1992;94.

National Task Force on the Prevention and Treatment of Obesity: Weight cycling. JAMA 1994;272:1196.

National Task Force on the Prevention and Treatment of Obesity: Very low calorie diets. JAMA 1993;270:967.

National Task Force on the Prevention and Treatment of Obesity: Research directions. Obesity Res 1994;2:571.

Neumark-Sztainer D. Excessive weight preoccupation. Nutr Today 1995;30:68.

Obarzanek E, et al. Resting metabolic rate of anorexia nervosa patients during weight gain. Am J Clin Nutr 1994;60:666.

Okamoto E, et al. High prevalence of overweight in inner-city school children. Am J Dis Child 1993;147:155.

Olmsted MP, et al. Rate and prediction of relapse in bulimia nervosa. Am J Psychiatry 1994;151:738.

Osterman J, et al. Serum cholesterol profiles during treatment of obese outpatients with a very low calorie diet: effect of initial cholesterol levels. Int J Obes 1992;216:49.

Paffenbarger RS, et al. The association of changes of physical activity level and other lifestyle characteristics with mortality among men. N Engl J Med 1993;328:538.

Pate RR, et al. Associations between physical activity and physical fitness in American children. Am J Dis Child 1990;144:1123.

Pate RR, Ross JG. The national children and youth fitness study II: factors associated with health-related fitness. J Phys Educ Recreation Dance 1987;58:93.

Pierce EF. Exercise dependence syndrome in runners. Sports Med 1994;18:149.

Pope HG Jr, Hudson H. Antidepressant drug therapy for bulimia: current status. J Clin Psychiatry 1986;47:339.

Prewitt ET, et al. Changes in body weight, body composition and energy in lean women fed high- and low-fat diets. Am J Clin Nutr 1991;54:304.

Rastam M, Gillberg C. The family background in anorexia nervosa: a population-based study. J Am Acad Child Adolesc Psychiatry 1991;30:283.

Ravussin E, Swinburn A. Pathophysiology of obesity. Lancet 1992;340:404.

Read N, et al. The role of the gut in regulating food intake in men. Nutr Rev 1994;52:1.

Reaven FM, et al. Insulin resistance and hyperinsulinemia in individuals with small, dense low density lipoprotein particles. J Clin Invest 1993;92:141.

Reiss D, et al. Bulimia nervosa: 5-year social outcome and relationship to eating pathology. Int J Eating Dis 1995;18:127.

Rink TJ. In search of a satiety factor. Nature 1994;372:406.

Rising R, et al. Decreased ratio of fat to carbohydrate oxidation with increasing age in Pima Indians. J Am Coll Nutr 1996;15:309.

Roberts SB, Greenberg AS. The new obesity genes. Nutr Rev 1996;54:41.

Robinson JI, et al. Redifining success in obesity intervention: the new paradigm. J Am Diet Assoc 1995;95:422.

Rocchini AP. Adolescent obesity and hypertension. Pediatr Clin North Am 1993;40:81.

Rumpler WV, et al. Energy-intake restriction and diet composition effects on energy expenditure in men. Am J Clin Nutr 1991;53:430.

Russell GFM, et al. An evaluation of family therapy in anorexia nervosa and bulimia nervosa. Arch Gen Psychiatry 1987;44:1047.

Salisbury JJ, et al. Refeeding, metabolic rate, and weight gain in anorexia nervosa: a review. Int J Eating Dis 1995;17:337.

Sallis JF. Epidemiology of physical activity and fitness in children and adolescents. Crit Rev Food Sci Nutr 1993;33:403.

Sasaki J, et al. A long-term aerobic exercise program decreases the obesity index and increases the high density cholesterol concentration in obese children. Int J Obesity 1987;11:339.

Schebendach J, et al. The use of indirect calorimetry in the nutritional management of eating disorders. Int J Eating Dis 1995;14:59.

Schlicker SA, et al. The weight and fitness status of United States children. Nutr Rev 1994;52:11.

Schotte DE, Stunkard AJ. The effects of weight reduction on blood pressure in 301 obese patients. Arch Intern Med 1990;150:1701.

Schwartz DM, Thompson MG. Do anorexics get well? Current research and future needs. Am J Psychiatry 1981;138:319.

Seim HC, Holtmeier KB. Effects of a six-week, low-fat diet on serum cholesterol, body weight, and body measurements. Fam Pract Res J 1992;12:411.

Serdula MK. Do obese children become obese adults? A review of literature. Prev Med 1993;22:167.

Siegel PZ, et al. Behavioral Risk Factor Surveillance, 1986–1990. MMWR 1991;40 (no. SS-4):1.

Sjostrom L. Morbidity of severely obese subjects. Mortality of severely obese subjects. Am J Clin Nutr 1992;55(suppl):508S, 516S.

Solanto MV, et al. Rate of weight gain of inpatients with anorexia nervosa under two behavioral contracts. Pediatrics 1994;93:989.

Sorenson TIA, et al. Childhood body mass index: genetic and familial environmental influences assessed in a longitudinal adoption study. Int J Obesity 1992;16:705.

Specker S, et al. Psychotherapy in subgroups of obese women with and without binge eating disorder. Compr Pyschiatry 1994;35:185.

Spitzer RL, et al. Binge eating disorder: its further validation in a multisite study. Int J Eating Dis 1993;13:137.

Staffieri, RR. A study of social stereotype of body image in children. J Pers Soc Psychol 1967;7:101.

Stevens SA. Weight loss intervention in phase I of the Trials of Hypertensive Prevention. Arch Int Med 1993;153:849.

Stewart DE. Reproductive functions in eating disorders. Ann Med 1992;24:287.

Strober M. Stressful life events associated with bulimia in anorexia nervosa: empirical findings and theoretical speculations. Int J Eating Dis 1984;3:3.

Stunkard AJ. Talking with patients. In: Stunkard AJ, Wadden TA, eds. Obesity: theory and therapy. 2nd. ed. New York: Raven Press, 1993.

Stunkard AJ. Eating patterns and obesity. Psychiatric Quest 1959;33:284.

Stunkard AJ, et al. The body mass index of twins who have been reared apart. N Engl J Med 1990;322:1483.

Stunkard AJ, et al. An adoption of human obesity. N Engl J Med 1986;314:193.

Sundgot-Borgen J. Nutrient intake of female elite athletes suffering from eating disorders. Int J Sport Nutr 1993;3:431.

Sutter E, Hawes MR. Relationship of physical activity, body fat, diet and blood lipid profile in youths 10–15 years. Med Sci Sports Exerc 1993;25:748.

Swift WJ, et al. Self-concept in adolescent anorexics. J Am Acad Child Psychiatry 1986;25:826.

Thiel A, et al. Obsessive compulsive disorder among patients with anorexia nervosa and bulimia nervosa. Am J Psychiatry 1995;152:72.

Timmerman MG, et al. Bulimia nervosa and associated alcohol abuse among secondary school students. J Am Acad Child Adolesc Psychiatry 1990;29:118.

Touyz SW, et al. Anorexia nervosa in males: a report of 12 cases. Aust N Z J Psychiatry 1993;27:512.

Turner MSJ, Shapiro C. The biochemistry of anorexia nervosa. Int J Eating Dis 1992;12:179.

U.S. Public Health Service. Prevalence of overweight among adolescents—United States, 1988–91. MMWR 1994;43:818.

U.S. Public Health Service. Binge eating disorder. Washington DC: National Institutes of Health, 1993.

Van Itallie TB, Kissileff HR. Physiology of energy intake: an inventory control model. Am J Clin Nutr 1988;42:914.

Van Itallie TB. Health implications of overweight and obesity in the United States. Ann Int Med 1985;103:983.

van Lenthe FJ, Kemper HCG, van Mechelen W. Rapid maturation in adolescence results in greater obesity in adulthood: The Amsterdam Growth and Health Study. Am J Clin Nutr 1996;64:18.

Vitousek K, Manke F. Personality variables and disorders in anorexia nervosa and bulimia nervosa. Abnormal Psych 1994;103:137.

Wadden TA, et al. A multicenter evaluation of a proprietary weight reduction program for treatment of obesity. Int J Obes 1990;14:135.

Walsh BT. Eating disorders, American Psychiatric Association DSM-IV Update: Task Force on the Diagnostic and Statistical Manual of Mental Disorders—Fourth Edition. January/February, 1990.

Weingarten HP. Stimulus control of eating: Implications for a two-factor theory of hunger. Appetite 1985;6:387.

Weintraub M. Long-term weight control study: conclusions. Clin Pharmacol Ther 1992;51:642.

Wilfley DE, et al. Group cognitive-behavioral therapy and group interpersonal psychotherapy for the non-purging bulimic: a controlled comparison. J Consul Clin Psychol 1993;61:296.

Williamson DF. "Weight cycling" and mortality: How do the epidemiologists explain the role of intentional weight loss? J Am Coll Nutr 1996;15:6.

Williamson DF, et al. Weight loss attempts in adults: goals, duration, and rate of weight loss. Am J Public Health 1992;82:1251.

Wing RR, et al. Effects of a very low-calorie diet on long-term glycemic control in obese type II diabetic subjects. Arch Intern Med 1991;151:1334.

Woodside DD. A review of anorexia nervosa and bulimia nervosa. Curr Prob Pediatr 1995;25:67.

Yaeger J, et al. American Psychiatric Association practice guidelines for eating disorders. Am J Psychiatry 1993;150:207.

Yanovski SZ. Binge eating disorder: current knowledge and future directions. Obesity Res 1993;1:306.

Yates A, et al. Overcommitment to sport: Is there a relationship to the eating disorders? Clin J Sport Med 1994;4:39.

Yates A. Current perspective on the eating disorders. II. Treatment, outcome, and research directions. J Am Acad Child Adol Psychiatry 1990;29:1.

Zachariasen RD. Oral manifestations of bulimia nervosa. Women and Health 1995;22:67.

Zelasko CJ. Exercise for weight loss: what are the facts? J Am Diet Assoc 1995;95:1414.

Zhang Y, et al. Positional cloning of the mouse obese gene and its human homologue. Nature 1994;372:425.

APPLICATION: Is It Weight, Fat, or Health?

Fred is a 30-year-old manager for a chain of hotels. He is 178 cm (70 in) in height, has a medium frame, and weighed 80 kg (170 lb) when he was 21. During high school and college he was active with part-time jobs and playing tennis or soccer. As his job responsibilities became more demanding, Fred had less time for exercice, and his weight began to creep up because he loved to eat. He noticed he often needed to buy new clothes, and he had begun to accumulate a closet full of things that were too tight. Now he weighs 95 kg (210 lb).

Last year Fred vowed to get physically fit and go on a diet. In order to lose weight he would skip breakfast and have a cup of yogurt for lunch. By dinner time he was ravenous, and later he would raid the refrigerator for snacks. He signed up to play tennis in a league but dropped out because he was embarrassed to be seen in a large pair of tennis shorts. Although Fred did lose a few pounds, he became increasingly frustrated with his semi-starvation/gorging diet pattern and regained the weight quickly. Now Fred is very self-conscious about his weight and sometimes avoids social activities because of it.

Fred's story is characteristic of millions of overweight and moderately obese adults who struggle to attain or maintain what is considered a "desirable" weight and whose lives become dominated by restrictive eating to control body weight. Although a combination of diet, exercise, and behavior modification can result in substantial success in achieving weight loss, only a small percentage of individuals who complete a comprehensive weight reduction pogram maintain that weight loss after five years (Wadden et al, 1992). Programs using these same techniques in a continuous care model similar to that used for other chronic conditions have resulted in maintenance of weight losses for a considerable period of time (Brownell and Rodin, 1994; Perri et al, 1992). However, the time demands and cost of such programs may limit the availability and scope of such dietary treatment (Berg, 1995).

Given the limited success of current weight loss attempts and given the measurable health benefits of even small weight losses (Kannel et al, 1996), what can health professionals do?

Traditional Approaches to Body Fatness

For decades obesity and overweight have been viewed as a deviation from normal, a problem with negative mental and physical health consequences, and one for which programs for prevention or treatment are required. Most frequently the methods used are dietary restriction and vigorous physical activity. A multibillion dollar weight-loss industry is supported by this approach to excess body fatness (National Task Force, 1994). Underlying this traditional approach to excess body fatness is an assumption that individuals can voluntarily control body fat and that those who fail to reduce or maintain an "acceptable" level are noncompliant and morally weak. Such an approach leads to stigmatization of obesity and the assumption that obese people do not care about being fat because, if they did, they would attempt to control it. However, Americans are trying to lose weight. At any one time, as many as 65 million may be dieting (Lustig, 1991).

Dieting requires external control that overrides the body's internal signals of hunger and satiety. This becomes problematic because the physiologic control mechanisms designed to protect the body from starvation are powerful. Negative calorie diets result in increased fuel mobilization, reduced energy expenditure, diminished lipolysis, and increased energy efficiency, the overall physiologic effect being conservation of energy and body mass—exactly opposite of the dieter's intent.

The psychological changes associated with weight loss diets are also self-defeating. Initially using willpower and self control, overweight individuals find that dieting works. They may be ebullient and active as weight is lost. However, as caloric restriction becomes prolonged, ebullience is replaced by peoccupation with food, food cravings, and the inability to continue food deprivation. As a result, many dieters develop binge eating patterns (Polivy and Herman, 1992). These binges are often precipitated by emotional stress for which binging brings only temporary relief. A pattern of self-denial and dietary restraint followed by binging is often established.

Thus, traditional approaches to body fitness are characterized by interventions with little likelihood of success. Nonetheless, as a society, we demand that obese persons attempt them anyway (Parham, 1996) and then tend to consider them failures when they are not successful.

The National Institutes of Health Conference on Methods for Voluntary Weight Loss and Control (1992) recommended increased research, education, and program development in the area of weight loss and maintenance. Advocates of new approaches to body fatness are promoting blame-free alternatives that emphasize the goals and health of the individual rather than weight loss.

Developing New Approaches to Fatness

- Eat in response to internal cues for hunger and satiety.
- Avoid restrictive dieting.
- Avoid binge eating.
- Recognize that there are no good or bad foods.
- Focus on psychological and physical health rather than appearance.
- Focus on self-acceptance—enjoy one's strengths and dispassionately view limitations or weaknesses.
- Develop self esteem.
- Use family and social support.
- Emphasize exercise that is within ability and enjoyed.
- Identify eating that is response to emotional or environmental factors.
- Develop alternatives to emotional eating responses.

A variety of new approaches to body fatness and treatment of obesity are being developed. Characteristics common to many nondieting programs are listed in the margin. A major advantage of this approach is that it diminishes emphasis on "dieting" and the frustration associated with failure to control eating behavior (Brownell and Wadden, 1992). An early nondiet approach that uses behavior modification strategies, longer treatments, and group support reported long-term success of weight control when emphasis was removed from calorie restriction and placed on normalizing eating habits (Foreyt and Goodrick, 1993).

Basic concepts of the new apraoches center on self-acceptance and nondieting. An important component of self-acceptance is self–size acceptance, Size acceptance rejects the negative concept of fatness, the assumption that obesity constitutes a major problem and that requires change. The basic premise of nondieting is to avoid perpetuation of the physiologic and psychological consequences of restrained eating. It focuses on adopting attidues and behaviors that enhance quality of life and eating in response to internal cues for hunger and satiety. In this context, some programs encourage modest losses of body weight.

These new approaches are especially helpful for binge eaters and other who feel their eating is out of control of guided by emotions or environmental factors rather than internal cues. Nondieting programs help individuals focus on health and well-being by breaking away from these old responses and developing new behaviors. A variety of methods are used to facilitate this approach, including psychologic, educational, cognitive, behavioral, and social techniques. Many programs use the techiques of traditional behavior modification approaches. In this case, however, the techniques are used to support physiologic response eating rather than control or restriction.

Are New Approaches to Body Fatness Successful?

Although nondieting approaches to body fatness are becoming increasingly popular, data regarding the succes of these techniques are limited. Traditional weight control programs are evaluated on the basis of loss of weight or fat, increases in physical fitness, and changes in blood pressure or levels of blood glucose or lipids. Nondieting emphasizes factors related to self esteem, eating behavior, and quality of life. Studies of these programs use scales that measure these parameters. Several short-term group programs have reported significant improvements in self acceptance (Omichinski and Harrison, 1995), eating style, dietary behavior, self esteem, physical activity (Carrier et al, 1994), preoccupation with food, assertion, body satisfaction, and body weight (Roughan et al, 1990), which were sustained at 24 (Roughan et al, 1990) and 36 months (Carrier et al, 1994) after treatment.

Most of the reports of nondieting programs have positive outcomes, which were maintained for more than a year. This approach may be very promising for individuals like Fred who have fallen into a restrictive eating/binging pattern. Compared to the traditional approaches, these programs are relatively inexpensive to operate and easy to initate because they can utilize available techniques. In addition, the nondieting approaches do not have physiologic and psychologic risks associated with chronic dieting. Weight loss is not usually a goal of these programs, but small changes may be a benefit of normalized eating patterns (Roughan et al, 1990), and modest weight loss can improve the risk profile for diabetes mellitus, hypertension, and coronary heart disease.

REFERENCES

Berg FM. Health Risks of Weight Loss, Hettinger, ND: Healthy Living Institute, 1995.

Brownell KD, Rodin J. The dieting maelstrom: is it possible and advisable to lose weight? Am Psychol 1994;49:781.

Brownell KD, Wadden TA. Etiology and treatment of obesity: understanding a serious, prevalent, and refractoy disorder. J Consult Clin Psychol 1992;60:505.

Carrier KM et al. Rethinking traditional weight management programs: a 3-year follow-up evaluation of a new approach. J Psychol 1994;128:517.

Foreyt JP, Goodrick GK. Weight management without dieting. Nutrition Today 1993;28:4.

Kannel WB et al. Effect of weight on cardiovascular disease. Am J Clin Nutr 1996;63:419S.

Lustig A. Weight loss programs: failing to meet ethical standards? J Am Diet Assoc 1991;91:1252.

National Institutes of Health Technology Assessment Conference Statement. Methods for voluntary weight loss and control. Bethesda MD: NIH, 1992.

National Task Force on the Prevention and Treatment of Obesity: Research directions. Obesity Res 1994;2:571.

Omichinski L, Harrison K. Reduction of dietary attitudes and practices after participation in a nondiet lifestyle program. J Can Diet Assoc 1995;56:81.

Parham ES. Is there a new weight paradigm? Nutr Today 1996;31:155.

Perri MG, et al. Improving the long-term management of obesity: theory, research and clinical guidelines. New York: Wiley, 1992.

Polivy J, Herman CP. Undieting: a program to help people stop dieting. Int J Eat Disord 1992;11:261.

Roughan P, et al. Long-term effects of a psychologically based group program for women preoccupied with body weight and eating behavior. Int J Obes 1990;14:135.

Wadden TA, et al. A multicenter evaluation of a proprietary weight reduction program for treatment of marked obesity. Arch Intern Med 1992;152:961.

CHAPTER 14

NUTRITION AND PHYSICAL ACTIVITY

Virginia is 68 years old and lives alone in a small town along the Eastern seaboard. She is the mother of three adult children and was recently widowed. She awakens this bright winter morning to the sound of muffled and intermittent scraping noises on the concrete outside her window. As she looks out the window, Virginia marvels at the beauty of the winter's first snow but she soon realizes that this gift of nature will require some work. Today, Virginia will not have time to read the morning paper as she normally does; today she will be shoveling snow from her 25-foot double driveway because she is expected at the hospital as a volunteer. Several years ago, before she began her water aerobics classes, Virginia would never have attempted to handle the physical challenge of shoveling snow. She would have had to cancel her plans. Now, she is more physically fit and will not only shovel her driveway but will also volunteer at the hospital *and* meet her friend for lunch and shopping!

Daily life in the industrialized world has become more sedentary, and an increasing body of evidence correlates sedentary lifestyles with elevated risks of chronic diseases, especially diabetes, obesity, cancer, and heart disease (Blair et al, 1989; Bouchard and Despres, 1995; National Institutes of Health Consensus Conference, 1996). The relationship between physical inactivity and chronic disease is so significant that Americans are strongly urged to become more active (Blair et al, 1996a; National Institutes of Health Consensus Conference, 1996; Phillips et al, 1996). Considerable health benefits may result from increases in activity. Some of these are improved lipoprotein profile, carbohydrate metabolism, blood pressure, body weight, and mortality rate, to name

a few. This chapter addresses the relationships between nutrition and physical activity in all individuals throughout all stages of the life span.

PHYSICAL FITNESS

■ What is physical fitness and how is it assessed?

■ What are the benefits of improved physical fitness?

■ What are some of the recommendations for improving physical fitness?

The set of characteristics or attributes that a body requires to perform the physical activities of daily life is

---

Contributed by Diane L. Habash.

known as **physical fitness** (American College of Sports Medicine, 1991). Some individuals are more "fit" than others and are capable of performing routine daily activities as well as unplanned activities of increased intensity and duration (such as shoveling snow, as in Virginia's case). On an individual basis, physical fitness can be viewed as a continuum. One extreme represents the attributes needed to perform only the routine daily tasks of living without any reserve for unplanned events; the other extreme represents attributes that are necessary to perform activities of daily life as well as unplanned events plus those required for participation in a competitive sport or activity.

Regardless of the level of physical fitness and whether an individual's daily activities involve sitting all day, jogging through the neighborhood, shoveling snow, planting a garden, moving furniture, competing in a marathon, or watching television, the attributes or components that make up physical fitness are similar for all individuals.

Components of Physical Fitness

The primary components of physical fitness include flexibility, muscle strength, muscle endurance, cardiorespiratory endurance, and body composition (Table 14–1). To estimate an individual's level of fitness, health professionals can measure each of these components for that person and compare those measurements to norms established as a result of data collected from large population groups. Suggestions can then be made for improving specific components of fitness for the purpose of reducing risk of chronic disease (American College of Sports Medicine, 1991).

Flexibility

Flexibility, or the range of motion around a joint, depends on muscle temperature, muscle viscosity (stiffness), and the distensibility, or give, of the ligaments and tendons associated with joints (Corbin, 1984). The most common test of flexibility, the "sit-and-reach" test, measures trunk flexion. This test determines the ability to bend at the waist and thus indicates lower back and hamstring flexibility (American College of Sports Medicine, 1991).

Flexibility is important to physical fitness because a person with a limited range of motion eventually has to reduce daily activities associated with the affected joint(s), which could result in total dependence on others. Aging is associated with a decline in flexibility. When stretching and warm-up exercises are used, flexibility can be improved by 20% to 50%, regardless of gender or age.

TABLE 14-1 Components of Physical Fitness	
Component	**Definition**
Flexibility	The range of motion around a joint
Muscle strength	The ability of a muscle to generate force or tension
Muscle endurance	The ability of a muscle to generate force or tension in a submaximal effort over a sustained period of time
Cardiorespiratory endurance	The ability to complete moderate- to high-intensity aerobic activity for more than a few minutes
Body composition	The percentage of the body composed of fat versus the percentage composed of lean mass

Muscle Strength

Muscle strength refers to the ability of a muscle to generate **force** or **tension** in a maximal effort. It depends on the anatomic location of the muscle, muscle size, speed of contraction, type of muscle action, and the flexibility of the joint associated with that particular muscle or muscle group (Knuttgen and Kraemer, 1987). As a result of these variables, tests used to measure muscle strength are diverse. For instance, one common strength test includes the use of a single movement such as a pull-up, while another involves lifting a maximal amount of weight with weight-lifting equipment for one repetition (1-repetition maximum or 1RM), and a third involves lifting a maximal weight throughout an entire range of motion on equipment that regulates and controls speed. The measure of an individual's muscle strength is best determined by using a combination of many methods (Knuttgen and Kraemer, 1987).

K E Y   T E R M S

physical fitness: the group of features needed for the body to perform physical activity
force or **tension:** the effort needed to resist or maintain a muscular movement

The significance of muscle strength in overall physical fitness is most obvious when an individual is suddenly required to lift or move a very heavy object. Improvements in muscle strength can be obtained by **resistance** or weight training, which progressively overloads the muscle (works the muscle against an increasing amount of opposing force). Resistance training improves not only muscle strength but also muscle endurance, a third component of physical fitness.

Muscle Endurance

Muscle endurance is the ability to generate force or perform work in a **submaximal** capacity over a sustained period of time until fatigue occurs. A test of muscle endurance measures the total number of repetitions of an exercise that can be completed within a timed interval, such as the 60-second sit-up or push-up test.

To improve muscle endurance, **calisthenics** and weight training are often suggested. A physically fit individual like Virginia would possess the muscle endurance to shovel several inches of snow from a driveway and still be capable of performing her usual daily activities.

Cardiorespiratory Endurance

Cardiorespiratory endurance is the one component of physical fitness that is familiar to most people. It represents the ability to perform moderate-to-high intensity activities for a prolonged period of time and, thus, relies on the efficiency of oxygen and carbon dioxide exchange at the lung and the muscle. The best estimator of cardiorespiratory endurance is obtained by measuring the maximum volume of oxygen consumed (VO_{2max}) during a graded exercise test to volitional fatigue or exhaustion. An example would be running on a treadmill set at 6 mph while the grade (slope) is increased 2% every 2 minutes until exhaustion.

However, measurement of maximal oxygen consumption is not practical in all individuals. Conveniently, scientists have validated correlations between maximal and submaximal heart rate, oxygen consumption, and performance in specific aerobic tests in order to predict VO_{2max}. Some of these tests, which include the 12-minute run and the 1-mile walk, can be more easily administered to various individuals or groups and do not require a maximal effort (American College of Sports Medicine, 1991). Improvements in cardiorespiratory endurance can be obtained by increasing the duration and frequency of aerobic exercise.

Body Composition

The final component of physical fitness, body composition, describes the amount and relative location of body fat and muscle. Body composition can be related to the risk of some chronic diseases—for instance, there is a correlation between abdominal obesity and increased risk of coronary heart disease (Pi-Sunyer, 1991). Body composition is typically defined in terms of a two-compartment model of fat versus fat-free or lean mass. The techniques most commonly used to measure body composition include anthropometry (fatfolds) and bioimpedance analyses. Many more sophisticated techniques exist; however, their use is often restricted to clinical and research populations.

In general, there are wide variations in percentage of body fat for adults; frequently used reference values are approximately 13% to 19% body fat for adult males and 19% to 25% body fat for adult females (Sizer and Whitney, 1994). These ranges of percentage of body fat for interpreting physical fitness should be used with care because body fat may vary depending on age, gender, genetic background, daily physical activity, and usual dietary intake.

Assessment of Physical Fitness

The American College of Sports Medicine (ACSM) (1991) suggests that fitness should be evaluated at least once before someone starts an exercise program. Health professionals, using the guidelines, tests, and recommendations established by the ACSM, would provide information on the current level of fitness and risk for chronic disease as well as some indication of the appropriate exercises needed for improvement (American College of Sports Medicine, 1991).

A comprehensive assessment of physical fitness may be quite extensive. It can include medical and activity histories and opinion questionnaires, a physical examination by a physician, an analysis of coronary artery disease risk profile, numerous diagnostic exercise tests (for the components of fitness as mentioned above), and perhaps advanced cardiac diagnostic tests such as coronary angiography, if needed (American College of Sports Medicine, 1991).

Benefits of Physical Fitness

An increase in daily physical activity promotes fitness by reducing the risk of chronic disease and by lowering mortality rates (Blair et al, 1989; Paffenbarger et al, 1986). In one 8-year epidemiologic study of over 13,000 people, those individuals who spent 30 minutes a day walking briskly 3 days per week significantly reduced their risk of dying from heart disease, cancer, and other causes compared to those who did not walk (Blair et al, 1989). In a recent follow-up of this study population, the authors concluded that low fitness levels were such great predictors of mortality that even the participants who smoked cigarettes but remained moderately active had reduced mortality rates (Blair et al, 1996). In a group of 17,000 male Harvard alumni, mortality rates were 21% lower for men who walked 9 miles per week compared to those who walked 3 miles or less per week (Paffenbarger et al, 1986).

Although increased physical activity improves health, which could be defined as the absence of disease, no single recommendation for increasing exercise or daily activity has been adopted. Instead, exercise recommendations have been made for enhancing health (i.e., lowering risk factors for chronic disease) and for enhancing fitness (i.e., increasing VO_{2max}, muscle strength, flexibility, and endurance) (American College of Sports Medicine, 1991; Pate et al, 1995).

For instance, the American College of Sports Medicine (1991) recommends that to improve health, one should participate in activities that use large muscle groups of the legs and trunk (such as walking, jogging, skating, climbing stairs, rowing, or cycling) 3 to 5 days each week for 15 to 60 minutes per day at a low-moderate intensity (American College of Sports Medicine, 1990). (Although this is described later in terms of heart rate, a general rule of thumb for low-moderate intensity exercise is that an individual is breathing harder during the exercise than at rest but is quite capable of carrying on a conversation.) Three brief 10-minute periods of moderate activity throughout the day have also been suggested as an alternative to one longer period of exercise (DeBusk et al, 1990).

To improve fitness, on the other hand, an increase in exercise intensity, frequency, and duration is recommended. This amounts to exercise involving large muscle groups at least five times per week for 15 to 60 minutes at a moderate-high intensity (American College of Sports Medicine, 1991). (At this intensity breathing rate is increased yet the individual should still be capable of some conversation.)

Whether the goal is to improve physical fitness or to enhance health, those who do exercise regularly may receive some or all of the following benefits:

- Improved cardiovascular function
- Increased strength
- Reduced body fat and increased lean body mass
- Improved blood lipid profile
- Decreased risk of chronic disease

- Restful sleep
- Improvement in measures of diabetes, obesity, or hypertension, which include decreased blood glucose, weight loss, and decreased blood pressure

Although increasing activity through structured exercise may result in many of the above benefits, some of these same benefits can be obtained by increasing the daily activities of normal life, such as taking the stairs instead of the elevator, walking instead of driving, gardening, washing the car, and actively playing with kids, to name a few.

Physical Inactivity

Despite the strong evidence that physical inactivity or a sedentary lifestyle is a risk factor for coronary heart disease, stroke, cancer, hypertension, and other chronic diseases, only 25% of U.S. adults in the late 1980s exercised at levels recommended to improve health, and only 10% exercised at levels intended for increasing cardiovascular fitness (Caspersen et al, 1986). Health professionals continue to express serious concern about the prevalence of sedentary life in the industrialized world (Blair et al, 1996a).

MUSCLE FIBERS AND THEIR ENERGY SYSTEMS

Participation in any physical activity, whether for enhancing health or for improving physical fitness, requires muscular work. The work that a muscle is able to complete depends on the type of muscle fiber involved, the availability of energy to fuel that muscular work, and how well the muscle has been trained to perform that work.

 KEY TERMS

resistance: an opposing force; in the case of resistance training it is typically a form of weight lifting in which muscles move against some force
submaximal: a level of exertion below maximal effort
calisthenics: exercises completed without the use of exercise equipment to increase heart rate and strength; examples are jumping jacks, sit-ups and push-ups

Danny is 14 years old and beginning the ninth grade at the end of this summer. He weighs 55 kg (120 lb) and is 158 cm (62 in) tall. He wants to play high school football in the fall and make the wrestling team in the winter. Just before school was dismissed for the summer, the high school football coaches met with potential players and explained the voluntary summer weight lifting and conditioning program. Danny is extremely eager to gain as much muscle as possible this summer, partly because he knows he will be stronger but also because he thinks it will look impressive and guarantee him a spot on the team. He has no idea what to expect during his 12 weeks of training.

Muscle Fiber Types

■ Of what are muscles composed and how do they enlarge?

■ How do weight training and aerobic training affect muscles?

■ What are reasonable expectations for improvements in strength and endurance with weight training and aerobic training?

Skeletal muscles are large bundles of **muscle fibers** that have been classified into one of three general fiber types: I, IIa, or IIb, based on structural and functional characteristics. These characteristics affect the strength, endurance, and speed with which a muscle contracts (Table 14–2).

Structurally, one characteristic that distinguishes muscle fiber types from one another is the variation in the concentration of **myoglobin**, a protein that "holds" oxygen for the muscle fiber. Other structural components of muscle fibers, such as the number of mitochondria and blood capillaries, also vary between muscle fiber types and are capable of influencing oxygen capacity as well as energy production in muscle fibers.

Functionally, muscle fibers are characterized by their ability to continue working and resist **fatigue**. In addition, the speed of **contraction** and the amount of force generated during a contraction are functional characteristics used to differentiate the various muscle fiber types. Many of these characteristics can be attributed to the availability of energy (ATP) in the muscle. Based on these characteristics, the three muscle fiber types are differentiated as follows:

1. *Type I fibers* are also called **slow-twitch**, **fatigue**-resistant, or slow-oxidative fibers. These fibers contain high amounts of myoglobin as well as many mitochondria and blood capillaries that make them appear red in color. Type I fibers rely on **aerobic** processes of ATP production such as the Krebs cycle (discussed later) and are not easily fatigued; however, they do not produce as much force or speed during their contraction as the other fibers. An example of muscles that contain many type I fibers is the postural muscles in the neck that hold the head upright.

2. *Type IIA fibers* are also called fast-twitch A, fatigue-resistant, or fast-oxidative fibers. Similar to type I fibers, these type IIA fibers contain high amounts of myoglobin as well as many mitochondria and are surrounded by many blood capillaries. These fibers appear red in color and use aerobic as well as **anaerobic** processes to produce ATP. Unlike the type I fibers, however, type IIA fibers have greater force and speed of contraction and are somewhat resistant to fatigue, but less so than type I fibers. The thigh

TABLE 14–2 Muscle Fibers and Their Structural and Functional Characteristics	
Fiber Type/Names	**Structural and Functional Characteristics**
TYPE I Slow-twitch Slow-oxidative Fatigue-resistant Red	Have very high amount of myoglobin and mitochondria, increased capillary density, slow velocity of contraction, appear red in color. Predominant use of oxidative processes for ATP production.
TYPE IIA Fast-twitch A Fast-oxidative Fatigue-resistant White	Have high amount of myoglobin and mitochondria, with many surrounding blood capillaries, so fibers appear red in color. Faster rate of ATP production so velocity of contraction is faster than type I. Somewhat less resistant to fatigue than type I fibers.
TYPE IIB Fast-twitch B Fast-glycolytic Fatigable White	Have little myoglobin, fewer mitochondria and blood capillaries than other muscle types so appearance is white. Relies on glycolytic- and phosphocreatine-derived sources of ATP, hence easily fatigued, but velocity of contraction is fast.

muscle is an example of a muscle with high numbers of type IIA fibers.

3. *Type IIB fibers* are also called fast-twitch B, fatigable, or fast-glycolytic fibers. These fibers contain less myoglobin and fewer capillaries than the other fibers and thus appear white. The speed and force of contraction in type IIb fibers are much greater than in the other two fiber types. Type IIb fibers contain fewer mitochondria and, therefore, must rely on anaerobic production of ATP. Their use of anaerobic processes suggests that these fibers will fatigue easily. Arm muscles contain a high number of type IIb fibers.

The examples of muscles noted above are those with a dominant type of muscle fiber. In reality, all skeletal muscles are a mixture of all three types, the proportion of which is genetically determined (McArdle et al, 1994). Interestingly, most sedentary individuals have a predominance (46–48%) of type I fibers. Trained elite athletes, on the other hand, have muscle fiber types that reflect their training (e.g., a prevalence of type IIb fibers with speed and strength training versus type I fibers with endurance training) (Saltin et al, 1977). It appears that fiber type may be altered in response to activity. However, further research describing the prevalence and time course of these changes is necessary (McArdle et al, 1994).

Regardless of muscle fiber type, muscle contraction requires energy in the form of ATP. The contractile proteins in muscle, actin and myosin, are unable to move without it, and the speed and force of contraction are greatest when ATP is most available. Like all cells, muscle cells obtain ATP through intracellular aerobic or anaerobic metabolic pathways. The actual pathways used to produce ATP in muscle depend on the fiber type, the nutrients available (fat, carbohydrate, or protein), and the intensity and duration of the muscular activity.

Aerobic and Anaerobic Energy Production Systems in Muscle Fibers

There are four potential sources of ATP within the cell. The use of ATP from the various sources occurs in an overlapping sequence during exercise, and the continued use of ATP from each source depends on the type of muscular activity as well as the supply of carbohydrates, fatty acids, or other nutrients (Fig. 14–1).

First, there is a small amount of free ATP available inside the cell, which is used to fuel the initial 2 to 3 seconds of strength or power types of activities. This source of ATP is very limited and is easily exhausted. In athletes, for example, the use of free ATP occurs in the first several seconds of a high jump, long jump, sprint, or lift. When this source of ATP is exhausted, the next most immediate source of ATP is derived from the molecule phosphocreatine (PC).

Phosphocreatine has a high energy phosphate group attached to it that can be used to convert ADP to ATP within

the cell. As with free ATP, phosphocreatine lasts for only 6 to 8 seconds and is easily exhausted. The phosphocreatine molecule can be remade after a period of rest. This source of energy, coupled with the free ATP (ATP-PC), provides a 100-meter sprinter with 98% of the energy to get to the finish line (about 10 to 12 seconds) (Table 14–3). Both sources of ATP are used when the muscle is in need of quick energy and when there is little time to use systems that require oxygen; thus, they are called anaerobic sources of ATP. Sports, such as football and basketball, require short bursts of speed and strength and depend upon these systems (see Table 14–3).

A third immediate source of ATP, also obtained from an anaerobic process, is called **glycolysis.** During this process, two pyruvate molecules are formed from the partial degradation of one glucose molecule, and ATP is produced quickly. However, the contribution of ATP from glycolysis lasts for only 1 to 2 minutes of a maximal effort (see Fig. 14–1). Athletes, who run 200 to 800 meters, swim 200 or more meters, run hurdles (see Fig. 14–2), or complete other events in 1 to 2 minutes rely primarily on glycolysis and the other systems of anaerobic ATP production. However, glycolysis is also used in events beyond 1 to 2 minutes for sports such as football, soccer, or basketball, where short bursts of intense activity are interspersed with longer periods of low-moderate activity that could last for 1 to 4 hours. These athletes rely on a highly developed glycolytic system for a "fast break," goal line defense, or touchdown run. The production of ATP from the glycolytic system becomes especially important in a

---

KEY TERMS

muscle fibers: individual muscle cells that are usually identified as Type I, IIa, or IIb

myoglobin: the protein in muscle that combines with or "holds" oxygen so that it is available to be used in aerobic oxidation of fuels

contraction: the shortening or lengthening of a muscle fiber, which results in the production or generation of force

slow-twitch: speed with which a type I fiber contracts

fatigue: a physical state in which one is unable to continue muscular work at the same intensity

aerobic: a metabolic process that requires oxygen to continue

anaerobic: a metabolic process that does not require oxygen

glycolysis: the breakdown of glucose to two pyruvate molecules

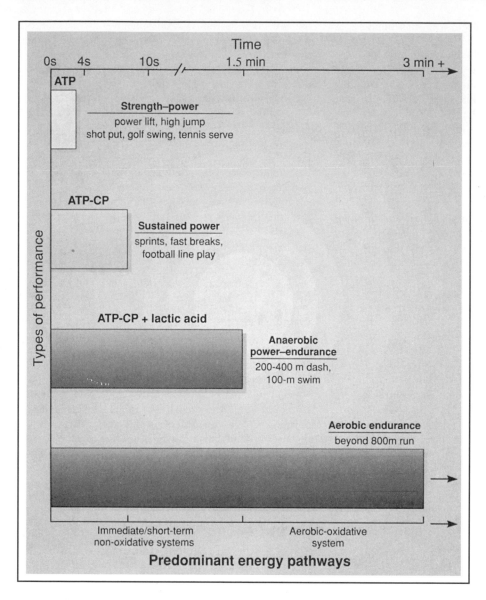

FIGURE 14–1. Predominant energy pathways. (From McArdle WD, et al. Exercise physiology, energy, and human performance. 3rd ed. Philadelphia: Lea & Febiger; 1991:424.)

team's final quarter of play when they are close to exhaustion yet must maintain speed and strength.

There are several limitations to glycolysis that make it necessary for an exercising muscle to seek additional ATP from yet a fourth system. First, for glycolysis to continue, its product (pyruvate) must not accumulate in the cell and must continue to be completely metabolized through the aerobic pathway of ATP production (discussed later). With limited use of the aerobic pathway, pyruvate is converted to lactic acid (LA), which can accumulate in the cell and eventually lower intracellular pH and impair muscle contraction. This is especially evident in exercising individuals who were previously sedentary, although it occurs to some degree in individuals of all fitness levels. Second, glycolysis requires a steady source of glucose. Sources of glucose might include glucose from the blood,

muscle and liver glycogen, and compounds such as some amino acids, glycerol, and lactic acid that the liver can remake into glucose in a process called **gluconeogenesis**. Many of these sources of glucose may be nearly exhausted after approximately 90 minutes of continuous exercise.

This fourth system of ATP production, which is used for exercise beyond 1 to 2 minutes, is the aerobic system known as the tricarboxylic acid cycle (or Krebs cycle). Unlike the other ATP producers, this system requires the presence of oxygen and mitochondria, produces relatively more ATP, and is less limited by the availability of a fuel source. Endurance athletic events and sports (see Table 14–3) that rely on the aerobic pathway include running (800 meters or more), swimming (200 meters or more), cross-country skiing, competitive cycling, and numerous others. Aerobic production of ATP is the source of ATP

TABLE 14–3 Popular Sports and Their Associated Energy Systems

Sports or Sport Activity	Percentage of Emphasis According to Energy Systems		
	ATP-PC and LA*	LA-O₂†	O₂‡
Baseball	80	20	—
Basketball	85	15	—
Fencing	90	10	—
Field hockey	60	20	20
Football	90	10	—
Golf	95	5	—
Gymnastics	90	10	—
Ice hockey			
forwards, defense	80	20	—
goalie	95	5	—
Lacrosse			
goalie defense, attack men	80	20	—
midfielders, man-down	60	20	20
Rowing	20	30	50
Skiing			
slalom, jumping, downhill	80	20	—
cross-country	—	5	95
pleasure skiing	34	33	33
Soccer			
goalie, wings, strikers	80	20	—
halfbacks or link men	60	20	20
Swimming and diving			
50 yd, diving	98	2	—
100 yd	80	15	5
200 yd	30	65	5
400, 500 yd	20	40	40
1500, 1650 yd	10	20	70
Tennis	70	20	10
Track and field			
100, 220 yd	98	2	—
field events	90	10	—
440 yd	80	15	5
880 yd	30	65	5
1 mile	20	55	25
2 miles	20	40	40
3 miles	10	20	70
6 miles (cross-country)	5	15	80
marathon	—	5	95
Volleyball	90	10	—
Wrestling	90	10	—

* Anaerobic (phosphagen system) (ATP-PC)
† Combination (lactic acid-oxygen) (LA-O₂)
‡ Aerobic (oxygen)

Adapted from Fox EL, Mathews DK. Interval training: conditioning for sports and general fitness. New York: Saunders College Publishing, 1974.

used to complete daily routine activities of living such as sitting, shoveling snow, walking up steps, weeding the garden, or raking leaves.

In summary, the production of ATP in a muscle fiber occurs in response to the need for energy and is related to the intensity and duration of the exercise, the type of muscle fiber involved in the exercise, and the availability of fuel (discussed later). Muscle fibers are classified by structural and functional features that generally relate to aerobic or anaerobic ATP production. For instance, Type I fibers have more mitochondria and more blood capillaries, which make them more capable of aerobic ATP production. Type IIb fibers have fewer mitochondria and blood capillaries but a greater concentration of glycolytic enzymes and thus greater anaerobic ATP production. Anaerobic production of ATP provides energy very quickly for brief, powerful muscle movements, usually lasting between 2 seconds and 2 minutes. Aerobic production of ATP produces energy for muscle movements of somewhat lower intensity that are sustained for a much longer period of time (beyond 2 minutes). For an elite athlete or a sedentary individual, the availability of these systems of energy production provides the versatility to meet the energy needs of the working muscle. Enhancing these energy production pathways is the key to improving some aspects of physical fitness.

Exercise Training and Enhancing Energy Production Systems

Athletes, coaches, and trainers develop training programs that enhance the energy production systems specific to their sport or event of interest. In other words, a sprinter, power lifter, or lineman on a football team will use resistance training to increase the anaerobic processes of ATP production because quick powerful bursts of energy are important for their sports performance. The opposite is true for a marathon athlete, who will run between 50 and 120 miles each week to enhance the aerobic oxidative system and aerobic endurance. However, as noted in Table 14–3, most sports require utilization of all systems of ATP production, thus, an individual may train both aerobically and anaerobically. Basketball, football, soccer, and ice hockey are examples of sports that require athletes to have quick start and stop movements, movements of

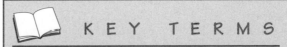

KEY TERMS

gluconeogenesis: a process in which some compound such as pyruvate, lactate, or an amino acid such as alanine is made into a glucose molecule

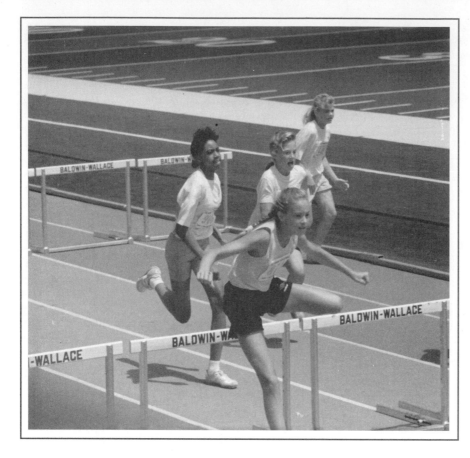

FIGURE 14–2. Glycolysis contributes energy for track athletes to jump hurdles. (Photo by Irv Mitchell)

enormous strength, and endurance to maintain these activities for a prolonged period of time.

For many sports, training regimens are individualized first for the athlete's level of fitness and second for performance of his or her specific sport. Muscles that are exercised and trained are not able to transfer their improvements to other muscles in the body (McArdle et al, 1994). For example, after 8 weeks of bicycle training, limited improvements in arm strength or running ability occur. The improvements that do occur are a result of enhanced energy production in the trained as opposed to the untrained muscles.

Aerobic Exercise Training

The basic requirement of an aerobic exercise training program for a sedentary individual is that the large muscles of the body must be exercised in a constant manner (as in walking, running, or cycling) for a minimum of 15 minutes three times per week at a moderate intensity (usually calculated as 60% to 80% of maximal heart rate; maximal heart rate = 220 minus age). In addition, warm-up (10 minutes) and cool-down periods (10–20 minutes) should accompany each exercise session. These recom-

mendations are based on large prospective and retrospective studies that determined that decreased rates of mortality from cardiovascular disease and cancer were associated with this minimal amount of weekly exercise (Blair et al, 1989; Blair et al, 1995; Blair et al, 1996a; Paffenbarger et al, 1986).

Certified exercise professionals use exercise tests to evaluate an individual's fitness and make recommendations based on the individual's fitness level and goals. The recommendation includes specifications of exercise type, frequency, duration, and intensity. To obtain the maximum benefit from an exercise training program, the frequency, duration, and intensity of exercise usually are gradually increased to suit the individual. Frequency increased from 3 to 5 times per week improves aerobic endurance slightly but may not necessarily offset the additional time invested by the individual (McArdle et al, 1994). Intensity of exercise, measured by heart rate and often difficult to prescribe and measure, is recommended to range from 60% to 80% of maximal heart rate (120–165 beats per minute); however, exercise at a lower intensity may initially be more appropriate for individuals who are extremely overweight (American College of Sports Medicine, 1991).

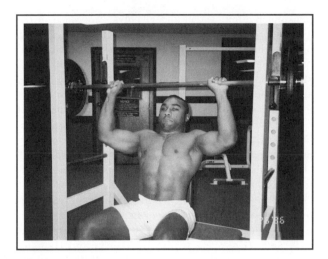

FIGURE 14–3. Muscle strength and size increase with resistance training. (Photo by Diane Habash)

Anaerobic Exercise Training

The premise of an anaerobic exercise training program is that strength will be increased by making the muscle work repeatedly to overcome resistance (see Fig. 14–3). This is often referred to as "overloading the muscle" and can be accomplished by altering either the resistance against which the muscle works, the number of repetitions completed, the speed of the repetition, or some combination of these. Three different methods of strength or resistance training can be used—isotonic, isometric, or isokinetic training. These methods differ from one another based on the length of the muscle when it contracts and whether the opposing force on the muscle remains the same throughout the entire range of motion.

Isotonic training, now referred to as weight training or dynamic resistance training, is completed when a muscle shortens or lengthens as it contracts. A common example is the bicep curl. In this situation, the bicep muscle must overcome the resistance of barbells, dumbbells, or an exercise machine to bring the weight from a nearly straight-arm position to the chest in a bent-arm position. Although this type of resistance training is the most popular and does improve strength, it may not be used for training some athletes because it may not imitate the movement or the strength requirement for their particular sport (McArdle et al, 1994).

Isometric training, sometimes called static exercise, occurs when the muscle is not allowed to shorten or lengthen while contracting. Male gymnasts who suspend their bodies in midair on the still rings use this form of resistance exercise. To expand the example of the bicep muscle, an individual would bend the arms at the elbow with the palms up, and a heavy weight (e.g., 35 lbs) would be supported using both hands but without the bicep

shortening (i.e., the weight would remain in the same horizontal position).

Isokinetic training is similar to weight training because the muscle shortens as it contracts; however, the speed with which the weight is moved and the force of resistance opposing the muscle remain the same throughout the entire range of motion (i.e., the movement is not faster or easier at any time during the lift). Isokinetic training is done with electronically sensitive, computer-aided equipment that is capable of setting, monitoring, and maintaining the speed and resistance against which the individual moves. Using the example of the bicep curl, when the individual begins the movement by bringing the weight toward the chest, the machine senses the speed and resistance of movement and then readjusts and maintains speed and resistance throughout the remainder of the curl.

A program of resistance training using these methods individually or in combination can be quite varied. In general, strength exercises should be completed two to three times per week, allowing time for rest and recovery. One program might include three sets of three to nine repetitions per set at a weight that ranges from 50% to 100% of the maximum weight that the person is able to lift in a single repetition. For example, an individual might lift 50% of maximum for the first set of nine repetitions, 75% of maximum for the second set, and 100% of maximum for as many repetitions as possible in the third set (usually one or two). As for aerobic exercise, any program to develop strength is adjusted for the individual who is lifting (American College of Sports Medicine, 1991).

To increase the size of the muscle, as a body builder might desire, resistance is greatly increased to near maximum while the number of repetitions is decreased. To obtain a greater increase in strength as opposed to the size of muscle, the resistance is lowered somewhat to 60% to 80% of maximum and the number of repetitions is increased. Danny, our aspiring teenage athlete, wants to increase both the size and the strength of his muscles; however, he would benefit first from increasing strength in order to obtain his primary goal of making the team. Additionally, Danny would be wise to avoid repeated lifts of 90% to 100% of maximum early in his training program due to the potential for damage to joints, tendons, and ligaments. Such injuries often require complete rest and could significantly lessen his chances of making the football team.

Adaptations and Results of Exercise Training

The changes and adaptations that occur in the body as a result of exercise training depend on the type of training completed, the state of physical fitness before training begins, and the intensity and duration of the exercise training. Sedentary individuals who participate in exericse training will have more significant adaptations to the training than individuals who complete the same exercise training program in a partially trained state (American College of Sports Medicine, 1991).

Aerobic Exercise Adaptations

Adaptations resulting from aerobic exercise are related to the transport and use of oxygen. The most significant change is that the volume of blood pumped from the heart with each beat is increased. To facilitate this adaptation, the wall of the left ventricle of the heart increases in thickness and its cavity enlarges in size to hold and pump more blood. Plasma volume also increases. These adaptations result in greater efficiency of the heart muscle and increased transport of oxygen to the body both during exercise and at rest. Other adaptations include improved oxygen uptake by the working muscle and increased ability to direct blood flow to the working muscle and away from areas that are less important during exercise, such as the gastrointestinal tract.

Other adaptations facilitate the use of oxygen. In all muscle fibers (especially Types I and IIa), mitochondria increase in size and number and the mitochondrial enzymes of the Krebs cycle increase in activity. These changes contribute to a greater capacity to oxidize fat and carbohydrate for production of ATP. Aerobic exercise also results in a reduction in systolic and diastolic pressures, increased lung volumes, an increased ability to dissipate body heat (or to cool more easily), and, over time, a reduction in the percentage of body fat.

The time of onset for these adaptations is variable, depending, to some extent, on the frequency, intensity, and duration of exercise training. For instance, after beginning an intense daily running program, plasma volume in a group of men increased 10% to 20% within 4 or 5 days of the start, and maximum oxygen uptake increased 15% to 30% within the first 6 months and 50% in the first 2 years (Saltin et al, 1977).

Anaerobic Exercise Adaptations

With an anaerobic exercise training program (resistance training), the adaptations that occur are usually related to the enhancement of anaerobic ATP production and neural responses (Sale et al, 1988). Therefore, enzymes of the phosphocreatine system and glycolysis increase in the ability to either recycle or produce ATP, respectively. Muscle fibers (type IIb) increase in cross-sectional area, contraction time decreases, and tendon and ligament strength increase. Capillary density and mitochondrial size and number appear to decrease because muscle fiber area increases. Another result of resistance training is that neural signaling to the trained muscles is greatly enhanced, which produces a much stronger and more powerful contraction.

Most individuals exhibit significant gains in strength after weight training three times per week for 6 to 8 weeks. However, a more sedentary individual has a greater potential for developing strength. The type of training, dynamic versus static, may result in strength increases of 11% and 20%, respectively (Duchateau and Hainaut, 1982). A genetic prevalence of type IIa and IIb fibers may also support training-related increases in strength (McArdle et al, 1994).

Strength can be improved with resistance training regardless of age. An average strength improvement of 174% was made in the leg extensor muscles (thigh muscles) of 10 subjects who were 90 years of age (Fiatarone et al, 1990). These men completed a weight training program 3 days per week for a period of 8 weeks that included three sets of leg extensions with seven to nine repetitions per set at 80% of the maximal weight they could lift. Although this level of improvement is greater than the 30% found in younger men and women (Duchateau and Hainaut, 1982) and in other studies of elderly men, the authors note that it does indicate that the potential for improvements in strength are significant. For our aspiring teenage athlete, Danny, a 30% to 70% improvement in strength, depending on the type of training, can be expected in a 2- to 3-month period (McArdle et al, 1991; Moritani and deVries, 1980).

NUTRIENTS THAT FUEL ATP PRODUCTION AND EXERCISE

An individual who must complete a physical task such as shoveling snow, running a race, or working an 8-hour construction job will have expectations about his or her performance that are likely related to physical attributes of strength, flexibility, and endurance. A critical factor influencing performance is the amount and type of fuel needed for providing the energy to complete the task.

The gun to start the race is up and ready to fire. The track is quiet. The athletes are conscious only of their beating hearts and the long wait for the gun. The gun sounds and they surge. Every muscle cell is required to move these athletes up and toward the finish, no matter the distance. As she reaches a sprint, Kristen remembers to stay relaxed. She nears the first turn of the track and the familiar rhythm of her practice drills comes to mind. She settles easily into her pace for the mile. She focuses on the track ahead and feels comfortable. She's not winded, she's sweating easily, and she has not been bothered by hunger since she began eating more regularly. Two months ago she did not feel this comfortable.

Back then Kristen was always hungry, yet she avoided food because she thought she was fat and that she would run faster if she lost weight. She routinely ate only 1200 to 1300 kcal a day and had become good at counting them. Eventually she became light-headed during practices and was unable to stay awake at night to do her homework. Sometimes she fell asleep in class. Even her running times were worse, despite a 5-lb weight loss. Luckily, she confided in her older brother, Justin, who convinced her that she needed to eat more to keep her muscles strong enough to compete.

Justin plays high school football, basketball, and lacrosse. As Justin watches his sister run on this hot afternoon he wonders if she drank enough water. He notices that her stride has not changed as she passes by him on her third of four laps around the track. Justin begins to remember the time he competed in the mile just after eating. He thought a candy bar would give him quick energy even though he was not hungry. Only after the race did he realize how the candy had made him feel sluggish and slow.

But here she was, striding now on the back stretch of her final lap. Only one competitor was between Kristen and the finish line. Justin wondered if she had the energy reserves to push her body to sprint past this last competitor. Could she increase her speed and find the endurance required to win? Many voices, including his, urged her toward the finish and she felt every aching muscle as her breathing increased in response to the demand for more oxygen. Could she hold this pace to the finish...?

■ How does an athlete's nutrition affect his or her fitness and performance?

■ What metabolic fuels are used for quick sprint activities versus endurance events?

■ Should athletes engaged in different sports eat distinctly different diets?

Carbohydrates, fats, and proteins are the macronutrient fuels that are oxidized by the working muscle to produce ATP. The relationship between nutrition and physical activity centers around the use and regulation of these fuels during physical work or exercise. Figure 14–4 identifies these fuels, pathways of energy production, and their metabolic products. Although each energy-yielding macronutrient is discussed individually, in reality energy is obtained simultaneously from these nutrients during physical work. The contribution of each pathway toward total energy production is regulated by intensity of effort, availability of fuels, the hormones responsive to exercise, diet, and the level of fitness of the individual.

Carbohydrates

In general, carbohydrates are the preferred fuel of a muscle during moderate- to high-intensity exercise (>50–60% maximal heart rate) because glucose is readily absorbed from blood, is available in the muscle cell as glycogen, and is a quick source of ATP (Bonen et al, 1989). However, the use of carbohydrates during physical activity also depends on other factors. For instance, the increase in some and decrease in other hormones, during exercise stimulates the degradation and use of stored carbohydrates. This effect is more pronounced as exercise continues beyond 30 minutes (Bonen et al, 1989) due to a relative rise in epinephrine, glucagon and glucocorticoids. End-products of glycolysis, pH, and oxygen availability can also regulate carbohydrate use. As glycolysis progresses through a series of enzymatic reactions, two molecules of pyruvic acid are produced. If there is sufficient oxygen in the cell and the concentration of hydrogen ion (H^+) is low, pyruvic acid is converted to acetyl-CoA and completely oxidized in the Krebs cycle. However,

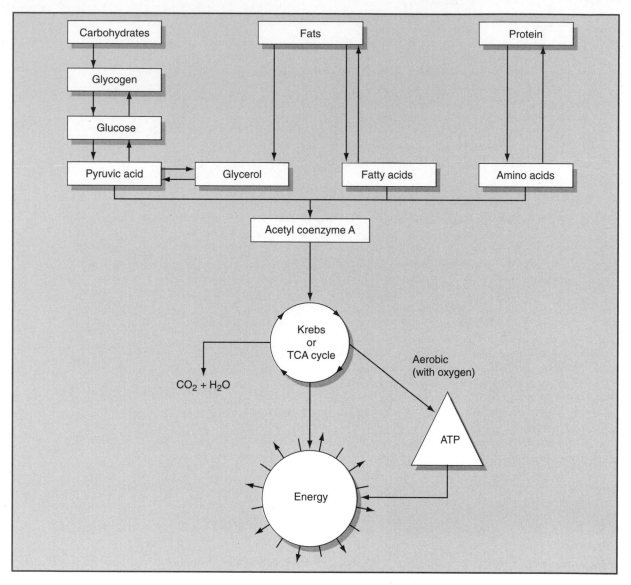

FIGURE 14–4. Oxidation processes to obtain ATP from nutrients: carbohydrate, protein, and fat.

with insufficient oxygen or even with sufficient oxygen but elevated H^+, pyruvic acid is converted to lactic acid (lactate), which accumulates in the cell and slows glycolysis. As glycolysis slows, less carbohydrate is used for fueling the physical activity, and performance in high-intensity exercise may be significantly impaired.

Lactate is normally produced during exercise, regardless of intensity. It is produced in greatest quantity during intense physical work when rapid movements of speed or strength are required or during prolonged (>60 minutes) moderate- to high-intensity exercise (Bonen et al, 1989; Stanley et al, 1988; McArdle et al, 1994). Lactate pro-

duced in the muscle cell enters the circulation, is taken up by the liver, is made into glucose, and is recirculated back to the muscle to be used. This form of gluconeogenesis, called the Cori cycle, occurs predominantly in sports in which glycolysis provides the energy for work (Stanley et al, 1988; Table 14–3).

Several other factors, such as fitness level and diet, have been shown to influence carbohydrate use during exercise. These are discussed in greater detail later in this chapter. The general sequence of carbohydrate utilization during exercise is illustrated in Figure 14–5. In this example, an endurance trained cyclist attempts to work at a

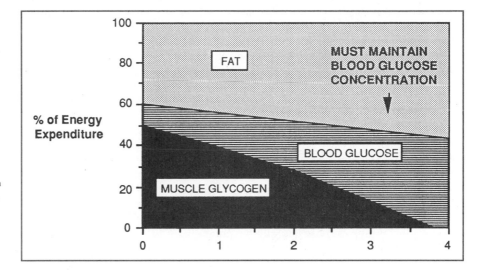

FIGURE 14–5. Glycogen depletion in cyclists. (Adapted from Coyle EF, Montain SJ. Carbohydrate and fluid ingestion during exercise: Are there trade-offs? Med Sci Sports Exerc 1992;24:671. Reprinted by permission of Williams & Wilkins.)

relatively high intensity (70% VO_{2max}) for as long as possible. Initially, when ATP is needed quickly, glucose derived from muscle glycogen is the primary carbohydrate contributor of energy as long as it is available. Muscle glycogen provides approximately 50% of the total energy in the early stages of this cyclist's work. As the availability of muscle glycogen declines, the use of blood glucose begins to increase. This glucose is obtained from the liver.

The contribution of glucose from hepatic sources comprises approximately 10% of the energy early in exercise but reaches 25% by 3 hours of cycling. As the level of liver-derived glucose begins to decline, performance at this intensity also eventually declines unless an exogenous source of glucose (i.e., ingestion of carbohydrate) is available.

During resistance exercise, blood glucose does not decline significantly after a 1-hour series of resistance exercises (Keul et al, 1978) and, in fact, it may actually increase slightly (Robergs et al, 1991). Carbohydrate ingestion just before and during resistance exercise could significantly increase insulin levels (Fahey et al, 1993), which may improve repletion of muscle glycogen stores and increase hypertrophy of the muscle. However, evidence regarding carbohydrate ingestion on performance during resistance exercise is conflicting (Jenkins et al, 1993; Lamb et al, 1990; Conley and Stone, 1996).

Fat

Fat is available to the muscle cell in the form of fatty acids in the blood or as intracellular triglycerides. Hormones secreted in response to exercise, such as norepinephrine, glucagon, and epinephrine, stimulate **lipolysis**, making fatty acids available for the muscle cell to oxidize for energy. To obtain ATP from fatty acids, the cell breaks fatty acids down into many two-carbon units and converts them to acetyl-CoA through **beta oxidation.** Once in the form of acetyl-CoA, carbons from the fatty acid molecule can progress through the aerobic oxidative system to yield many ATP. However, for fatty acids to be made into acetyl-CoA and used for energy, there must be a carbohydrate-derived compound available. Oxaloacetate, the link to oxidation in the Krebs cycle, is required to combine with acetyl-CoA, and thus one often hears the phrase "fat burns in the flame of carbohydrate." A source of carbohydrate, then, must be present to oxidize fat, which can be a challenge for an athlete participating in a competitive endurance sport.

The glycerol molecule, which is a part of a triglyceride, can be converted to glucose by the liver and made available for glycolysis. The amount of glucose available from

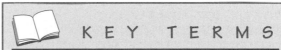

K E Y   T E R M S

lipolysis: the breakdown of a triglyceride into three fatty acids and a glycerol molecule
beta oxidation: the process in which a fatty acid is broken down into 2-carbon units that enter the Krebs cycle and are oxidized to yield ATP

this conversion is small and is not capable of sustaining intense activity.

Endurance exercise training enhances the use of fat as an exercise fuel because it increases the number, size, and activity of mitochondria and their enzymes as well as the deposition of intramuscular stores of triglycerides. As a result, some individuals have suggested that endurance athletes should consume diets high in fat in order to "load" these intramuscular stores and improve performance; however, this has not been verified scientifically (Clarkson, 1996). On the other hand, with resistance exercise the increased concentration of free fatty acids in the blood (Conley and Stone, 1996) could potentially elevate total fat oxidation, resulting in a decrease in body fat. More research is required to better understand the contribution of fat as a fuel during exercise and with the various types of exercise training.

Protein

Proteins are not a preferred fuel at rest or during short-term exercise. However, during endurance exercise, or when the intake of energy or carbohydrate before endurance exercise is low, proteins may contribute from 5% to 15% of the energy needs (Lemon and Mullin, 1980; Meredith et al, 1989).

For proteins to serve as fuels in the muscle cell, they must be degraded into their constituent amino acids, and the nitrogen must be removed and excreted in urea. The remaining carbons can be converted to glucose by the liver or can be oxidized in the Krebs cycle of muscle mitochondria. During exercise, alanine (and other amino acids that have been converted by the working muscles to alanine) is released into the blood, taken up by the liver, and converted to glucose. This specific gluconeogenic process, identified as the glucose-alanine cycle, can contribute as much as 60% of the liver's glucose output during exercise (Felig and Wahren, 1971). Excessive use of protein during exercise, which has occured in the early weeks of intense strength training and during high-intensity endurance training, may compromise nitrogen balance (Tarnopolsky et al, 1988) and be quite costly for an athlete.

ADAPTATIONS IN FUEL METABOLISM WITH EXERCISE TRAINING

The pathways used to produce energy from carbohydrate, fat, and protein are interconnected, which enhances the adaptability of ATP production and facilitates a response to changes in metabolism (see Fig. 14–4). For instance, during rest, when energy is predominantly supplied by fatty acids, nutrients that are not used for fuel can be used

for accretion of body protein, triglycerides, or glycogen. When an individual engages in physical activity, the sources used as fuels are altered compared to those used in the resting state. In the case of the competetive cyclist, he or she obtains a greater proportion (60%) of energy from carbohydrates and less from fat (40%) during exercise (Coyle and Montain, 1992).

Improvements in physical fitness result in adaptations in the use of carbohydrates, fat, and protein. With exercise training, muscle cells begin to use fatty acids in greater proportions even at high intensities, thus conserving stored carbohydrate and slowing the onset of fatigue (Saltin et al, 1977). In addition, fatigue is also delayed as glycolytic adaptations and the processing of lactic acid improve.

For instance, exercise intensities, in general, must reach 55% to 65% of VO_{2max} in untrained individuals and approximately 80% of VO_{2max} in trained individuals before lactate accumulation in the blood impairs performance (McArdle et al, 1994). After aerobic exercise training, an individual produces less absolute lactate at any relative intensity and is capable of improved performance. This adapation is a result of metabolic improvements in fat utilization, lactate and alanine-derived gluconeogenesis in the liver, and more efficient oxygen delivery, uptake, and utilization at the muscle. Nutrition and exercise scientists have studied these adaptations and have learned to exploit them to enhance exercise performance.

Enhancing Performance with Nutrient Fuels

A classic study of diet and human performance was conducted to determine the effect of varying carbohydrate intake on running performance (Astrand, 1968). Several days before a timed treadmill run, three groups of runners were fed diets of high fat (94% calories from fat), medium carbohydrate (55% of calories from carbohydrates), or high carbohydrate (83% of calories from carbohydrate). Figure 14–6 shows that a high-carbohydrate diet greatly improved the endurance time and consequently improved performance significantly (Astrand, 1968). This study laid the groundwork for the current concept of "carbohydrate loading," in which muscle cells, forced to store more glycogen before exercise, experience a delay in the onset of fatigue during endurance exercise.

For athletes who compete in events that last less than 60 minutes or for those who participate in resistance exercise, a high-carbohydrate diet (55–60% or more of total energy) is sufficient to replete carbohydrate stores (McArdle et al, 1994) and increase insulin (Fahey et al, 1993), which promotes both glycogen and protein synthesis. Very little information is available regarding the use of carbohydrate loading in resistance trained athletes (Conley and Stone, 1996).

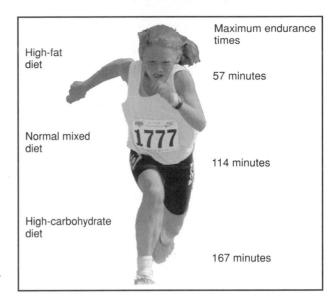

High-fat diet

Normal mixed diet

High-carbohydrate diet

Maximum endurance times

57 minutes

114 minutes

167 minutes

FIGURE 14–6. The effect of diet on exercise endurance. (Data from Astrand P. Something old and something new . . . very new. Nutr Today 1968:9. Photo by Kurt Fisher.)

The basic concept of carbohydrate loading involves depletion of muscle glycogen by exhaustive exercise and consumption of a high-fat, low-carbohydrate diet (60–120g/d) followed by repletion of glycogen stores with a high-carbohydrate diet (55% or more) and low-intensity exercise. Some methods of carbohydrate loading may not be safe and have resulted in abnormal heart rhythms and ankle edema (McArdle et al, 1994). A safe method of carbohydrate loading begins with a 90-minute bout of high-intensity exercise (85% of VO_{2max}) completed 6 days before the day of competition (Sherman et al, 1981). The athlete should exercise for the next 2 days at the same intensity but for half the time (40 minutes). After days 2 and 3, there should be 2 days of even less exercise (20 minutes/day), and finally a day of rest just before competition. Carbohydrate intake, on the other hand, should be increased from 50% of calories on the first 3 days to 70% of total calories daily until competition (Sherman et al, 1981).

Other suggestions for increasing carbohydrate stores in the body, maintaining blood glucose, and delaying the onset of fatigue during exercise include:

- Eating a high-carbohydrate diet every day (55–60% kcal as carbohydrate, or between 300 and 600 g/d for most athletes, or 10g/kg body weight).
- Ingesting carbohydrate liquids during endurance exercise because this form is better absorbed. Ingesting 30 to 60 g per hour or 200 g once after 90 minutes of exercise.
- Replacing carbohydrates within 30 minutes of the end of exercise. Eating 50 to 75 g of carbohydrate every 2 hours after exercise or until 500 g has been consumed.

VITAMINS, MINERALS, WATER, AND PERFORMANCE

■ Do athletes have increased vitamin and mineral requirements because they exercise?

■ Does vitamin and mineral supplementation enhance exercise performance?

■ What is the importance of hydration to performance? How is good hydration achieved?

Vitamins, minerals, and water are essential nutrients for the human body in intense activity or at complete rest. The work of vitamins and minerals would have little meaning without the appropriate volume of water and electrolyte concentrations inside, outside, and between the cells. Figure 14–7 illustrates at what point water-soluble vitamins and minerals are required in the metabolism of carbohydrate, fat, protein, and ultimately the production of energy. Because the production of energy is essential for athletes, adequacy of all vitamins and minerals in the diet is imperative. This is most evident for elite athletes who train for long periods of time every day.

Water-Soluble Vitamins

Economos et al (1993) evaluated the dietary intake of over 900 athletes who trained at least 90 minutes per day and competed in either aerobic (distance running, cycling, nordic skiing, swimming, rowing, or triathlons) or anaerobic (weight lifting, bodybuilding or throwing field) sports. They found that the athletes who consumed less than 45

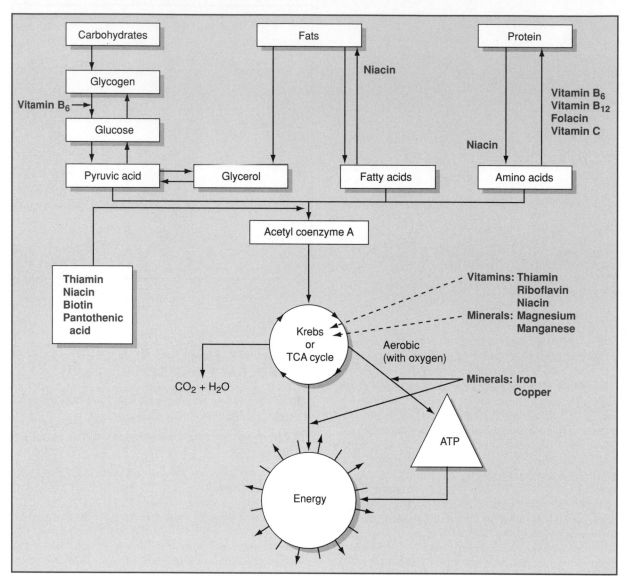

FIGURE 14–7. The integration of vitamins and minerals in metabolism.

kcal/kg/d (i.e., 2000 kcal/d for females and 2100 kcal/d for males) had intakes less than 70% of RDA for vitamin B_{12} and several minerals. If energy consumption was greater than 2600 kcal/d in females and 3500 kcal/d in males, thiamin, riboflavin, and pyridoxine were less than 70% of the RDA, which may indicate a higher intake of calories from fat and simple sugars.

Most research studies indicate that as long as the athlete is eating at least 45 to 50 kcal/kg/d there is little need for vitamin supplementation (Tiidus and Houston, 1995; van der Beek, 1985; Economos et al, 1993). Only one exception involving riboflavin in young female athletes has been noted (Belko et al, 1983). Interestingly, regardless of the

level of energy intake, most of the 900 elite athletes studied (80–100% female and 60–80% male) used a daily multivitamin supplement (Economos et al, 1993).

Because it is well known that vitamins are important in energy production, many individuals may claim that megadosing with vitamins (or minerals) enhances performance. For athletes who eat a well-balanced diet, there is little research to support this claim (Hickson 1989, Lukaski 1994, Weight et al, 1988). However, with insufficient energy intake it is conceivable that marginal deficiencies may result in impaired performance (McDonald and Keen, 1988; van der Beek, 1985). For instance, after an 8-week dietary restriction of thiamin, riboflavin, pyridoxine, and ascorbic acid in six healthy men, there was a 16% decrease in aerobic power and a 24% decrease in the anaerobic threshold (an indicator of lactic acid accumulation) (van der Beek, 1985). The authors could not attribute these changes to any one of these vitamins, however.

The research conducted on vitamin supplementation in athletes is not easy to interpret. Vitamin status of the athlete before supplementation may not have been adequately measured (Hickson, 1989), and it may be unclear whether exercise produced a change in the required amount, distribution, or metabolism of such vitamins as riboflavin, niacin, pyridoxine, and pantothenic acid (Hickson, 1989; Benardot et al, 1993). For instance, some researchers do not account for the **hemoconcentration** that occurs with exercise. In addition, although studies of supplementation with thiamin, niacin, pyridoxine, and cobalamin in athletes do not indicate any benefit to performance (Benardot et al, 1993; Burke and Read, 1989), folate, biotin, pantothenic acid, and riboflavin have not been studied individually for their effect on performance (Benardot et al, 1993).

Vitamin C may elicit some benefit for the well-fed athlete during recovery from exercise by slowing the peroxidative damage of exercise and subsequently decreasing the loss of contractile function (Jakeman and Maxwell, 1993). This benefit, though, is not evident in all exercise studies using ascorbic acid supplementation (Dekkers et al, 1996).

Fat-Soluble Vitamins

Whether exercise increases the requirement for a specific fat-soluble vitamin is difficult to answer, primarily because these vitamins are easily stored in body fat, which is in good supply even in thin athletes. Likewise, assessing the effect of supplementation on performance is equally difficult because it is a challenge to produce even a marginally deficient state (van der Beek, 1985; Tiidus and Houston, 1995). Although supplementation with fat-soluble vitamins D and K does not appear to enhance performance in athletes (Weight et al, 1988; Burke and Read, 1989; Hickson and Wolinsky, 1989; Economos et al, 1993; van der Beek, 1985), there is some debate over the effect of supplementation with vitamins A and E.

Vitamin A is known to have a role in glycogen synthesis, yet there was no effect on aerobic exercise performance in humans after a 6-month depletion diet. This is thought to be due to the large storage of vitamin A in the liver (van der Beek, 1985). Vitamin E, an important antioxidant, seems to reduce oxidative damage in exercising rats (Robertson et al, 1990; Tiidus and Houston, 1995) and may be important for avoiding or recovering from some forms of exercise-induced muscle damage in humans (Dekkers et al, 1996); however, this is still controversial (Jakeman and Maxwell, 1993).

During exercise, especially aerobic exercise, there is a normal increase (approximately 20-fold) in the amount of oxygen circulated to working cells (Dekkers et al, 1996). All but about 5% of this oxygen combines with hydrogen to produce water (McArdle et al, 1994). The small percentage of oxygen that does not combine with hydrogen instead forms **superoxides** and eventually hydrogen peroxide (H_2O_2) or other **free radicals**, which can be very destructive to a cell. The oxidative damage of free radicals can result in leaky mitochondria and cell membranes, damaged genes and DNA, and general destruction of cellular proteins including cytochrome Q in the electron transport chain (Sizer and Whitney, 1994; McArdle et al, 1994).

In humans, performance after vitamin E supplementation was not improved in swimmers, cyclists, or athletes who completed eccentric exercise (proven to be the most damage-inducing type of muscular work where the muscle contracts while lengthening, as in downhill running) (Robertson et al, 1990; Cannon et al, 1990; Tiidus and Houston, 1995). However, athletes who cycled at an altitude greater than 2700 m demonstrated an improvement in endurance time and anaerobic threshold (an indicator of fatigue) after supplementation with vitamin E (Tiidus and Houston, 1995; Simon-Schnauss and Pabst, 1988). To date, the most significant contribution of vitamin E seems to be associated with the recovery of strength after exercise-induced damage to the muscle although further investigation is warranted.

In summary, vitamin supplements, which are consumed by a majority of athletes (Economos et al, 1993), are probably not necessary as long as the athlete is consuming an adequate diet (Benardot et al, 1993).

Minerals

The research related to the mineral requirements of athletes suggests that, as with vitamins, those who consume an adequate energy intake will have adequate stores of

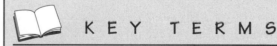

KEY TERMS

hemoconcentration: decrease in volume of plasma as water shifts during exercise; results in increased concentrations of RBCs, hormones, and other blood constituents

superoxides: oxygen-containing molecules that are free radicals

free radicals: unstable molecules with unpaired electrons in their outer shells that are trying to combine with other molecules to satisfy their electron configuration.

minerals (Burke and Read, 1989; Economos et al, 1993). However, with an energy intake lower than approximately 45 kcal/kg/d, elite endurance athletes who exercised at least 90 minutes per day had low intakes of iron, zinc, copper, magnesium, and calcium (Economos et al, 1993).

Exercise, especially endurance exercise, may elevate requirements for minerals, based on either an increased loss from the body in sweat or urine or an increase in their metabolism during exercise (Economos et al, 1993; McDonald and Keen, 1988; Hickson et al, 1989). An adequate well-balanced energy intake should be sufficient to meet the increased requirements (Economos et al, 1993; Burke and Read, 1989).

Sports performance, depending on how it is measured, may not be enhanced with mineral supplementation (Burke and Read, 1989; McDonald and Keen, 1988). For instance, women who consumed 135 mg/d of zinc had an increase in isokinetic strength (Krotkiewski et al, 1982), yet rats who were zinc deficient for 3 weeks could perform equally well on a treadmill compared to a zinc-sufficient group of rats (McDonald and Keen, 1988), and blood levels of zinc in trained or untrained men did not correlate with VO_{2max} (Lukaski et al, 1983). These inconsistent research results are common for minerals, probably because of the variety of experimental designs and performance tests (McDonald and Keen, 1988; Economos et al, 1993). In addition, supplementation of one mineral may impair the absorption and metabolism of a second mineral (McDonald and Keen, 1988).

The minerals that have received the most attention in the literature and that are most likely to affect athletes, their health, and perhaps their sports performance are calcium and iron.

Calcium

Calcium intakes of athletes have been found to be below the RDA (Benardot et al, 1989; Nelson et al, 1986; Economos et al, 1993). Most susceptible to the effects of low calcium status are female athletes involved in rigorous endurance training with 17% percent or less body fat and a dietary calcium intake less than the RDA. Female athletes with these risk factors may experience **athletic amenorrhea** and **stress fractures**. The bone density of these athletes may be so poor that it resembles that of a 70-year-old woman (Goulding, 1986; Sizer and Whitney, 1994). The hormonal shifts that result in amenorrhea may not be entirely compensated for by an increase in dietary calcium. Some recommend hormone replacement therapy along with a decrease in training and a dietary intake of 1500 mg/d calcium (Benardot et al, 1993).

Iron

Athletes may have difficulty maintaining adequate iron status for several reasons. Athletes lose iron through sweat and blood losses associated with their sport, such as the small amount of hemorrhaging that occurs in the feet of runners every day. Athletes expend more energy and thus have an increased demand for the iron-containing proteins of the electron transport chain (Sizer and Whitney, 1994). Athletes may have both poor absorption and poor intake of iron (Benardot et al, 1989). Finally, female athletes lose iron monthly during their menstrual cycle (Haymes, 1987).

Three levels of iron deficiency in athletes have been described, ranging from the mildest to the most severe. These include (1) iron depletion, which is a reduction in serum ferritin (<12–20 μg/L), (2) iron deficiency erythropoiesis, or an elevation in protoporphyrin, the protein that binds iron to facilitate erythropoiesis (>1.8 mmol/L), and, (3) iron deficiency anemia, defined as hemoglobin values less than 14 g/dl in men and 12 g/dl in women (McDonald and Keen, 1988; Weight, 1993; Clarkson, 1990).

Some of the difficulty in diagnosing iron deficiency anemia has been due to the hemodilution of the blood that accompanies endurance exercise training, resulting in falsely low hemoglobin values (Casoni et al, 1985). This condition has been identified as a pseudoanemia or "false anemia" and continues to be reported as "sports anemia," which some suggest is a misnomer (Eichner, 1988; Weight, 1993). The incidence of iron deficiency anemia in athletes has been severely overstated due to this hemodilution problem (Weight, 1993; Clarkson, 1990) and is actually no different from that in the general public when athletes consume balanced diets (Weight, 1993). Female athletes and those who purposely restrict energy intake, such as gymnasts and wrestlers, are predisposed to low iron stores.

Dietary recommendations for increasing iron absorption include consuming meat, fish, or poultry three to four times per week; increasing consumption of iron-fortified breads, cereals, and grains; and consuming foods high in vitamin C. In addition, foods that inhibit iron absorption, such as tea, coffee, and bran, should be consumed in moderation (Benardot et al, 1993). Iron supplementation has been recommended in some cases of iron deficiency anemia (Eichner, 1988), but improved sports performance has been observed only during submaximal and not maximal exercise (McDonald and Keen, 1988).

Water

The importance of water to performance can never be stressed enough to an athlete or any active person, regardless of age or skill level. Sixty percent of the body is made of water and a 5% depletion of body water could have serious consequences (Benardot et al, 1993). The primary functions of water during activity are to transport nutrients in the blood, to participate in metabolic reactions, and, most importantly, to cool the body. This cooling effect of water occurs as the heat produced during exercise is dissipated through the blood and eventually to the skin, where sweat is produced. The amount of heat produced during sustained vigorous exercise is enough to raise core body temperature (i.e., that of the deep tissues) by approximately 1°C every 5 minutes (McArdle et al, 1991).

Adequate cooling is essential during exercise because the body can tolerate an increase of only about 5°C before sports performance is impaired (McArdle et al, 1991). Heat dissipation is especially critical in a hot humid environment when the body's ability to sweat is reduced. Physically active individuals participating in outdoor activities on humid days such as mowing the lawn, weeding the garden, or playing a game of baseball should be aware of the need to keep the body hydrated and cool. Likewise, athletes in long endurance events such as marathons (26.2 miles) and ultramarathons (50 or more miles), as well as other long sporting events that allow intermittent rest, such as football and soccer, must address these same issues.

Excessive sweating in the heat can also result in the loss of electrolytes such as sodium, potassium, and chloride, which influence fluid concentration in and around cells (Benardot et al, 1993). With excess loss of sweat and electrolytes, core body temperature may increase (Hiller et al, 1989; Noakes et al, 1990). Athletes with elevated core body temperatures may experience decreased performance as well as **heat exhaustion** and **heat stroke**.

In fact, numerous studies, using body weight as a marker of water loss, have demonstrated that a decrease in body weight of 1% to 3% during a bout of exercise can significantly increase the risk of poor performance (Sawka et al, 1984; Armstrong et al, 1985). The typical amount of water lost during activity was demonstrated in controlled experiments in which football athletes, dressed in full uniform, lost 1.8% of their body weight after 30 minutes of exercise (Matthews et al, 1969), while marathon athletes lost as much as 6% to 10% of their body weight during the 2- to 4-hour race (Pugh et al, 1966). These differences may be related to intensity and duration of exercise as well as hydration level prior to the start of exercise.

Fluid Replacement

One of the first recommendations for fluid replacement is that athletes should never begin practice or competition in a poorly hydrated state. This can be avoided if the athlete drinks fluids before the event. In addition, an athlete should determine his or her usual change in body weight associated with practice or competition and should replace fluids lost during the practice or competition so that there is no weight change as a result of exercise (Benardot et al, 1993).

However, some sports may not allow time for fluid replacement. In this case, a general recommendation is that for each pound of weight lost during practice or competition, an athlete should consume 1 pint (16 oz, or 2 cups)

of fluid as soon as possible. Ideally, an athlete should drink 4 to 8 oz every 15 to 30 minutes during the game or event. It has been suggested that for every pound of weight lost above the 3% limit, an additional 2 cups of fluid should be consumed (Benardot et al, 1993).

The type of beverage to drink and perhaps the temperature of the fluid consumed by the athlete depend on the event, environmental conditions, and personal preferences. Most athletes may want to drink cool water, others prefer cold water, and still others want room temperature water because they have abdominal cramping with cold water. Carbohydrate-electrolyte replacement beverages are recommended when exercise continues for more than 60 to 90 minutes (Benardot et al, 1993). For athletes who exercise for less than 60 minutes, either plain water or a carbohydrate-electrolyte beverage serves the purpose of cooling the body; personal preference is usually the deciding factor.

Sports Drinks

Exercise or activity that occurs over a long period of time (>60 minutes) or in a hot, humid environment is likely to result in the production of 1 to 1.5 L of sweat per hour (Noakes et al, 1988; Hickson et al, 1989). In addition to fluid, sodium, potassium, and chloride are also lost in sweat (Benardot et al, 1993). Replacement of minerals lost during 1 to 2 hours of moderate exercise can be easily accomplished with usual food intake. However, athletes who are active in hot conditions for a few hours may lose up to 12 g of salt, and the use of a carbohydrate-electrolyte replacement beverage may be necessary (Coleman, 1988).

Table 14–4 lists numerous fluid-replacement beverages and compares the type and percentage of carbohydrate and concentration of electrolytes. Electrolytes in sports

K E Y T E R M S

athletic amenorrhea: the cessation of the menstrual cycle usually brought on by low body fat and excessive athletic training
stress fractures: fractures or breaks in bones resulting from stress related to exercise
heat exhaustion: a state of dehydration in which body fluids have been depleted and body temperature may be slightly elevated (<40°C [104°F]). Fluid replacement is necessary.
heat stroke: a dangerous and acute reaction to the increase of body temperature. Symptoms include dizziness, weakness, cessation of sweating, confusion, body temperature >40°C (104°F) and perhaps loss of consciousness. Medical intervention is necessary.

TABLE 14-4 Common Fluid-Replacement Beverages

Beverages	Flavors	CHO Type	% CHO	Na/8 oz (mg)	K/8 oz (mg)	Other Vitamins/ Minerals	Osmolality
Gatorade (Quaker Oats Co)	Many	Sucrose/ glucose	6	110	25	Cl, P	320–360
Gatorade Light	Many	Glucose	2.5	80	25	Trace	200
Quickick (Cramer Products, Inc)	Many	Fructose/ sucrose	4.7	116	23	Ca, Cl, P	305
Sqwincher (Univ Prod, Inc)	Many	Glucose/ fructose	6.8	60	36	Vit C, Cl, P, Ca, Mg	470
Exceed (Ross Labs)	Lemon/ lime, orange	Glucose polymer/ fructose	7.2	50	45	Ca, Mg, P, Cl	250
PowerBurst (PowerBurst Corp)	Many	Fructose	6.0	35	55	Vit B, C, A, E; Cl; Mg; Ca; pantothenic acid; folic acid; biotin	433
Body Fuel 450 (Vitex Foods, Inc)	Orange	Maltodextrin/ fructose	4.2	80	20	P; Cl; Fe; vit A, B, C	210
10-K (Bev Prod, Inc)	Many	Sucrose, glucose, fructose	6.3	52	26	Vit C, Cl, P	350
Mountain Dew Sport (PepsiCo, Inc)	Regular	High fructose Corn syrup/ sucrose	10	60	40	Vit C, Cl, Ca	674
Soft drinks	Many	High fructose Corn syrup/ sucrose	10.2–11.3	9.2–28	Trace	P	600–715
Diet soft drinks	All	None	0	0–25	Low	P	<50
Fruit juice	Many	High fructose/ sucrose	11–15	0–15	61–150	P; vit C, A, B; Ca; Fe	690–890
Water	—	—	0	Low	Low	Low	10–20

Adapted from Gatorade Thirst Quencher, copyright 1990, Quaker Oats Company.

drinks, specifically sodium and potassium, are most beneficial because they are needed to maintain intra- versus extracellular fluid balance. Ingesting them will not necessarily prevent the muscle cramping often thought to be associated with prolonged exercise in the heat; however, one advantage to a glucose-salt drink, during or after an event, is that a weak salt solution enhances glucose absorption (Coleman, 1988) and consumption of fluids is improved with a flavored sports drink. As suggested earlier in this chapter, sports performance during exercise that lasts longer than 60 minutes has been enhanced with the ingestion of glucose before the onset of fatigue (Coggan and Coyle, 1987) because endogenous sources of glucose and liver and muscle glycogen cannot maintain blood glucose levels. With exercise lasting less than 60 minutes, there may be no benefit to these drinks.

The carbohydrates in these drinks are supplied predominantly in the form of glucose; however, some beverages contain sucrose, fructose, maltodextrin, or **glucose polymer**. The latter are not as sweet in taste and may be preferred by some athletes; however, when provided in concentrations of 10%, glucose polymers may inhibit fluid absorption.

Care should be taken not to consume a concentrated beverage during an endurance event in the heat when the beverage could be too concentrated and draw water into the gastrointestinal system. In addition, drinking a beverage with excessive caffeine may bring on or increase dehydration. Other beverages consumed during exercise by some recreational athletes, including beer and other alcoholic drinks, are dangerous because alcohol dehydrates the body and impairs performance.

DIET RECOMMENDATIONS FOR ATHLETES

■ What should an athlete eat and drink in the hours and moments before competition or practice?

■ Can an athlete improve recovery from an intense workout by consuming specific foods?

Most of the guidelines for planning the diet of an athlete have been formulated from research data specific to endurance athletes; limited nutrition-related work has been completed with resistance athletes (Benardot et al, 1993). However, individuals of varying fitness and activity levels, such as recreational or weekend athletes, can benefit from the application of these concepts because they are based on recommendations and guidelines from the Food Guide Pyramid and Dietary Guidelines that were presented in Chapter 1.

Training Diet

No one diet or meal plan is perfect for every athlete. There are general concepts that should be followed, but no magical diet.

Energy

Athletes of any fitness level require fuel to perform their activity. The amount required varies depending on age, gender, body mass, and body composition, as well as type, duration, and intensity of the activity (Burke and Read, 1989). In general, a range of 3000 to 6000 kcal/d has been recommended for most athletes except those attempting to lose or gain weight (Burke and Read, 1989; Benardot et al, 1993). Most endurance athletes report that they consume about 45 to 50 kcal/kg/d, or 2500 to 5000 kcal/d.

Total energy requirement for an athlete can be calculated by adding the energy required for his or her activity to the RDA for energy (25 to 35 kcal/kg/d). Tabular data that provide an estimate of the energy expended for various sports are available for calculating specific energy needs of athletes (McArdle et al, 1991).

A balanced and complete dietary intake may be easily accomplished by using the guidelines set up by the Food Guide Pyramid (page 12). Table 14–5 lists the approximate number of servings required from each food group along with a menu for a diet of 2000 versus 4000 kcalories. Although attempting to obtain a sufficient number of servings from each food group in the pyramid ensures balance, some athletes find that it is very difficult to eat this much food while maintaining time for training as well as other commitments. It is easy to see why many athletes who require even 3000 kcal/d take daily vitamin, mineral, and energy supplements.

Because carbohydrates are the preferred fuel of working muscles and because performance and endurance are enhanced with adequate stores of carbohydrate, it has been recommended that athletes consume 55% to 70% of their energy intake from carbohydrates, with 10% of this from simple sugars (Sizer and Whitney, 1994; Benardot et al, 1993; American Dietetic Association, 1993). However, this level of carbohydrate intake is difficult and perhaps unrealistic to attain. In a recent review of various studies of dietary intakes of athletes, Hawley and co-workers (1995) found that most athletes consumed only 45% to 50% of their 2000 to 4000 kcalories from carbohydrates.

The amount of dietary protein required by an athlete is often misunderstood and even controversial (Lemon, 1994; Sizer and Whitney, 1994). Most recommendations are to obtain about 0.8 g/kg/d, or 10% to 12% of total calories from protein (National Research Council, 1989). However, some athletes who are involved in intense strength and endurance training may require slightly more, or 1.0 to 2.0 g/kg/d (Benardot et al, 1993; Lemon, 1994). Most Americans consume well above the RDA, so it is usually not a concern for an athlete to obtain a greater level of protein intake (Benardot et al, 1993; Lemon, 1994; Lamb and Wardlaw, 1991). Of course, these recommendations are based on assumptions of adequate intake of energy and high-quality proteins.

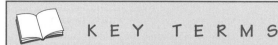

K E Y   T E R M S

glucose polymer: chains of glucose molecules attached to each other; also called maltodextrins. They provide a decreased sweetness in sports drinks and may appeal to some athletes.

TABLE 14–5 Number of Servings Required for 2000 kcal and 4000 kcal Diets

2000 kcal diet	4000 kcal diet
10 servings of starch	20 servings of starch/breads
4 servings of vegetables	7 servings of vegetables
5 servings of fruit	10 servings of fruit
6 ounces of meat	10 ounces of meat
3 servings of milk	6 servings of milk
7 servings of fat	11 servings of fat

MENU

BREAKFAST

1½ c apple juice	3 c apple juice
1 c oatmeal + butter	1½ c oatmeal + margarine
1 slice toast + 1 T jelly	2 slices toast + 2 T jelly
1 c milk	1 banana

MID-MORNING SNACK

1½ c orange juice	2 c orange juice + bagel

LUNCH

2 slices bread	4 slices bread (4 st)
2 oz turkey	4 oz turkey
1 oz cheese	½ sliced tomato
2 T low-fat mayonnaise	4 T low-fat mayonnaise
½ c baby carrots	2 oz cheese
½ c pretzels	1 c baby carrots
1 c milk	12 gingersnaps
	2 c milk

DINNER

3–4 oz chicken breast	6–8 oz chicken breast
1 c noodles + butter	1 c noodles + butter
1 c green beans	1½ c green beans
1 c salad	2 c salad
3 T low-fat salad dressing	5 T low-fat salad dressing
Iced tea	Iced tea

SNACK

½ c low-fat frozen yogurt	1 c low-fat frozen yogurt
½ c sliced peaches	1 c sliced peaches
1 slice angel food cake	1 slice angel food cake

Proteins of high quality include meat, eggs, milk, and cheese, or a combination of these and dried beans, nuts, and seeds for the various types of vegetarians. Many athletes are convinced that they need additional protein (Slavin et al, 1988), and a high proportion of athletes use protein powders and supplements, which are not recommended as the best quality source of protein (Philen et al, 1992). Their mix of amino acids may not be absorbed as well as amino acids from foods, and their concentrations of all the amino acids may not support growth and repair as well as food proteins. Additionally, manufacturers lure individuals into purchasing protein supplements with sensational advertising, much of which has not been scientifically verified (Lemon, 1994; Williams, 1993).

Fat obtained from the diet should be about 30% or less of total kcal intake. Ideally, saturated, polyunsaturated, and monounsaturated fatty acids should each represent about 10% of the total fat intake. Eating lean meats and drinking low-fat milk helps to ensure that athletes can obtain good sources of protein while they limit saturated fat intake.

In summary, athletes who obtain adequate energy for their activity level from a variety of all foods, as suggested by the Dietary Guidelines and the Food Guide Pyramid, are likely to obtain adequate nutrients to support their sport performance.

Pre-Event Foods

Twenty to 30 years ago many coaches and trainers believed that the meal eaten just before competition should be composed of high-protein foods such as steak and eggs. With research completed since then, we now know that high-carbohydrate meals are more advisable because carbohydrate stores in the body, once refilled, prolong the onset of fatigue and promote performance during exercise (Coggan and Coyle, 1987).

The purpose of the pre-event meal is multifaceted. It should prevent symptoms of hypoglycemia such as lightheadedness and fatigue before the event, decrease hunger, provide energy for working muscles and fluid for hydration, and fit the personal preferences and habits of the athlete (Benardot et al, 1993). The pre-event meal should be easy to digest and should not remain in the stomach for longer than 3 to 4 hours. If an athlete is prone to gastrointestinal distress from either a nervous stomach or the intake of high-fiber foods, the pre-event meal should be adjusted with this in mind. Foods that cause distress should be excluded from the diet on the day of competition or even the day before competition. Identification of these foods and food preferences can be accomplished with a training log in which the athlete records foods and beverages that may cause gastrointestinal distress.

The timing of the competition and the type of sport influence the timing of the pre-event meal and the volume of food ingested. For morning competition, the athlete should eat 1 to 2 hours before the event. A small meal of cereal and milk, toast with jelly, or a liquid carbohydrate that is easily digested and not high in fat is appropriate. Ingesting a high-carbohydrate dinner the night before competition is very important for the morning athlete because liver glycogen is nearly depleted after an overnight fast.

Athletes such as runners who are sensitive to food movement in the stomach during exercise may want to eat foods that are rapidly absorbed. Cyclists, on the other hand, may not be as sensitive to food movement in the stomach and thus can consume different quantities and types of foods (Benardot et al, 1993).

Afternoon athletic events allow an athlete to eat a breakfast with more carbohydrates. One suggestion is 4 to 5 pancakes, or about 600 kcal (Benardot et al, 1993). Regardless of the time of day, it is important that athletes drink plenty of fluids before an event in order to maintain hydration.

Athletes preparing for evening competition can use the beginning of the day to refill their carbohydrate stores from the previous day and to become properly hydrated. Both breakfast and lunch should be high-carbohydrate meals, which could be followed by a light snack 1 to 2 hours before competition. Recommended energy content of these meals ranges from 600 to 1000 kcal, with 60% to 70% carbohydrate and approximately 45% to 50% of the carbohydrate from complex carbohydrate (Benardot et al, 1993). A typical pre-event meal for some athletes is 2 cups of spaghetti with 1 cup meat sauce, a salad with 2 dinner rolls, and a glass of milk or juice (approximately 1000 kcal).

Eating candy, as our track athlete Justin did, or drinking sweet beverages within 45 minutes of the start of exercise or a competitive event may cause feelings of sluggishness and premature fatigue in some individuals. This has been attributed to the release of insulin and the corresponding uptake of glucose from the blood. It has been suggested that avoiding these types of foods would benefit the athlete; however, this has recently become controversial (Lamb and Wardlaw, 1991). The athlete should experiment with pre-event foods or beverages (1 to 2 cups of a 10% to 20% carbohydrate beverage) to determine if his or her performance is adversely affected due to the intake of simple sugars within 45 minutes of exercise.

Foods During Competition

Athletes who perform moderate to intense exercise for more than 60 minutes benefit from carbohydrate consumption during competition. Studies of cyclists have indicated that endurance performance was increased by 18% when 1 g carbohydrate/kg body weight was consumed after 60 to 90 minutes of exercise (Coggan and Coyle, 1987).

During intense exercise some athletes may not prefer to consume anything but water; however, sports drinks with sugar concentrations less than 8% are usually well tolerated, taste good, and offer advantages such as the maintenance of blood glucose and replacement of fluid and electrolytes. Some of these beverages are listed in Table 14–4.

Although blood flow to the abdominal organs is decreased during exercise and although absorption is 60% to 70% of normal, some endurance athletes such as cyclists and ultramarathoners can also eat solid and semi-solid foods while exercising. Carbohydrate gels and fruit/grain bars are currently popular methods for carbohydrate ingestion during exercise.

Currently, no specific dietary information is available for improving performance of resistance athletes during exercise (Conley and Stone, 1996).

Post-Event Foods

Recent research has indicated that, without adequate consumption of carbohydrate after exercise, glycogen stores and endurance in subsequent events are hindered (Ivy, 1988). Many athletes do not feel like eating after exercise; however, it has been demonstrated that consumption of a carbohydrate beverage (50–100 g carbohydrate or 200–400 kcal) within 2 hours of the event aids recovery of muscle glycogen. Additionally, a high-carbohydrate meal within 4 hours after the event is recommended (Benardot et al, 1993; Ivy, 1988).

Suggestions for high-carbohydrate foods that provide 50 to 100g carbohydrate within the first 2 hours after exercise include one or several of the following:

- 1 bagel (36 g carbohydrate, 187 kcal)
- 1 oz raisins (22 g carbohydrate, 84 kcal)
- 8-oz orange juice (27 g carbohydate, 112 kcal)
- 1 banana (27 g carbohydrate, 104 kcal)
- 1 low-fat granola bar (22 g carbohydrate, 110 kcal)
- 3 c air-popped popcorn (18 g carbohydrate, 93 kcal)
- 1 c pasta (40 g carbohydrate, 197 kcal)
- 1 c yogurt with fruit (43 g carbohydrate, 230 kcal)
- 1 large apple (32 g carbohydrate, 212 kcal)

Individuals who exercise regularly and are highly active, as well as those who are competitive athletes, benefit from balanced nutrition and exercise training habits. Using sound principles of nutrition to consume adequate fluid, eating nutrient-dense foods, and satisfying energy requirements improves endurance and performance during exercise and enhances recovery after exercise.

NUTRITION CONCERNS FOR ATHLETES ACROSS THE LIFE SPAN

■ Do age, gender, and level of physical fitness affect nutrition requirements for athletes?

■ Are ergogenic aids useful for athletes for enhancing performance? Who uses them?

Athletes and their nutrition requirements cannot be made into a "one size fits all" program. Just as nutrition requirements are varied across the life span, the nutrition requirements of athletes are also varied.

Child Athletes

Many young children are participating in sports and athletic competitions today at very early ages. Some begin gymnastics, skating, and dance practice at the age of 2 or 3 years. Once in school, at age 5 or 6, many children join soccer, baseball or football leagues (Fig. 14–8). The opportunities to participate in sports are endless, and as children become more involved in sports, it is imperative to provide nutrition guidance to them and their parents (Steen, 1994).

Several physiologic aspects of children's bodies may affect their training and sports nutrition. They have lower peak strength or power per kg body weight compared to adults (Inbar and Bar-Or, 1986) but similar or, perhaps, in some cases, greater maximal aerobic power per kg body weight (Bar-Or, 1995). This implies that they may have low performance in sprinting or jumping events but they are able to achieve steady state quickly at the start of aerobic work and are capable of faster recovery than adults (Bar-Or, 1995).

The ability of children to sweat is low compared to adults, for reasons still unknown (Benardot et al, 1993; Steen, 1994; Bar-Or, 1995). A child has a greater relative surface area than an adult, which implies increased energy production per kg body weight and thus greater insensible heat loss. These factors, along with a decreased ability to acclimatize to a hot environment (Bar-Or, 1995), result in increased requirements to maintain hydration and core body temperature. Thus, hydration before, during, and after a game or an event is crucial.

Hydration in children can be maintained in a fashion similar to that in adults. It has been recommended that children drink approximately 1.5 to 2 cups of fluid before exercise and 0.5 to 1.0 cups every 15 minutes as exercise progresses (Benardot et al, 1993; Meyer and Bar-Or, 1994). Some researchers found that providing flavored water resulted in increased consumption of fluid by young athletes, especially with grape flavor compared to orange or apple (Meyer et al, 1994).

Because children have a greater relative body surface area than adults and because children are growing, their energy requirements (kcal/kg body weight) are much greater (47–55 kcal/kg) compared to adults (25–35 kcal/kg). Athletic children may require energy above these levels (Freedson et al, 1981). In addition, children are less efficient at athletic movements than adults, suggesting they may waste energy (Freedson et al, 1981). However, as in other areas related to the young athlete, the research lags behind that for adults (Bar-Or, 1995), and an exact estimation of energy needs is difficult.

Dietitians in the field of pediatric sports nutrition suggest that children who participate in exercise may have caloric requirements that are 500 to 1500 kcalories above the 1800 to 2200 kcalories suggested by the RDA (Jennings and Nelson-Steen, 1993). Some suggest kcalories alloted for exercise should be based on exercise intensity, which can be quite subjective (Benardot et al, 1993). One additional suggestion is to monitor body weight during the training and competitive seasons and adjust energy intake accordingly (Benardot et al, 1993).

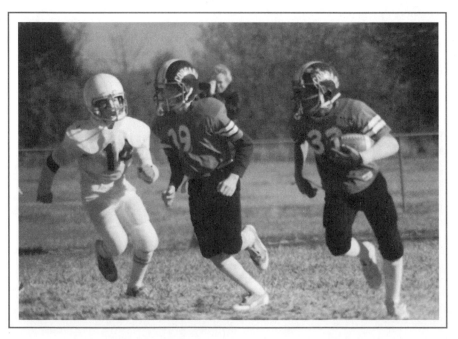

FIGURE 14–8. Young athletes participating in football sports league.

At any rate, parents, coaches, and trainers are urged to become aware of the specific nutrition needs of young athletes (American Dietetic Association, 1996a) and to provide a healthy and safe sports environment. Additional research is necessary to better understand the requirements for pediatric sports nutrition.

Adolescent Athletes

The physiologic requirements of adolescent growth and maturity greatly influence a teenager's nutrition requirements, as described in Chapter 7. The incorporation of one or more sports or activities into an already busy lifestyle may increase requirements for energy and some nutrients. It is likely that a balanced diet can have its most significant impact at this time of the life span, yet studies suggest that poor dietary intakes are the norm (Calabrese, 1985; Risser et al, 1988; Benardot and Czerwinski, 1991).

One major nutritional concern for the adolescent athlete is total energy intake (Benardot and Czerwinski, 1991). Energy needs can be determined as basal needs plus estimates of energy expenditure from charts with energy costs for many athletic activities (McArdle et al, 1991). In general, adolescent female athletes require a total of 2500 to 3500 kcal/d, while males require 3000 to 6000 kcal/d. However, with excessive pressure to be thin, more athletes find themselves in a situation similar to that of Kristen, the track athlete described earlier in this chapter, who selectively and sometimes drastically decrease energy intake to lose weight and body fat.

Athletes who often participate in weight loss practices are involved in weight classification sports such as wrestling or appearance sports such as gymnastics, dance, and figure skating (Benardot et al, 1993). Neither they nor their coaches may know that such practices decrease performance.

Roemmich and Sinning (1996) studied the anthropometry and strength changes in a group of high school wrestlers during training, the competitive season, and post-season. These wrestlers admitted repeated use of restricted energy and fluid intake in order to compete in a lower weight class. In comparison to a control group who participated in the same resistance training, they found that, during the competitive season, the wrestlers had a significant decrease in strength that was only partially explained by lack of lean tissue accretion. Interestingly, both strength and lean tissue increased post-season, which the authors attributed to more normal nutrition (Roemmich and Sinning, 1996).

It is exceedingly important to help adolescents understand changes associated with growth and help them learn to focus on good health and reasonable weights for their bodies. This is no easy task, and some adolescent athletes, especially in sports sensitive to leanness, can experience eating disorders such as anorexia nervosa, bulimia nervosa, binge eating disorder, or a subclinical classification of an eating or weight disorder now known as anorexia athletica (Sundgot-Borgen, 1994). Anorexia athletica is characterized by an obsession with body weight and fat and the impression that severe caloric restriction coupled with excessive daily exercise and perhaps some binging and purging will produce the desired body weight, even if weight loss is not warranted (Sundgot-Borgen, 1994).

The prevalence of such disorders in teenage athletes is difficult to detect because there are many variables to consider, such as type of sport, length of season, and method of measuring eating or weight disorder. It is estimated that from <1% to more than 39% of female athletes experience an eating or weight disorder of some type (Sundgot-Borgen, 1994). Less is known about the prevalence of these disorders in male athletes; however, one group found that 11% of wrestlers surveyed admitted to vomiting to lose weight (Steen and McKinney, 1991).

Another concern for the adolescent athlete is the increased demand for the proteins myoglobin and hemoglobin. Many vitamins and minerals are required for protein synthesis; iron, however, is especially in demand. Normal losses of iron through the menstrual cycle and during contact sports in which bruising and some bleeding may occur elevate iron requirements for teens (Risser et al, 1988; Rowland et al, 1987). One study indicated that 25% of female athletes and 12% of male athletes had iron deficiency (serum ferritin levels less than 12 g/dL) (Rowland et al, 1987). Recommendations to improve iron levels in teens include eating adequate amounts of meat, fish, and poultry as well as a source of vitamin C. Iron supplements have been suggested for some adolescent athletes after an evaluation of serum ferritin and hemoglobin levels (Benardot et al, 1993).

Female adolescent athletes who are significantly underweight, with less than 17% body fat, who may have low estrogen levels as well as low calcium intake, and who participate in endurance events may not only suffer low bone density and stress fractures while competing but may also be setting the stage for poor bone density and other bone-related disorders such as osteoporosis later in life (Benardot et al, 1993). Recommendations for these athletes include increasing calcium intake to 1400 to 1500 mg/d and obtaining a medical evaluation for hormone status and bone density (Benardot et al, 1993). Depending on the outcome of the medical evaluation, it may be necessary for these athletes to drastically decrease training and receive estrogen therapy in order to restore proper bone density.

A final influence on the nutrition of adolescent athletes is that, like other athletes, they are interested in improving performance at almost any cost. They are easily convinced that some nutrients possess a magic ability to improve performance or perhaps increase the size of their muscles. These types of products are generally characterized as **ergogenic aids** and are discussed in greater detail in the Application at the end of this chapter. Few of these products have been tested in an unbiased scientific fashion, yet millions of dollars are spent on them each year in hopes of achieving what good nutrition, regular exercise training, and some mental discipline can accomplish.

In addition, certainly more dangerous and definitely illegal, many adolescent athletes begin to learn about and use anabolic steroids to build strength or to bulk up their muscles (Buckley et al, 1988). Middleman and DuRant (1996), in their recent review of anabolic steroid use, estimated that 1 million Americans spend over $100 million per year on black market anabolic steroids. Their review suggests that 4% to 11% of male and 0.5% to 2.9% of female adolescents in the United States have used anabolic steroids.

Anabolic steroids, sometimes called anabolic-androgenic steroids, are derivatives of testosterone, which is the predominant male hormone responsible for masculinizing the male body. Easily obtained on the black market, the hormone derivatives come in the form of intramuscular injections, transdermal patches, oral tablets, or nasal sprays (Yesalis and Bahrke, 1995). Athletes traditionally use them in repeating 6- to 12-week cycles. Because there are many derivatives, they may take more than one steroid at a time in a procedure called "stacking." Dosages used by athletes depend on the sport. Endurance athletes may use near-physiologic doses (7 mg/d), sprinters may use 1 to 2 times this amount, and those interested in greatly increasing strength and bulk may use 10 to 100 times this amount (Yesalis and Bahrke, 1995).

Use of anabolic steroids increases skeletal muscle mass, strength, and protein synthesis and decreases body fat (Yesalis and Bahrke, 1995; Middleman and DuRant, 1996). However, there are numerous potential side effects, some of which can be severe, such as testicular atrophy, aggressive behavior, mood swings, premature closure of bone growth plates, acne, alopecia, hypertension, abnormalities in cholesterol metabolism, liver dysfunction, kidney and prostate tumors (Lamb, 1989; Middleman and DuRant, 1996), and perhaps even cardiomyopathy and cerebrovascular accident (Mochizuki and Richter, 1988).

Adolescent athletes must face the nutrition challenges associated with growth and the increased activity of their chosen sport. Likewise, adolescence is a time when a person is learning, experiencing, and being influenced by family, friends, school, and society in general. Because all of these factors can potentially influence their nutrition, it is beneficial for these athletes to have reliable parents, coaches, trainers, and even dietitians to assist them in achieving a healthy balance and understanding of their bodies' best nutrition (American Dietetic Association, 1996b).

Adult and Older Athletes

The peak of fitness and performance for most people occurs between the late teens and early thirties (Benardot et al, 1993; Evans, 1992). After 30, there is usually a gradual decline in several metabolic and physiologic markers of fitness, including cardiorespiratory values, flexibility, strength, lean body mass, and bone density (Benardot et al, 1993). Current issues of investigation during these adult years are whether regular exercise delays this normal decline and whether exercise training can reverse these declines (Fiatarone et al, 1990; Evans, 1992).

Recently, resistance exercise research in older men and women has demonstrated that resistance training can result in increased strength in the trained muscles, muscle area, and, more applicably for nursing home residents, the walking speed of these individuals (Fiatarone et al, 1990; Fontera et al, 1988). Although some studies of resistance-trained elderly men or women have not reported the same level of improvement (most likely due to differences in amount and frequency of weight lifted), the data strongly suggest that age-related declines in lean tissue and strength can be reversed with training (Fiatarone et al, 1990; Evans, 1992). Interestingly, detraining resulted in a 32% loss of maximum strength in just 4 weeks (Fiatarone et al, 1990).

The two nutrition issues that may affect resistance-trained elderly are adequacy of protein and energy intake. The study conducted by Fiatarone and co-workers suggested that men who were supplemented with approximately 560 kcals and 90 g protein per day had significantly greater gains in muscle mass than those who did not recieve supplements (Fiatarone et al, 1990; Evans, 1992). Additional research with noninstitutionalized older athletes is warranted.

In general, however, nutrition concerns for older athletes involve not only normal nutrition but also the nutrition associated with chronic diseases such as diabetes, atherosclerosis, hypertension, cancer, and obesity. Adequate and balanced nutrition may delay the onset and progression of these diseases, and key nutrition issues must be individualized and focused on the athletic goals without losing sight of any predisposition to chronic diseases.

Most nutritional recommendations for individuals over 50 have been extrapolated from the data for younger adults. Because limited data are available for this age group and since there is great diversity and heterogeneity in this population, nutrition requirements must be considered individually (Hegsted et al, 1989). In addition, in many older adults who use both prescription and over-the-counter medications, the impact of drug-nutrient intake and utilization is beginning to be recognized. The effects of exercise under these circumstances are relatively unknown but warrant investigation (Benardot et al, 1993).

Exercise is beneficial for adults because it decreases risk factors for cardiovascular disease such as lowering serum total cholesterol, LDL cholesterol, and triglycerides while it raises HDL cholesterol (Tran and Weltman, 1985). It also increases insulin sensitivity and improves glucose tolerance, which may prevent or delay the onset of type II diabetes (Rosenthal et al, 1983). Additionally, exercise contributes to weight maintenance and, as noted earlier, delays muscle loss in the aging athlete.

Protein requirements may be elevated above 0.8 g/kg/d for endurance athletes of all ages. Vitamin requirements are not elevated for the older adult, but little is known about these requirements for the older athlete (Garry et al, 1982). Most sports-related nutrition requirements for athletes over the age of 50 are based on principles of nutrition discussed previously with the additional considerations of age and medical condition.

Pregnant and Lactating Athletes

In the last 30 years, women have made tremendous achievements in the world of athletics. One consequence of such achievements is that more women will choose to remain competitive for a longer period of time, which may encompass their reproductive years.

Women experience numerous physiologic changes during pregnancy and lactation (see Chapter 8), which may influence or be influenced by their physical activity. Numerous reviews have addressed the effects of exercise on factors associated with maternal and fetal health; however, there is very little nutrition information available for the pregnant or lactating athlete (Benardot et al, 1993; Sternfeld et al, 1995; McMurray et al, 1993; Lokey et al, 1991; Cohen, 1991; Gorski, 1985; Revelli, 1992).

Pregnancy

Major changes that occur during pregnancy may affect the pregnant woman's ability to exercise. Some of these include an increase in body weight, which alters the center of gravity and, ultimately, balance, and an increase in blood volume, which increases the amount of blood ejected by the heart and potentially affects blood pressure, heat distribution for the fetus, and, perhaps, oxygen availability in the blood (Kulpa et al, 1987; Clapp and Dickstein, 1984; Clapp et al, 1987).

Many of the effects of exercise during pregnancy are not well understood. For instance, a decrease in maternal blood glucose after 30 to 40 minutes of aerobic exercise (Clapp et al, 1987) may or may not result in low fetal blood glucose values (McMurray et al, 1993). Uterine blood flow does appear to be reduced during exercise; however, it does not seem to have a detrimental effect on the fetus because the natural improvement in oxygen uptake coupled with the elevated maternal cardiac output are sufficient compensation for both the exercising muscles and the fetus (Sady and Carpenter, 1989). Further research of the

effect of exercise at higher intensities and for longer duration is warranted (Cohen, 1991).

The American College of Obstetricians and Gynecologists (1985) has established guidelines for women who choose to exercise during pregnancy and postpartum (Table 14–6). Benefits of exercise during pregnancy have been documented in many research studies. They include a positive self-image (Jarski and Trippett, 1990; Hall and Kaufmann, 1987), maintenance of aerobic fitness (Wolfe et al, 1989; Sady and Carpenter, 1989), shorter labor and quicker, easier delivery (Jarski and Trippett, 1990), and more vaginal deliveries and fewer surgical interventions (Wolfe et al, 1989; Clapp, 1990).

There are also several potential benefits from exercise during pregnancy that have not been unequivocally proven by research. For instance, there is some suggestion that exercise during pregnancy may (Hall and Kaufmann, 1987; Wolfe et al, 1989) or may not (Kulpa et al, 1987) improve Apgar scores of infants. Birth weight may not be reduced as a result of maternal exercise (Hall and Kaufmann, 1987; Kulpa et al, 1987); however, this has not been found in every study (Clapp, 1990). The composition and pattern of weight, especially fat, gained during pregnancy may be reduced with exercise (Jarski and Trippett, 1990); however, this has not yet been adequately evaluated (Wolfe et al, 1989; Jarski and Trippett, 1990).

The Sports and Cardiovascular Nutritionists Practice Group (SCAN) of the American Dietetic Association recommends that women who exercise throughout pregnancy should:

- Obtain sufficient energy to sustain growth of the fetus as well as the physcial activity of the mother
- Obtain liberal amounts of fluid before, during, and after exercise to prevent dehydration
- Follow the recommendations of their physician and those of the American College of Obstetricians and Gynecologists during their pregnancy regarding exercise.

Lactation

After pregnancy, regardless of lactation status, many women begin to exercise and reduce energy intake to lose the weight retained as a result of pregnancy. Health pro-

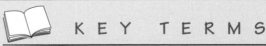

KEY TERMS

ergogenic aids: a term that implies "energy-producing" or "energy-giving" but in fact has not been proven as such for products with which it is associated

TABLE 14-6 Recommendations for Exercise in Pregnancy and Postpartum

For women who do not have any additional risk factors for adverse maternal or perinatal outcome, the following recommendations have been made:

1. During pregnancy, women can continue to exercise and derive health benefits even from mild-to-moderate exercise routines. Regular exercise (at least three times per week) is preferable to intermittent activity.

2. Women should avoid exercise in the supine position after the first trimester. Such a position is associated with decreased cardiac output in most pregnant women; because the remaining cardiac output will be preferentially distributed away from splanchnic beds (including the uterus) during vigorous exercise, such regimens are best avoided during pregnancy. Prolonged periods of motionless standing should also be avoided.

3. Women should be aware of the decreased oxygen available for aerobic exercise during pregnancy. They should be encouraged to modify the intensity of their exercise according to maternal symptoms. Pregnant women should stop exercising when fatigued and not exercise to exhaustion. Weight-bearing exercises may under some circumstances be continued at intensities similar to those prior to pregnancy throughout pregnancy. Non-weight-bearing exercises such as cycling or swimming will minimize the risk of injury and facilitate the continuation of exercise during pregnancy.

4. Morphologic changes in pregnancy should serve as a relative contraindication to types of exercise in which loss of balance could be detrimental to maternal or fetal well-being, especially in the third trimester. Further, any type of exercise involving the potential for even mild abdominal trauma should be avoided.

5. Pregnancy requires an additional 300 kcal/d in order to maintain metabolic homeostasis. Thus women who exercise during pregnancy should be particularly careful to ensure an adequate diet.

6. Pregnant women who exercise in the first trimester should augment heat dissipation by ensuring adequate hydration, appropriate clothing, and optimal environmental surroundings during exercise.

7. Many of the physiologic and morphologic changes of pregnancy persist 4–6 weeks postpartum. Thus, prepregnancy exercise routines should be resumed gradually based on a woman's physical capability.

From American College of Obstetricians and Gynecologists. Exercise during pregnancy and the postpartum period. Technical Bulletin No 189. Washington, DC, ACOG © February 1994.

fessionals have cautioned women who are lactating to restrict weight loss to < 2 kg/mo (Dewey and McCrory, 1994) to ensure adequate milk quality and quantity.

The research completed to date indicates that women who do not restrict energy intake but participate in submaximal aerobic exercise 3 to 5 days per week may lose up to 3.5 kg over a 12- to 14-week training period without stopping lactation (Habash and Mitchell, 1994) and without having a negative effect on the volume or composition of breast milk (Lovelady et al, 1990). On the other hand, when energy intake was restricted to 1800 kcal/d in a group of sedentary lactating women, mean weight loss was 4.8 ± 1.2 kg in 10 weeks and lactation was not affected (Dusdieker et al, 1994). No studies have assessed the combination of increased activity and restricted energy intake on body weight and lactation status in new mothers. In addition, only one study has measured infant acceptability of breast milk after maximal exercise (Wallace et al, 1992). These authors found that maximal exercise, specifically a treadmill test of VO_{2max}, did decrease infant acceptability of breast milk at 10 and 30 minutes after the test. All other studies have evaluated the effect of the specific experimental condition by noting no compromise in infant growth (Lovelady et al, 1990; Habash and Mitchell, 1994).

Although more research is needed, current nutritional recommendations for exercising lactating women include (1) obtaining sufficient kilocalories for exercise above the daily energy needs to sustain lactation, as discussed in Chapter 10, and (2) increasing fluid intake by approximately 3 8-oz glasses per day to ensure adequate hydration (Benardot et al, 1993).

In conclusion, scientists and health professionals continue to justify the importance of increased activity and balanced nutrition for our everyday lives. Whether an individual is 90 or 9, whether they are elite marathoners or budding gymnasts, a complementary balance of nutrition and exercise improves performance at any stage of the life span.

CONCEPTS TO REMEMBER

▶ Physical fitness is defined as the set of attributes required to perform physical activity, including flexibility, muscular strength and endurance, cardiorespiratory endurance, and body composition.

▶ Exercise in which large muscle groups of the back and legs are used continuously for at least 15 minutes three times per week are beneficial for lowering the risk of chronic diseases such as cardiovascular disease, obesity, and diabetes.

▶ Muscle fibers respond to specific exercise training by adapting either aerobic or anaerobic energy production.

▶ All nutrients play an important role in the total performance of an athlete, regardless of age.

▶ A high daily intake of carbohydrates (55–70% of total energy) improves the aerobic endurance performance of an athlete.

▶ Working muscles prefer to use glucose as their primary fuel source, especially at higher intensities of work.

▶ Aerobic exercise training enhances the use of fatty acids and improves performance by sparing endogenous carbohydrate stores.

▶ Resistance exercise training enhances lean body mass accretion and sustains or improves bone density.

▶ The best way to build more muscle is to eat a well-balanced diet and exercise or overload the muscle with some form of resistance training.

▶ Athletes experience decreased performance if not properly hydrated.

▶ Ergogenic aids are not likely to enhance performance and may actually impair it.

▶ Use of anabolic steroids is illegal and risky for the long-term health of the athlete.

▶ Individuals of all ages and fitness levels benefit from regular exercise, especially if it is coupled with a well-balanced diet.

References

American College of Sports Medicine. Guidelines for exercise testing and prescription. 4th ed. Philadelphia: Lea & Febiger, 1991.

American College of Sports Medicine. Position statement: The recommended quantity and quality of exercise for developing and maintaining cardiorespiratory and muscular fitness in healthy adults. Med Sci Sports Exerc 1990;22:265.

American Dietetic Association. Timely statements. Nutrition guidance for child athletes in organized sports. J Am Diet Assoc 1996a;96:610.

American Dietetic Association. Timely statements. Nutrition guidance for adolescent athletes in organized sports. J Am Diet Assoc 1996b;96:611.

American Dietetic Association and Canadian Dietetic Association. Position statement: nutrition for physical fitness and athletic performance for adults. J Am Diet Assoc 1993;93:691.

American College of Obstetricians and Gynecologists. Exercise during pregnancy and the postnatal period. Washington, DC: 1985.

Armstrong LE, et al. Influence of diuretic-induced dehydration on competitive running performance. Med Sci Sports Exerc 1985;17:456.

Astrand P. Something old and something new...very new. Nutr Today 1968;June:9.

Bar-Or O. The young athlete: some physiological considerations. J Sports Sci 1995;13:S31.

Belko AZ, et al. Effects of exercise on riboflavin requirements of young women. Am J Clin Nutr 1983;37:509.

Benardot D, ed. Sports nutrition. A guide for the professional working with active people. 2nd ed. Chicago: American Dietetic Association, 1993.

Benardot D, et al. Nutrient intake in young, highly competitive gymnasts. J Am Diet Assoc 1989;89:401.

Benardot D, Czerwinski C. Selected body composition and growth measures of junior elite gymnasts. J Am Diet Assoc 1991;91:29.

Blair SN, et al. Physical activity, nutrition, and chronic disease. Med Sci Sports Exerc 1996a;28:335.

Blair SN, et al. Physical fitness and all-cause mortality. A prospective study of healthy men and women. JAMA 1989;262:2394.

Blair SN, et al. Changes in physical fitness and all-cause mortality. A prospective study of healthy and unhealthy men. JAMA 1995;273:1093.

Blair SN, et al. Influences of cardiorespiratory fitness and other precursors on cardiovascular disease and all-cause mortality in men and women. JAMA 1996b;276:205.

Bonen A, et al. Carbohydrate metabolism in skeletal muscle: an update of current concepts. Int J Sports Med 1989;10:385.

Bouchard C, Despres JP. Physical activity and health: atherosclerotic, metabolic, and hypertensive diseases. Res Quar Exer Sport 1995;66:268.

Buckley WE, Yesalis CE III, Friedl KE, Anderson WA, Streit AL, Wright JE. Estimated prevalence of anabolic steroid use among male high school seniors. JAMA 1988;260:3441.

Burke LM, Read RSD. Sports nutrition: approaching the nineties. Sports Med 1989;8:80.

Calabrese LH. Nutritional and medical aspects of gymnastics. Clin Sports Med 1985;4:23.

Cannon JG, et al. Acute phase response in exercise: interactions of age and vitamin E on neutrophils and muscle enzyme release. Am J Physiol 1990;259:R1214.

Casoni I, et al. Reduced hemoglobin concentration and red cell hemoglobinization in Italian marathon and ultramarathon runners. Int J Sports Med 1985;6:176.

Caspersen CJ, et al. Status of the 1990 physical fitness and exercise objectives: evidence from the NIHS. Pub Health Rep 1986;101:587.

Clapp JF. Thermoregulatory and metabolic responses to jogging prior to and during pregnancy. Med Sci Sports Exerc 1987;19:124.

Clapp JF. The course of labor after endurance exercise during pregnancy. Am J Obstet Gynecol 1990;163:1799.

Clapp JF, Dickstein S. Endurance exercise and pregnancy outcome. Med Sci Sports Exerc 1984;16:556.

Clapp JF, et al. Maternal physiologic adaptations to early human pregnancy. Am J Obstet Gynecol 1988;159:1456.

Clarkson PM. Tired blood: iron deficiency in athletes and effects of iron supplementation. Gatorade Sports Science Institute. Sports Science Exchange, September 1990.

Clarkson PM. Nutrition for improved sports performance. Current issues on ergogenic aids. Sports Med 1996;6:393.

Coggan AR, Coyle EF. Reversal of fatigue during prolonged exercise by carbohydrate infusion or ingestion. J Appl Physiol 1987;63:5.

Cohen GC. Exercise in pregnancy. Gatorade Sports Science Institute. Sports Science Exchange, March 1991.

Coleman E. Sports drink update. Gatorade Sports Science Institute. Sports Science Exchange, August 1988.

Conley MS, Stone MH. Carbohydrate ingestion/supplementation for resistance exercise and training. Sports Med 1996;21:7.

Corbin CB. Flexibility. Clin Sports Med 1984;3:101.

Coyle EF, Montain SJ. Carbohydrate and fluid ingestion during exercise: Are there trade-offs? Med Sci Sports Exerc 1992;24:671.

DeBusk RF, et al. Training effects of long versus short bouts of exercise in healthy subjects. Am J Cardiol 1990;65:1010.

Dekkers JC, et al. The role of antioxidant vitamins and enzymes in the prevention of exercise-induced muscle damage. Sports Med 1996;21:213.

Dewey KG, McCrory MA. Effects of dieting and physical activity on pregnancy and lactation. Am J Clin Nutr 1994;59(Suppl):446S.

Duchateau J, Hainaut K. Isometric or dynamic training: differential effect on mechanical properties of a human muscle. J Appl Physiol 1982;6:296.

Dusdieker LB, et al. Is milk production impaired by dieting during lactation? Am J Clin Nutr 1994;59:833.

Economos CD, et al. Nutrition practices of elite athletes: practical recommendations. Sports Med 1993;16:381.

Eichner ER. "Sports anemia": poor terminology for a real phenomenon. Gatorade Sports Science Institute. Sports Science Exchange, August 1988.

Evans WJ. Exercise, nutrition, and aging. J Nutr 1992;122:796.

Fahey TD, et al. The effects of intermittent liquid meal feeding on selected hormones and substrates during intense weight training. Int J Sport Nutr 1993;3:67.

Felig P, Wahren J. Amino acid metabolism in exercising man. J Clin Invest 1971;50:2703.

Fiatarone MA, et al. High-intensity strength training in nonagenarians: effects on skeletal muscle. JAMA 1990;263:3029.

Fontera WR. Strength conditioning in older men: skeletal muscle hypertrophy and improved function. J Appl Physiol 1988;64:1038.

Freedson PS, et al. Energy expenditure in prepubescent children: influence of sex and age. Am J Clin Nutr. 1981;34:1827.

Garry PJ, et al. Nutritional status in a healthy elderly population: vitamin C. Am J Clin Nutr 1982;36:332.

Gorski J. Exercise during pregnancy: maternal and fetal responses. A brief review. Med Sci Sports Exerc 1985;17:1985.

Goulding A. Athletic amenorrhoea: a risk factor for osteoporosis in later life? N Z Med J 1986;99:765.

Habash DL, Mitchell MC. Exercise training in postpartum women: changes in body mass index, percent body fat, and body fat distribution [abstract]. Annual Meeting of the American College of Nutrition. Atlanta, GA. October, 1994.

Hall DC, Kaufmann DA. Effects of aerobic and strength conditioning on pregnancy outcomes. Am J Obstet Gynecol 1987;157:1199.

Hawley JA, et al. Nutritional practices of athletes: are they sub-optimal? J Sport Sci 1995;13:S75.

Haymes EM. Nutritional concerns: need for iron. Med Sci Sports Exerc 1987;19:S197.

Hegsted DM. Recommended dietary intakes of elderly subjects. Am J Clin Nutr 1989;50:1190.

Hickson JF, Wolinsky I. Nutrition in exercise and sport. Boca Raton, FL: CRC Press, 1989.

Hiller WDB. Dehydration and hyponatremia during triathlons. Med Sci Sports Exerc 1989;21:S219.

Inbar O, Bar-Or O. Anaerobic characteristics in male children and adolescents. Med Sci Sports Exerc 1986;18:264.

Ivy JL. Muscle glycogen synthesis after exercise: effect of time of carbohydrate ingestion. J Appl Physiol 1988;64:1480.

Jakeman P, Maxwell S. Effect of antioxidant vitamin supplementation on muscle function after eccentric exercise. Eur J Appl Physiol 1993;67:426.

Jarski RW, Trippett DL. The risks and benefits of exercise during pregnancy. J Fam Pract 1990;30:185.

Jenkins DG, et al. The influence of dietary carbohydrates on performance of supramaximal intermittent exercise. Eur J Appl Physiol 1993;67:309.

Jennings D, Nelson-Steen S, eds. Sports nutrition for the child athlete. Chicago: American Dietetic Association, 1993.

Knuttgen HG, Kraemer WJ. Terminology and measurement in exercise performance. J Appl Sports Sci Res 1987;1:1.

Krotkiewski M, et al. Zinc and muscle strength. Acta Physiol Scand 1982;116:309.

Kuel J, et al. The effect of weight lifting exercise on heart rate and metabolism in experienced weightlifters. Med Sci Sports Exerc 1978;10:13.

Kulpa PJ, et al. Aerobic exercise in pregnancy. Am J Obstet Gynecol 1987;156:1395.

Lamb DR. Abuse of anabolic steroids in sport. Gatorade Sports Science Institute. Sports Science Exchange, April 1989.

Lamb DR, et al. Dietary carbohydrate and intensity of interval swim training. Am J Clin Nutr 1990;52:1058.

Lamb DR, Wardlaw G. Sports nutrition. Nutri-News. St. Louis: Mosby-Year Book 1991.

Lemon PWR, Mullin JP. Effect of initial muscle glycogen levels on protein catabolism during exercise. J Appl Physiol 1980;48:624.

Lemon WR. Dietary protein and amino acids with exercise: are more better? Gatorade Sports Science Institute. Sports Science Exchange, November 1994.

Lokey, et al. Effects of physical exercise on pregnancy outcomes: a meta-analytic review. Med Sci Sports Exerc 1991;23:1234.

Lovelady CA, et al. Lactation performance of exercising women. Am J Clin Nutr 1990;52:103.

Lukaski HC. Micronutrients (magnesium, zinc, and copper): are mineral supplements needed for athletes? Gatorade Sports Science Institute, November 1994.

Lukaski HC, et al. Maximum oxygen consumption as related to magnesium, copper, and zinc nutriture. Am J Clin Nutr 1983;37:407.

Matthews DK, et al. Physiological responses during exercise and recovery in a football uniform. J Appl Physiol 1969;26:611.

McArdle WD, et al. Exercise physiology, energy, and human performance. 3rd ed. Philadelphia: Lea & Febiger; 1991.

McArdle WD, et al. Essentials of exercise physiology. Philadelphia: Lea & Febiger, 1994.

McDonald R, Keen CL. Iron, zinc, and magnesium nutrition and athletic performance. Sports Med 1988;5:171.

McMurray RG, et al. Recent advances in understanding maternal and fetal responses to exercise. Med Sci Sports Exerc 1993;25:1305.

Meredith CN, et al. Dietary protein requirements and body protein metabolism in endurance-trained men. J Appl Physiol 1989;66:2850.

Meyer F, et al. Hypohydration during exercise in children: Effect on thirst, drink preferences, and rehydration. Int J Sports Nutr 1994;4:22.

Meyer F, Bar-Or O. Fluid and electrolyte loss during exercise: the pediatric angle. Sports Med 1994;18:4.

Middleman AB, DuRant RH. Anabolic steroid use and associated health risk behaviours. Sports Med 1996;21:251.

Mochizuki RM, Richter KJ. Cardiomyopathy and cerebrovascular accident associated with anabolic-androgenic steroid use. Physician and Sportsmed 1988;16:109.

Moritani T, deVries HA. Potential for gross muscle hypertrophy in older men. J Gerontol 1980;35:672.

National Institutes of Health Consensus Conference. Physical activity and cardiovascular health. JAMA 1996;276:241.

National Research Council. Recommended dietary allowances. 10th ed. Washington, DC: National Academy Press, 1989.

Nelson ME, et al. Diet and bone status in amenorrheic runners. Am J Clin Nutr 1986;43:910.

Noakes TD, et al. The incidence of hyponatremia during prolonged ultraendurance exercise. Med Sci Sports Exerc 1990;22:165.

Noakes TD, et al. The danger of inadequate water intake during prolonged exercise: a novel concept revisited. Eur J Appl Physiol 1988;57:210.

Paffenbarger RS Jr, et al. Physical activity, all-cause mortality, and longevity of college alumni. N Engl J Med 1986;314:605.

Pate RR, et al. Physical activity and public health. A recommendation from the Centers for Disease Control and Prevention and the American College of Sports Medicine. JAMA 1995;273:402.

Philen RM, et al. Survey of advertising for nutritional supplements in health and bodybuilding magazines. JAMA 1992;268:1008.

Phillips WT, et al. Lifestyle activity. Current recommendations. Sports Med 1996;22:1.

Pi-Sunyer FX. Health implications of obesity. Am J Clin Nutr 1991;53:1595S.

Pugh LCGE, et al. Rectal temperatures, weight losses and sweat rates in marathon running. J Appl Physiol 1966;21;1251.

Revelli A, et al. Exercise and pregnancy: a review of maternal and fetal effects. Obstet Gynecol Surv 1992;47:355.

Risser WL, et al. Iron deficiency in female athletes: its prevalence and impact on performance. Med Sci Sports Exerc 1988;20:116.

Robergs RA, et al. Muscle glycogenolysis during differing intensities of weight-resistance exercise. J Appl Physiol 1991;70:1700.

Robertson JD. Influence of vitamin E supplementation on muscle damage following endurance exercise. Int J Vitam Nutr Res 1990;60:171.

Roemmich JN, Sinning WE. Sport-seasonal changes in body composition, growth, power and strength of adolescent wrestlers. Int J Sports Med 1996;17:92.

Rosenthal M, et al. Demonstration of a relationship between level of physical training and insulin-stimulated glucose utilization in normal humans. Diabetes 1983;32:408.

Rowland TW, et al. Iron deficiency in adolescent endurance athletes. J Adolesc Health Care 1987;8:322.

Sady SP, Carpenter MW. Aerobic exercise during pregnancy. Sports Med 1989;7:357.

Sale DG, et al. Neural adaptation to resistance training. Med Sci Sports Exerc 1988;20:S135.

Saltin B, et al. Fiber types and metabolic potentials of skeletal muscles in sedentary man and endurance runners. Ann N Y Acad Sci 1977;301:3.

Sherman WM, et al. Effect of exercise-diet manipulation on muscle glycogen and its subsequent utilization during performance. Int J Sport Nutr 1981;2:114.

Simon-Schnauss I, Pabst H. Influence of vitamin E on physical performance. Int J Vitam Nutr Res 1988;58:49.

Sizer FS, Whitney EN. Nutrition and physical activity. In: Sizer F and Whitney E, eds. Nutrition concepts and controversies. 6th ed. Minneapolis, MN: West Publishing Co., 1994:357.

Slavin JL, et al. Amino acid supplement: beneficial or risky? Physician and Sports Med 1988;16:221.

Stanley WC, et al. Glucose and lactate interrelations during moderate-intensity exercise in humans. Metabolism 1988;37:850.

Steen SN. Nutrition for young athletes: Special considerations. Sports Med 1994;17:152.

Steen SN, McKinney S. Nutrition assessment of college wrestlers. Phys Sportmed 1991;14:100.

Sternfeld B, et al. Exercise during pregnancy and pregnancy outcome. Med Sci Sports Exerc 1995;35:634.

Sundgot-Borgen J. Eating disorders in female athletes. Sports Med 1994;17:176.

Tarnopolsky M, MacDougall D, Atkinson S. Influence of protein intake and training status on nitrogen balance and lean body mass. J Appl Physiol 1988;64:187.

Tiidus PM, Houston ME. Vitamin E status and response to exercise training. Sports Med 1995;20:12.

Tran ZV, Weltman A. Differential effects of exercise on serum lipid and lipoprotein levels seen with changes in body weight: a meta-analysis. JAMA 1985;254:919.

van der Beek EJ. Vitamins and endurance training: Food for running or faddish claims? Sports Med 1985;2:175.

Wallace JP, et al. Infant acceptance of postexercise breast milk. Pediatrics 1992;89:1245.

Weight LM. 'Sports anaemia,' does it exist? Sports Med 1993;16:1.

Weight LM, et al. Vitamin and mineral status of trained athletes including the effects of supplementation. Am J Clin Nutr 1988;47:186.

Williams MH. Nutritional supplements for strength trained athletes. Gatorade Sports Science Institute. Sports Science Exchange, 1993.

Wolfe LA, et al. Prescription of aerobic exercise during pregnancy. Sports Med 1989;8:273.

Yesalis CE, Bahrke MS. Anabolic-androgenic steroids. Current issues. Sports Med 1995;19:326.

APPLICATION: Are Ergogenic Aids Enhancers of Sports Performance?

Steve Lacey would be starting his final year at tight end for a Division I college football team. It was the middle of the summer and the team was scheduled to begin the most grueling practice sessions of the season, known as "three-a-days." None of the athletes relished the work ahead of them, but they knew they would be better prepared for their competition.

Steve has additional concerns. He wants to play professional football, but he is considered, by some standards, to be small for his position. He weighs 109 kg (240 lb) and is 193 cm (76 in) in height. Although he has fully recovered from a knee injury suffered late in last year's season, Steve is looking for ways to make sure he stays healthy and in top shape.

Last year when he was rehabilitating his knee, he started to drink protein shakes at night "to help build strength and muscle" in his injured leg. Now he is drinking these shakes three times a day and has recently begun to take ginseng because he heard it would make him feel good. He was thinking about trying creatine supplements again, too, since he had used them in his freshman year. Steve is not sure what to do.

All athletes want to be stronger, faster, or bigger than their opponents, and many of them will try anything that gives them a competitive edge. Despite a lack of scientific proof, some professional athletes have admitted to spending more than $150 per week on nutrition-related substances known as "ergogenic" (work producing) aids in order to stay at the top of their game (Kanter et al, 1991a). The use of nutritional substances to enhance performance may be increasing since anabolic steroids have been banned by many athletic regulatory agencies.

A list of ergogenic aids, their advertising claims, and available scientific support is given in Table 14A–1. In general, advertisers claim these substances can accomplish one or more of the following: (1) build strength and lean muscle mass, (2) enhance endurance and energy production, or (3) improve the chemical environment of the muscle so that it can either work harder and longer or recover more easily.

In many cases, advertisers cite impressive-looking journal citations to support their claims. Many of these scientific citations do not support the actual claim or may have serious flaws in design. Often the advertiser uses results from studies of individuals who are not athletes but may have a marginal nutritional status. In addition, some claims rely on results from animal research (Williams, 1995; Clarkson, 1996; Eichner, 1989; Kris-Etherton, 1989; Lamb and Wardlaw, 1991; Smith et al, 1982). From the limited testing completed thus far, few nutritional substances have been found to improve sports performance except under very specific conditions (Williams, 1995; Clarkson, 1996).

Protein powders and amino acid supplements are some of the most popular ergogenic aids used by athletes (Slavin et al, 1988). Research has indicated that protein requirements for endurance and strength athletes should range from 1.0 to 2.0 g/kg/d (Lemon et al, 1981; Lemon et al, 1984; Tarnopolsky et al, 1988), which is slightly higher than the RDA of 0.8 g/kg/d for healthy individuals (National Research Council, 1990) but is easily obtained in the typical American diet (Benardot et al, 1993). Most athletes eat approximately 16% of total calories from protein (Brotherhood, 1984). The football player, Steve, described above reported to the team dietitian that his dinner consisted of 2 chicken breasts, 4 cups of milk, 2 cups of mashed potatoes, 2 rolls, 1 cup of corn and a bowl of ice cream which, the dietitian calculated, was about 106 g protein or about 50% of the recommended amount for strength athletes. In total, Steve's usual daily intake was 25% above the 2 g/kg/d recommendation and the dietitian suggested that supplements were not necessary.

Individual amino acids such as arginine and ornithine have been shown to enhance the release of growth hormone and, subsequently, lean mass, but not necessarily in well-nourished athletes. One advertiser used this claim because lean mass increased in a population of poorly-nourished Crohn's patients supplemented with arginine (Smith et

TABLE 14A–1 Ergogenic Aids: Advertisers' Claims and Scientific Evidence

Ergogenic Aid	Claim of Advertiser	Scientific Evidence
Protein powders	Muscle growth, weight gain	Usual dietary intake provides extra amount needed
Individual amino acids: lysine/arginine, aspartates, ornithine/tyrosine	Stimulate release of human growth hormone (HGH) and insulin, which facilitates muscle growth	Serum HGH may increase; no proof muscle growth is stimulated
Creatine	Increases body mass; increase in strength, power	Some evidence for ability to perform repeated high-intensity work with sufficient rest; more research needed
Carnitine	Increases use of fat; spares muscle glycogen; increases endurance	Research inconsistent
Inosine	Increases oxygen delivery; improves strength	No data to support claim
Chromium	Assists insulin; increases lean mass	Most research inconsistent; need controlled studies
Magnesium	Increases muscle growth and strength	No data to support claim
Boron	Increases testosterone and growth	No proof of increased growth
Vitamin B_{12}	Stimulates muscle growth	No studies completed
Antioxidants (C, E, beta carotene)	Prevent muscle damage from high-intensity exercise	Some data to support claim; need controlled studies
Medium chain triglycerides	Increase thermic effect and fat loss	No data to support claim
Omega 3 fatty acids	Stimulates HGH; increase muscle	No data to support claim
High-fat diet	Spares use of muscle glycogen	Insufficient data available
Glycerol	Induces hyperhydration	Controlled research needed
CoEnzyme Q_{10} (CoQ_{10})	Boosts ATP production	Limited supportive data
Dihydroxyacetone pyruvate	Enhanced endurance time	Limited supportive data
Phosphates	Increase endurance	Need controlled research
Ginseng	Stimulate central nervous system; increase stamina, improve VO$_{2\ max}$	Data inconsistent; more research needed
Yohimbine and gamma oryzanol	Plant extracts that stimulate testosterone and HGH release	No data to support claim
Smilax	Increases serum testosterone; increases muscle growth/strength	No data to support claim
Caffeine	Improves high-intensity effort	Data still inconsistent
Sodium bicarbonate	Buffers lactic acid; delays fatigue	Some supportive data
Bee pollen	Mix of bee saliva/plant nectar/pollen; increases energy/fitness	No data to support claim
Brewer's yeast	Product of beer brewing used to increase energy	No data to support claim
Gelatin	Protein from collagen; improves muscle contraction	No data to support claim
Kelp	Vitamin/mineral increases energy	No data to support claim
Pangamic acid	Increases delivery of oxygen	No data to support claim
Octacosanol	Alcohol isolate from wheat germ; increases energy and performance	No data to support claim
Royal jelly	Substance fed to queen bee by worker bees; increases strength	No data to support claim
Superoxide dismutase	Enzyme to decrease peroxidation	No data to support claim

Data from Benardot et al, 1993; Kanter, 1991b; Kris-Etherton, 1989; Williams, 1993; Williams, 1995.

al, 1982). Most athletes do not realize that for a 70-kg man to obtain this supposed benefit he may have to ingest 18 g/day of arginine, at a cost of about $10 a day (Slavin et al, 1988). Good food would be a better investment.

Caffeine is one ergogenic aid that has been shown to enhance endurance performance in runners by 44% (Graham and Spriet, 1991); however, any amount above a habitual intake (7 mg/kg or approximately 4 cups coffee or 10 cola drinks per day) is considered illegal by the International Olympic Committee (Clarkson, 1996). Caffeine delays central fatigue (volitional fatigue) and increases the availability and use of free fatty acids during exercise, thus sparing carbohydrate (Spriet, 1994). A significant disadvantage to caffeine ingestion is that it can cause dehydration, which results in decreased performance.

Creatine and bicarbonate are two other substances ingested, especially by strength athletes, to provide a faster recycling of the phosphocreatine molecule (for more energy) and a delay in fatigue, respectively (Balsom et al, 1994; Horswill, 1995). Although some success may have been obtained in exercising animals and small groups of athletes, neither supplement has improved performance consistently in humans (Clarkson, 1996).

There is serious hesitation in regard to the other ergogenic aids that have received some scientific scrutiny (Clarkson, 1996). For instance, diets high in fat may delay endogenous carbohydrate use by increasing intracellular fat stores of the muscle; some (Muoio et al, 1994) but not all (Sherman and Leenders, 1995) studies have demonstrated an improvement in endurance. Two major issues conflict in this argument. First, many endurance athletes eat less carbohydrate (and thus more fat) than recommended (45–50% of energy as opposed to 60–70%), which some suggest is the reason that a higher fat diet would benefit endurance (Hawley et al, 1995). Secondly, many health professionals have difficulty suggesting a diet of 38% fat in light of the potential chronic effects on body composition and cardiovascular health (Clarkson, 1996). Further investigation of fat loading and exercise performance is warranted.

A more recent ergogenic aid, carnitine, is gathering attention despite limited scientific evidence. It is supposed to improve fatty acid oxidation in muscle, spare muscle glycogen, and delay fatigue (Clarkson, 1996; Heinonen, 1996), yet most of the research has not demonstrated these effects (Williams, 1995) and some data suggest that carnitine may increase muscle glycogen use (Eichner, 1989; Williams, 1995).

In short, although few substances have been shown to have "work producing" effects and none have been tested for safety, athletes are investing a great deal of money and trust in claims listed by the maufacturer. For these as well as other reasons scientists and athletic trainers have strongly suggested that the usage of these substances be discontinued (Clarkson, 1996; Eichner, 1989; Kanter, 1991b).

REFERENCES

Balsom PD, Soderlund K, Ekblom B. Creatine in humans with special reference to creatine supplementation. Sports Med 1994;18:268.

Benardot D, ed. Sports nutrition: A guide for the professional working with active people. 2nd ed. Chicago: American Dietetic Association, 1993.

Brotherhood JR. Nutrition and sports performances. Sports Med 1984;1:350.

Clarkson PM. Nutrition for improved sports performance. Current issues on ergogenic aids. Sports Med 1996;6:393.

Eichner ER. Ergolytic drugs. Gatorade Sports Science Institute. Sports Science Exchange, June 1989.

Graham T, Spriet L. Performance and metabolic responses to a high caffeine dose during prolonged exercise. J Appl Physiol 1991;71:2292.

Hawley JA, et al. Nutritional practices of athletes: Are they sub-optimal? J Sports Sci 1995;13:S75.

Heinonen OJ. Carnitine and physical exercise. Sports Med 1996;2:109.

Horswill CA. Effects of bicarbonate, citrate, and phosphate loading on performance. Int J Sports Nutr 1995;5:S111.

Kanter M, et al. Ergogenic aids: the athletic trainer's perspective. Gatorade Sports Science Institute. Sports Science Exchange Roundtable. Fall, 1991a.

Kanter M, et al. Ergogenic aids: the scientist's perspective. Gatorade Sports Science Institute. Sports Science Exchange Roundtable. Winter, 1991b.

Kris-Etherton PM. The facts and fallacies of nutritional supplements for athletes. Gatorade Sports Science Institute. Sports Science Exchange, August, 1989.

Lamb DR, Wardlaw G. Sports nutrition. Nutri-News. St. Louis: Mosby-Year Book, 1991.

Lemon P, Nagle F. Effects of exercise on protein and amino acid metabolism. Med Sci Sports Exerc 1981;13:141.

Lemon P, et al. The importance of protein for athletes. Sports Med 1984;1:474.

Muoio DM, et al. Effect of dietary fat on metabolic adjustments to maximal VO_2 and endurance in runners. Med Sci Sports Exerc 1994;26:81.

National Research Council. National Academy of Sciences. Recommended dietary allowances. 10th ed. Washington, DC, 1989.

Sherman WM, Leenders N. Fat loading: the next magic bullet? Int J Sports Nutr 1995;5:S1.

Slavin JL, et al. Amino acid supplements: Beneficial or risky? Physician and Sports Med 1988;16:221.

Smith JL, et al. Increased ureagenesis and impaired nitrogen use during infusion of a synthetic amino acid formula: a controlled trial. N Engl J Med. 1982;306:1013.

Spriet L. Caffeine and performance. Gatorade Sports Science Institute. Sports Science Exchange. November 1994.

Tarnopolsky MA, et al. Influence of protein intake and training status on nitrogen balance and lean body mass. J Appl Physiol 1988;64:187.

Williams MH. Nutritional supplements for strength trained athletes. Gatorade Sports Science Institute. Sports Science Exchange 1993;6(6).

Williams MH. Nutritional ergogenics in athletics. J Sport Sci 1995;13:S63.

CHAPTER 15

NUTRITION OF PERSONS WITH DEVELOPMENTAL DELAYS AND DISABILITIES

Nutritional Needs, Concerns, and Risk
  Factors
Nutrition Screening, Assessment,
  Intervention, and Monitoring

Summary
Concepts to Remember

Frank is a 23-year-old male who has a diagnosis of mild spastic cerebral palsy and moderate mental retardation. He is ambulatory and does not use assistive devices with any gross motor activities. He has satisfactory vision but is severely hearing impaired and nonverbal. Signing has been used to communicate with him since he was very young, and he interacts effectively using the technique. Frank resides with his parents and a 25-year-old brother. He participates in sheltered employment in conjunction with a day program for persons with developmental disabilities. In addition to receiving vocation training, he receives support in the area of behavior management through that program.

Frank receives professional health care through a family medicine practice, with referral to specialists as the need is indicated. His only surgeries have been to remove his adenoids and place tubes in his ears and to correct curvature of his spine. He has a history of behavioral outbursts and has received a variety of psychotropic medications in the past. Currently he receives no prescription medications. His mother describes him as being chronically constipated and estimates that he has one hard, dry bowel movement, with difficulty, approximately every other week unless he receives a laxative. Frank is 65 in (165 cm) tall and weighs 86 lb (39 kg). He weighed 98 lb (44.5 kg) 6 months ago but lost approximately 15 lb (6.8 kg) over a period of several weeks of intense food refusal, and his weight has remained near that lower level. Current measurements of triceps and subscapular skinfolds and mid-upper arm circumference are all below the fifth percentile of general population reference data. His hemoglobin level was recently determined to be 11.8 g/dl, which also is low for a male his age. The weight loss, from a weight that was already low for his stature, is of major concern to his parents, work supervisors, behavior management specialists, and the health professionals who work with him.

A major factor contributing to Frank's poor nutritional status, as reflected by his low hemoglobin, low weight for stature, and weight loss, is his extremely limited food acceptance, in terms of both quantity and variety. His mother reports that weight loss first became an issue with Frank when he received Ritalin at approximately 10 years of age. Reduction in appetite is a commonly reported side effect of that medication, which also may lead to slight reduction in height growth. (Scheduling meals to coincide with times of lowest medication effects and periodically discontinuing the medication have been suggested as means of minimizing those effects.) Although Frank received the medication for only a short time, his family believes that is when problems related to his acceptance of food began. They report that his food acceptance has ranged from moderate to low since that time, with low intakes sometimes attributed to effects of various other psychotropic medications and some-

Contributed by Betty Kozlowski.

times occurring when he was receiving no medications. For several years, his family responded to his reduced food intake by having foods they thought he was most likely to accept readily available. Gradually, his range of food acceptance and the quantities of food he consumed declined, while the intensity with which he expressed his food "intentions" increased.

Frank's family concurs with other care providers that more aggressive and consistent intervention measures than have been taken in the past are needed to improve his food acceptance and nutritional status. Evaluations by an occupational therapist have confirmed that Frank's oral sensory motor functioning and his self-feeding skills are more than adequate to support adequate intake of foods with a wide variety of textures. Further studies revealed no swallowing problems or other physical conditions that would be expected to adversely affect either his intake of food or his body's utilization of it. Evaluation by a dietitian revealed that, while Frank's diet includes some high-calorie foods of low nutrient density, the primary limiting factors are overall low intake and limited variety. His intake is inadequate in calories, fluid, fiber, and most nutrients. His weight status and low hemoglobin level are consistent with his diet, which also is probably contributing to his constipation. Utilizing intake goals and recommendations from the dietitian concerning foods of high nutrient and energy density, psychologists have begun working with Frank and his parents and with other personnel at the day program in which he participates to develop and consistently implement behavioral intervention measures to help Frank improve his intake. While it is too soon to know whether satisfactory intake will be achieved through these means, Frank's early responses to attempted changes have been encouraging. However, he has had many years to "fine tune" his pattern of intake control and to develop nutritional deficits, and the level of change that care providers consider desirable may come slowly. A daily multivitamin and mineral supplement has been recommended to help meet Frank's needs as behavioral change is being attempted. As active members of the intervention team, the primary care physician and dietitian will continue to monitor Frank's diet and nutritional status and work with Frank, his family, the psychologists, and other team members to promote improved nutrition.

■ Identify four criteria of a developmental disability, as defined in federal legislation.

■ How do "developmental delay" and "special health needs" differ from "developmental disability"?

■ Identify five causes or risk factors for developmental delay or disability. Identify two factors that have resulted in major changes in the population of persons with developmental disabilities in recent decades.

■ Describe major changes that have occurred in services for persons with developmental delays and disabilities during the last half of the twentieth century. Discuss implications of these changes in relation to nutrition services.

Interrelated nutrition and feeding problems, such as those described for Frank, occur in many persons with developmental disabilities. Although feeding problems and nutritional risk often are not alleviated even when they are identified early and anticipatory guidance and ongoing coordinated interdisciplinary support are provided, adverse effects often can be minimized and nutritional needs met through means that promote individual development and increase mealtime enjoyment for individuals with disabilities, their families, and other care providers. Inclusion of nutrition services as a central component of person/family-centered, culturally competent, community-based, coordinated care is becoming a reality for increasing numbers of persons with developmental delays and disabilities. However, many more persons in this population than currently receive nutrition services could benefit from them. These key concepts for services have been defined in a position paper of the American Dietetic Association (1995).

Persons with developmental delays and disabilities are as diverse with respect to their health and developmental characteristics, including those related to nutrition and feeding, as they are in other regards. Some persons in this population show delays or deficits in cognitive development but have health characteristics, physical development, feeding characteristics, and nutritional needs that are well within normal ranges for the general population. Other persons, with widely varying levels of cognitive functioning, have complex medical problems and altered nutritional needs in combination with physical, neuromotor, and behavioral characteristics that increase the complexity of their needs. Health and development may be compromised or survival may be threatened by nutritional problems that require scientifically and technologically complex interventions, or the needed intervention may be as basic as making adequate food available. As a group, persons with developmental delays and disabilities are at increased nutritional risk because of a wide range of biologic, psychosocial, and environmental factors. Because nutrition is one of the many variables that affect health, developmental potential, and the extent to which that potential is realized, it is critical for all people to have access to appropriate nutrition. At the same time, it must be appreciated that people have many needs in addition to those related to nutrition and feeding. Nutrition and feeding must be viewed within the context of other needs and priorities.

Definitions

According to the Developmental Disabilities Assistance and Bill of Rights Act of 1990, Public Law 101–496:

> The term *"developmental disability"* means a severe, chronic disability of a person 5 years of age or older which is attributable to a mental or physical impairment or combination of mental and physical impairments; is manifested before the person attains age twenty-two; is likely to continue indefinitely; results in substantial functional limitations in three or more of the following areas of major life activity: (i) self-care, (ii) receptive and expressive language, (iii) learning, (iv) mobility, (v) self-direction, (vi) capacity for independent living, and (vii) economic sufficiency; and reflects the person's need for a combination and sequence of special, interdisciplinary, or generic care, treatment, or other services which are of lifelong or extended duration and are individually planned and coordinated, except that such term, when applied to infants and young children means individuals from birth to age 5, inclusive, who have substantial developmental delay or specific **congenital** or acquired conditions with a high probability of resulting in developmental disabilities if services are not provided.

Congress reported there were more than three million persons with developmental disabilities in the United States in 1990 (Developmental Disabilities Assistance and Bill of Rights Act of 1990, Sec. 101). That figure represented between 1% and 2% of the population.

The meaning is less consistent from one user to another when the terms "developmental delay," "special health needs," or "special needs" are used than when the term "developmental disability" is applied. All of these terms are commonly used to refer to overlapping but not synonymous segments of the population. **"Developmental delay"** refers to development that is below accepted developmental norms. Delays sometimes are overcome or remain so mild as to be of little consequence. In other instances, they are preliminary to the diagnosis of developmental disability. States have developed definitions of developmental delay to use in conjunction with their respective early intervention programs and services, many of which serve children at biologic or environmental risk as well as those with identified delay or disability. It has been estimated that 10% of children would benefit from those services (Baker et al, 1993). The terms **"special needs"** and **"special health needs"** are used in relation to the pediatric population to encompass serious physical, cognitive, developmental, learning, or emotional problems or disabilities; social or socioeconomic disadvantage; or other conditions that may increase the vulnerability of particular children (Aday, 1992). Approximately 10% to 15% of the pediatric population, including many children with developmental delays or disabilities, are considered to have special health needs (Baer et al, 1991).

Etiologies

Many biologic and environmental factors have been identified as causes of developmental delays and disabilities, but many disorders continue to result from unknown causes. Some disorders, such as inborn errors of metabolism, Duchenne muscular dystrophy, and fragile X syndrome are hereditary. Other disorders, such as Down syndrome, and myelomeningocele, are the result of alterations that occur preconceptionally or early in embryonic development. Still other disorders are the result of intrauterine factors, such as exposure to infections, alcohol or other drugs, lead, or other harmful agents. Fetal malnutrition, complications associated with prematurity, and obstetric complications with full-term infants are also risk factors for developmental disabilities, as are such postnatal events as physical trauma from accidents or child abuse; poisoning from lead or other agents; infections such as viral encephalitis, meningitis, and human immunodeficiency virus; and environmental deprivation (Crocker, 1989; Baer et al, 1991).

Although medical advances and improvements in health care have reduced the prevalence of many risk factors in recent decades, other risk factors have emerged, and many changes have occurred in the population of persons who have developmental delays and disabilities. Acquired immunodeficiency syndrome, prenatal exposure to alcohol and other drugs, and child maltreatment are examples of risk factors that have become of increasing concern (American Dietetic Association, 1995). The prognosis has dramatically improved for infants of very low birth weight, but long-term impairments continue to be more prevalent among them than among infants of higher birth weights (King et al, 1992). Survival rates of persons with many types of disorders have increased, resulting in larger groups of older persons with those disorders, and the population of persons dependent on medical technology has expanded (American Dietetic Association, 1995).

Services and Supports

Major changes have occurred in services and supports for persons with developmental disabilities and their families during the second half of the twentieth century. Federal legislation has promoted development of services and supports, including increased preparation of professionals, to improve health and developmental outcomes. Strong parent/consumer and professional voices and legislative initiatives have embodied principles of normalization, interdependence, and self determination, and have contributed to the integration of large numbers of persons with developmental disabilities into the mainstream of public education, health care, employment, recreation, and community living, with services and supports provided as needed to promote quality of life in the least restrictive environment. Legislation expresses a commitment for persons with developmental disabilities to achieve full integration into the community and society (Developmental Disabilities Assistance and Bill of Rights Act of 1994 [Public Law 103–230]). Through the Americans with Disabilities Act (Public Law 101–336), civil rights protection has been extended to people who are discriminated against because of their physical or mental handicaps (American Dietetic Association, 1992).

Occupancy of large state-operated residential facilities for persons with developmental disabilities in the United States declined by almost two-thirds over a 26-year period, from approximately 195,000 in 1967 to 71,000 in 1993 (Smith and Gettings, 1993). Concurrent increases occurred in the numbers of persons living at home with their families and in small group homes, supervised apartments, and intermediate care facilities for people with mental retardation (ICF/MR), and the movement toward integration into the community continues. New community-based programs are developing for persons with medical and behavioral conditions that present complex management challenges, once thought to justify continued operation of the large public residential facilities (Ziring, 1991).

With the integration of persons with developmental disabilities into the community and expanded societal commitment to meeting their needs, service providers in many settings have become increasingly involved with the provision of services to this population. Improved basic health care and advances in health technology have altered morbidity and mortality rates and expanded the adolescent, adult, and elderly segments of this population. These include persons whose needs, in order to achieve or maintain satisfactory nutritional status, range from complex medical intervention to basic health care, homemaker services, food preparation assistance, basic nutrition knowledge, or financial assistance. Nutrition professionals need skills in coordination and collaboration, as well as nutrition knowledge and skills, if community-based comprehensive care of the highest quality is to be provided.

Since the passage of Public Law 94–142, The Education for All Handicapped Children's Act of 1975, free public education in the least restrictive setting has been mandated for all children, ages 6 to 21 years, despite disability. Child nutrition programs funded by the U.S. Department of Agriculture are required to provide special meals at no additional charge to children who have medical certification that disabilities restrict their diets. In addition, the dining area must be accessible for children with disabilities, and special feeding equipment must be provided if needed. Attention is being directed to these regulations and laws nationally, and effort is being made through workshops, training materials, and revised instructions and guidance from the USDA to improve the utilization of these important resources (American Dietetic Association, 1995; Cloud, 1994; Gandy et al, 1991; Yadrick and Sneed, 1994).

It is widely accepted today that appropriate developmental support reduces the occurrence of developmental delays and disabilities in infants and children who are at high biologic or environmental risk and minimizes the consequences of diagnosed disabilities. One piece of legislation that specifically addresses the development of services for very young children was enacted in 1986 as Part H of the Education of the Handicapped Act Amendments, Public Law 99–457, and is now encompassed in the Individuals with Disabilities Education Act, or IDEA (Public Law 102–119). Systems of service are evolving around concepts of family-centered, community-based, culturally competent, coordinated, comprehensive care, which are central to this legislation and to the legislation of other health-related programs, such as maternal and child health programs. These concepts differ from many service

KEY TERMS

congenital: conditions that are present at, and usually before, birth

developmental delay: development that is below accepted developmental norms; definitions used in conjunction with early intervention programs vary from one state to another

special needs and **special health needs:** terms used particularly in relation to the pediatric population to encompass serious physical, cognitive, developmental, learning, or emotional problems or disabilities; social or socioeconomic disadvantage; or other conditions that may increase the vulnerability of particular individuals

practices of the past, and their implementation often necessitates new ways of functioning for agencies, programs, and individual service providers (Lichtenwalter et al, 1993). Strong collaboration and coordination must occur within and between disciplines involved in all aspects and levels of care in order to promote the delivery of appropriate services to children and their families. Care coordination, or "case management," is required to pull together primary, secondary, and tertiary levels of care from health, social, educational, and family resources. Family-centered care reaffirms families as the primary guardians of their children's well-being and development (Fenichel, 1991) and acknowledges them as equal partners with professionals. Services are built on identified family needs and family perceptions of their needs, and with appreciation of family goals and aspirations. The role of professionals shifts away from primary decision-making to collaboration and partnership with families and with other service providers (Venn et al, 1992).

Nutritionists are among the personnel identified in Part H of the Individuals with Disabilities Act as qualified to provide early intervention services. Because many children with developmental delay or disability are at high nutritional risk, it is important for nutritionists and dietitians to be members of interdisciplinary service teams with families and other health, education, and social service providers and for nutritional needs to be addressed as a part of family-centered, community-based, culturally competent, coordinated care. The critical role of nutrition in preventive and habilitative services to children with disabilities and their families has been recognized for many years at the federal level in maternal and child health programs (Egan and Oglesby, 1991). This is reflected in the support provided by the Maternal and Child Health Bureau for nutrition services for children with special health needs and for training nutrition professionals to work with this population, including funding since the late 1960s for nutrition training in University-Affiliated Programs. Nevertheless, major needs continue to exist for the enhancement of nutrition services to children with developmental delays and disabilities (Baer et al, 1991; Hine et al, 1989; Bayerl et al, 1993; American Dietetic Association, 1992; American Dietetic Association, 1995).

NUTRITIONAL NEEDS, CONCERNS, AND RISK FACTORS

■ Describe examples of alterations in physical size or growth that occur in persons with developmental disabilities. Identify one diagnosis with which each is commonly associated, and discuss nutrition implications.

■ Discuss major factors that alter energy needs of many persons with developmental disabilities and factors that complicate the assessment of those needs.

■ Why are energy needs of persons with developmental disabilities often expressed in relation to their height?

■ Although individual differences always exist, persons with some disorders (e.g., Prader-Willi syndrome) show much more similarity in their nutrition-related characteristics and apparent nutritional needs than do persons with other disorders (e.g., cerebral palsy). Why? What are some characteristeristics of disorders that contribute to the similarities or differences? Discuss implications in relation to nutrition assessment and intervention.

■ Discuss evidence of body composition differences in persons with selected diagnoses. What are the implications of these differences with respect to using equations that contain anthropometric variables for estimating basal metabolic rate or body composition?

■ What are the major nutritional implications associated with anticonvulsant medications and psychotropic medications?

■ Identify major factors that contribute to the occurrence of feeding problems in persons with developmental delays and describe how diet and nutrition are likely to be affected. Identify circumstances that lead to the initiation of tube feeding.

■ Discuss psychosocial factors that may increase nutritional risk of persons with developmental disabilities.

Although many persons with developmental delays and disabilities do not differ nutritionally from the general population, many others are affected by a wide range of factors that alter their nutritional needs or increase the difficulty of meeting their needs. Major factors, which often occur in combination with one another and in association with problems related to other areas of the person's health or development, can be grouped into several broad categories (Table 15–1).

Much of the difficulty associated with determining the nutritional needs of persons with developmental delays and disabilities and meeting those needs revolves around a triad of altered physical size, growth, and/or body composition; altered activity patterns, energy cost of activity, and energy needs; and altered feeding characteristics. Deviations in any one of those areas from characteristics of nondisabled, healthy individuals complicate attempts to ensure that satisfactory nutrition is being achieved. When deviations in all three areas occur together, as is common in this population, the development of appropriate nutrition and feeding recommendations often hinges on evaluating the extent to which those deviations are interrelated. Other factors listed in Table 15–1 may occur alone or in combination with these factors and must also be taken into account.

Altered Nutritional Needs

Alterations in nutritional needs may result from many causes. Those most commonly seen with this population

TABLE 15–1 Major Factors That Alter Nutritional Needs, Complicate Assessment of Nutritional Needs, or Increase Nutritional Risk of Persons with Developmental Delays or Disabilities

A. Altered nutritional needs
   1. Altered physical size, growth, and energy needs
      a. Decreased linear growth
      b. Low weight for stature
      c. High weight for stature
      d. Altered energy needs
   2. Effects of medications
   3. Chronic constipation
   4. Other factors
      a. Stress of illness or surgery
      b. Metabolic or gastrointestinal disorders
      c. Other complex medical conditions

B. Food allergies or intolerances

C. Altered feeding characteristics
   1. Physical characteristics and health of mouth area
   2. Neuromotor factors
   3. Behaviors
   4. Tube feeding

D. Increased demands on time, energy, and financial and emotional resources

E. Inadequate information and support

though limited, support clinical impressions that body composition also is altered with many disorders. Nutritional assessment and development of nutritional recommendations will be greatly facilitated when the effects of various dietary manipulations, exercise regimens, and other treatments, as well as effects of various disorders per se, on the relative amounts of body fat and lean body mass are known.

Physical growth and development account for a major component of nutrient and energy needs during infancy, childhood, and adolescence, and serve as key indicators of the adequacy of nutritional intakes. Low weight for stature is often one of the first clinical signs of undernutrition and, in children, this is followed by reduced linear growth when nutritional deficits are prolonged or severe. However, many variables in addition to nutrition influence size and growth, and adequate nutrition does not ensure that physical development will occur in accordance with reference data for the general population (Garn and Weir, 1971; Roche, 1979). Holm (1994) described deviations in physical size and growth in this population according to their association with familial short stature or slow maturation, conditions of primary prenatal onset (genetic disorders and syndromes of unknown etiology), conditions of secondary prenatal onset (intrauterine infections, drug exposure), or conditions of perinatal or postnatal onset (chronic infections, endocrine disorders, metabolic diseases, major organ defects, and severe neurologic impairment).

Although particular patterns of physical size and growth are characteristic of certain disorders, variations occur among individuals within diagnostic groupings. Careful monitoring of growth, body weight, and nutrition is needed to ensure that nutrition is appropriate for growth potential to be realized, adequate weight to be achieved and maintained, and, when obesity is characteristic, to ensure that energy intake is adequately (but not excessively) restricted while satisfactory intake of nutrients occurs. Because body composition and stature often differ from those of the general population, energy needs of persons with developmental disabilities are often expressed in relation to the person's height rather than his or her age, "ideal body weight," or other conventions more commonly used with the general population. Nutritional needs must be evaluated on a person-by-person basis. Diet, biochemical, and other clinical parameters must be considered along with diagnosis, physical size, and growth in evaluating the adequacy of the individual's intake. Assessing the relative contribution of nutrition to deviations in physical size and growth presents a major challenge to professionals who work with this population.

include altered physical size, growth, or energy needs; effects of medications; chronic constipation; stress of illness or surgery; metabolic or gastrointestinal disorders; or other complex medical conditions. Therefore, the appropriateness of quantities of nutrients recommended for the general population must be evaluated on a person-by-person basis. As is always the case, objective data strengthen that evaluation.

Many forms of "meganutrient therapy" have been proposed for treatment of behavioral and cognitive disorders, physical characteristics, and other manifestations in persons with developmental disabilities. Except in the presence of nutritional deficiencies or with selected metabolic disorders, the effectiveness of these treatments has not been established. Well-designed, controlled studies have not supported the efficacy of megadose supplementation with multivitamins and/or minerals in the treatment of cognitive disabilities or attention deficit disorders (Kozlowski, 1992).

Alterations in Physical Size, Growth and Energy Needs

Deviations in physical size and growth rate from those of the general population are common among persons with developmental delays and disabilities. Available data, al-

DECREASED LINEAR GROWTH Decreased linear growth is common among persons with many disorders of known and unknown etiologies. Down syndrome, Prader-Willi syndrome, Cornelia de Lange syndrome, Williams syndrome, Rett syndrome, and fetal alcohol syndrome are examples of disorders with which reduced growth in height or length is characteristic (Holm, 1994), even when identified nutritional needs have been met. Reduced linear growth is also common among persons with myelomeningocele (Ekvall, 1993b) and cerebral palsy (Kozlowski, 1990), although the variation in growth among persons with these diagnoses is greater, and the relative contribution of nutrition versus other factors is more difficult to evaluate than with the syndromes listed above. Ambulation and participation in other weight-bearing activity, as well as the underlying defects that influence ability to perform these activities, may influence linear growth and may be particularly significant in cerebral palsy and myelomeningocele. All of the factors listed in Table 15–1 must be considered in ruling out inadequate nutrition as a contributing factor to short stature.

LOW WEIGHT FOR STATURE   Low weight for stature is one of the primary reasons persons with developmental delays and disabilities are referred for nutrition assessment and intervention. Two disorders with which low weight for stature is commonly associated are Rett syndrome and cerebral palsy.

Rett Syndrome   **Rett syndrome** is a disorder in which deterioration in functioning follows apparently normal early development and leads to severe mental and physical impairment. The disorder appears only in females and has an estimated occurrence of 1 in 10,000 to 1 in 15,000 females (Perry, 1991). Etiology is unknown, although the pattern of occurrence suggests that it is genetic (Holm, 1994). The presence of a metabolic disorder, possibly related to carbohydrate metabolism, has been suggested but not yet established (Haas et al, 1986). Developmental stagnation beginning between 6 and 18 months of age is followed by rapid developmental regression, loss of expressive language, loss of purposeful hand use, and severe psychomotor retardation. Severe seizure activity is common. Wasting is often described as a major concern, but obesity has been reported (Pipes and Holm, 1993). Little is known about the nutrient and energy needs of persons with the disorder. Although instances of undernourished appearance despite good appetites and relatively high calorie intakes have been described (Rice and Haas, 1988), appetite also may be poor and calorie intake very low in persons with this disorder.

Growth data of a girl with Rett syndrome are presented in Figure 15–1 (pages 424–427). Head circumference data for the period birth to 3 years were not available, but the measurement value at age 6 years was more than 2 standard deviations below the mean of general population reference data. The parents of this child reported that she was feeding herself at 2 years of age but had totally stopped by 2.5 years. Note that the most dramatic decline in her weight status occurred between the ages of 4 and 5 years. She showed little interest in eating, and the behavioral approach that was introduced to increase her food acceptance met with limited success. Minimal improvement

in weight gain occurred even after the initiation of nutrition and feeding intervention at age 6 years.

As occurred with this child, attempts are often made to promote weight gain in girls with Rett syndrome by increasing their overall caloric intake. Varying levels of success have been reported. Some success also has been reported in achieving weight gain with a ketogenic diet, which was first tried for control of seizures that were resistant to anticonvulsant medication. Long-term implications of using the ketogenic diet, which is very high in fat, are not known, and it is viewed as a temporary measure (Rice and Haas, 1988). Severe neurologic deficit, an underlying metabolic disorder, or both have been proposed as possible contributing factors to the growth retardation exhibited by persons with Rett syndrome (Holm, 1994).

Cerebral Palsy   **Cerebral palsy** is a general designation for a group of disorders of motor control and posture. The prevalence is approximately 2 per 1000 among children in the United States (Newacheck and Taylor, 1992). Cerebral palsy results from permanent, nonprogressive brain abnormalities that may originate prenatally, **perinatally**, or in early childhood. Manifestations vary widely. The location, severity, and timing of insult to the brain determine the muscle tone pattern and the severity and distribution of motor abnormalities throughout the body. Muscle tone may be decreased or increased, or it may fluctuate. **Hypertonicity** and stereotyped, limited movement characterize **spasticity**, which is present in more than half of cases of cerebral palsy. Part or all of the body may be affected. **Dyskinesia** refers to involuntary, extraneous motor activity that increases with stress or exertion. **Athetosis** is the most common form of dyskinesia. Seizures occur in approximately 35% to 45% of persons with cerebral palsy. Disorders related to speech, hearing, vision, behaviors, and learning are also common, as is some degree of mental retardation (Schangenbacher, 1985; Wilson, 1984; Healy, 1990).

Many factors contribute to physical size deviations in persons with cerebral palsy. Extremely low weight for stature and low values for other anthropometric indices are most common in persons who have severe motor dysfunction and feeding problems (Krick and Van Duyn, 1984; Thommessen et al, 1991; Stallings et al, 1993a). Low weight is more common in persons with athetosis, but may occur in as many as 50% of children with spastic cerebral palsy (Shaddix, 1991). Reduced body cell mass has been attributed to muscle atrophy from disease and low physical activity (Berg, 1970; Berg and Isaksson, 1970), but inadequate nutrient and energy intakes may also be contributing factors (Bandini et al, 1991; Pipes and Glass, 1993; Stallings et al, 1993a). Triceps fat appears to be more depleted than subscapular fat, which also is seen in children with some forms of malnutrition (Spender et al, 1988; Stallings et al, 1993a; Stallings et al, 1993b). Increases in weight for stature have been documented in association with increases in nutrient and energy intake, particularly with the initiation of tube feeding

(Sanders et al, 1990; Isaacs et al, 1994). Some data showing increases in triceps skinfolds also have been presented (Isaacs et al, 1994). Additional information concerning changes in body fat and muscle mass would be extremely useful in evaluating this weight gain. The fact that weight gain in children may be accompanied by increased length growth and often has been preceded by very low intakes for long periods of time indicates that, at least to some extent, it reflects improved nutrition status. Unless increases in lean body mass occur along with increases in body fat, however, obesity will be present at lower weight-for-stature percentiles than if lean body mass also increases.

Variations in voluntary and involuntary activity patterns, in the energy costs of activity, and in growth and body size characteristics are all factors that contribute to the wide range of energy needs that exists among individuals with cerebral palsy. Based on a study of children between the ages of 5 and 12 years who were considered to be adequately nourished, one group of investigators reported the intake of the children who had mild to moderate motor dysfunction but were ambulatory as 13.9 kcal/cm of height and of those who were nonambulatory as 11.1 kcal/cm of height (Culley and Middleton, 1969). Many professionals use those figures as starting points when planning or evaluating intakes of children with cerebral palsy. For comparison, the Recommended Dietary Allowance for children of comparable age is approximately 15 to 16 kcal/cm of height (National Research Council, 1989). Some professionals derive an estimate of basal energy needs and then add calories according to muscle tone and estimated needs for activity and growth (Krick et al, 1992; Cloud, 1993). Because basal energy needs are related to lean body (or fat-free) mass, which is likely to be altered with cerebral palsy, the limitations of applying general population equations for calculating basal needs to persons with cerebral palsy without considering differences in lean body mass should be recognized. One group of investigators concluded that neither the FAO/WHO equation developed for normal children nor two equations published specifically for use with children who have cerebral palsy yielded estimates of energy needs similar to those derived from indirect calorimetry (Sridhar et al, 1995). Another group, also using indirect calorimetry, concluded that resting metabolic rate per unit of fat-free mass was elevated in their subjects with athetoid cerebral palsy but that fat-free mass, as estimated from anthropometric measurements, was lower in their subjects with cerebral palsy than in those who did not have the disorder (Johnson et al, 1996). Energy needs for activity and growth (including catch-up) also are highly variable and difficult to estimate. While it is hoped that research will yield more satisfactory guides than currently exist for deriving estimates of energy needs of persons with cerebral palsy, individual evaluation will continue to be a critical part of the process.

HIGH WEIGHT FOR STATURE The consequences of excessive body fat are often particularly serious for persons with developmental disabilities. Negative health and social implications that are associated with obesity in nondisabled persons are superimposed on health risks and social barriers related to other aspects of disabling conditions. In addition, excessive weight may compromise the ability of persons who have movement disorders to perform activities and thereby decrease their activity levels, increase their risk for obesity, and potentially decrease the level of independence they are able to achieve. Excessive weight also increases the difficulty of providing physical support to persons who require it.

The incidence of obesity appears to be higher among adults with mental retardation than among the general population. Based on anthropometric criteria used with the general population, the incidence has been found to be higher among females than males with mental retardation; higher among persons functioning in the mild to moderate range than in the severe to profound range of mental retardation; and, within levels of mental retardation, higher among persons living in family settings, group homes or intermediate care facilities than in institutions. In one recent study of persons with mental retardation, 55% of the subjects who lived in family settings were classified as obese, compared with 16% in institutions; of those with severe to profound mental retardation, 64% of females living in family settings versus 30% in institutions were classified as obese (Rimmer et al, 1993).

Different criteria must be used to define obesity in some

KEY TERMS

Rett syndrome: degenerative disorder of unknown etiology, recognized only in females; apparently normal early development followed by severe mental and physical impairment, including severe movement disorder, severe seizure activity, loss of expressive language, loss of purposeful hand use

cerebral palsy: general designation for group of disorders of motor control and posture; results from permanent, nonprogressive brain abnormalities that may originate prenatally, perinatally, or in early childhood

perinatal: weeks shortly before and after birth

hypertonicity: excessive muscle tone

spasticity: hypertonicity; seen with stereotyped, limited movements in the most common type of cerebral palsy

dyskinesia: involuntary, extraneous motor activity that increases with stress or exertion; seen in some types of cerebral palsy

athetosis: most common form of dyskinesia; characterized by involuntary slow, writhing movements, especially in wrists and hands

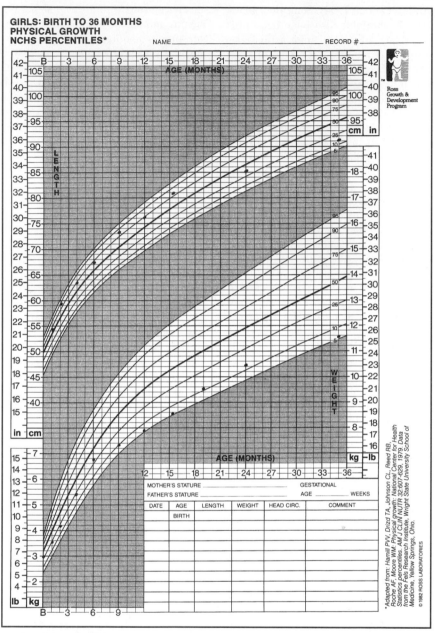

FIGURE 15–1. Height (or length) and weight data of a girl with Rett syndrome are plotted in relation to general population reference data in these four charts (National Center for Health Statistics, 1978). Her parents reported that this child's food acceptance became a gradually worsening problem after age 2 years.

persons with developmental disabilities than with the general population. Differences in body segment ratios (e.g., proportion of height, that is, trunk versus leg length), fat to lean body mass ratios, and distributions of fat on the body are associated with some disorders. As illustrated below, those differences may decrease the accuracy of body fat estimates that are derived by applying general population anthropometric criteria to this population. In addition, amounts of body fat that are desirable for some persons with developmental disabilities (e.g., persons with severe neuromotor dysfunction) may be lower than for the general population.

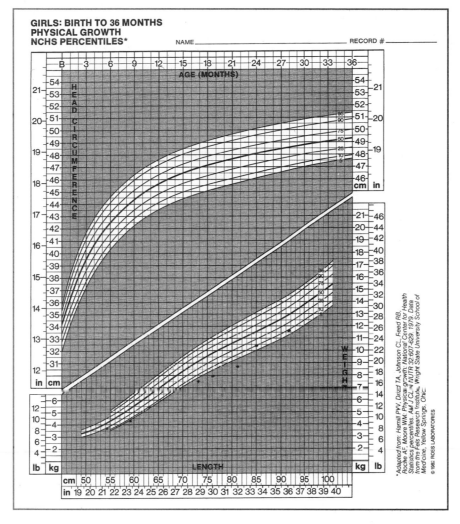

FIGURE 15–1 *Continued*

Figure continued on following page

Many factors contribute to the occurrence of obesity in persons with disabilities, as in the general population. The tendency toward excessive weight gain is particularly strong with some disorders. Down syndrome, Prader-Willi syndrome and myelomeningocele are three disorders with which obesity is commonly associated. Obesity also presents substantial problems in some persons with spastic cerebral palsy, especially in the teenage years and beyond.

Down Syndrome Down syndrome is the most commonly recognized chromosomal disorder with which mental retardation is associated. It occurs in approximately 1 in 700 births worldwide (Hayes and Batshaw, 1993). Trisomy 21 (the presence of extra chromosome 21)

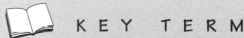

KEY TERM

Down syndrome: most commonly recognized chromosomal abnormality with which mental retardation is associated; involves chromosome 21, most common form being trisomy 21; additional common features include short stature, short hands with wide space between first and second digits, congenital heart disease, hypotonia, upward slant to eyes; excessive weight for length common after early childhood

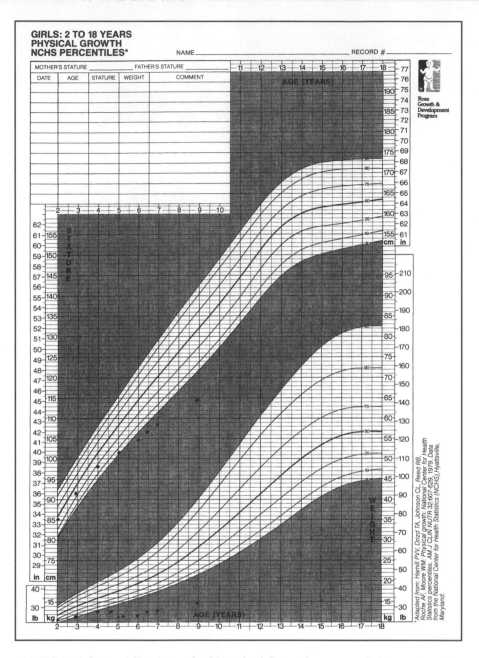

FIGURE 15–1 *Continued.* Note that weight of this girl with Rett syndrome was nearly the same at ages 3 and 6 years, but slightly higher at age 4. Nutrition intervention efforts, initiated at age 6 years, were accompanied by some improvement in food intake but only slight weight gain. Weight, stature, and weight for stature remained substantially below the fifth percentiles of reference data.

accounts for about 95% of the cases, with mosaics (trisomy 21 only in some cells) and translocations involving chromosome 21 accounting for the remainder. The occurrence increases substantially with increasing maternal age. Some degree of mental retardation, reduced muscle tone, and short stature is characteristic of the disorder (Blackman, 1990). Congenital cardiovascular malforma-

tions are present about 50% of the time (Martin et al, 1989). These malformations, together with **hypotonia** and a weak suck, which also are common, may result in inadequate food intake during infancy. With developmental progression and treatment of heart disorders or other medical complications, caloric intake relative to need typically increases. Excessive weight for length is often pre-

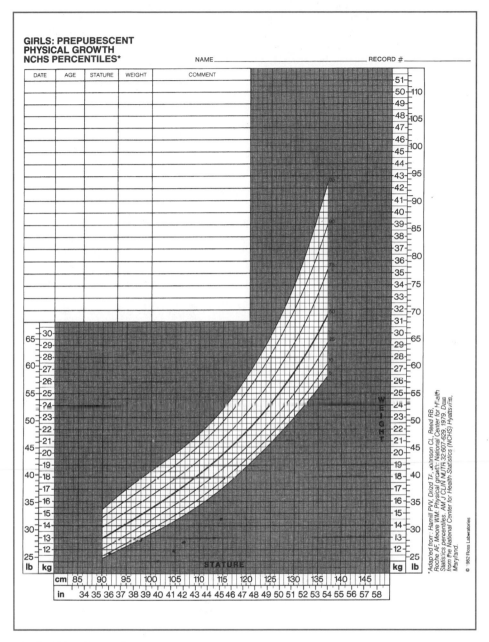

FIGURE 15–1 *Continued*

sent by the age of 3 years, and increased risk for obesity continues throughout life for many persons with Down syndrome (Cronk, 1978). Hypothyroidism and other forms of thyroid dysfunction are substantially more common than in the general population, and the prevalence apparently increases with age (Pueschel and Bier, 1992). Hypothyroidism can contribute to obesity and short stature.

Although a tendency toward obesity may be present in persons with Down syndrome, weight for stature is often maintained within general population normal limits through physical activity; careful monitoring of weight,

growth, and diet; and implementation of dietary change as the need is indicated. Energy needs vary in relation to activity and health characteristics. Because height is reduced, total energy need is often lower than for other per-

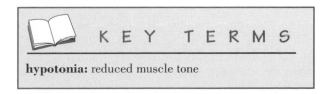

hypotonia: reduced muscle tone

sons of comparable chronologic age even if the need per centimeter of height is not reduced.

Prader-Willi Syndrome   Problems related to weight status characteristically change dramatically between infancy and early childhood in persons with **Prader-Willi syndrome**. Inadequate weight gain typically occurs during infancy, sometimes to the point that tube feeding is required. This is replaced by a very strong tendency toward development of obesity beginning in early childhood and continuing throughout the remainder of the life span (Pipes, 1990). Both extremes of weight status can have life-threatening consequences, and their prevention and treatment present some of the greatest management challenges associated with the disorder (Cassidy, 1984). An abnormality related to chromosome 15 can almost always be detected with Prader-Willi syndrome (Holm, 1994). Hypotonia, developmental delays, food-seeking and gorging behaviors, and other physical and behavioral factors that result in obesity are characteristic of the disorder, which occurs in 1 in 10,000 to 1 in 25,000 live births (Pipes, 1990). Most success with weight management has been described with early implementation of environmental controls and behavior management techniques across persons and locations to control food intake in combination with physical activity for energy expenditure and close professional monitoring and encouragement. Calorie requirements for persons with this syndrome vary from one individual to another. However, intakes of 8 to 9 kcal/cm of height have been found generally to yield slow weight loss and 10 to 11 kcal/cm, or approximately two-thirds of the Recommended Dietary Allowance for energy, to maintain appropriate weight and support growth (Holm and Pipes, 1976; Pipes and Glass, 1993).

Fat-free mass appears to be reduced in persons with Prader-Willi syndrome. Basal metabolic rate per unit of fat-free mass does not appear to be altered. Probably reflecting the lower fat-free mass, basal metabolic rate does appear to be reduced in relation to body weight, body surface area, height, weight, and age. Equations based on various combinations of those variables, which are commonly used to estimate basal metabolic rate for the general population, overestimate measured values for subjects with this syndrome. In addition, estimates of body fat derived from skinfold measurements do not agree with those derived using other techniques, which is consistent with the impression that body fat distribution is altered in Prader-Willi syndrome (Schoeller et al, 1988).

Myelomeningocele   With **myelomeningocele**, a defect in development toward the end of the first prenatal month causes the spinal cord to protrude into a sac at some place along the spine. This results in varying degrees of muscle weakness and paralysis in the trunk and lower body, with lesions higher on the spinal column causing greater paralysis. Excessive weight gain and reduced stature are commonly associated with this disorder. Energy needs vary widely because there is wide variation in the extent of the muscle weakness and paralysis. The needs generally are lower, both absolutely and per centimeter of height, than for age- and gender-matched peers in the general population (Dustrude and Prince, 1990; Ekvall, 1993b). Lean body mass and, therefore, resting metabolic rate appear to be reduced. Increases in energy expenditure necessary to perform some tasks may be offset by decreased time spent in activity. Fat distribution is altered, with relatively greater amounts of fat on the lower extremities (Bandini et al, 1991).

Approximately 2500 infants are born in the United States each year with myelomeningocele or other forms of neural tube defects, and it has been estimated that an additional 1500 fetuses with these disorders are aborted. Evidence has been presented in recent years that supplementation with folic acid during the **periconceptional period** is associated with reduced incidence of these birth defects, although the mechanisms involved are not yet known. This led to an announcement in the United States in 1996 of plans for enriched flour to be fortified with folic acid. The measure is intended to increase intake of folate by women in their childbearing years, and, it is hoped, to reduce the occurrence of neural tube defects without promoting excessive intake of the vitamin by other segments of the population (Hine, 1996).

ALTERED ENERGY NEEDS   Resting energy expenditure and energy for activity are major components of energy needs. Differences in growth account for some differences in energy needs in persons with developmental disabilities. Differences in body composition affect resting energy expenditure, and also may affect the amount of energy expended in activity by either increasing or decreasing the burden and the efficiency of movement. When movement disorders are present, mechanical efficiency, intensity, or duration of activity may be altered, thereby affecting energy needs (Fig. 15–2). Differences in intensity or duration of activity may also be related to behavioral characteristics, as in persons with attention deficit hyperactivity disorder. Medications; stresses of illness and surgery; cardiovascular, respiratory, and endocrine disorders; and other medical conditions are examples of additional factors that affect energy needs.

Effects of Medications

Medication use is very widespread among persons with developmental disabilities. Requirements for energy or specific nutrients may be altered by medication use, or more general effects on nutrient intakes or nutrition status may result from effects on appetite, metabolism, elimination or activity level (Table 15–2). Many persons receive multiple medications concurrently and for long periods of time, which generally increases the likelihood that nutrition-related effects will be clinically significant. The implications are even greater when nutrition status is already

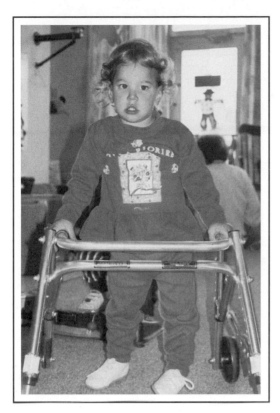

FIGURE 15–2. When movement disorders are present, mechanical efficiency, intensity, and/or duration of activity may be altered, thereby affecting energy needs.

stressed by inadequate or excessive nutritional intakes or by effects of physical anomalies, disease, or surgery (Roe, 1985).

Based on data from a variety of sources (Aman and Singh, 1988), it has been estimated that 20% to 40% of persons residing in institutions, intermediate care facilities for persons with mental retardation, and group homes, and 6% to 18% of children with developmental disabilities who reside in the community receive anticonvulsant medications (Aman M, personal communication, 1995). Use is most prevalent among persons with the most severe handicapping conditions, many of whom are nonambulatory and among whom feeding problems also are most common. Increased requirements for folic acid, vitamin D, and calcium by persons receiving phenytoin, phenobarbital, and carbamazepine have been extensively described. Effects of other anticonvulsants on these nutrients and of these and other anticonvulsants on many other nutrients have been reported, but remain less well established. Weight gain or loss may occur secondary to changes in appetite or energy expenditure. Persons receiving anticonvulsants should be considered at overall increased nutritional risk, and at particular risk with respect to folate, vitamin D, and calcium. Anticipatory guidance and moni-

toring of diet and biochemical parameters should occur in persons receiving these medications. Prophylactic use of nutrient supplements is controversial because vitamin D intoxication can occur and because some reports have been presented of increased seizure activity with folate administration (Kozlowski, 1990). Roe (1985) pointed out that folate deficiency can cause neurologic deficits and recommended that hematologic and biochemical monitoring accompany supplementation if it is required to meet the folate needs of persons receiving anticonvulsants.

Approximately 27% of 1000 adults included in a recent survey of community residential placements were receiving one or more psychotropic drugs, with neuroleptic drugs the most commonly used (Aman et al, 1995). Similar figures have been reported in the last decade from several other studies (Aman and Singh, 1988). Use of medications for seizure control or treatment of behavioral disorders is prevalent among these same individuals. Many of the psychotropic drugs cause dry mouth, constipation, and effects on appetite, which may have nutritional consequences (Roe, 1985; Roe, 1989; Gray and Gray, 1989). Stimulant medications such as methylphenidate and dextroamphetamine are used in combination with behavioral measures for treating attention deficit hyperactivity disorder in children. Loss of appetite, reduction in food intake, and a slowing of growth may accompany use of these drugs. Timing food presentation to take advantage of peak appetite, which is within the first 30 minutes or 4 to 6 hours after administration of the stimulant drugs, has been suggested (Lucas, 1993). The growth of children and the weight status and nutrient and energy intakes of persons of any age who are receiving psychotropic drugs should be monitored.

Possible nutritional consequences should be considered with the use of any medication. In addition to those just mentioned, medications used by many persons with de-

---

  K E Y   T E R M S

Prader-Willi syndrome: syndrome characterized by low weight gain in infancy followed by obesity by early childhood and continuing thereafter, mental retardation, and abnormal food seeking and gorging behavior

myelomeningocele: defect in development in first prenatal month causes spinal cord to protrude into sac at some place along spine; results in varying degrees of weakness and paralysis in trunk and lower body, with higher lesions causing greater paralysis; excessive weight gain is common

periconceptional period: weeks shortly before and following conception

TABLE 15–2 Medication Effects with Nutritional Implications

Medications*	Effects	References
ANTICONVULSANTS		
Phenytoin (Dilantin), Phenobarbital, primidone (Mysoline), carbamazepine (Tegretol)	Decreased folate in serum, red cells, cerebrospinal fluid; may lead to megaloblastic anemia	Roe, 1985; Roe, 1989; Deb, 1994
Phenytoin (Dilantin), phenobarbital, carbamazepine (Tegretol), possibly others	Depressed vitamin D status; may lead to rickets or osteomalacia; effect may be exacerbated by non-ambulation	Roe, 1985; Roe, 1989; Ala-Houhala et al, 1986; Lamberg-Allardt et al, 1990
Carbamazepine (Tegretol), primidone (Mysoline)	Depressed biotin status	Kraus, 1985; Kraus, 1988; Said, 1989
Phenytoin (Dilantin)	Gum hypertrophy may alter eating ability	Chambers, 1982; Roe, 1985
Valproic acid (Depakene)	Reduced serum carnitine	Roe, 1989
General	Constipation, diarrhea, nausea, vomiting, altered appetite	Roe, 1989
PSYCHOTROPICS		
NEUROLEPTICS		
Thioridazine (Mellaril), chlorpromazine (Thorazine), fluphenazine (Prolixin), thiothixene (Navene), trifluoperazine (Stelazine)	Dry mouth, constipation, weight gain	Roe, 1989; Gray and Gray, 1989
Haloperidol (Haldol)	Dry mouth, loss of appetite, nausea, vomiting, constipation, diarrhea	Physicians Desk Reference, 1995
HETEROCYCLIC ANTIDEPRESSANTS		
Amitriptyline (Elavil), desipramine (Norpramin), doxepin (Sinequan), fluoxetine (Prozac), imipramine (Trofranil), nortriptyline (Pamelor), trazodone (Desyrel)	Dry mouth, constipation, increase in appetite, weight gain (except with fluoxetine)	Gray and Gray, 1989
MONAMINE OXIDASE INHIBITORS		
Phenelzine (Nardil), tranylcypromine (Parnate)	Dry mouth, constipation, weight gain (with phenelzine), vitamin B_6 deficiency; neurotoxicity may occur with tryptophan intake, acute hypertension with tyramine intake	Gray and Gray, 1989
LITHIUM	Nausea, vomiting, loose stools, thirst, abdominal pains; weight gain from edema, increased food intake, or altered carbohydrate metabolism; excretion increased by caffeine or sodium	Gray and Gray, 1989
CNS STIMULANTS		
Methylphenidate (Ritalin), dextroamphetamine (Dexedrine), pemoline (Cylert)	Reduced appetite; slowing of weight gain; may lead to reduced height growth	Lucas, 1993
LAXATIVES	Chronic use may result in loss of fat-soluble vitamins (mineral oil), malabsorption, mineral depletion, gastrointestinal side effects; weight loss	Roe, 1989
ANTACIDS		
Aluminum hydroxide (Amphojel, Di-Gel, Maalox, Mylanta)	Hypophosphatemia, bone demineralization with abuse of medication	Roe, 1989
Sodium bicarbonate (Alka-Seltzer)	High intake reduces folate absorption	Roe, 1989
H-2 RECEPTOR ANTAGONISTS†		
Cimetidine (Tagamet)	Can induce vitamin B_{12} deficiency	Roe, 1989
Famotidine (Pepcid)	Possible vitamin B_{12} depletion	Roe, 1989

*Trade names in parentheses.
†Reduce acid toxicity of reflux.

velopmental delays and disabilities that may directly or indirectly affect their nutritional status include laxatives, antacids, medications to reduce acid toxicity of reflux, and antibiotics (Brizee, 1992; Kozlowski, 1990; American Dietetic Association, 1992; Roe, 1989).

Chronic Constipation

Persons with cerebral palsy, myelomeningocele, Rett syndrome, Down syndrome, and many other disorders commonly experience chronic constipation. Hard, dry stools that are eliminated with difficulty may be the result of many different factors, including inadequate intake of fluid and fiber, effects of medications, decreased physical activity, altered muscle tone, repeated failure to respond to physical signals of the need to defecate, and failure to establish a bowel routine.

Other Factors Affecting Nutritional Needs

Although it is beyond the scope of this section to describe in detail the other factors listed in Table 15–1 as altering nutritional needs, they should be recognized as affecting many persons in this population. Illness or surgery increases the individual's nutritional needs, and often adversely affects appetite and food intake. Without nutrition intervention, recovery time may be extended and a downward spiraling effect on the person's health may develop. Increasing numbers of people who have complex medical problems, including those dependent on medical technologies, are living in the community and presenting new challenges with respect to their needs for nutrition services. When metabolic or gastrointestinal disorders or other complex medical conditions are present, nutrition and feeding recommendations must be formulated by nutritionists with specialized areas of expertise working in collaboration with physicians. Improved health care has increased the life span of people with many different kinds of developmental disabilities who need age-appropriate health care, including nutritional guidance, as they face developmental changes and health risks at all stages of the life cycle.

Food Allergies and Intolerances

Food allergies are immunologically mediated adverse food reactions, whereas **food intolerances** are adverse reactions that are not proven to be immunologic in nature and may be idiosyncratic, pharmacologic, metabolic, or toxic reactions (Atkins, 1986). With the exception of selected metabolic disorders, these reactions are not known to be more common among persons with developmental delays or disabilities than among the general population. However, when disorders are present for which a cause or effective treatment has not been identified, individuals or their families sometimes hope that identification of offending food substance(s) may hold the key. Suspected allergy or intolerance should be called to the attention of a physician for evaluation according to techniques accepted by established medicine. Special attention is necessary to ensure that substances confirmed or highly suspected as offenders are eliminated from the diet, while also assuring that nutritional needs are met and unnecessary restrictions are not placed on the individual.

Adverse food reactions have been hypothesized for many years to be a cause of negative behaviors. The idea was popularized in the 1970s in response to a proposal by Feingold (1975) that certain food substances were major causes of hyperactive behavior in children. Although the proposal was not made specifically in relation to children with developmental delay or disability, it attracted the attention of many care providers involved with this population as well as those involved with typically developing children. Salicylates occurring naturally in foods, such as almonds, tomatoes, apricots, peaches, cucumbers, oranges, nectarines, apples, and berries, were suggested first as being primary offending substances, and then certain food additives and preservatives were added to the list. The term "defined diets" was adopted to refer to various modifications of the Feingold diet (Office for Medical Applications of Research, NIH, 1982). Well-designed double-blind studies have failed to provide evidence that dietary substances are major causes of what is now referred to as **attention deficit hyperactivity disorder** (ADHD). However, some evidence has been provided that the hyperactive behavior of a small percentage of children with ADHD, particularly children of preschool age, improves on a "defined diet" (Office for Medical Applications of Research, NIH, 1982; Lipton and Mayo, 1983; Kanerek and Marks-Kaufman, 1991). Compliance with other more established forms of intervention and close attention to maintaining overall nutritional quality of the diet is recommended if dietary intervention trials for ADHD are implemented.

The idea that sugar intake promotes hyperactive behavior in children has been widely expressed by parents, teachers, and others. The Feingold diet was relatively low in sugar, and, when other substances for which claims had been made failed to be confirmed as major causative factors for hyperactivity, sugar was suggested as a possible culprit (American Council on Science and Health, 1987; Hershey Foods Corp, 1992). In addition, a group of investigators found a correlation between reported prior sugar intake and destructive-aggressive and restless behaviors in a group of hyperactive children 4 to 7 years old. Reported prior sugar intake was also correlated with total body movement in the children who were not hyperactive

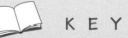

KEY TERMS

food allergy: immunologically mediated adverse food reaction

food intolerance: adverse reactions to food that are not proven to be immunologic; may be idiosyncratic, pharmacologic, metabolic, or toxic

attention deficit hyperactivity disorder (ADHD): clinical diagnosis in children; involves extended presence of inattention, impulsivity, hyperactivity

(Prinz et al, 1980). Although causal relationships are not confirmed by correlational data, the data were translated as such in the popular media. Results of numerous subsequent studies have not supported the hypothesis that either chronic high sugar consumption or acute sugar loading is a clinically significant cause of increased activity or disruptive behavior in children (Kanarek and Marks-Kaufman, 1991; Anderson, 1991; Kruesi et al, 1987; Rapoport, 1986). Rather, it has been suggested that carbohydrate consumption may have a calming effect, brought about by increased brain serotonin levels, if the environment allows the internal effect to be expressed (Anderson, 1991).

Altered Feeding Characteristics

Feeding problems in many persons with developmental disabilities complicate the process of establishing and maintaining feeding and eating routines that meet their nutritional needs and promote their personal-social, cognitive, and motor development. Feeding problems may result from delayed maturation, abnormal development, or a combination of the two. They may be secondary to physical or behavioral factors related to illness or disease. Many feeding problems are behaviorally based or include strong behavioral components. Characteristics of the caregiving environment may contribute to the development of feeding problems. Without effective intervention, feeding problems add stress to relationships with care providers and often lead to nutritional, developmental, and social compromise. Feeding problems are major contributors to the high nutritional risk of persons with developmental delays and disabilities (Morris and Klein, 1987; Lane and Cloud, 1988; Kozlowski et al, 1989; Kozlowski, 1990; Pipes and Glass, 1993).

Physical Characteristics and Health of Mouth Area

Physical characteristics of the mouth area alter feeding and eating for some individuals. Examples include cleft lip or palate, high arched palate, and malocclusion. Excessive growth of gum tissue often occurs as a side effect of the anticonvulsant medication phenytoin, and it may interfere with functional chewing. In addition, oral hygiene and health are adversely affected by many feeding problems or undesirable feeding practices, and this often leads to the development of conditions that further impede feeding. Prolonged use of a nursing bottle; lack of oral stimulation from hard, crunchy foods; inadequate clearing of the mouth; frequent exposure of the teeth to foods throughout the day; pooling of refluxed stomach contents in the mouth; nutritional deficiencies; inadequate professional dental care; and inadequate oral hygiene contribute to the occurrence of tooth decay and periodontal disease. Pain

and tooth loss associated with these conditions may cause the person to resist eating many foods.

Neuromotor Factors

Delays and abnormalities in neuromotor development affect feeding in many different ways. Abnormalities of muscle tone, reflex development, or responses to sensory stimulation may adversely affect the ability of the individual to assume or maintain positioning that is needed for eating; take food to the mouth; suck, drink from a cup, chew, or swallow; or focus on eating (Kozlowski et al, 1989; Kozlowski, 1990). **Tonic bite** is one abnormal reflex that can interfere with feeding. It is a forceful bite, elicited from contact with the teeth or gums, that is difficult for the person to release. **Tongue thrust** is a forceful protrusion of the tongue from the mouth, and is much stronger than the movements associated with infantile suckling. Children with low muscle tone, including many with Down syndrome, exhibit **exaggerated tongue protrusion**. Rhythmic motion of the tongue is retained, but protrusion is exaggerated (Morris and Klein, 1987). Persons with hypersensitivity may have very guarded responses that limit food textures or temperatures they will accept. Those with a lowered threshold to sensory information may be easily distracted and require a quiet environment with minimal distraction in order to focus on eating. Some people exhibit hyposensitivity in relation to taste, smell, or touch. This may reduce their interest in eating or result in poor food clearance from the mouth. Food may be lost from the mouth because of exaggerated tongue protrusion, hyposensitivity, or poor lip closure, as illustrated by the child with Down syndrome in Figure 15–3. Problems with biting, chewing, or swallowing may result from abnormal oral sensory motor characteristics, and they typically cause texture progression to be delayed. Reflux and aspiration are additional examples of problems that interfere with feeding and eating. Any of these problems may cause the feeding–eating process to be very slow and tiring, and nutritional and developmental aspects may suffer as a result. Feelings of frustration on the part of caregivers or the person with the disability may pave the way for feeding to become emotionally charged and for behavioral characteristics that further complicate feeding to develop (Morris and Klein, 1987; Kozlowski et al, 1989; Kozlowski, 1990; Pipes and Glass, 1993).

Behaviors

Behavioral aspects of feeding and eating may be altered whether or not oral sensory motor problems are present. Progression in feeding skill development is delayed in some persons, as are other areas of their development, but follows the same sequence as in typically developing individuals. Care providers sometimes need assistance in recognizing signs that an individual is developmentally ready

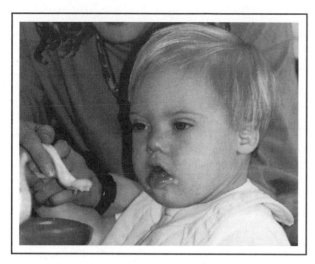

FIGURE 15–3. As illustrated by this child with Down syndrome, food may be lost from the mouth because of hyposensitivity, exaggerated tongue protrusion, or poor lip closure.

to progress from one feeding stage to the next, such as from eating strained foods to eating foods with slightly coarser texture, from being bottle-fed to drinking from a cup, or from being fed entirely by someone else to progressing toward independent spoon feeding. Progression is likely to be met with greater resistance if opportunities are not presented at the time the person becomes developmentally ready (Pipes and Glass, 1993). Alternatively, caregivers sometimes need assistance in recognizing that a person is not developmentally ready for feeding progression, even though he or she has reached or passed the chronologic age at which the progression typically occurs.

Noncompliant or maladaptive behaviors that adversely affect feeding may also be present. Parents and other care providers sometimes use food and feeding as ways of expressing affection or concern and need assistance in setting nutritionally and developmentally appropriate limits. Persons who have control over few aspects of their lives may quickly learn to control many aspects of feeding. For example, noncompliant behavior can be the reason a person does not drink from a cup or has a narrow range of food intake, although oral sensory motor problems can also cause either. Ruminating or gagging may be behavioral, but they also may have other causes, which should always be evaluated.

Feeding problems rarely have a single cause. Rather, multiple factors contribute. Efforts should be made to identify causes of the problems, and this usually is best accomplished through interdisciplinary team evaluation.

Tube Feeding

Some form of tube feeding becomes necessary, either supplementally or to provide total nutrition, when ade-

quate nutrition cannot be achieved by other means. Oral feeding is encouraged unless it jeopardizes the person's health or safety or requires unreasonable expenditures of time and energy. Parenteral nutrition is used if the gastrointestinal tract must be bypassed completely. Much more commonly, sources of nutrients are delivered by tube into the gastrointestinal tract. The need for tube feeding may last from a few days to a lifetime, and the anticipated duration is one of the factors taken into account in deciding the form of tube feeding that will be used. In persons with developmental delays and disabilities, orogastric, nasogastric, and gastrostomy feeding are the most common forms of tube feeding. Establishing orogastric or nasogastric tube feeding does not involve surgery, and one of these forms of tube feeding is often used when use is expected to be of short duration. **Gastrostomy** feeding is used when non-oral feeding is expected to be of longer duration. A surgical procedure to reduce the likelihood of gastroesophageal reflux often is performed in conjunction with the surgery necessary to establish gastrostomy feeding.

If the conditions that created the need for tube feeding can be resolved and other conditions that interfere with oral feeding do not arise, use of the tube can be reduced or eliminated. However, many persons who have been tube fed for long periods of time or at very early ages oppose the transition to oral feeding. The transition often occurs very slowly. Behavioral and oral sensory motor factors may contribute to the resistance. As discussed later in this chapter (see Intervention), facilitating the transition to oral feeding is one of many important reasons for oral sensory motor treatment to occur along with tube feeding. Collaborative effort of caregivers and an interdisciplinary team of professionals is often needed to promote satisfactory nutrition, food acceptance patterns, and oral sensory motor functioning (Blackman and Nelson, 1985; Morris and Klein, 1987; Glass and Lucas, 1990; Smith and Pederson, 1990; Schauster and Dwyer, 1996).

 K E Y   T E R M S

tonic bite: abnormal reflex involving forceful bite, elicited from contact with teeth or gums, which is difficult for person to release; can interfere with feeding
tongue thrust: forceful protrusion of tongue from mouth; much stronger than infantile suckling movement
exaggerated tongue protrusion: exaggerated protrusion of tongue with rhythmic motion of tongue retained, as seen in many children with hypotonia
gastrostomy: surgical creation of artificial opening into the stomach

Increased Demands on Time, Energy, and Financial and Emotional Resources

The needs of persons for extraordinary support related to any aspect of their health or development are likely to create emotional and financial stress. Because of the multitude of concerns facing them, persons with developmental disabilities and their families or other care providers may need assistance that will enable them to direct adequate time, energy, and financial resources to nutrition and feeding. This may include assistance with respite care, homemaking services, health care, or other support services, as well as food, formula, or special equipment.

Inadequate Information and Support

Nutritional risk is reduced when (1) health and education professionals, family members, other care providers, and, to the extent feasible, the person with disabilities have adequate knowledge, skills, and resources related to nutrition and feeding; and (2) the information and resources are applied to day-to-day practices and to the provision of appropriate nutrition screening, assessment, intervention, and support. Awareness of the nutrition risks and problems of persons with developmental disabilities has increased in recent years, as has the number of professionals with knowledge and clinical skills in nutrition and feeding as it applies to this population. Although greater numbers of people in this population and their care providers are receiving services related to nutrition and feeding than in the past, the needs of many continue to be unrecognized or inadequately addressed. Individuals, their families, and other care providers need guidance and support in the prevention, recognition, and management of nutrition-related problems throughout the life span. Health promotion and nutrition education must be included as components of supported community living as these living opportunities continue to expand nationally and increasing emphasis is placed on consumer choice (Rimmer et al, 1994).

Knowledge and skills needed for nutritional assessment and treatment of persons with developmental disabilities vary from being the same as with nondisabled persons to being much more complex. Advances in technology and treatment modalities, changes in philosophies of care, and changes in funding have resulted in persons with much more complex medical conditions receiving services in a greater variety of settings than was the case even a few years ago. Professionals, whether generalists or specialists, must continually expand and update their knowledge related to this population. The role of the nutrition professional is to support, not supplant, the role of the family (Baer et al, 1991). Whether nutrition and feeding recommendations are developed in a primary care setting in the person's geographic area of residence or in a tertiary center many miles away, implementation typically needs to occur at home and in educational and work settings. Therefore, it is critical that education and support be provided to persons who can be key players in this implementation. That group often includes the individual, family members, and personnel from educational and employment settings. Dietitians and other community-based professionals play important roles in providing or contributing to that education, assisting with implementation and monitoring, and, thus, contributing to family-centered, community-based, coordinated, culturally competent care. Research is needed to expand the information base concerning nutrition of this population, but the health of many individuals can be improved by expanded application of information that is currently available.

Feeding and mealtimes fulfill cultural and social functions in addition to providing nutrition. Positive mealtime experiences can promote interaction and attachment and provide opportunities for the development of cognitive, motor, communication, and social skills. However, nutrition and feeding also can be the source of many stressors for persons with developmental delay or disabilities, their families and friends, and other persons with whom they have contact during eating. Difficulties in feeding, extremely long feeding times, failure of children to grow according to expectations, failure for desired health outcomes to be achieved, or inability to implement recommendations for dietary change may cause persons with disabilities, their families, and other care providers to question their own skills and develop feelings of inadequacy. Lack of sensitivity can result in service approaches that worsen the problems. By responding to and respecting the values, lifestyles, resources, desires, and needs of persons with disabilities, their families, and other care providers, and working collaboratively with them, professionals provide support that reduces stress and helps to enhance responses to the needs of persons with developmental disabilities (Morris and Klein, 1987; Kozlowski et al, 1989; Baer et al, 1991; American Dietetic Association, 1992; Venn et al, 1992; American Dietetic Association, 1995).

NUTRITION SCREENING, ASSESSMENT, INTERVENTION AND MONITORING

■ Describe the major areas addressed in nutritional assessment of this population. Identify differences from nutritional assessment of the general population.

■ Describe factors that complicate anthropometric assessment. Identify alternative measurement techniques and alternative anthropometric parameters that sometimes can be substituted for those more commonly used with the general population. Discuss differences in interpretation of anthropometric data compared with procedures used in interpreting data from the general population.

■ How may dietary assessment need to differ from that typically conducted with the general population?

■ Identify three nutrition-related problems often addressed in dietary recommendations for individuals in this population. In addition to specific dietary constituent(s) of primary concern, identify factors that must be taken into account in development of dietary recommendations.

■ Identify groups of professionals who often have expertise in feeding assessment.

■ Describe major areas addressed in feeding assessments. What are advantages of interdisciplinary nutrition-feeding assessments with this population? What are disadvantages or limitations?

■ With respect to nutrition services, what are advantages or benefits of comprehensive, coordinated interdisciplinary service approaches that are individual- and family-centered, community based, comprehensive, and culturally competent, versus more traditional service approaches?

■ Why are monitoring and reassessment important aspects of nutrition service?

Screening

Screening for nutrition-related problems provides an entree for anticipatory guidance, which can prevent some potential problems from arising. When the need is indicated, nutritional assessment can occur and intervention plans can be developed. Screening can be performed by trained members of the interdisciplinary team using criteria developed by the nutritionist or registered dietitian. Nutrition screening should begin in infancy and occur on an ongoing basis throughout life.

Assessment

Major areas addressed in nutritional assessments of persons with developmental delays and disabilities are listed in Table 15–3. The extent to which the respective areas are addressed and the manner in which that occurs should be tailored to the characteristics of the individual and his or her support system. In the absence of feeding problems, complex medical problems, or diagnoses with specific nutritional or physical growth implications, nutritional assessment may differ little from that conducted with persons of similar age who do not have disabilities. When more severe or complex problems are present, input may be needed from a wide range of professionals, including

TABLE 15–3 Major Areas Addressed in Nutritional Assessment of Persons with Developmental Delays or Disabilities
Health, social and developmental histories
Clinical/medical
Anthropometric
Biochemical
Dietary
Feeding

some with highly specialized areas of expertise. The assessment is best accomplished as an interdisciplinary activity. Examples of professionals whose expertise may be needed to complement that of the nutritionist include occupational and physical therapists, speech pathologists, psychologists, special educators and early intervention specialists, nurses, dentists, dental hygienists, social workers, primary care physicians, and a variety of medical specialists. The use of community-based primary nutrition services for assessment of clients who have no complicating conditions enhances access to services. Resources for specialized assessments are usually located in specialty clinics or tertiary care settings. Strong linkages between these settings and community-based health, education, vocational, and social services are needed to promote continuity of care and contribute to a coordinated system of comprehensive, community-based, culturally competent, person- and family-centered care (American Dietetic Association, 1995). Clinical criteria and indicators for nutrition services for persons ages 10 years and older with developmental disabilities and feeding problems are available from the American Dietetic Association (Posthauer et al, 1993).

Health, Social, and Developmental Histories

Many persons with developmental disabilities have very complex histories. Even at very young ages, they may have received or currently be receiving many different kinds of services in many different locations. In addition to interviewing the individual and/or other persons such as parents, spouse, friend, supported living providers, or other primary care providers as part of the nutritional assessment process, review of extensive records and discussions with other service providers are often very useful. Background information may be available about diagnosis, medical or social complications, nutrition or feeding problems and interventions, physical growth patterns of children and adolescents and weight patterns of adults, past and current services, strengths of the person's primary support system, and resources for accessing health and nutrition services and food. Using this information helps to avoid unnecessary duplication of tests and contributes to the assessment of the person's current physical size characteristics, feeding practices, nutrition status, and apparent nutritional needs. It also facilitates the development of recommendations and the delivery of integrated services that are person/family centered, culturally competent, coordinated, and comprehensive.

Clinical and Medical Assessment

Input from a variety of medical specialists may be needed, particularly in assessments of persons with complex medical conditions, to evaluate the contribution of nutritional factors to the occurrence of health problems and also to evaluate the implications of various conditions with respect to diet and feeding recommendations (Kozlowski, 1990). Examination should always be conducted for possible clinical signs of malnutrition. Particular attention should be paid to possible signs of dehydration in persons who have communication difficulties or feeding problems and to signs of deficiencies of nutrients affected by medications the person is receiving. The mouth area should be examined for structural characteristics and evidence of disease, including nursing bottle mouth, that could have nutrition or feeding implications. Evaluation for swallowing disorders, aspiration, esophagitis, or gastroesophageal reflux may be indicated if the person is having feeding problems or shows signs of discomfort that could be related to eating. **Videofluoroscopy** is used extensively as a component of interdisciplinary feeding assessments to gain information about swallowing and the safety of oral feeding of persons who have neurologic disorders (Fox, 1990; Morton et al, 1993). Radiographic techniques are used for evaluating characteristics of the skeleton, such as bone quality, bone age, or maturation pattern. Bone age, which is determined by radiographic assessment of either the wrist-hand area or the knee, is a better indicator of biologic maturity than is chronologic age (Roche, 1979). Information about bone age or maturation pattern is sometimes used, for example, in syndrome identification and to help to elucidate physical growth deviation, and may contribute to the nutritional assessment. Information about bone quality may be useful in evaluating nutritional status, effects of some anticonvulsant medications, and presence of diseases such as osteoporosis. Conditions for which nondisabled persons of comparable chronologic or biologic age would be evaluated, such as cardiovascular disease risk, diabetes, and cancer, must also be taken into account. Review of elimination patterns often reveals needs for dietary change or medical treatment.

Anthropometric Assessment

Anthropometric data are a key component of nutritional assessment of persons with developmental disabilities and

are particularly useful when data are available from measurements repeated over time. Serial profiles of accurate anthropometric data provide an objective basis for evaluating growth of children and generally provide one of the best indications of their nutrition status. With adults and children, serial data for weight, length, or stature, skinfolds, and various body circumferences provide objective means of quantifying changes in weight, weight for stature, and indirect indications of body composition and body fat distribution. Patterns of change in these variables often reveal the timing of significant events related to health or nutrition. When viewed in conjunction with information from other aspects of the assessment, anthropometric data can serve as key indicators of the need for and the effects of nutrition interventions.

Behaviors, physical deformities, or neuromotor characteristics of some persons with developmental disorders complicate the process of making anthropometric measurements, and sometimes make it impossible for measurement techniques used with the general population to be applied. In addition to more commonly used equipment, chair scales, bed scales, adult-sized length measuring boards, and calipers for measuring knee height are useful with some subjects. Measurements should be performed by skilled personnel using accurately calibrated, appropriately maintained equipment and techniques as near to those recommended for use with the general population as is feasible. Any difficulty encountered in performing a measurement and any deviation from standard measuring techniques should be documented. Even small measurement errors can lead to large errors in conclusions drawn from them, and some measurements cannot be performed accurately with some subjects. Professional judgment must be applied in determining whether a measurement is appropriate with a particular subject. If subject behavior is the complicating factor, techniques for improving compliance can sometimes be identified by care providers who are accustomed to interacting with the individual or by behavior management specialists.

Length or stature often presents the greatest measurement challenge with this population. Measurement of length is recommended through age 2 years, and stature, which is 1 to 2 cm shorter than the recumbent measurement, is usually measured thereafter if the individual can be satisfactorily positioned. Many persons must continue to be measured in a recumbent position, and even that is not feasible with persons who have physical deviations such as scoliosis or severe contractures. Physical or occupational therapists can sometimes suggest techniques that facilitate satisfactory measurement positioning of individuals who have slight contractures, but alternatives to traditional length or stature measurement techniques are often needed. If any uncertainty exists regarding procedures that should be followed to ensure that physical injury does not occur to the person being measured (e.g., length measurement of person who has dislocated hips), physicians or therapists should be consulted. When measurement of stature or total length cannot be accomplished, body segments sometimes can be measured as indicators of linear growth attainment, depending on characteristics of the individual. These measurements include crown-rump length, sitting height, arm span, upper arm length, knee height, and lower leg length. Techniques for performing these measurements have been described in detail (Belt-Niedbala, 1986; Martin et al, 1988; Spender et al, 1989; Pipes and Glass, 1993). Crown-rump length and arm span, two of the measurements that are often referenced for use with this population and with which nutrition students may not be familiar, are briefly described here.

For accurate measurement of **crown-rump length** or **sitting height**, the trunk and neck of the subject must be straight. Crown-rump length, the recumbent counterpart of sitting height, is measured using a length measuring board. The subject is positioned by two or more examiners as for length measurement, except that the subject's legs are raised by an examiner so that the thighs are at a 90-degree angle to the flat surface of the length measuring board. The moveable perpendicular piece of the measuring board is slid firmly against the subject's buttocks. A third examiner is often needed to hold the subject's trunk in alignment. The distance from crown to rump is read from the measuring board (Martin et al, 1988).

Arm span is the distance between the tips of the longest fingers of each hand with both arms extended maximally at the level of the shoulders and the back pressed against a flat surface. It is highly correlated with stature and is sometimes assumed to approximate stature; however, the ratio of arm span to stature apparently varies with age, gender, and race (Martin et al, 1988). According to one method that has been described for this measurement, a calibrated steel rod is held by two examiners against the subject's upper back and the backs of his or her outstretched arms (Pipes and Glass, 1993). Alternatively, the subject may stand with the back against a flat wall, arms outstretched and palms facing forward, with a measuring tape against the wall at shoulder height. Distance between the tips of the longest fingers is read from the tape (Martin et al, 1988). Either method requires a compliant subject who does not have upper extremity contractures or deformity. The measurement may be useful with persons who have myelomeningocoele (Belt-Niedbala et al, 1986) or for estimating young adult stature of elderly persons who have experienced stature loss or whose length or stature cannot be accurately measured (Martin et al, 1988).

When subjects have contractures or other conditions that preclude the measurements listed above, attempts are sometimes made to measure the lengths of the head, neck, trunk, and lower extremities, and the sum of the segment lengths is used as an estimate of total body length. Accuracy and reliability are, at best, difficult to achieve in total body length estimates derived in this manner with subjects who have no conditions that complicate measure-

ment, and they become increasingly less likely to be achieved as contractures or skeletal deformities increase. Any linear measurement of individuals who have upper and lower extremity contractures and spinal curvature is subject to question, and the high potential for error in measurements taken under those circumstanstances should be recognized.

Information regarding general physical characteristics, health status, and medical diagnoses and their implications relative to growth and physical development should influence the examiner's selection of anthropometric measurements to perform on a particular individual, and must be integrated with information from other components of the nutrition assessment in evaluating anthropometric data. Information regarding bone age may be particularly useful in the evaluation of growth and nutrition status of children whose stature is outside general population normal limits relative to chronologic age. For example, stature that is short for a child's chronologic age may be consistent with biologic age if bone age is depressed, and the child is likely to have more time for catch-up growth to occur than if bone age is advanced. Differences in growth rate, height attainment, body segment length ratios, total body weight, and distribution patterns and proportions of fat and muscle are characteristic of some disorders. For

KEY TERMS

videofluoroscopy: technique used to videotape modified barium swallow studies, which are performed to assess oral and pharyngeal phases of swallowing; such factors as transit time and presence of aspiration are evaluated by observing response to small amounts of barium mixed with small amounts of food or beverage

crown-rump length: recumbent counterpart of sitting height; measured in first 3 years of life and later when subject cannot be positioned for sitting height; measured with subject positioned on length measuring board as for length measurement, except that thighs are at 90-degree angle to surface of board and sliding perpendicular board is positioned firmly against buttocks

sitting height: composite measure that includes trunk, neck, and head; measurement of distance from seating surface to superior point on head with subject in sitting position according to standard protocol

arm span: distance between the tips of the longest fingers of each hand with both arms extended maximally at the level of the shoulders and the back pressed against flat surface; highly correlated with stature

example, arm and leg lengths are decreased relative to trunk length in persons with Down syndrome (Cronk, 1992). Differences in body fat distribution are characteristic of Prader-Willi syndrome. Failure to take such differences into account can lead to inaccurate interpretation of anthropometric data relative to nutrition status. As described earlier, error is likely to be introduced if equations for estimating body composition are applied to population groups for whom they have not been validated. Equations using a combination of skinfold measurements, which had been validated with persons who did not have the syndrome, underestimated the percent of body weight that was fat in subjects with Prader-Willi syndrome by 16% compared with estimates based on stable isotope techniques (Schoeller et al, 1988). Comparison of skinfold measurements with reference data for specific sites, such as triceps or subscapular skinfolds, and comparison of values obtained over time can be useful in helping to monitor fat deposition at the respective sites even if the data do not provide an indication of total body fat or lean body mass. For example, one might question what benefit was being derived from forcing increased calories into a child whose length for age was below the 5th percentile of reference data if the increase resulted in subscapular and triceps skinfolds greater than the 95th percentile and no increase in length percentile, even though weight for stature was only at the 15th percentile.

Interpretation of anthropometric data may involve comparison with general population reference data, comparison of data collected for the individual over time, and, when available, comparison with disorder-specific reference data. Monitoring data for the individual in relation to general population reference data and for the individual in relation to him- or herself can be useful when the data are appropriately interpreted (Chumlea, 1989; Kozlowski, 1990). At the minimum, data for children should be plotted on National Center for Health Statistics (NCHS) general population growth charts of weight and length or stature for age and weight for length (National Center for Health Statistics, 1978). Incremental growth charts also are available (Roche and Himes, 1980; Guo et al, 1991). Plotting data gives a picture of relative growth velocity of a child and provides additional information that is useful in the nutritional assessment. Head circumference measurements for children through age 3 years are usually plotted on NCHS charts, and charts from other sources are used thereafter. Diagnosis-specific charts also are used when available. General population data from various surveys of NCHS are available to use as references for heights, weights, and sitting heights of adults, and for triceps and subscapular skinfolds and mid-upper arm circumferences of children and adults (National Center for Health Statistics, 1981; Frisancho, 1990). Sources of reference data for less commonly measured variables have been listed by Lohman and co-workers (1988). When anthropometric data are outside normal limits for the general

population or change substantially in percentile ranking, assistance with interpretation should be sought from a physician or other professional with expertise in the area of growth deviation assessment.

Whenever they are available, diagnosis-specific reference data should be used in combination with reference data for the general population. Growth charts for length or stature and weight are available for Down syndrome (Cronk et al, 1988), and stature charts are available for Prader-Willi syndrome (Holm, 1988). Reference data also are available for several other less commonly occurring disorders (Saul et al, 1988). Skinfold reference data for various disorders are not generally available. When syndrome-specific charts are used, measurements also should be compared with general population data. Even the reference data for children with Down syndrome were developed from small, nonrandom samples, and values at outer percentiles may represent pathologic conditions (Cronk and Anneren, 1992). Help with the interpretation of data regarding deviations in growth and physical development of persons with disorders should be sought from professionals with expertise in that area.

Biochemical Assessment

Biochemical assessment, like other aspects of the nutritional assessment, should be tailored to the characteristics of the individual. In addition to variables that are monitored in the general population, such as cholesterol in adults and hemoglobin or hematocrit in children and adults, one or many tests may be ordered because of such factors as nutrient–drug interactions, overall low food intake, exclusion of particular food groups or nutrients from the diet, the presence of disease known to increase nutritional risk, or the presence of clinical signs of malnutrition. For example, biochemical monitoring of status with respect to calcium, vitamin D, and folacin is often recommended for persons receiving long-term treatment with certain anticonvulsant medications (Roe, 1985; Kraus et al, 1988; Roe, 1989). Laboratory tests are also used for detecting and monitoring inborn errors of metabolism.

Dietary Assessment

Dietary information is collected in much the same manner as in nutritional assessment of non-disabled persons, with the exception that more persons may be needed to serve as informants. As much information as possible should be elicited from the person with the disability and additional information obtained from adults who are most knowledgeable concerning that person's food intake. In addition to family members and friends, this may include teachers, therapists, nurses, daycare providers, supported living providers, employers, and job coaches and other workshop personnel. If a nutrition problem is suspected, it may be necessary to obtain detailed records of intake from several different persons and settings. The most complete information usually is obtained from a combination of interview, diet records, and direct observation. Attention to details of recipes, feeding schedules, and food provided versus food actually consumed is particularly important. Information should be elicited regarding nutrient supplements, including special formulas, which may be viewed by informants as "medicine" and thus not included with nutrition information unless specifically elicited.

Information regarding nutrient and energy intake should be evaluated in relation to information obtained from other aspects of the nutritional assessment and with consideration of factors such as altered activity levels, altered physical growth potential, nutrient–drug interactions, and apparent nutritional deficiencies that may cause the person's needs to differ from those of the general population. While Recommended Dietary Allowances (National Research Council, 1989) are often used as reference points in evaluating vitamin, mineral and protein intakes, limitations of this approach in relation to special population groups should be recognized. Sound professional judgement must be applied in integrating information from the total evaluation to arrive at dietary recommendations for the individual.

Feeding Assessment

Diet and feeding must be considered together when assessing the nutrition status of persons with developmental disabilities. When feeding development is delayed or performance is abnormal, interdisciplinary assessment with the expertise of other disciplines to complement that of the nutritionist is highly desirable. Many occupational therapists, physical therapists, and speech pathologists have expertise in assessing motor, sensory, and oral motor aspects, whereas psychologists are most likely to have expertise in conducting in-depth assessment of behavioral aspects of feeding. Some nurses and child development specialists also have expertise in assessment of behavioral aspects of feeding, including caregiver–child interactions during feeding. Observations of eating/feeding and interactions surrounding the activity, with and without intervention from therapists, often provide insights that are valuable for all team members in their assessment of the problem(s) and development of recommendations for the individual. Observations made in the client's usual environment, including home, school, or work settings, have many advantages but often are not feasible. When site visits cannot be made, videotaping of feeding/eating sessions sometimes can be arranged. Alternatively, and probably most commonly practiced, observations may be carried out in clinic settings. Team observation of the person eating independently or with feeding assistance, as "usually" practiced, is often followed by questioning and testing by one or more team members of various parameters related to feeding. Behaviors observed include conditions that

evoke positive and negative reactions from the person being fed and caregiver responses; expressions of food preferences, hunger, satiety, readiness for the "next bite," and caregiver responses to those cues; responses to presentation of food and feeding attempts (dependent feeder); other interactions during feeding/eating; and responses to other factors in the environment (e.g., noise).

Oral motor functioning of most people is facilitated by positioning with their hips and knees flexed, head and trunk in midline, and feet supported. Positioning is observed for stability, comfort, and appropriateness for maximizing feeding skills and behaviors. Positions assumed by care providers are observed for ease in providing feeding support needed by the person who is being fed and ease in promoting appropriate social interaction with that person. Other factors evaluated include equipment needed for feeding; ability of individuals to take food and feeding equipment to their mouths; responses to foods with various flavors, textures, temperatures, and consistencies; general body tone and movement; presence of normal and abnormal reflexes; characteristics of oral-facial structures, including condition of the teeth; jaw, lip, and tongue control; oral motor patterns related to sucking, biting, chewing, and swallowing; and responses to noise and other environmental stimuli (Morris and Klein, 1987; Kozlowski et al, 1989; Kozlowski, 1990). Dental hygienists make a valuable contribution to the assessment by evaluating the adequacy of home and professional dental care and providing suggestions for dental hygiene and oral stimulation. Approaches used in feeding assessments have been extensively described (Morris and Klein, 1987; Kozlowski et al, 1989; Cloud and Bergman, 1991; Padgett, 1992; O'Neil, 1993; Pipes and Glass, 1993). A Developmental Feeding Tool from the University Affiliated Program of The University of Tennessee, Memphis (Smith et al, 1982) can serve as a guide to feeding observations of children.

Intervention

As indicated previously, concerns and needs for services are likely to exist in relation to many areas of the health and development of persons with developmental disabilities, not just in relation to nutrition. In addition, the expertise of more than one professional is often needed to address nutrition-related problems. The development of person- and family-centered, culturally competent, community-based, coordinated, interdisciplinary service systems means that individuals, family members, and other primary care providers and professionals work together as a team to address common goals in a unified way. A written plan is developed in which prioritized goals and objectives are stated and means are identified for addressing them. Optimal service practices provide support to individuals and their families while also respecting and reinforcing their rights to make choices regarding services, supports, and treatment modalities. Strengths of current practices should be reinforced, and plans for intervention with respect to problems that are identified should be developed in partnership with the individual, family members, and/or primary care providers, and in collaboration with other agencies, programs and professionals. Goals and objectives should be incorporated into the person's individualized service plan. Because many persons may be involved in implementation of the plan, it is crucial for recommendations to be clearly stated. Anticipatory guidance should be provided, and plans for follow-up should be established.

Care coordination reduces the likelihood that incompatible recommendations regarding a particular problem will be provided from different sources or that major problems will go unaddressed. For example, without care coordination, a WIC dietitian might provide one set of recommendations to a family, a hospital dietitian who sees the child in a neonatal intensive care follow-up clinic might provide a second set, and a dietitian working in a clinic for children with cerebral palsy might provide a third set . . . none of which might reach the occupational therapist who is developing a feeding program for the child in an early intervention program. When the nutrition professional becomes a team member and nutrition recommendations become part of a bigger plan, awareness and understanding of the recommendations by other professionals is heightened and avenues are created for obtaining assistance with implementation and monitoring. For example, the classroom teacher may become a key player in reinforcing family attempts to implement dietary recommendations made by the dietitian, food service personnel may adapt school breakfast and lunch to meet the child's special needs and promote implementation of the recommendations, or the school nurse may agree to weigh a child weekly and report the results to the hospital dietitian as efforts are under way to achieve weight gain in a severely malnourished child. Parents of children with disabilities have indicated greater satisfaction with ongoing services from dietitians who are part of a healthcare team than from dietitians who function separate from a team (Bonam et al, 1993). Throughout all aspects of service, including coordination and collaboration, it is imperative that the individual's confidentiality rights be protected and that information be requested or transmitted only with written consent from persons who are legally authorized to give it.

The nutrition care plan may include recommendations for medical or dental treatment; behavioral intervention; positioning, equipment, techniques or schedules for feeding; texture, temperature, variety, or quantities of foods, formulas or supplements; and training to enable individuals, their parents, or other caregivers to implement recommendations (Kozlowski, 1990). Identification of sources of financial assistance, respite care, or assistance with obtaining or preparing food also may be needed.

Dietary recommendations should be developed by the dietitian in collaboration with the person who has the disability, family members, supported living providers, and other team members to ensure that individual food preferences, family dietary patterns, available resources, and readiness to implement changes are reflected in the recommendations. Changes in diet or feeding techniques, while offering the potential for long-term benefits, are sometimes met with resistance from the individual and result in temporary worsening of the problem they are intended to treat. Nutritional habilitation attempts often are most successful if they begin with changes the person is expected to tolerate well before proceeding to diet or feeding changes to which he or she is more resistant, but that are necessary for meeting long-term goals.

The diet should be planned to meet nutritional needs and optimize functioning, including feeding development and independence. Nutrient amounts and proportions in relation to one another; calorie level and distribution from carbohydrate, fat and protein; fluid needs; and fiber intake should be taken into account. Special allowance should be made for nutrient–drug interactions or other special needs revealed by the assessment.

If oral sensory motor feeding problems are present, dietary recommendations should be developed in accordance with consistencies, textures, temperatures, and volumes of intake determined by the therapist to be appropriate for the individual. Nutrient- and energy-dense foods are often indicated for the person with feeding problems who needs to gain weight. Commercially available formulas, fortified puddings, and instant breakfast drinks are beneficial for some clients. Needs can often be met by fortifying foods from the family diet. Examples of energy-dense foods often recommended for increasing calories are listed in Table 15–4. Care is necessary to maintain a reasonable distribution of calories from carbohydrate, protein, and fat in the diet within a volume that is reasonable for the individual to consume and that also meets fluid needs.

Dietary measures for weight maintenance or reduction are similar to those recommended for persons without disabilities, with those for children taking into account nutrient needs to maintain growth. As with the general population, preferred weight reduction programs include increased activity as well as changes in diet.

Dietary measures for treatment of constipation are also similar to those recommended for other individuals (Ekvall, 1993a). Care must be taken to ensure that fluid intake is adequate and that increases in fiber and fluid intake do not compromise intakes of energy sources and other nutrients, which may already be marginal or inadequate in persons with feeding impairments. The American Health Foundation has suggested that dietary fiber intake equivalent to the child's age plus 5 g per day may be an appropriate goal between the ages of 3 and 20 years. Intakes of 25 to 35 g of fiber per day, together with adequate fluid, energy, and nutrients has been recommended for

TABLE 15–4 Examples of Foods Used for Increasing Caloric Density of Diets

Food	Amount	Approximate Calories*
Banana	½ medium	50
Peaches, pears (canned, heavy syrup)	¼ c	45
Sweet potato	¼ c mashed	85
Refried beans	¼ c	70
Avocado	¼ medium	75
Wheat germ	1 tbsp	25
Peanut butter	1 tbsp	95
Egg, cooked plain	Large	75
Meat, commercial infant or junior	3.5 oz	90–140
Evaporated milk, whole	Fluid ounce	40
Nonfat dry milk	1 tbsp	25
Fluid milk, whole (3.3% fat)	Fluid ounce	20
Cheddar	½ oz	55
Cream cheese	1 tbsp (½ oz)	50
Sour cream	1 tbsp	25
Whipping cream, heavy	1 tbsp	50
Vegetable oil	1 tbsp	120
Margarine, mayonnaise	1 tbsp	100
Jelly	1 tbsp	50

* Values rounded to nearest 5 calories.

Data from Pennington JA. Bowes and Church's Food Values of Portions Commonly Used. 16th ed. Philadelphia: JB Lippincott, 1994.

persons 20 years of age and older (Williams, 1995). The need for caution in the use of high-fiber foods for children has been expressed, and high fiber diets are not recommended for children under the age of 1 year (Haben-Bartz, 1994; Committee on Nutrition, American Academy of Pediatrics, 1985). If dietary and other measures to treat constipation are not successful and the physician determines that laxatives are necessary, administration should be timed to minimize adverse nutritional effects.

When tube feeding is indicated, appropriate commercial formula can often be identified for use. Products also are available for adjusting the nutrient and energy content to "customize" formulas, or blenderized feedings can be home-prepared. Convenience, defined composition, and microbiologic considerations often weigh in favor of commercial formulas, while cost, desire to include foods from family meals, and other psychological factors may be rea-

sons for choosing to home-prepare tube feedings. Many factors need to be taken into account in choosing a formula, including the age and size of the individual, medical condition, gastrointestinal functioning, food intolerances, volume tolerance, nutrient and energy requirements, fluid requirements, osmolality, size and type of tube, method of administration, expense, availability, ease of preparation, caregiver support, and preferences of the individual and/or primary care providers (Smith and Pederson, 1990; Klein and Delaney, 1994). Feeding methods and schedules should be established with physician consultation, taking into account the physical and developmental characteristics of the individual and means of optimizing his or her functioning. Practicality for all persons involved also must be considered. Various combinations of continuous drip and bolus tube feedings and oral feeding are most satisfactory for different individuals. If encouraging oral intake is a goal, the tube feeding schedule must be arranged in a way that allows the individual opportunity to develop some sensation of hunger. Expecting someone to eat a hearty breakfast by mouth at 6 a.m. if the continuous drip overnight tube feeding ended at 5 a.m. is not reasonable.

A program of oral sensory motor treatment is usually recommended in conjunction with tube feeding. It may be designed to promote oral health, promote oral sensory motor development, minimize loss of oral motor functioning, or promote social interaction. The input of therapists and dental hygienists or dentists is particularly valuable in developing recommendations for oral stimulation activities appropriate for the individual. Age-appropriate items that can be safely mouthed, such as teething rings, pacifiers, and toys for children, can provide oral stimulation, as can tooth brushing and washing the face and lips. Continuation of oral feeding is generally recommended unless it is unsafe for the individual, even if the level of intake is nutritionally insignificant. Nutrients and calories from the oral feedings should not be overlooked when arriving at tube feeding recommendations.

Guidelines concerning implementation, monitoring, and discontinuation of tube feeding are available (Morris and Klein, 1987; Sondel and Knickmeyer, 1989; Rombeau and Caldwell, 1990; Howard, 1990; Smith and Pederson, 1990; Glass and Lucas, 1990; American Dietetic Association, 1992; Klein and Delaney, 1994; Schauster and Dwyer, 1996). Team collaboration, including the individual and/or care providers from home and educational settings, physician(s), a dietitian, and an occupational, physical, or speech therapist, is highly desirable. Nurses often play key roles in tube feeding, and they also are critical members of the team. The input of behavior management specialists may be needed to address issues that often arise in relation to tube feeding, which range from resisting its use to resisting its discontinuation when oral feeding appears to be physically appropriate. Monitoring of tube feeding is essential to assure appropriateness of the diet, feeding, and oral motor regimens in relation to changing needs of the individual and his or her support system.

Monitoring and Reevaluation

Monitoring and periodic reassessment are critical aspects of nutrition service. They provide opportunities to evaluate the appropriateness and effectiveness of recommendations and care plans, reinforce efforts of clients and their care providers, recognize positive changes that have occurred, update recommendations, and provide anticipatory guidance. Achieving goals is often a long-term process, and small steps along the way need to be acknowledged. Individuals and circumstances change, and progress itself means that recommendations become outdated. Through early identification of problems or risks, development and implementation of effective care plans, monitoring and periodic reassessment, and the provision of anticipatory guidance, health and performance are supported and benefits are derived by individuals and their families.

SUMMARY

Persons with developmental delays or disabilities are susceptible to the same factors that place other persons at nutrition risk and to additional factors less commonly seen in the general population. Growth patterns and physical size characteristics that differ from those of the general population are common, and evaluating the nutritional implications of these differences is a major complicating factor in nutrition assessment and estimation of nutritional needs. Movement disorders and behavioral characteristics that affect efficiency, intensity, and duration of activity also have a major influence on dietary recommendations and how they differ from recommendations for the general population. Medications, metabolic and gastrointestinal disorders, and other medical conditions or treatments may alter nutrition needs and may also affect food intake. Additional factors that increase nutrition risk include feeding problems; excessive demands on time, energy, and financial and emotional resources; and inadequate knowledge and skills of individuals with developmental disabilities and their care providers.

Nutrition assessment and intervention often are strengthened by interdisciplinary team activity, with nutrition professionals working in partnership with individuals with disabilities, family members, or other primary care providers, and with other health, education, and social service providers. Services should contribute to integrated systems of comprehensive, community-based support that is person- and family-centered and culturally competent. Integrated systems of comprehensive community-based support for persons with developmental delays

and disabilities and their families challenge professionals to expand their knowledge bases and to function in ways that differ from many service practices of the past.

CONCEPTS TO REMEMBER

▶ Developmental delays and disabilities have a wide range of causes, manifestations, and consequences, many of which place individuals at increased nutritional risk.

▶ The occurrence of developmental delays and disabilities in infants and children who are at high biologic or environmental risk is reduced and the consequences of disabilities are minimized through early identification and the provision of appropriate services and supports, including appropriate nutritional support.

▶ Improved quality of life is promoted for persons with developmental delays or disabilities when adequate supports are provided in the least restrictive manner. In contrast with institutional service practices of earlier decades, current service delivery strategies are to provide supports in integrated community settings.

▶ A combination of specialized and generic services from many agencies and professionals is often required. Individualized service approaches should contribute to integrated systems of comprehensive, community-based support that is person and family centered and culturally competent.

▶ Integration of persons with developmental disabilities into the mainstream of public education, health care, employment, recreation, and other aspects of community living challenges professionals to expand their own knowledge bases and to function in ways that differ from traditional service practices.

▶ All persons with developmental delays and disabilities should have access to appropriate nutrition services and supports.

▶ Optimal service practices provide support to individuals and their families, while also respecting and reinforcing their rights to make choices relative to services, supports, and treatment modalities.

▶ Differences in growth patterns, physical size characteristics, and energy needs for activity alter the nutritional needs of many persons with developmental disorders and are major complicating factors in nutrition assessment. Difficulty associated with interpreting these differences and determining nutritional needs contributes to the high nutritional risk of this population.

▶ Additional factors that increase nutritional risk include feeding problems; effects of medications; stresses of illness or medical interventions; metabolic and gastrointestinal disorders and other complex medical conditions; excessive demands on time, energy, and financial and emotional resources; and inadequate knowledge and skills of individuals and their care providers.

▶ Nutritional assessment and intervention often are strengthened by interdisciplinary team functioning, with nutrition professionals working in partnership with individuals and their families and with other health, education, and social service providers.

References

Aday LA. Health insurance and utilization of medical care for chronically ill children with special needs. Advance Data from the Centers for Disease Control/ National Center for Health Statistics. DHHS publication (PHS) 92–1250, 1992.

Ala-Houhala M, et al. Long-term anticonvulsant therapy and vitamin D metabolism in ambulatory pubertal children. Neuropediatrics 1986;17:212.

Aman MG, Sarphare G, Burrow WH. Psychotropic drugs in group homes: prevalence and relation to demographic/psychiatric variables. Am J Ment Retard 1995;99:500.

Aman MG, Singh NN. Patterns of drug use, methodological considerations, measurement techniques, and future trends. In: Aman MG, Singh NN, eds. Psychopharmacology of the developmental disabilities. NY: Springer-Verlag, 1988:1.

American Council on Science and Health. Diet and behavior. Summit, NJ: 1987.

American Dietetic Association. Manual of clinical dietetics. 4th ed. Chicago: American Dietetic Association, 1992.

American Dietetic Association. Nutrition in comprehensive program planning for persons with developmental disabilities. J Am Diet Assoc 1992;92:613.

American Dietetic Association. Nutrition services for children with special health needs. J Am Diet Assoc 1995;95:809.

Anderson GH. Facts and myths about sugar. Contemp Nutr 1991;16(1).

Atkins FM. Food allergy and behavior: definitions, mechanisms and a review of the evidence. Nutr Rev 1986;44(Suppl).104.

Baer MT, et al. Children with special health care needs. In: Sharbaugh CO, ed. Call to action. Better nutrition for mothers, children, and families. Washington, DC: National Center for Education in Maternal and Child Health, 1991:191.

Baker SS, et al. Common oral motor and gastrointestinal/nutritional problems in children referred to early intervention programs. Semin Pediatr Gastroenterol Nutr 1993;4:3.

Bandini LG, et al. Body composition and energy expenditure in adolescents with cerebral palsy or myelodysplasia. Pediatr Res 1991;29:70.

Bayerl CT, et al. Nutrition issues of children in early intervention programs: primary care team approach. Semin ediatr Gastroenterol Nutr 1993;4:11.

Belt-Niedbala BJ, et al. Linear growth measurement: a comparison single arm length and arm span. Dev Med Child Neurol 1986;28:319.

Berg K. Effect of physical activation and of improved nutrition on the body composition of school children with cerebral palsy. Acta Paediatr Scand Suppl 1970;204:53.

Berg K, Isaksson B. Body composition and nutrition of school children with cerebral palsy. Acta Paediatr Scand Suppl 1970;204:41.

Blackman JA. Down syndrome. In: Medical aspects of developmental disabilities in children birth to three. 2nd ed. Rockville, MD: 1990:107.

Blackman JA, Nelson CLA. Reinstating oral feedings in children fed by gastrostomy. Clin Ped 1985;8:434.

Bonam SB, et al. Defining nutrition service needs for children with special health care needs: focus group approach. Top Clin Nutr 1993;8:79.

Brizee L. Drug-nutrient interactions-concerns for children with special health care needs. Nutr Focus Child Spec Health Care Needs 1992;7(6):1.

Cassidy SB. Prader-Willi syndrome. Curr Prob Pediatr 1984;14:1.

Chambers DW. Patient motivation and education. In: Stewart RE et al, eds. Pediatric dentistry: Scientific foundations and clinical practice. St. Louis: CV Mosby, 1982:630.

Chumlea WC. Assessing growth and nutritional status of children who are chronically ill or handicapped. In: Ekvall SM, Stevens F, eds. Nutritional needs of the handicapped/chronically ill child. Manual 3. Cincinnati, OH: University Affiliated Cincinnati Center for Developmental Disorders, 1989:11.

Cloud HH. Developmental disabilities. In: Queen PM, Lang CE, ed. Handbook of pediatric nutrition. Gaithersburg, MD: Aspen, 1993:400.

Cloud HH. Role of school food service in providing nutrition for children with special needs. Top Clin Nutr 1994;9:47.

Cloud HH, Bergman J. Eating/feeding problems of children: the team approach. Nutr Focus Child Special Health Care Needs 1991;6(6):1.

Committee on Nutrition, American Academy of Pediatrics. Pediatric nutrition handbook. Elk Grove, IL: American Academy of Pediatrics, 1985:99.

Crocker AC. The spectrum of medical care for developmental disabilities. In: Rubin IL, Crocker AC, eds. Developmental disabilities. Delivery of medical care for children and adults. Philadelphia: Lea & Febiger, 1989:10.

Cronk CE. Growth of children with Down's syndrome: birth to age 3 years. Pediatrics 1978;61:564.

Cronk C, et al. Growth charts for children with Down syndrome;1 month to 18 years of age. Pediatrics 1988;81:102.

Cronk CE, Anneren G. Growth. In: Pueschel SM, Pueschel J, eds. Biomedical concerns in persons with Down syndrome. Baltimore: Paul H. Brookes, 1992:19.

Culley WJ, Middleton TO. Caloric requirements of mentally retarded children with or without motor dysfunction. J Pediatr 1969;75:380.

Deb S. Effect of folate metabolism on the psychopathology of adults with mental retardation and epilepsy. Am J Ment Retard 1994;98:717.

Developmental Disabilities Assistance and Bill of Rights Act, 1990. PL 101–496.

Dustrude A, Prince A. Provision of optimal nutrition care in myelomeningocele. Top Clin Nutr 1990;5:34.

Education of All Handicapped Children Act of 1975, PL 94–142, 89 Stat 773 (codified as amended as 20 USC § 1401).

Education of the Handicapped Act Amendments of 1986, PL99–457, 100 Stat. 1146. Congressional Record Vol. 132, 1986.

Egan MC, Oglesby AC. Nutrition services in the maternal and child health program: a historical perspective. In: Sharbaugh CO, ed. Call to action: better nutrition for mothers, children and families. Washington, DC: National Center for Education in Maternal and Child Health, 1991:73.

Ekvall SW. Constipation and fiber. In: Ekvall SW, ed. Pediatric nutrition in chronic diseases and developmental disorders. Prevention, assessment, and treatment. New York: Oxford University Press, 1993a:301.

Ekvall SW. Myelomeningocele. In: Ekvall SW, ed. Pediatric nutrition in chronic diseases and developmental disorders. Prevention, assessment, and treatment. New York: Oxford University Press, 1993b:107.

Feingold BF. Why your child is hyperactive. New York: Random House, 1975.

Fenichel E. Health Focus Group of the National Early Childhood Technical Assistance System (NEC*TAS). Promoting the health of infants and toddlers through Part H of the Individuals with Disabilities Education Act. Arlington, VA: National Center for Clinical Infant Programs, 1991.

Fox CA. Implementing the modified barium swallow evaluation in children who have multiple disabilities. Infants and Young Children 1990;3:67.

Frisancho AR. Anthropometric standards for the assessment of growth and nutritional status. Ann Arbor: University of Michigan Press, 1990.

Gandy LT, et al. Serving children with special health care needs: nutrition services and employee training needs in the school lunch program. J Am Diet Assoc 1991;91:1585.

Garn SM, Weir HF. Assessing the nutritional status of the mentally retarded. Am J Clin Nutr 1971;24:853.

Glass RP, Lucas B. Making the transition from tube feeding to oral feeding. Nutr Focus Children Special Health Care Needs 1990; 5(6):1.

Gray GE, Gray LK. Nutritional aspects of psychiatric disorders. J Am Diet Assoc 1989;89:1492.

Guo S, et al. Reference data on gains in weight and length during the first two years of life. J Pediatr 1991;119:355.

Haas RH, et al. Therapeutic effects of a ketogenic diet in Rett syndrome. Am J Med Genet 1986;24:225.

Haben-Bartz A. Dietary fiber and the child. Dietetics in Developmental and Psychiatric Disorders Newsletter 1994;12:1.

Hayes A, Batshaw ML. Down syndrome. Pediatr Clin North Am 1993;40:523.

Healy A. Cerebral palsy. In: Blackman JA, ed. Medical aspects of developmental disabilities in children birth to three. Rockville, MD: Aspen, 1990:59.

Hershey Foods Corporation. Hyperactivity: is candy causal? Top Nutr Food Safety, Summer 1992.

Hine RJ. What practitioners need to know about folic acid. J Am Diet Assoc 1996;96:451.

Hine RJ, et al. Early nutrition intervention services for children with special health care needs. J Am Diet Assoc 1989;89:1636.

Holm VA. Appendix A: Growth charts for Prader-Willi syndrome. In: Greensway LR, Alexander PC, eds. Management of Prader-Willi syndrome. New York: Springer-Verlag, 1988.

Holm VA. Growth in children with developmental disabilities. Nutr Child Spec Health Care Needs 1994;9(2):1.

Holm VA, Pipes PL. Food and children with Prader-Willi syndrome. Am J Dis Child 1976;130:1063.

Howard LJ. Parenteral and enteral nutritional therapy. In: Wilson JD et al, eds. Harrison's principles of internal medicine. 12th ed. New York: McGraw-Hill, 1990:434.

Individuals with Disabilities Education Act, PL 102–119, 105 Stat. 587. Congressional Record Vol. 137, 1991.

Isaacs JS, Georgeson KE, Cloud HH, Woodall N. Weight gain and triceps skinfold fat mass after gastrostomy placement in children with developmental disabilities. J Am Diet Assoc 1994;94:849.

Johnson RK, et al. Athetosis increases resting metabolic rate in adults with cerebral palsy. J Am Diet Assoc 1996;96:145.

Kanarek RB, Marks-Kaufman R. Nutrition and behavior. New perspectives. New York: Van Nostrand Reinhold, 1991.

King EH, et al. Risk factors for developmental delay among infants and toddlers. Children's Health Care 1992;21:39.

Klein MD, Delaney TA. Feeding and nutrition for the child with special needs. Tucson, AZ: Therapy Skill Builders, 1994.

Kozlowski BW. Cerebral palsy. In: Gines D, ed. Nutrition management in rehabilitation. Rockville, MD: Aspen, 1990:7.

Kozlowski BW. Megavitamin treatment of mental retardation in children: a review of effects of behavior and cognition. J Child Adol Psychopharmacol 1992;2:307.

Kozlowski BW, et al. Nutrition and feeding problems of children with developmental disabilities. Columbus, OH: Nisonger Center Videotape Production, Ohio State University, 1989.

Kraus K-H, et al. Biotin status of epileptics. Ann NY Acad Sci 1985;447:297.

Kraus K-H, et al. Effect of long-term treatment with antiepileptic drugs on vitamin status. Drug-Nutr Interact 1988;5:317.

Krick J, Murphy PE, Markham JFB, Shapiro BK. A proposed formula for calculating energy needs of children with cerebral palsy. Dev Med Child Neurol 1992;34:481.

Krick J, Van Duyn. The relationship between oral-motor involvement and growth: a pilot study in a pediatric population with cerebral palsy. J Am Diet Assoc 1984;84:555.

Kruesi M, et al. Effects of sugar and aspartame on aggression and activity in children. Am J Psychiatry 1987;144:11.

Lamberg-Allardt C, et al. Vitamin D status of ambulatory and nonambulatory mentally retarded children with and without carbamazepine treatment. Ann Nutr Metab 1990;34:216.

Lane SJ, Cloud HH. Feeding problems and intervention: an interdisciplinary approach. Top Clin Nutr 1988;3:23.

Lichtenwalter L, et al. Providing nutrition services to children with special health care needs in a community setting. Top Clin Nutr 1993;8:75.

Lipton MA, Mayo JP. Diet and hyperkinesis—update. J Am Diet Assoc 1983;83:132.

Lohman TG, et al, eds. Anthropometric standardization reference manual. Champaign, IL: Human Kinetics Books, 1988.

Lucas B. Stimulant medication. In: Pipes PL, Trahms CM, eds. Nutrition in infancy and childhood. St. Louis: CV Mosby, 1993:155.

Martin AD, et al. Segment lengths. In: Lohman TG, Roche AF, Martorell R, eds. Anthropometric standardization reference manual. Champaign, IL: Human Kinetics Books, 1988:9.

Martin GR, et al. Prevalence of heart disease in trisomy 21: an unbiased population. Pediatr Res 1989;25:225A.

Morris SE, Klein, MD. Pre-feeding skills. Tucson, AZ: Therapy Skill Builders, 1987.

Morton RE, et al. Videofluoroscopy in the assessment of feeding disorders of children with neurological problems. Dev Med Child Neurol 1993;35:388.

National Center for Health Statistics, Centers for Disease Control. NCHS growth curves for children, birth–18 years. Washington, DC: US Government Printing Office, 1978. [Series 11,165. DHEW publication (PHS) 78 1650.]

National Center for Health Statistics, Centers for Disease Control. Basic data on anthropometric measurements and angular measurements of the hip and knee joints for selected age groups 1–74 years of age. Washington, DC: US Government Printing Office, 1981. [Series 11, 219. DHEW publication (PHS) 81 1669.]

National Research Council. Recommended dietary allowances. 10th ed. Washington, DC: National Academy Press, 1989.

Newacheck PW, Taylor WR. Childhood chronic illness: prevalence, severity, and impact. Am J Public Health 1992;82:364.

Office for Medical Applications of Research, National Institutes of Health. Consensus conference. Defined diets and childhood hyperactivity. JAMA 1982;248:290.

O'Neil SM. Management of mealtime behaviors. In: Pipes PL, Trahms CM, eds. Nutrition in infancy and childhood. St. Louis: CV Mosby, 1993: 344.

Padgett D. Behavior management of feeding problems. Nutr Focus Child Spec Health Care Needs 1992;7(1):1.

Perry A. Rett syndrome: a comprehensive review of the literature. Am J Ment Retard 1991;966:275.

Physicians' desk reference. Oradell, NJ: Medical Economics, Co, Inc, 1994.

Pipes P. Prader-Willi syndrome and Rett syndrome. Nutr Focus Child Spec Health Care Needs 1990;5(2):1.

Pipes PL, Glass RP. Developmental disabilities and other special health care needs. In: Pipes PL, Trahms CM, eds. Nutrition in infancy and childhood. St. Louis: CV Mosby, 1993:344.

Pipes P, Holm V. Rett syndrome. In: Ekvall SW, ed. Pediatric nutrition in chronic diseases and developmental disorders. Prevention, assessment, and treatment. New York: Oxford University Press, 1993:161.

Posthauer ME, et al, eds. Clinical criteria and indicators for nutrition services in developmental disabilities, psychiatric disorders, and substance abuse. Chicago: The American Dietetic Association, 1993.

Prinz Rj, et al. Dietary correlates of hyperactive behavior in children. J Consult Clin Psychol 1980;48:760.

Pueschel SM, Bier JB. Endocrinologic aspects. In: Pueschel SM, Pueschel J, ed. Biomedical concerns in persons with Down syndrome. Baltimore: Paul H. Brookes, 1992:259.

Rapoport JL. Diet and hyperactivity. Nutr Rev 1986;44(Suppl):158.

Rice MA, Haas RH. The nutritional aspects of Rett syndrome. J Child Neurol 1988;3:S35.

Rimmer JH, et al. Prevalence of obesity in adults with mental retardation: implications for health promotion and disease prevention. Ment Retard 1993;31:105.

Rimmer JH, et al. Cardiovascular risk factor levels in adults with mental retardation. Am J Ment Retard 1994;98:510.

Roche AF. Growth assessment in handicapped children. Diet Curr 1979;6(5):1.

Roche AF, Himes JH. Incremental growth charts. Am J Ment Retard 1980;33:2041.

Roe DA. Drug-induced nutritional deficiencies. Westport, CT: AVI Publishing Co, 1985.

Roe DA. Handbook of drug and nutrient interactions. Chicago: The American Dietetic Association, 1989.

Rombeau JL, Caldwell MD, eds. Enteral and tube feeding. 2nd ed. Philadelphia: WB Saunders, 1990.

Said HM, et al. Biotin transport in the human intestine: inhibition by anticonvulsant drugs. Am J Clin Nutr 1989;49:127.

Sanders KD, et al. Growth response to enteral feeding by children with cerebral palsy. J Parenter Enteral Nutr 1990,14:23.

Saul RA, et al. Growth references from conception to adulthood. Supplement No. 1. Proceedings of the Greenwood Genetics Center. Clinton, SC: Jacobs Press, 1988.

Schangenbacher KE. Diagnostic problems in pediatrics. In: Clark PN, Allen AS, eds. Occupational therapy for children. St. Louis: CV Mosby, 1985:94.

Schauster H, Dwyer J. Transition from tube feedings to feedings by mouth in children: preventing eating dysfunction. J Am Diet Assoc 1996;96:277.

Schoeller DA, et al. Energy expenditure and body composition in Prader-Willi syndrome. Metabolism 1988;37:115.

Shaddix TE. Nutritional implications in children with cerebral palsy. Nutr Focus Child Spec Health Care Needs 1991;6(2).

Smith BC, Pederson, AL. Nutrition focus—tube feeding update. Nutr Focus Child Spec Health Care Needs. 1990;5(5).

Smith GA, Gettings RM. Medicaid's ICF/MR program: Present status and recent trends. Alexandria, VA: National Association of State Directors of Developmental Disabilities Services, 1993.

Smith MAH, et al. Developmental feeding tool. In: Feeding management for a child with a handicap. Memphis, TN: Boling Child Development Center, University of Tennessee Center for Health Sciences, 1982:69.

Sondel S, Knickmeyer M. Nutrition for your gastrostomy-fed child: a parent handbook. Madison, WI: University of Wisconsin Hospital and Clinics, Department of Food and Nutrition and Pediatric Pulmonary Center, 1989.

Spender QW, et al. Fat distribution in children with cerebral palsy. Ann Human Biol 1988;15:191.

Spender QW, et al. Assessment of linear growth of children with cerebral palsy: use of alternative measures to height or length. Dev Med Child Neurol 1989;31:206.

Sridhar SN, et al. Comparison of energy expenditure of cerebral palsy children with predicted energy expenditure. J Am Diet Assoc 1995; 95:A-61.

Stallings VA, et al. Nutrition-related growth failure of children with quadriplegic cerebral palsy. Dev Med Child Neurol 1993a;35:126.

Stallings VA, et al. Nutritional status and growth of children with diplegic or hemiplegic cerebral palsy. Dev Med Child Neurol 1993a;35: 997.

Thommessen M, et al. The impact of feeding problems on growth and energy intake in children with cerebral palsy. Eur J Clin Health 1991;45:479.

Venn ML, et al. Feeding and nutritional issues. In: Bailey DB, Wolery M, eds. Teaching infants and preschoolers with disabilities. New York: Macmillan, 1992:441.

Williams C. Importance of dietary fiber in childhood. J Am Diet Assoc 1995;95:1140.

Wilson JM. Cerebral palsy. In: Campbell SK, ed. Pediatric neurologic physical therapy. New York: Churchill Livingstone, 1984:353.

Yadrick K , Sneed J. Nutrition services for children with developmental disabilities and chronic illnesses in education programs. J Am Diet Assoc 1994;94:1122.

Ziring P. The knowledge base of health care for youth and adults with developmental disabilities. In: Eklund E, ed. Health care for youth and adults with developmental disabilities: Policies and partnerships. Proceedings of a conference. Silver Springs, MD: American Association of University Affiliated Programs for Persons with Developmental Disabilities, 1991:45.

Suggested Resources

Baer MT, et al, comps. Nutrition strategies for children with special needs. Los Angeles: Center for Child Development, Children's Hospital of Los Angeles, 1991.

CARE: Special nutrition for kids. Montgomery: Alabama State Department of Education, Child Nutrition Programs, Federal Administrative Services, 1993.

Ekvall SW, ed. Pediatric nutrition in chronic diseases and developmental disorders. Prevention and treatment. New York: Oxford University Press, 1993.

Cines DJ, ed. Nutrition management in rehabilitation. Rockville, MD: Aspen, 1990.

Klein MD, Delaney TA. Feeding and nutrition for the child with special needs. Handouts for parents. Tucson, AZ: Therapy Skill Builders, 1994.

Kozlowski BW, et al. Nutrition and feeding problems of children with developmental disabilities. Columbus, OH: Nisonger Center Videotape Production, Ohio State University, 1989.

Morris SE, Klein MD. Pre-feeding skills. A comprehensive resource for feeding development. Tucson, AZ: Therapy Skill Builders, 1987.

Rokusek C, Heinrichs E, eds. Nutrition and feeding for persons with special needs. A practical guide and resource manual. 2nd ed. Vermillion, SD: South Dakota Department of Education and Cultural Affairs, 1992.

US Department of Agriculture Food and Nutrition Service, Southeast Regional Office and University of Alabama at Birmingham, Department of Nutrition Sciences and Sparks Clinic. Meeting their needs. Training for child nutrition program personnel serving children with special needs. Atlanta: US Department of Agriculture Food and Nutrition Service, 1993.

APPLICATION: A Case for Nutrition Intervention

In the preceding chapter, many variables that increase the nutritional risk of persons with developmental disabilities are described. Approaches for prevention, identification, and treatment of nutrition-related problems also are discussed. The case description presented here illustrates many of those points. In addition to presenting information about the child and the nutrition and feeding intervention that occurred, comments are made about additional information that would have been useful in assessing the child's growth and nutritional status, positive and negative aspects of some occurrences, difficulties that were encountered, and alternative courses of action that might have been taken.

Bill was the first child of a couple who were in their early 20s when he was born. His father was employed full-time outside the home and his mother was a full-time homemaker. Pregnancy, labor, and delivery were uncomplicated, and Bill was born at 40 weeks gestation. His birth weight of 6.9 lb (3.14 kg) and length of 20 in (50.8 cm) were near the respective 50th percentiles of National Center for Health Statistics (NCHS) reference data (Fig. A15–1). Breast-feeding was established without difficulty, and he and his mother were discharged from the hospital when Bill was 3 days old. At 17 days, he became irritable, developed a fever, and began having seizures. He was diagnosed as having bacterial meningitis and was hospitalized for 3 weeks for treatment of the infection and associated complications. During the hospitalization, he received total parenteral nutrition for 10 days and then received his mother's milk from a bottle for several days before returning to breast-feeding. At discharge, Bill's weight was at the 5th percentile and his length was in the 10th to 25th percentile range of reference data for children his age (see Fig. A15–1). He was receiving anticonvulsant medication for seizure control and was described as showing muscle weakness, particularly on his right side. In addition, he was cortically blind. Referral to the early intervention program in his county of residence provided a channel through which Bill's parents could learn about and gain access to developmental services and supports.

The central nervous system damage that Bill experienced as a result of the meningitis, although not progressive, became increasingly apparent in the weeks that followed, and the diagnosis of cerebral palsy was made. He showed little progress in developing head and trunk control, and he exhibited abnormal muscle tone and abnormal reflex development. A therapist with the early intervention program began working with him and his parents and suggesting activities for his parents to carry out. His developmental progress was slow, but he did turn his head toward noises and appeared to recognize the voices of people with whom he spent the most time. Medical records indicate that his mother tried feeding cereal to him at 4 months, but that he had trouble taking it. It was also indicated that she wanted to begin weaning him at 6 months but he had difficulty with all forms of feeding except breast-feeding. Evaluation by a therapist with expertise in feeding, followed by the development of feeding recommendations and monitoring of feeding progression, would have been desirable. Monitoring of his diet and growth by a dietitian, working in collaboration with the therapist and with Bill's physician, also would have been desirable. However, coordinated professional input related to his nutrition and feeding did not occur at this point.

Data from Bill's medical records and records kept by his parents concerning his weight, length, and head circumference at various ages are presented in Figure A15–1. His intake of breast milk supported rapid weight gain for several months. His weight quickly rose from the 5th percentile, to which it had dropped during his hospitalization, to the 50th percentile, where it remained until he was 6 months old. While his length was increasing during that time, the rate of change compared with that of other children declined, and his measurement values gradually dropped to lower percentiles. By the time he was 7 months old, his length was near the 5th percentile. While supporting laboratory data would be useful in characterizing his nutritional status, the weight gain data and description of his intake during that time indicate that at least his calorie needs were being met between the ages of 2 and 6 months. This suggests that the early decline in

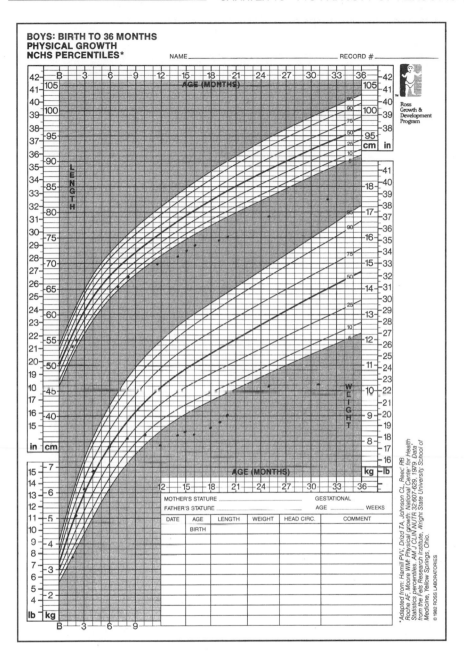

FIGURE A15-1. Height, weight, and head circumference data for Bill, plotted in relation to general population reference data.   *Figure continued on following page*

his relative rate of length growth probably reflected factors other than nutrition, including his neuromuscular damage. Note from the charts that weight and length data were not systematically recorded for the same measurement dates, as would have been desirable for monitoring his growth and evaluating weight gain in relation to length. Nevertheless, it is apparent that his weight gain outpaced his growth in length during the early months. Head circumference data are not available for the first 7 months, but it was reported that his head circumference was within normal limits at birth. At 7 months, his

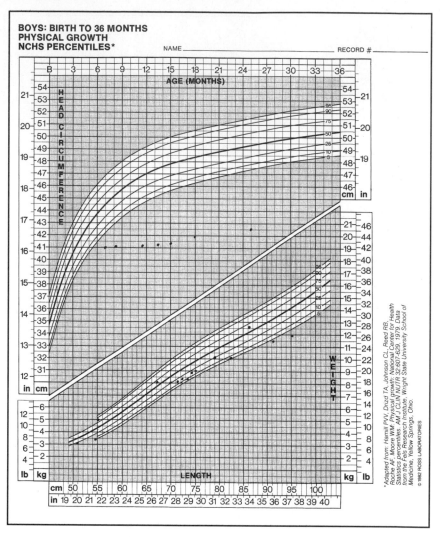

FIGURE A15–1 *Continued*

head circumference was below the 5th percentile of reference data. Reflecting the insult that had occurred to his brain, head circumference measurements remained essentially the same between ages 7 months and 15 months, and showed little increase thereafter.

Major changes occurred in Bill's growth pattern and in his nutrition over the next several months. Medical records indicate he was experiencing constipation and showing increasing evidence of neuromuscular involvement. By the time he was 7 months old, his mother was pregnant. Although she wanted to wean Bill from breast-feeding, he refused to take a bottle, was unable to drink from a cup, and had difficulty taking food from a spoon. A great deal of effort was necessary to get even small quantities of food into him through spoon feeding. Bill was enrolled in the WIC program and continued to receive developmental stimulation and therapy through an early intervention program. His mother needed more assistance in responding to Bill's nutrition and feeding problems than was provided through those programs, but referral for further assistance did not occur for several months. Earlier referral might have prevented some of the feeding difficulties and apparent nutritional deficits that occurred, as well as the physical and emotional stress related to his feeding that Bill's mother experienced. A note was made in

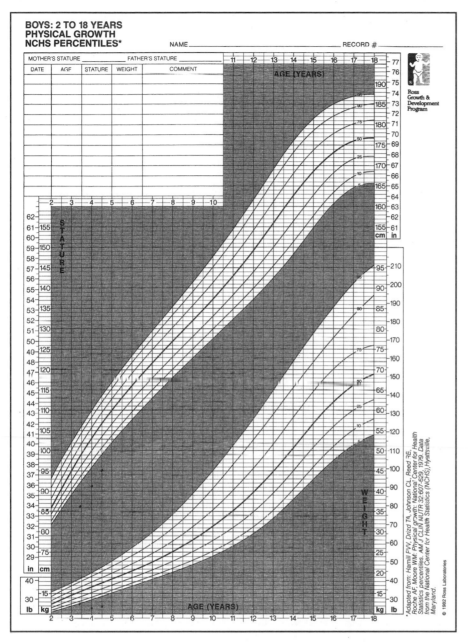

FIGURE A15–1 *Continued*

Bill's WIC record when he was 12 months old that he had gained no weight in 5 months. By that time, his weight had dropped from the 50th to below the 5th percentile. While he had continued to grow in length, the rate of change relative to that of other infants had declined, and his length, like his weight, was below the 5th percentile.

When Bill was 14 months old, a physician referred him for an interdisciplinary nutrition and feeding assessment in a clinic that specialized in services for children with developmental disabilities. While his mother was anxious to receive assistance, the baby was due in 3 weeks and circumstances were less than ideal for initiating intensive nutrition–feeding intervention. Progress often comes slowly and requires substantial input of time and energy of care providers, especially with problems as severe as Bill's, and there was no reason to believe that his situation would be an exception. However, changes in Bill's nutrition and feeding needed to occur quickly, and intervention was initiated. Because Bill had poor postural control, which enhances oral motor problems in many persons with cerebral palsy, the occupational therapist instructed his mother in how to position him to achieve stability with his hips flexed and his head and trunk supported in midline. She also suggested equipment and techniques for placing the spoon in Bill's mouth to minimize his bite reflex. It was difficult to differentiate between the behavioral and oral sensory motor aspects of Bill's refusal of a nursing bottle, and suggestions related to both areas were offered. While it was clear that Bill's intake of calories, fluid, and essentially all nutrients needed to increase, achieving that through oral feeding was contingent on either finding ways to enhance his oral sensory motor functioning and increase his acceptance of a nursing bottle, or initiating tube feeding, which was rejected by his parents as an option. Nutritionally desirable food choices were identified, including a combination of formula and age- and developmentally-appropriate nutrient and energy-dense choices. Consideration was also given to possible nutritional implications of anticonvulsant medications. Dietary recommendations were consistent with the guidelines for introducing new foods (varieties, not textures) that are generally given for typically developing infants. Actual physical assistance in the home with feeding Bill would have been desirable, but his mother continued to be the primary feeder. Bill's weight remained essentially unchanged for approximately 3 months as attention was divided between him and the new baby. Gradually, when Bill was between 18 and 20 months of age, his weight began to move upward toward the 5th percentile but his length did not. From a health and nutrition standpoint, more rapid change would have been desirable. Certainly, potential benefits of tube feeding during the period when weight gain was not occurring could be stated. However, an alternative might have been for more assistance with feeding Bill to have been provided to the family.

Feeding remained very difficult. Bill was lost to follow-up by the interdisciplinary nutrition–feeding clinic for several months. He was referred by his physician for nutrition evaluation in another location, and recommendations were made for Bill to receive a concentrated formula, with margarine and glucose polymer added to further increase the caloric density. Attention focused on calorie intake rather than overall nutritional value of his diet. At 25 months, his mother returned with him to the interdisciplinary nutrition-feeding clinic. His weight of 22.5 lb (10.2 kg), although still below the 5th percentile of reference data for boys his age, was at the 25th percentile in relation to his length. Additional anthropometric data would have been useful in evaluating his weight status. Recommendations for dietary change included some reduction in caloric density, with increased attention to overall nutrient intake and increased fluid intake. Extensive feeding evaluation was performed to determine changes that had occurred, identify possible contraindications of various forms of feeding, and develop updated feeding recommendations. Drinking was more difficult for Bill than eating pureed foods, although neither was easy, and ensuring adequate fluid intake was a major challenge. Promoting feeding development continued to be balanced with short-term and long-term goals for meeting nutritional needs. Laboratory data would have been useful for better defining his nutrition status.

At age 3 years, Bill began attending a center-based developmental program. The teachers there agreed with Bill's parents that feeding and nutrition were major concerns, and relevant goals and objectives were included in his individualized plan. When Bill returned to the interdisciplinary clinic for evaluation at age 40 months, he and his mother were accompanied by one of his teachers and a therapist. Although he only attended the developmental program for half days, a system had been developed whereby he received breakfast at home; a second breakfast and lunch at school; and a second lunch, dinner, and one or two snacks at home. The fact that he was accepting food at all of those times, and actually showing some pleasure in it, illustrates a benefit often seen from small frequent feedings. While the increased attention was apparently one of the benefits for Bill, endurance may be another factor. Many people stop eating not because they are full, but because they become too tired to eat any more at one sitting. Bill's meals at school were used as times for the therapist to work with him, and intake of texture-modified table foods was emphasized. The feeding program at school incorporated recommendations received by Bill's mother at previous nutrition–feeding clinic visits, and updates and progress reports were sent home with Bill by his teachers and his therapist. Because a nutritionist was not available at the developmental center, much of the clinic visit focused on updating nutrition recommendations, reviewing the composition of his diet at school, and identifying foods that were preferable selections from a nutritional perspective. Although Bill had only been attending the program for a few months, great improvement with respect to both his nutrition and his feeding was evident. For the first time in over 2 years, Bill's weight had reached the 5th percentile of reference data for boys his age. While praising all of the parties for the progress that had occurred, it was also pointed out that his length was parallelling but had not reached the 5th percentile, and weight for length was in the 50th to 75th percentile range. A plan was developed for monitoring his length and weight to assure that Bill did not become obese! This was of particular concern since Bill has severe neuromuscular impairment and needs extensive assistance with movement.

When Bill was approximately 3.5 years of age, surgery was performed on both of his legs. This resulted in casting of his legs and extended absence from the developmental center. His interest in eating declined and weight loss occurred. Six months later, his mother reported that she was pleased to finally see some progress with his eating but that he still had not returned to his presurgery status. At 4 years 3 months, his mother and teachers reported that he was experiencing increased amounts of ill time, which was having a negative impact on his feeding. They commented that just as he would begin to get his appetite back, he would become ill and his interest in eating would again decline. In part reflecting weight loss that he experienced around the time of the surgery and also reflecting his reduced interest in eating, his weight at age 4 years 6 months was below the level it had reached a year earlier. Over the next few months, increases in his weight occurred.

Bill's nutrition and feeding problems are far from being resolved. Means that appear to be generally pleasurable, although laborious, for him and his care providers have been established for providing him with nutritional intake that is much more nearly adequate than was the case earlier in his life. However, the response to his last surgery from a weight and appetite standpoint suggests that his status continues to be precarious, and raises questions of what can be done to better prepare him for periods of stress or increased nutritional needs. As some problems related to Bill's nutrition and feeding have decreased, others have appeared. Although indications of the need for anticipatory guidance and support appeared when Bill was very young, many months passed and major problems developed before effective intervention was achieved. The greatest signs of progress were seen when coordination and collaboration evolved among home, school, and an evaluation center. Many questions remain unanswered and many alternative courses of action can be identified. It is likely that meeting Bill's nutrition and feeding needs will present an ongoing challenge.

APPENDICES

APPENDIX 1A Estimated Sodium, Chloride, and Potassium Minimum Requirements of Healthy Persons*

Age	Weight (kg)	Sodium (mg)*†	Chloride (mg)*†	Potassium (mg)‡
MONTHS				
0–5	4.5	120	180	500
6–11	8.9	200	300	700
YEARS				
1	11.0	225	350	1000
2–5	16.0	300	500	1400
6–9	25.0	400	600	1600
10–18	50.0	500	750	2000
>18§	70.0	500	750	2000

Reprinted with permission from Recommended Dietary Allowances, 10th ed., © 1989 by the National Academy of Sciences. Published by National Academy Press.

* No allowance has been included for large, prolonged losses from the skin through sweat.

† There is no evidence that higher intakes confer any health benefit.

‡ Desirable intakes of potassium may considerably exceed these values (~3500 mg for adults).

§ No allowance included for growth. Values for those below 18 years assume a growth rate at the 50th percentile reported by the National Center for Health Statistics and averaged for males and females.

APPENDIX 1B Estimated Safe and Adequate Daily Dietary Intakes of Selected Vitamins and Minerals

Category	Age (yrs)	Vitamins	
		Biotin (μg)	Pantothenic Acid (mg)
Infants	0–0.5	10	2
	0.5–1	15	3
Children and adolescents	1–3	20	3
	4–6	25	3–4
	7–10	30	4–5
	11+	30–100	4–7
Adults		30–100	4–7

Category	Age (yrs)	Trace Elements*				
		Copper (mg)	Manganese (mg)	Fluoride (mg)	Chromium (μg)	Molybdenum (μg)
Infants	0–0.5	0.4–0.6	0.3–0.6	0.1–0.5	10–40	15–30
	0.5–1	0.6–0.7	0.6–1.0	0.2–1.0	20–60	20–40
Children and adolescents	1–3	0.7–1.0	1.0–1.5	0.5–1.5	20–80	25–50
	4–6	1.0–1.5	1.5–2.0	1.0–2.5	30–120	30–75
	7–10	1.0–2.0	2.0–3.0	1.5–2.5	50–200	50–150
	11+	1.5–2.5	2.0–5.0	1.5–2.5	50–200	75–250
Adults		1.5–3.0	2.0–5.0	1.5–4.0	50–200	75–250

Reprinted with permission from Recommended Dietary Allowances, 10th ed., © 1989 by the National Academy of Sciences. Published by National Academy Press.

* Since the toxic levels for many trace elements may be only several times the usual intakes, the upper levels for the trace elements given in this table should not be habitually exceeded.

APPENDIX 2 Recommended Nutrient Intakes (RNIs), Canada, 1990, Based on Age, Energy, and Body Weight Expressed as Daily Rates

Age	Sex	Energy (kcal)†‡	Weight (kg)	Thiamin (mg)	Riboflavin (mg)	Niacin (NE)*	n-3 PUFA† (g)	n-6 PUFA† (g)	Protein (g)	Vit. A (RE)‡	Vit. D (µg)	Vit. E (mg)	Vit. C (mg)	Folate (µg)	Vit. B₁₂ (µg)	Calcium (mg)	Phosphorus (mg)	Magnesium (mg)	Iron (mg)	Iodine (µg)	Zinc (mg)
MONTHS																					
0–4§	Both	600	6.0	0.3	0.3	4	0.5	3	12‖	400	10	3	20	50	0.3	250‖	150	20	0.3#	30	2#
5–12	Both	900	9.0	0.4	0.5	7	0.5	3	12	400	10	3	20	50	0.3	400	200	32	7	40	3
YEARS																					
1	Both	1100	11	0.5	0.6	8	0.6	4	19	400	10	3	20	65	0.3	500	300	40	6	55	4
2–3	Both	1300	14	0.6	0.7	9	0.7	4	22	400	5	4	20	80	0.4	550	350	50	6	65	4
4–6	Both	1800	18	0.7	0.9	13	1.0	6	26	500	5	5	25	90	0.5	600	400	65	8	85	5
7–9	Male	2200	25	0.9	1.1	16	1.2	7	30	700	2.5	7	25	125	0.8	700	500	100	8	110	7
7–9	Female	1900	25	0.8	1.0	14	1.0	6	30	700	2.5	6	25	125	0.8	700	500	100	8	95	7
10–12	Male	2500	34	1.0	1.3	18	1.4	8	38	800	2.5	8	25	170	1.0	900	700	130	8	125	9
10–12	Female	2200	36	0.9	1.1	16	1.1	7	40	800	2.5	7	25	180	1.0	1100	800	135	8	110	9
13–15	Male	2800	50	1.1	1.4	20	1.4	9	50	900	5	9	30	150	1.5	1100	900	185	10	160	12
13–15	Female	2200	48	0.9	1.1	16	1.2	7	42	800	5	7	30	145	1.5	1000	850	180	13	160	9
16–18	Male	3200	62	1.3	1.6	23	1.8	11	55	1000	5	10	40**	185	1.9	900	1000	230	10	160	12
16–18	Female	2100	53	0.8	1.1	15	1.2	7	43	800	2.5	7	30**	160	1.9	700	850	200	12	160	9
19–24	Male	3000	71	1.2	1.5	22	1.6	10	58	1000	2.5	10	40**	210	2.0	800	1000	240	9	160	12
19–24	Female	2100	58	0.8	1.1	15	1.2	7	43	800	2.5	7	30**	175	2.0	700	850	200	13	160	9
25–49	Male	2700	74	1.1	1.4	19	1.5	9	61	1000	2.5	9	40**	220	2.0	800	1000	250	9	160	12
25–49	Female	2000	59	0.8	1.0	14	1.1	7	44	800	2.5	6	30**	175	2.0	700	850	200	13	160	9
50–74	Male	2300	73	0.9	1.3	16	1.3	8	60	1000	5	7	40**	220	2.0	800	1000	250	9	160	12
50–74	Female	1800	63	0.8†	1.0†	14†	1.1†	7†	47	800	5	6	30**	190	2.0	800	850	210	8	160	9
75+	Male	2000	69	0.8	1.0	14†	1.0	7	57	1000	5	6	40**	205	2.0	800	1000	230	9	160	12
75+	Female‡‡	1700	64	0.8†	1.0†	14†	1.1†	7†	47	800	5	5	30**	190	2.0	800	850	210	8	160	9
PREGNANCY (ADDITIONAL)																					
1st Trimester		100		0.1	0.1	0.1	0.05	0.3	5	100	2.5	2	0	300	1.0	500	200	15	0	25	6
2nd Trimester		300		0.1	0.3	0.2	0.16	0.9	20	100	2.5	2	10	300	1.0	500	200	45	5	25	6
3rd Trimester		300		0.1	0.3	0.2	0.16	0.9	24	100	2.5	2	10	300	1.0	500	200	45	10	25	6
Lactation (additional)		450		0.2	0.4	0.3	0.25	1.5	20	400	2.5	3	25	100	0.5	500	200	65	0	50	6

From Recommended Nutrient Intakes for Canadians, Bureau of Nutritional Sciences, Ottawa, 1990.
Reproduced with the permission of the Minister of Public Works and Government Services, Canada, 1997.
*NE = Niacin equivalents.
†PUFA = polyunsaturated fatty acids.
‡RE = Retinol equivalents.
§Protein is assumed to be from breast milk and must be adjusted for infant formula.

‖Infant formula with high phosphorus should contain 375 mg calcium.
#Breast milk is assumed to be the source of the mineral.
**Smokers should increase vitamin C by 50%.
††Level below which intake should not fall.
‡‡Assumes moderate physical activity.

APPENDIX 3A Norms for Triceps Fatfold (mm) from the Second National Health and Nutrition Examination Survey

Sex and Age	Percentile								
	5th	10th	15th	25th	50th	75th	85th	90th	95th
MALE									
6–11 months	6.5	7.0	7.0	8.0	10.0	12.0	14.0	15.0	16.0
1 year	6.5	7.0	7.5	8.5	10.0	12.0	13.0	14.0	15.5
2 years	6.0	7.0	7.0	8.0	10.0	12.0	13.0	14.5	15.0
3 years	6.5	7.0	7.5	8.0	9.5	11.5	12.5	13.0	15.0
4 years	6.0	6.5	7.0	7.5	9.0	11.0	12.0	13.0	15.0
5 years	5.5	6.0	6.5	7.0	8.0	10.5	11.5	12.5	14.5
6 years	5.0	5.5	6.0	6.5	8.0	10.5	12.0	13.0	17.5
7 years	5.0	5.5	6.0	6.5	8.5	11.0	12.0	15.0	17.5
8 years	5.5	6.0	6.0	7.0	9.0	12.0	16.5	17.0	22.0
9 years	5.0	5.0	6.0	7.0	9.0	12.5	16.0	19.0	23.0
10 years	5.0	6.0	6.5	7.5	11.0	16.5	20.0	22.0	26.0
11 years	4.5	5.5	6.0	7.5	10.5	17.0	22.0	25.0	30.0
12 years	5.0	6.0	6.0	8.0	11.0	15.0	18.0	21.5	26.5
13 years	5.0	5.5	6.0	7.0	9.0	12.5	16.5	20.5	22.5
14 years	4.0	5.0	5.5	6.0	9.0	13.0	15.0	17.0	23.0
15 years	5.0	5.0	6.0	6.0	7.5	11.0	14.5	18.0	22.0
16 years	4.5	5.0	5.5	6.5	8.0	13.0	18.5	20.5	25.5
17 years	4.0	4.5	5.0	5.5	7.0	10.5	12.5	15.0	18.0
18 years	4.0	5.0	5.0	6.0	9.5	14.5	17.5	19.0	22.5
18–24 years	4.5	5.0	6.0	6.5	10.0	15.0	17.5	20.0	24.5
25–34 years	4.5	5.5	6.5	7.5	11.5	16.5	20.0	23.0	26.0
35–44 years	5.0	6.0	7.0	9.0	12.5	17.0	20.0	23.0	27.0
45–54 years	5.5	6.5	7.0	9.0	12.0	16.5	20.0	22.0	25.5
55–64 years	5.0	6.0	7.5	9.0	12.0	16.0	19.5	21.5	25.5
65–74 years	5.0	6.0	7.0	8.0	11.5	16.0	18.5	21.0	25.0
FEMALE									
6–11 months	6.5	7.0	7.0	8.0	10.0	11.5	12.5	13.0	14.5
1 year	6.0	7.0	7.5	8.0	10.5	12.0	13.5	15.0	16.5
2 years	6.0	7.0	7.5	8.0	10.5	12.5	13.5	15.0	16.0
3 years	6.0	7.0	7.0	8.0	10.0	12.0	12.5	13.5	16.5
4 years	6.0	6.5	7.5	8.0	10.0	12.0	13.0	14.0	15.5
5 years	6.0	7.0	7.5	8.5	10.5	12.5	14.0	14.5	16.0
6 years	6.0	7.0	7.5	8.0	10.0	12.0	14.5	16.0	18.5
7 years	6.0	7.0	7.5	9.0	10.5	13.0	15.0	18.0	20.0
8 years	6.0	6.5	7.0	8.5	11.0	14.0	16.0	18.0	21.0
9 years	7.0	7.5	8.5	10.0	13.0	16.0	20.0	23.0	27.0
10 years	7.0	8.0	8.0	10.0	13.5	18.0	21.0	22.5	24.5
11 years	8.0	8.5	9.0	11.0	14.0	19.5	21.5	23.0	29.5
12 years	7.5	8.0	9.0	11.5	13.5	18.5	21.5	23.0	27.0
13 years	6.0	7.5	9.0	10.5	15.0	19.0	22.0	25.0	30.0
14 years	8.0	10.0	10.5	12.0	17.0	21.5	25.0	29.5	32.0
15 years	8.5	9.5	10.0	11.5	16.5	20.5	24.5	26.0	32.1
16 years	11.0	11.5	12.0	14.0	18.0	23.0	27.0	30.5	33.1
17 years	9.5	11.0	11.5	14.0	20.0	24.5	26.5	28.5	34.5
18 years	11.0	12.0	12.5	14.0	18.0	23.5	27.0	32.5	35.0
18–24 years	10.0	11.5	12.5	15.0	19.0	25.0	29.5	32.0	37.0
25–34 years	10.0	13.0	14.0	16.5	22.0	29.0	33.5	36.6	43.5
35–44 years	12.0	14.5	16.5	19.5	25.0	32.6	37.0	40.5	44.5
45–54 years	12.5	15.0	17.0	20.5	27.0	34.0	38.0	40.5	45.0
55–64 years	12.0	15.0	17.5	21.0	26.5	33.0	37.0	40.0	43.6
65–74 years	12.0	14.5	16.5	19.0	25.0	31.0	35.0	37.6	42.0

From Anthropometric Reference Data and Prevalence of Overweight, United States, 1976–80. Vital and Health Statistics Series 11, No 238, National Center for Health Statistics, US Department of Health and Human Services, 1987.

Sex and Age	Percentile								
	5th	10th	15th	25th	50th	75th	85th	90th	95th
MALE									
6–11 months	4.0	5.0	5.0	5.5	6.0	7.5	8.0	8.5	9.0
1 year	4.0	4.5	5.0	5.0	6.5	7.5	8.0	9.0	10.5
2 years	3.5	4.0	4.0	5.0	5.5	7.0	7.5	9.0	10.0
3 years	4.0	4.0	4.0	4.5	5.5	6.5	7.0	7.5	9.0
4 years	3.5	3.5	4.0	4.0	5.0	6.0	7.0	7.5	9.0
5 years	3.0	3.5	4.0	4.0	5.0	6.0	6.5	7.0	8.0
6 years	3.5	3.5	4.0	4.0	5.0	6.0	8.0	10.0	16.0
7 years	3.5	4.0	4.0	4.0	5.0	6.0	7.0	7.5	11.5
8 years	3.5	4.0	4.0	4.5	5.0	6.5	8.0	11.0	21.0
9 years	3.5	4.0	4.0	4.5	6.0	7.0	10.0	12.0	15.0
10 years	4.0	4.0	4.5	5.0	6.0	9.5	11.5	17.0	22.0
11 years	4.0	4.0	4.5	5.0	6.5	10.0	17.5	25.0	31.0
12 years	4.0	4.5	4.5	5.0	6.5	10.0	15.5	19.0	22.5
13 years	4.0	4.5	5.0	5.0	7.0	9.0	13.0	15.0	24.0
14 years	4.5	5.0	5.5	6.0	7.0	9.0	12.0	13.5	20.0
15 years	5.0	5.5	6.0	6.0	7.5	10.0	12.0	16.0	24.5
16 years	5.0	6.0	6.5	6.5	9.0	12.5	14.5	21.5	25.0
17 years	5.5	6.0	6.5	7.0	8.5	11.5	14.0	17.0	20.5
18 years	6.0	7.0	7.0	8.0	10.0	14.0	16.0	18.0	24.0
18–24 years	6.5	7.0	7.5	8.5	11.5	16.0	20.0	23.0	30.0
25–34 years	7.0	8.0	9.0	10.0	15.0	22.0	25.5	29.0	34.0
35–44 years	7.0	8.5	10.0	12.0	17.0	24.0	28.0	30.5	37.0
45–54 years	7.5	9.0	10.0	12.5	18.0	25.0	29.0	31.0	36.0
55–64 years	7.5	9.0	10.0	12.5	18.0	24.0	27.0	30.0	34.5
65–74 years	7.0	8.0	9.5	11.0	16.0	23.0	27.5	30.5	35.1
FEMALE									
6–11 months	4.5	5.0	5.0	5.5	6.5	7.5	8.0	9.0	10.0
1 year	4.0	4.0	5.0	5.0	6.5	8.0	8.5	9.5	10.5
2 years	4.0	4.5	4.5	5.0	6.0	7.5	8.5	9.5	11.0
3 years	3.5	4.0	4.5	5.0	6.0	7.0	8.0	9.0	11.0
4 years	3.5	4.0	4.5	5.0	5.5	7.0	8.0	9.0	10.5
5 years	4.0	4.0	4.5	5.0	5.5	7.0	8.0	10.0	12.0
6 years	4.0	4.0	4.0	5.0	6.0	7.5	9.0	10.5	14.0
7 years	3.5	4.0	4.0	4.5	6.0	7.5	9.0	12.0	16.5
8 years	3.5	4.0	4.5	5.0	6.0	8.0	10.5	12.0	15.0
9 years	4.0	5.0	5.0	5.5	7.0	9.5	13.0	21.0	29.0
10 years	4.5	5.0	5.0	6.0	8.0	13.5	18.0	19.5	23.0
11 years	4.5	5.0	5.5	6.5	8.0	12.0	17.0	22.0	29.0
12 years	5.0	5.5	6.0	6.5	9.0	13.0	17.0	22.0	29.0
13 years	4.5	5.5	6.0	7.0	9.5	14.0	17.5	20.0	29.0
14 years	6.0	6.5	7.0	7.5	10.5	16.0	22.0	26.0	31.0
15 years	6.0	7.0	7.5	8.5	10.5	16.0	20.5	22.5	27.5
16 years	6.5	7.5	8.5	9.5	12.0	16.5	23.5	26.0	36.6
17 years	6.5	7.0	8.0	9.5	13.0	19.5	27.0	29.0	37.0
18 years	7.0	7.5	8.0	10.0	13.0	18.5	22.0	27.5	34.5
18–24 years	7.0	7.5	8.0	10.0	13.0	20.5	26.0	31.0	38.0
25–34 years	7.0	8.0	8.5	10.5	16.0	27.0	33.5	38.0	45.0
35–44 years	7.0	8.5	10.0	12.0	19.0	31.0	36.6	40.1	46.5
45–54 years	7.0	10.0	11.0	14.5	22.0	32.5	37.5	40.5	47.6
55–64 years	7.5	9.0	11.0	13.5	22.0	32.0	37.0	41.0	47.0
65–74 years	7.0	8.5	10.0	13.0	21.0	30.0	35.0	37.1	43.0

From Anthropometric Reference Data and Prevalence of Overweight, United States, 1976–80. Vital and Health Statistics Series 11, No 238, National Center for Health Statistics, US Department of Health and Human Services, 1987.

APPENDIX 3C Percentiles for Upper Arm Circumference and Estimated Upper Arm Muscle Circumference of Whites in the United States Health and Nutrition Examination Survey I, 1971 to 1974*

Age Group	Arm Circumference (mm)							Arm Muscle Circumference (mm)						
	5th	10th	25th	50th	75th	90th	95th	5th	10th	25th	50th	75th	90th	95th
MALE														
1–1.9	142	146	150	159	170	176	183	110	113	119	127	135	144	147
2–2.9	141	145	153	162	170	178	185	111	114	122	130	140	146	150
3–3.9	150	153	160	167	175	184	190	117	123	131	137	143	148	153
4–4.9	149	154	162	171	180	186	192	123	126	133	141	148	156	159
5–5.9	153	160	167	175	185	195	204	128	133	140	147	154	162	169
6–6.9	155	159	167	179	188	209	228	131	135	142	151	161	170	177
7–7.9	162	167	177	187	201	223	230	137	139	151	160	168	177	190
8–8.9	162	170	177	190	202	220	245	140	145	154	162	170	182	187
9–9.9	175	178	187	200	217	249	257	151	154	161	170	183	196	202
10–10.9	181	184	196	210	231	262	274	156	160	166	180	191	209	221
11–11.9	186	190	202	223	244	261	280	159	165	173	183	195	205	230
12–12.9	193	200	214	232	254	282	303	167	171	182	196	210	223	241
13–13.9	194	211	228	247	263	286	301	172	179	196	211	226	238	245
14–14.9	220	226	237	253	283	303	322	189	199	212	223	240	260	264
15–15.9	222	229	244	264	284	311	320	199	204	218	237	254	266	272
16–16.9	244	248	262	278	303	324	343	213	225	234	249	269	287	296
17–17.9	246	253	267	285	308	336	347	224	231	245	258	273	294	312
18–18.9	245	260	276	297	321	353	379	226	237	252	264	283	298	324
19–24.9	262	272	288	308	331	355	372	238	245	257	273	289	309	321
25–34.9	271	282	300	319	342	362	375	243	250	264	279	298	314	326
35–44.9	278	287	305	326	345	363	374	247	255	269	286	302	318	327
45–54.9	267	281	301	322	342	362	376	239	249	265	281	300	315	326
55–64.9	258	273	296	317	336	355	369	236	245	260	278	295	310	320
65–74.9	248	263	285	307	325	344	355	223	235	251	268	284	298	306
FEMALE														
1–1.9	138	142	148	156	164	172	177	105	111	117	124	132	139	143
2–2.9	142	145	152	160	167	176	184	111	114	119	126	133	142	147
3–3.9	143	150	158	167	175	183	189	113	119	124	132	140	146	152
4–4.9	149	154	160	169	177	184	191	115	121	128	136	144	152	157
5–5.9	153	157	165	175	185	203	211	125	128	134	142	151	159	165
6–6.9	156	162	170	176	187	204	211	130	133	138	145	154	166	171
7–7.9	164	167	174	183	199	216	231	129	135	142	151	160	171	176
8–8.9	168	172	183	195	214	247	261	138	140	151	160	171	183	194
9–9.9	178	182	194	211	224	251	260	147	150	158	167	180	194	198
10–10.9	174	182	193	210	228	251	265	148	150	159	170	180	190	197
11–11.9	185	194	208	224	248	276	303	150	158	171	181	196	217	223
12–12.9	194	203	216	237	256	282	294	162	166	180	191	201	214	220
13–13.9	202	211	223	243	271	301	338	169	175	183	198	211	226	240
14–14.9	214	223	237	252	272	304	322	174	179	190	201	216	232	247
15–15.9	208	221	239	254	279	300	322	175	178	189	202	215	228	244
16–16.9	218	224	241	258	283	318	334	170	180	190	202	216	234	249
17–17.9	220	227	241	264	295	324	350	175	183	194	205	221	239	257
18–18.9	222	227	241	258	281	312	325	174	179	191	202	215	237	245
19–24.9	221	230	247	265	290	319	345	179	185	195	207	221	236	249
25–34.9	233	240	256	277	304	342	368	183	188	199	212	228	246	264
35–44.9	241	251	267	290	317	356	378	186	192	205	218	236	257	272
45–54.9	242	256	274	299	328	362	384	187	193	206	220	238	260	274
55–64.9	243	257	280	303	335	367	385	187	196	209	225	244	266	280
65–74.9	240	252	274	299	326	356	373	185	195	208	225	244	264	279

From Frisancho AR: New norms of upper limb fat and muscle areas for assessment of nutritional status. Am J Clin Nutr 1981;34:2540. © Am J Clin Nutr. American Society for Clinical Nutrition.

* Percentiles are not yet available for the black population for upper arm circumference or arm muscle circumference.

Age Group	Arm Muscle Area Percentiles (mm²)							Arm Fat Area Percentiles (mm²)						
	5th	20th	25th	50th	75th	90th	95th	5th	10th	25th	50th	75th	90th	95th
MALE														
1–1.9	956	1,014	1,133	1,278	1,447	1,644	1,720	452	486	590	741	895	1,036	1,176
2–2.9	973	1,040	1,190	1,345	1,557	1,690	1,787	434	504	578	737	871	1,044	1,148
3–3.9	1,095	1,201	1,357	1,484	1,618	1,750	1,853	464	519	590	736	868	1,071	1,151
4–4.9	1,207	1,264	1,408	1,579	1,747	1,926	2,008	428	494	598	722	859	989	1,085
5–5.9	1,298	1,411	1,550	1,720	1,884	2,089	2,285	446	488	582	713	914	1,176	1,299
6–6.9	1,360	1,447	1,605	1,815	2,056	2,297	2,493	371	446	539	678	896	1,115	1,519
7–7.9	1,497	1,548	1,808	2,027	2,246	2,494	2,886	423	473	574	758	1,011	1,393	1,511
8–8.9	1,550	1,664	1,895	2,089	2,296	2,628	2,788	410	460	588	725	1,003	1,248	1,558
9–9.9	1,811	1,884	2,067	2,228	2,657	3,053	3,257	485	527	635	859	1,252	1,864	2,081
10–10.9	1,930	2,027	2,182	2,575	2,903	3,486	3,882	523	543	738	982	1,376	1,906	2,609
11–11.9	2,016	2,156	2,382	2,670	3,022	3,359	4,226	536	595	754	1,148	1,710	2,348	2,574
12–12.9	2,216	2,339	2,649	3,022	3,496	3,968	4,640	554	650	874	1,172	1,558	2,536	3,580
13–13.9	2,363	2,546	3,044	3,553	4,081	4,502	4,794	475	570	812	1,096	1,702	2,744	3,322
14–14.9	2,830	3,147	3,586	3,963	4,575	5,368	5,530	453	563	786	1,082	1,608	2,746	3,508
15–15.9	3,138	3,317	3,788	4,481	5,134	5,631	5,900	521	595	690	931	1,423	2,434	3,100
16–16.9	3,625	4,044	4,352	4,951	5,753	6,576	6,980	542	593	844	1,078	1,746	2,280	3,041
17–17.9	3,998	4,252	4,777	5,286	5,950	6,886	7,726	598	698	827	1,096	1,636	2,407	2,888
18–18.9	4,070	4,481	5,066	5,552	6,374	7,067	8,355	560	665	860	1,264	1,947	3,302	3,928
19–24.9	4,508	4,777	5,274	5,913	6,660	7,606	8,200	594	743	963	1,406	2,231	3,098	3,652
25–34.9	4,694	4,963	5,541	6,214	7,067	7,847	8,436	675	831	1,174	1,752	2,459	3,246	3,786
35–44.9	4,844	5,181	5,740	6,490	7,265	8,034	8,488	703	851	1,310	1,792	2,463	3,098	3,624
45–54.9	4,546	4,946	5,589	6,297	7,142	7,918	8,458	749	922	1,254	1,741	2,359	3,245	3,928
55–64.9	4,422	4,783	5,381	6,144	6,919	7,670	8,149	658	839	1,166	1,645	2,236	2,976	3,466
65–74.9	3,973	4,411	5,031	5,716	6,432	7,074	7,453	573	753	1,122	1,621	2,199	2,876	3,327
FEMALE														
1–1.9	885	973	1,084	1,221	1,378	1,535	1,621	401	466	578	706	847	1,022	1,140
2–2.9	973	1,029	1,119	1,269	1,405	1,595	1,727	469	526	642	747	894	1,061	1,173
3–3.9	1,014	1,133	1,227	1,396	1,563	1,690	1,846	473	529	656	822	967	1,106	1,158
4–4.9	1,058	1,171	1,313	1,475	1,644	1,832	1,958	490	541	654	766	907	1,109	1,236
5–5.9	1,238	1,301	1,423	1,598	1,825	2,012	2,159	470	529	647	812	991	1,330	1,536
6–6.9	1,354	1,414	1,513	1,683	1,877	2,182	2,323	464	508	638	827	1,009	1,263	1,436
7–7.9	1,330	1,441	1,602	1,815	2,045	2,332	2,469	491	560	706	920	1,135	1,407	1,644
8–8.9	1,513	1,566	1,808	2,034	2,327	2,657	2,996	527	634	769	1,042	1,383	1,872	2,482
9–9.9	1,723	1,788	1,976	2,227	2,571	2,987	3,112	642	690	933	1,219	1,584	2,171	2,524
10–10.9	1,740	1,784	2,019	2,296	2,583	2,873	3,093	616	702	842	1,141	1,608	2,500	3,005
11–11.9	1,784	1,987	2,316	2,612	3,071	3,739	3,953	707	802	1,015	1,301	1,942	2,730	3,690
12–12.9	2,092	2,182	2,579	2,904	3,225	3,655	3,847	782	854	1,090	1,511	2,056	2,666	3,369
13–13.9	2,269	2,426	2,657	3,130	3,529	4,081	4,568	726	838	1,219	1,625	2,374	3,272	4,150
14–14.9	2,418	2,562	2,874	3,220	3,704	4,294	4,850	981	1,043	1,423	1,818	2,403	3,250	3,765
15–15.9	2,426	2,518	2,847	3,248	3,689	4,123	4,756	839	1,126	1,396	1,886	2,544	3,093	4,195
16–16.9	2,308	2,567	2,865	3,248	3,718	4,353	4,946	1,126	1,351	1,663	2,006	2,598	3,374	4,236
17–17.9	2,442	2,674	2,996	3,336	3,883	4,552	5,251	1,042	1,267	1,463	2,104	2,977	3,864	5,159
18–18.9	2,398	2,538	2,917	3,243	3,694	4,461	4,767	1,003	1,230	1,616	2,104	2,617	3,508	3,733
19–24.9	2,538	2,728	3,026	3,406	3,877	4,439	4,940	1,046	1,198	1,596	2,166	2,959	4,050	4,896
25–34.9	2,661	2,826	3,148	3,573	4,138	4,806	5,541	1,173	1,399	1,841	2,548	3,512	4,690	5,560
35–44.9	2,750	2,948	3,359	3,783	4,428	5,240	5,877	1,336	1,619	2,158	2,898	3,932	5,093	5,847
45–54.9	2,784	2,956	3,378	3,858	4,520	5,375	5,964	1,459	1,803	2,447	3,244	4,229	5,416	6,140
55–64.9	2,784	3,063	3,477	4,045	4,750	5,632	6,247	1,345	1,879	2,520	3,369	4,360	5,276	6,152
65–74.9	2,737	3,018	3,444	4,019	4,739	5,566	6,214	1,363	1,681	2,266	3,063	3,943	4,914	5,530

From Frisancho AR: New norms of upper limb fat and muscle areas for assessment of nutritional status. Am J Clin Nutr 1981;34:2540. © Am J Clin Nutr. American Society for Clinical Nutrition.

*Percentiles are not yet available for the black population for arm fat areas.

PERSONAL INFORMATION, HABITS

1. When were you born? _____ / _____ / _____
   Month   Day   Year

2. How old are you? _____ years

3. Sex: 1 ___ Male   2 ___ Female

4. Race or ethnic background:
   1 ___ White, not of Hispanic origin   4 ___ American Indian/Alaskan native
   2 ___ Black, not of Hispanic origin   5 ___ Asian
   3 ___ Hispanic   6 ___ Pacific Islander

5. Please circle the highest grade in school you have completed:
   1 2 3 4 5 6 7 8 9 10 11 12   13 14 15 16+

6. What is your marital status?   1 ___ Single   3 ___ Widowed
                                   2 ___ Married   4 ___ Divorced/Separated

7. How many times have you moved or changed residences in the last ten years? ___ times

8. Have you smoked at least 100 cigarettes in your entire life? 1 ___ No   2 ___ Yes   **If Yes,**

> IF YES: About how old were you when you first started smoking cigarettes fairly regularly?
> _____ years old
>
> On the average of the entire time you smoked, how many cigarettes did you smoke per day?
> _____ cigarettes per day
>
> Do you smoke cigarettes now? 1 ___ No   2 ___ Yes
>   IF NO: How old were you when you stopped smoking? _____ years old
>   IF YES: On the average, about how many cigarettes a day do you smoke now? _____ cigarettes

9. Have you ever smoked a pipe or cigars regularly? 1 ___ No   2 ___ Yes   **If Yes,**

> IF YES: For how many years? _____ years
>   About how much? _____ pipes or cigars per _____
>   (day or week)
>   1   2

10. During the past year, have you taken any vitamins or minerals?
    1 ___ No   2 ___ Yes, fairly regularly   3 ___ Yes, but not regularly   **If Yes,**

> What do you take fairly regularly?   # of PILLS per DAY, WEEK,
>   etc.
> *Multiple Vitamins*
>   One-a-day type   _____ pills per _____
>   Stress-tabs type   _____ pills per _____
>   Therapeutic, Theragran type _____ pills per _____   How many milligrams
> *Other Vitamins*   or IUs per pill?
>   Vitamin A   _____ pills per _____ ➞ _____ IU per pill
>   Vitamin C   _____ pills per _____ ➞ _____ mg per pill
>   Vitamin E   _____ pills per _____ ➞ _____ IU per pill
>   Calcium or dolomite _____ pills per _____ ➞ _____ mg per pill
> Other (What?) 1 ___ Yeast 2 ___ Selenium 3 ___ Zinc 4 ___ Iron 5 ___ Beta-carotene
>   6 ___ Cod liver oil 7 ___ Other _____
> Please list the brand of multiple vitamin/mineral you usually take: _____

Appendix continued on following page

11. Are you on a special diet?

1 ____ No   2 ____ Weight loss   3 ____ For medical condition   4 ____ Vegetarian   5 ____ Low salt
6 ____ Low cholesterol   7 ____ Weight gain

12. How often do you eat the following foods from *restaurants* or *fast food places?*

RESTAURANT FOOD	1 Almost every day	2 2-4 times a week	3 Once a week	4 1-3 times a month	5 5-10 times a year	6 1-4 times a year	7 Never, or less than once a year
Fried chicken							
Burgers							
Pizza							
Chinese food							
Mexican food							
Fried fish							
Other foods							

13. This section is about your *usual* eating habits. Thinking back over the past year, how often do you usually eat the foods listed on the next page?

First, check (√) whether your usual serving size is small, medium or large. (A small portion is about one-half the medium serving size shown, or less; a large portion is about one-and-a-half times as much, or more.)

Then, put a NUMBER in the most appropriate column to indicate *HOW OFTEN,* on the average, you eat the food. You may eat bananas *twice a week* (put a 2 *in the "week"* column). If you never eat the food, check "Rarely/Never." Please DO NOT SKIP foods. And please BE CAREFUL which column you put your answer in. It will make a big difference if you say "Hamburger once a day" when you mean "Hamburger once a week"!

Some items say "in season." Indicate how often you eat these just in the 2-3 month time when that food is in season. (Be careful about overestimating here.)

Please look at the *example* below. This person

1) eats a medium serving of cantaloupe once a week, in season.

2) has ½ grapefruit about twice a month.

3) has a small serving of sweet potatoes about 3 times a year.

4) has a large hamburger or cheeseburger or meat loaf about four times a week.

5) never eats winter squash.

EXAMPLE:

	Medium Serving	Your Serving Size S M L			How often? Day	Week	Month	Year	Rarely/Never
Cantaloupe (in season)	¼ medium		✔			1			
Grapefruit	(½)		✔				2		
Sweet potatoes, yams	½ cup	✔						3	
Hamburger, cheeseburger, meat loaf	1 medium					4.			
Winter squash, baked squash	½ cup								✔

PLEASE GO TO NEXT PAGE

	Medium Serving	Your Serving Size			How often?				
FRUITS & JUICES		S	M	L	Day	Week	Month	Year	Rarely/Never
EXAMPLE – Apples, applesauce, pears	(1) or ½ cup		✓			**4**			
Apples, applesauce, pears	(1) or ½ cup								
Bananas	1 medium								
Peaches, apricots (canned, frozen or dried, whole year)	(1) or ½ cup								
Peaches, apricots, nectarines (fresh, in season)	1 medium								
Cantaloupe (in season)	¼ medium								
Watermelon (in season)	1 slice								
Strawberries (fresh, in season)	½ cup								
Oranges	1 medium								
Orange juice or grapefruit juice	6 oz. glass								
Grapefruit	(½)								
Tang, Start breakfast drinks	6 oz. glass								
Other fruit juices, fortified fruit drinks	6 oz. glass								
Any other fruit, including berries, fruit cocktail	½ cup								
VEGETABLES		S	M	L	Da	Wk	Mo	Yr	Nv
String beans, green beans	½ cup								
Peas	½ cup								
Chili with beans	¾ cup								
Other beans such as baked beans, pintos, kidney beans, limas	¾ cup								
Corn	½ cup								
Winter squash, baked squash	½ cup								
Tomatoes, tomato juice	(1) or 6 oz.								
Red chili sauce, taco sauce, salsa picante	2 Tblsp. sauce								
Broccoli	½ cup								
Cauliflower or brussel sprouts	½ cup								
Spinach (raw)	¾ cup								
Spinach (cooked)	½ cup								
Mustard greens, turnip greens, collards	½ cup								
Cole slaw, cabbage, sauerkraut	½ cup								
Carrots, or mixed vegetables containing carrots	½ cup								
Green salad	1 med. bowl								
Salad dressing, mayonnaise (including on sandwiches)	2 Tblsp.								
French fries and fried potatoes	¾ cup								
Sweet potatoes, yams	½ cup								
Other potatoes, including boiled, baked, potato salad	(1) or ½ cup								
Rice	¾ cup								
Any other vegetable, including cooked onions, summer squash	½ cup								
Butter, margarine or other fat on vegetables, potatoes, etc.	2 pats								
MEAT, FISH, POULTRY & MIXED DISHES		S	M	L	Da	Wk	Mo	Yr	Nv
Hamburgers, cheeseburgers, meat loaf	1 medium								
Beef—steaks, roasts	4 oz.								
Beef stew or pot pie with carrots, other vegetables	1 cup								
Liver, including chicken livers	4 oz.								
Pork, including chops, roasts	2 chops or 4 oz.								
Fried chicken	2 sm. or 1 lg. piece								
Chicken or turkey, roasted, stewed or broiled	2 sm. or 1 lg. piece								
Fried fish or fish sandwich	4 oz. or 1 sand.								
Tuna fish, tuna salad, tuna casserole	½ cup								
Shell fish (shrimp, lobster, crab, oysters, etc.)	(5) ¼ cup or 3 oz.								
Other fish, broiled, baked	4 oz.								
Spaghetti, lasagna, other pasta with tomato sauce	1 cup								
Pizza	2 slices								
Mixed dishes with cheese (such as macaroni and cheese)	1 cup								

Appendix continued on following page

	Medium Serving	Your Serving Size			How often?				
		S	M	L	Day	Week	Month	Year	Rarely/Never
LUNCH ITEMS		S	M	L					
Liverwurst	2 slices								
Hot dogs	2 dogs								
Ham, lunch meats	2 slices								
Vegetable soup, vegetable beef, minestrone, tomato soup	1 med. bowl								
Other soups	1 med. bowl								
BREADS / SALTY SNACKS / SPREADS		S	M	L	Da	Wk	Mo	Yr	Nv
Biscuits, muffins, burger rolls (incl. fast foods)	1 med. piece								
White bread (including sandwiches), bagels, etc., crackers	2 slices, 3 cracks								
Dark bread, including whole wheat, rye, pumpernickel	2 slices								
Corn bread, corn muffins, corn tortillas	1 med. piece								
Salty snacks (such as chips, popcorn)	2 handfuls								
Peanuts, peanut butter	2 Tblsp.								
Butter on bread or rolls	2 pats								
Margarine on bread or rolls	2 pats								
Gravies made with meat drippings, or white sauce	2 Tblsp.								
BREAKFAST FOODS		S	M	L	Da	Wk	Mo	Yr	Nv
High fiber, bran or granola cereals, shredded wheat	1 med. bowl								
Highly fortified cereals, such as Product 19, Total, or Most	1 med. bowl								
Other cold cereals, such as Corn Flakes, Rice Krispies	1 med. bowl								
Cooked cereals	1 med. bowl								
Sugar added to cereal	2 teaspn.								
Eggs 1 egg = small,	2 eggs = medium								
Bacon	2 slices								
Sausage	2 patties or links								
SWEETS		S	M	L	Da	Wk	Mo	Yr	Nv
Ice cream	1 scoop								
Doughnuts, cookies, cakes, pastry	1 pc. or 3 cookies								
Pumpkin pie, sweet potato pie	1 med. slice								
Other pies	1 med. slice								
Chocolate candy	small bar, 1 oz.								
Other candy, jelly, honey, brown sugar	3 pc. or 1 Tblsp.								
DAIRY PRODUCTS		S	M	L	Da	Wk	Mo	Yr	Nv
Cottage cheese	½ cup								
Other cheeses and cheese spreads	2 slices or 2 oz.								
Flavored yogurt	1 cup								
Whole milk and bevs. with whole milk (not incl. on cereal)	8 oz. glass								
2% milk and bevs. with 2% milk (not incl. on cereal)	8 oz. glass								
Skim milk, 1% milk or buttermilk (not incl. on cereal)	8 oz. glass								
BEVERAGES		S	M	L	Da	Wk	Mo	Yr	Nv
Regular soft drinks	12 oz. can or bottle								
Diet soft drinks	12 oz. can or bottle								
Beer	12 oz. can or bottle								
Wine	1 med. glass								
Liquor	1 shot								
Decaffeinated coffee	1 med. cup								
Coffee, not decaffeinated	1 med. cup								
Tea (hot or iced)	1 med. cup								
Lemon in tea	1 teaspn.								
Non-diary creamer in coffee or tea	1 Tblsp.								
Milk in coffee or tea	1 Tblsp.								
Cream (real) or Half-and-Half in coffee or tea	1 Tblsp.								
Sugar in coffee or tea	2 teaspn.								
Artifical sweetener in coffee or tea	1 packet								
Glasses of water, not counting in coffee or tea	8 oz. glass								

From National Cancer Institute, Division of Cancer Prevention and Control, National Institutes of Health

APPENDIX 4 One-Month Increments in Recumbent Length and Weight From Age 1 to 12 Months*

Age (months)	Recumbent Length (cm/month)		Weight (kg/month)	
	Boys	Girls	Boys	Girls
1–2	3.88	3.54	1.28	1.12
2–3	2.85	2.70	0.85	0.76
3–4	2.35	2.28	0.66	0.61
4–5	2.05	2.03	0.55	0.52
5–6	1.83	1.83	0.48	0.45
6–7	1.68	1.68	0.43	0.41
7–8	1.55	1.57	0.38	0.37
8–9	1.45	1.47	0.35	0.34
9–10	1.37	1.39	0.33	0.32
10–11	1.30	1.32	0.31	0.30
11–12	1.24	1.26	0.29	0.28

From Roche AF, Shumei G, Moore MWM. Weight and recumbent length from 1 to 12 months of age: Reference data for 1-mo increments. Am J Clin Nutr 1989;49;599. © Am J Clin Nutr. American Society for Clinical Nutrition.

*Increments represent the 50th percentile from the Fels Longitudinal Study of Infants.

APPENDIX 5 Nutrient Content of Breast Milk and Commercial Infant Formulas

Nutrient Source	Breast Milk	Similac	Enfamil	S.M.A.	Gerber
Protein		Casein	Reduced mineral whey, casein	Demineralized whey, casein	Nonfat milk
Fat		Soy oil, coconut oil, corn oil	Soy oil, coconut oil	Oleo; soybean, safflower, and coconut oils	Soy oil, coconut oil
Carbohydrate		Lactose	Lactose	Lactose	Lactose
Linoleic Acid (% kcal)	6–15	16	13	13	12
NUTRIENTS PER DECILITER—NORMAL DILUTION					
Energy (kcal)	67	68	67	67	67
Protein (g)*	1.1 (6–8)	1.5 (9)	1.5 (9)	1.5 (9)	1.5 (9)
Fat (g)*	3.9 (56)	3.6 (48)	3.8 (50)	3.6 (48)	3.6 (48)
Carbohydrate (g)*	7.2 (38)	7.2 (43)	6.9 (41)	7.2 (43)	7.1 (43)
Vitamin A (IU)	223	200	207	240	200
Vitamin D (IU)	22	40	42	42	40
Vitamin E (IU)	0.2	2	2	1	2
Vitamin C (mg)	4.0	5.5	5.5	5.8	6.0
Thiamin (μg)	21.0	65	53	71	67
Riboflavin (μg)	3.5	10	11	11	10
Niacin (mg) (equiv.)	0.15	0.7	0.8	1.0	0.7
Pyridoxine (μg)	0.02	40	42	40	40
Vitamin B_{12} (μg)	0.09	0.15	0.16	0.11	0.16
Folate (μg)	8.5	10	10.5	5.3	10
Calcium (mg)	52	51	46	44	50
Phosphorus (mg)	28	39	31.7	33	38
Magnesium (mg)	3.5	4	4	5	3.3
Iron (mg)	0.03	Trace	Trace	Trace	Trace
Zinc (mg)	0.12	0.5	0.5	0.37	0.5
Copper (μg)	24	60.0	63.4	48	60
Iodine (μg)	11	10	6.8	7	5.3

*% kilocalories in parentheses.

Good Start	Prosobee	Isomil	Nutramigen	Progestimil
Hydrolyzed, reduced-mineral whey	Soy protein	Soy protein	Casein hydrolysate	Casein hydrolysate
Palm, safflower, and coconut oil.	Soy oil	Coconut oil, soy oil	Corn oil	Corn oil, medium-chain triglycerides
Lactose, corn syrup	Corn syrup solids	Corn syrup solids, sucrose	Modified tapioca starch, sucrose	Corn syrup solids, modified tapioca starch
8	12	16	21	13
67	67	68	67	68
1.6 (9)	2.0 (12)	2.0 (12)	1.9 (11)	1.9 (11)
3.4 (46)	3.1 (48)	3.6 (48)	2.7 (35)	2.8 (35)
7.4 (45)	7.1 (40)	6.8 (40)	9.4 (54)	9.4 (54)
200	210	203	210	250
40	42.0	41.0	42.0	51.0
8	2.2	2.0	2.1	2.5
5.3	6.0	5.5	5.5	7.9
40	52.0	41.0	52.0	52.0
9	63.0	61.0	63.0	63.0
0.5	0.8	0.9	0.8	0.8
40	42.0	41.0	42.0	42.0
0.17	0.2	0.3	0.2	0.2
6	11.0	10.0	10.6	10.6
42	63.0	71.0	63.0	63.0
24	50.0	51.0	42.0	42.0
4.5	7.4	5.1	7.4	7.4
Trace	1.3	1.2	1.3	1.3
0.5	0.5	0.5	0.5	0.5
53	63.0	51.0	63.0	63.0
5.6	7.0	10.0	4.8	4.8

APPENDIX 6 Recommended Nutrient Levels of Infant Formulas (per 1000 kcal)

Nutrient	Range	
	Lowest Adequate	Not to Exceed*
Protein (g)	1.8[†]	4.5[†]
Fat (g)	3.3 (30% of Cal)	6 (54% of Cal)
Including essential fatty acid (linoleate) (mg)	300 (2.7% of Cal)	
Vitamins		
A (IU)	250 (75 μg)[‡]	750 (225 μg)[‡]
D (IU)	40 (1 μg)[§]	100 (2.5 μg)[§]
K (μg)[‖]	4	—
E (IU)	0.7 (0.5 mg)[¶] at least 0.7IU (0.5 mg)/g linoleic acid	—
C (ascorbic acid) (mg)	8	—
B$_1$ (thiamine) (μg)	40	—
B$_2$ (riboflavin) (μg)	60	—
B$_6$ (pyridoxine) (μg)	35.0 (15 μg/g of protein)	—
B$_{12}$ (μg)	0.15	—
Niacin (μg)	250 (or 0.8 mg niacin equivalents)	—
Folic acid (μg)	4	—
Panthotenic acid (μg)	300	—
Biotin (μg)	1.4[#]	—
Choline (mg)	7[#]	—
Inositol (mg)	4[#]	—
Minerals**		
Calcium (mg)	60[††]	—
Phosphorus (mg)	30[††]	—
Magnesium (mg)	6	—
Iron (mg)	0.15	2.5[‡‡]
Iodine (μg)	5	25
Zinc (mg)	0.5	—
Copper (μg)	60	—
Manganese (μg)	5	—
Sodium (mg)	60 (5.8 mEq)	60 (17.5 mEq)
Potassium (mg)	80 (13.7 mEq)	200 (34.3 mEq)
Chloride (mg)	55 (10.4 mEq)	150 (28.3 mEq)
Selenium (μg)[§§]	3	—

*Where no upper limit is given, toxicity is not well defined; massive excesses may have adverse consequences.
[†] At least nutritionally equivalent to casein quality recommended as outlined in Statement: Commentary on breast feeding and infant formulas, including proposed standards for formulas. *Pediatrics* 1976;57:278–285.
[‡] Retinol equivalents.
[§] Cholecalciferol.
[‖] Any vitamin K added shall be in the form of phylloquinone.
[¶] d-Alpha tocopherol equivalents.
[#] Average present in milk-based formulas; should be included in this amount in other formulas.
**Formula should be made with water low in fluoride and in any case contain less than 45 μg/100 kcal. For explanation, see Committee on Nutrition Statement: Fluoride Supplementation. *Pediatrics* 1986;77:758–761.
[††] Calcium to phosphorus ratio should be no less than 1.1 nor more than 2.
[‡‡] Prudence indicates that there should be an upper limit on iron. If formula is labeled "infant formula with iron," it must contain not less than 1 mg/100 kcal.
[§§] Selenium is not included in 1987 recommendations. The level that causes toxicity is very narrow.
Used with permission of the American Academy of Pediatrics from *Pediatric Nutrition Handbook*, 3rd edition, 1993, pp. 360–361.

APPENDIX 7A Girls: Prepubescent; Physical Growth NCHS Percentiles

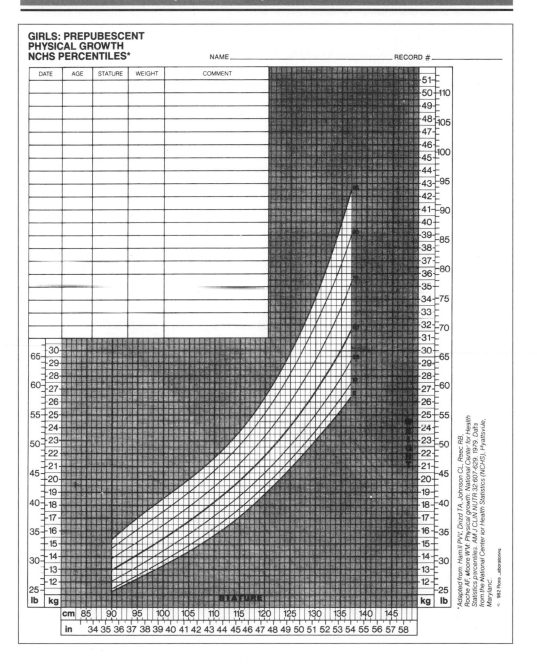

GIRLS: PREPUBESCENT PHYSICAL GROWTH NCHS PERCENTILES*

NAME _____   RECORD # _____

*Adapted from: Hamill PVV, Drizd TA, Johnson CL, Reec RB, Roche AF, Moore WM. Physical growth: National Center for Health Statistics percentiles. AM J CLIN NUTR 32:607-629, 1979. Data from the National Center for Health Statistics (NCHS), Hyattsville, Maryland.

© 1982 Ross Laboratories

APPENDIX 7B Boys: Prepubescent; Physical Growth NCHS Percentiles

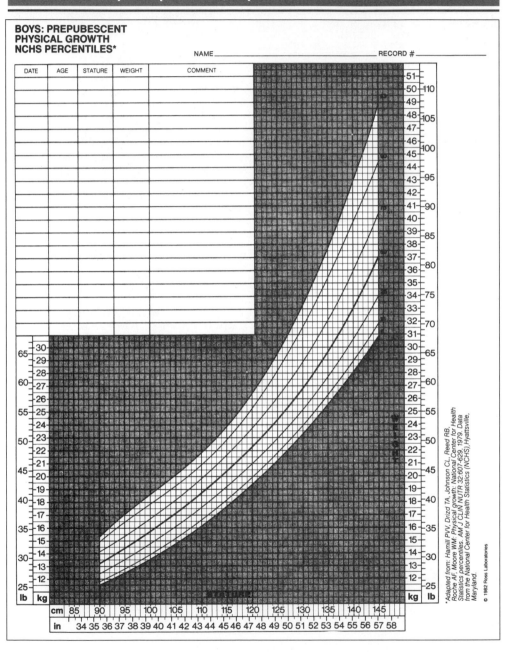

BOYS: PREPUBESCENT
PHYSICAL GROWTH
NCHS PERCENTILES*

NAME _____ RECORD # _____

DATE	AGE	STATURE	WEIGHT	COMMENT

*Adapted from: Hamill PVV, Drizd TA, Johnson CL, Reed RB, Roche AF, Moore WM: Physical growth: National Center for Health Statistics percentiles. AM J CLIN NUTR 32:607-629, 1979. Data from the National Center for Health Statistics (NCHS), Hyattsville, Maryland.

© 1982 Ross Laboratories

APPENDIX 8 Percentiles for Weight for Height of Youths Aged 12 to 17 Years (Weight in kg of Youths Aged 12 Years at Last Birthday)

Sex and Height	n	N	$\bar{X}$	s	$s_{\bar{x}}$	5th	10th	25th	50th	75th	90th	95th
MALE												
Under 130 cm	5	15	*	*	*	*	*	*	*	*	*	*
130.0–134.9 cm	4	8	*	*	*	*	*	*	*	*	*	*
135.0–139.9 cm	34	111	32.50	3.741	0.727	26.6	27.6	30.2	31.6	34.7	37.7	39.4
140.0–144.9 cm	80	241	34.28	3.635	0.601	28.1	30.0	31.8	34.1	36.5	38.6	40.7
145.0–149.9 cm	123	386	39.27	6.243	0.615	32.1	33.2	35.7	38.2	40.9	46.1	52.5
155.0–154.9 cm	156	513	42.90	6.314	0.480	34.9	36.1	38.2	42.1	46.0	51.6	56.3
155.0–159.9 cm	135	432	47.35	7.551	0.769	38.3	39.4	41.9	46.2	50.5	57.4	61.9
160.0–164.9 cm	65	201	50.82	8.735	1.388	42.1	42.7	44.9	48.4	56.0	61.1	67.1
165.0–169.9 cm	29	88	55.75	8.811	2.031	43.3	46.4	49.0	54.4	59.9	68.3	76.6
170.0–174.0 cm	8	21	62.37	4.503	1.993	54.0	58.1	60.1	61.0	66.0	69.1	69.5
175.0–179.9 cm	3	10	*	*	*	*	*	*	*	*	*	*
100.0 101.9 cm	1	2	*	*	*	*	*	*	*	*	*	*
185.0–189.9 cm	—	—	—	—	—	—	—	—	—	—	—	—
190.0–194.9 cm	—	—	—	—	—	—	—	—	—	—	—	—
195.0 cm and over	—	—	—	—	—	—	—	—	—	—	—	—
FEMALE												
Under 130 cm	—	—	—	—	—	—	—	—	—	—	—	—
130.0–134.9 cm	3	10	*	*	*	*	*	*	*	*	*	*
135.0–139.9 cm	12	44	29.41	3.372	0.914	25.0	25.0	26.4	28.9	32.1	34.1	34.2
140.0–144.9 cm	32	116	38.30	7.314	1.194	28.8	30.6	33.3	36.8	41.4	49.2	55.1
145.0–149.9 cm	72	258	39.78	6.205	0.975	31.8	32.8	35.5	38.5	42.8	48.3	50.6
150.0–154.9 cm	147	517	44.00	7.421	0.677	34.4	35.8	38.9	42.8	47.4	52.9	57.4
155.0–159.9 cm	144	525	48.74	8.369	0.714	37.9	39.2	43.0	46.8	53.8	60.7	63.5
160.0–164.9 cm	95	336	53.06	8.010	0.658	42.5	43.9	47.2	51.1	57.2	65.6	69.6
165.0–169.9 cm	31	117	54.89	7.022	1.384	43.9	47.1	50.4	53.1	59.7	64.5	71.3
170.0–174.9 cm	11	42	63.66	14.501	6.214	48.7	50.1	50.8	56.7	82.2	86.0	86.1
175.0–179.9 cm	—	—	—	—	—	—	—	—	—	—	—	—
180.0–184.9 cm	—	—	—	—	—	—	—	—	—	—	—	—
185.0–189.9 cm	—	—	—	—	—	—	—	—	—	—	—	—
190.0–194.9 cm	—	—	—	—	—	—	—	—	—	—	—	—
195.0 cm and over	—	—	—	—	—	—	—	—	—	—	—	—

From National Center for Health Statistics: Height and Weight of Youths 12–17 Years, United States. In Vital and Health Statistics, Series 11, no. 124. Health Services and Mental Health Administration. Washington, DC, US Government Printing Office, 1973.

Note: n = sample size; N = estimated number of youths in population in thousands; $\bar{X}$ = mean; s = standard deviation; $s_{\bar{x}}$ = standard error of the mean.

Table continued on following page

APPENDIX 8 Percentiles for Weight for Height of Youths Aged 12 to 17 Years *Continued* (Weight in kg of Youths Aged 13 Years at Last Birthday)

Sex and Height	*n*	*N*	$\bar{X}$	*s*	$s_{\bar{x}}$	Percentile						
						5th	10th	25th	50th	75th	90th	95th
MALE												
Under 130 cm	—	—	—	—	—	—	—	—	—	—	—	—
130.0–134.9 cm	2	5	*	*	*	*	*	*	*	*	*	*
135.0–139.9 cm	6	25	32.62	5.624	7.716	27.2	27.6	28.9	31.0	34.9	43.1	43.2
140.0–144.9 cm	18	56	36.54	5.852	1.607	30.0	30.5	32.1	36.1	39.2	41.7	53.2
145.0–149.9 cm	65	204	39.03	5.270	0.662	32.4	33.9	36.1	37.9	41.2	44.5	46.4
150.0–154.9 cm	99	312	42.58	6.724	0.865	34.8	36.2	37.9	41.0	45.5	49.4	61.0
155.0–159.9 cm	131	421	47.27	7.482	0.717	37.8	39.2	41.7	45.8	51.1	58.7	61.7
160.0–164.9 cm	125	393	53.01	9.324	0.916	41.5	43.7	46.9	50.4	58.2	64.4	72.5
165.0–169.9 cm	91	285	55.92	8.560	0.833	46.3	47.5	49.3	53.6	59.4	69.0	75.0
170.0–174.9 cm	63	215	62.01	10.362	1.033	51.2	51.6	53.7	60.1	67.0	76.0	85.0
175.0–179.9 cm	19	68	67.92	12.085	3.428	56.3	57.9	60.1	63.3	70.3	88.3	89.0
180.0–184.9 cm	5	15	*	*	*	*	*	*	*	*	*	*
185.0–189.9 cm	—	—	—	—	—	—	—	—	—	—	—	—
190.0–194.9 cm	—	—	—	—	—	—	—	—	—	—	—	—
195.0 cm and over	—	—	—	—	—	—	—	—	—	—	—	—
FEMALE												
Under 130 cm	—	—	—	—	—	—	—	—	—	—	—	—
130.0–134.9 cm	1	3	*	*	*	*	*	*	*	*	*	*
135.0–139.9 cm	—	—	—	—	—	—	—	—	—	—	—	—
140.0–144.9 cm	15	51	37.13	7.317	2.259	26.6	27.5	30.5	36.7	40.1	44.5	56.1
145.0–149.9 cm	47	165	42.23	6.880	0.888	34.7	35.6	38.2	40.5	44.2	53.6	57.6
150.0–154.9 cm	98	329	44.32	7.029	0.787	35.6	36.5	39.2	42.9	47.3	53.7	57.9
155.0–159.9 cm	152	499	49.75	8.757	0.699	39.1	39.9	43.8	48.4	53.8	61.0	65.9
160.0–164.9 cm	156	515	53.16	8.399	0.522	41.2	43.9	47.7	52.2	57.0	63.8	68.5
165.0–169.9 cm	86	284	58.17	9.125	0.921	46.2	47.4	52.2	58.1	61.5	69.3	76.2
170.0–174.9 cm	24	87	58.11	13.209	2.343	46.2	47.1	48.4	52.9	65.3	68.6	96.8
175.0–179.9 cm	3	10	*	*	*	*	*	*	*	*	*	*
180.0–184.9 cm	—	—	—	—	—	—	—	—	—	—	—	—
185.0–189.9 cm	—	—	—	—	—	—	—	—	—	—	—	—
190.0–194.9 cm	—	—	—	—	—	—	—	—	—	—	—	—
195.0 cm and over	—	—	—	—	—	—	—	—	—	—	—	—

From National Center for Health Statistics: Height and Weight of Youths 12–17 Years, United States. In Vital and Health Statistics, Series 11, no. 124. Health Services and Mental Health Administration. Washington, DC, US Government Printing Office, 1973.

Note: *n* = sample size; *N* = estimated number of youths in population in thousands; $\bar{X}$ = mean; *s* = standard deviation; $s_{\bar{x}}$ = standard error of the mean.

APPENDIX 8 Percentiles for Weight for Height of Youths Aged 12 to 17 Years *Continued* (Weight in kg of Youths Aged 14 Years at Last Birthday)

Sex and Height	n	N	$\bar{X}$	s	$s_{\bar{x}}$	Percentile						
						5th	10th	25th	50th	75th	90th	95th
MALE												
Under 130 cm	—	—	—	—	—	—	—	—	—	—	—	—
130.0–134.9 cm	—	—	—	—	—	—	—	—	—	—	—	—
135.0–139.9 cm	2	7	*	*	*	*	*	*	*	*	*	*
140.0–144.9 cm	3	13	*	*	*	*	*	*	*	*	*	*
145.0–149.9 cm	11	42	40.51	1.829	0.644	36.9	38.6	39.6	40.6	42.0	42.5	42.7
150.0–154.9 cm	45	135	43.63	6.277	1.182	36.2	37.0	39.0	41.4	48.0	51.7	55.3
155.0–159.9 cm	83	261	47.42	7.822	0.872	37.7	38.7	41.8	46.1	51.2	58.0	62.7
160.0–164.9 cm	96	299	52.28	6.785	0.584	42.5	44.0	47.5	52.1	56.3	61.5	65.1
165.0–169.9 cm	134	432	58.07	9.416	1.054	47.7	49.3	51.6	55.4	62.3	70.6	75.7
170.0–174.9 cm	144	435	62.37	11.516	1.095	49.7	51.0	55.0	59.4	65.6	79.2	86.3
175.0–179.9 cm	71	228	65.54	9.704	1.306	50.9	55.1	58.5	64.7	69.9	74.5	84.0
180.0–184.9 cm	25	81	72.44	13.011	2.298	59.6	60.0	65.1	69.4	77.0	83.0	94.3
185.0–189.9 cm	3	9	*	*	*	*	*	*	*	*	*	*
190.0–194.9 cm	1	3	*	*	*	*	*	*	*	*	*	*
195.0 cm and over	—	—	—	—	—	—	—	—	—	—	—	—
FEMALE												
Under 130 cm	—	—	—	—	—	—	—	—	—	—	—	—
130.0–134.9 cm	—	—	—	—	—	—	—	—	—	—	—	—
135.0–139.9 cm	1	2	*	*	*	*	*	*	*	*	*	*
140.0–144.9 cm	2	6	*	*	*	*	*	*	*	*	*	*
145.0–149.9 cm	17	52	42.00	5.879	1.683	32.0	35.3	36.3	42.3	47.5	49.5	51.1
150.0–154.9 cm	64	196	48.26	6.797	0.926	37.7	39.2	42.5	47.9	53.3	55.9	58.8
155.0–159.9 cm	157	508	51.35	7.705	0.520	41.2	43.4	46.3	49.6	55.6	62.2	64.3
160.0–164.9 cm	186	603	54.59	8.810	0.707	43.0	45.0	48.4	53.0	59.7	66.7	70.7
165.0–169.9 cm	114	372	58.46	10.185	0.955	45.9	47.5	52.1	56.8	61.8	70.5	76.4
170.0–174.9 cm	36	121	64.37	15.821	2.814	49.2	52.1	56.2	59.8	70.5	72.9	99.4
175.0–179.9 cm	7	28	61.33	5.496	2.620	51.7	52.0	57.7	59.8	64.6	70.2	70.6
180.0–184.9 cm	2	7	*	*	*	*	*	*	*	*	*	*
185.0–189.9 cm	—	—	—	—	—	—	—	—	—	—	—	—
190.0–194.9 cm	—	—	—	—	—	—	—	—	—	—	—	—
195.0 cm and over	—	—	—	—	—	—	—	—	—	—	—	—

From National Center for Health Statistics: Height and Weight of Youths 12–17 Years, United States. In Vital and Health Statistics, Series 11, no. 124. Health Services and Mental Health Administration. Washington, DC, US Government Printing Office, 1973.

Note: n = sample size; N = estimated number of youths in population in thousands; $\bar{X}$ = mean; s = standard deviation; $s_{\bar{x}}$ = standard error of the mean.

Table continued on following page

APPENDIX 8 **Percentiles for Weight for Height of Youths Aged 12 to 17 Years** *Continued*
(Weight in kg of Youths Aged 15 Years at Last Birthday)

Sex and Height	n	N	$\bar{X}$	s	$s_{\bar{x}}$	Percentile						
						5th	10th	25th	50th	75th	90th	95th
MALE												
Under 130 cm	—	—	—	—	—	—	—	—	—	—	—	—
130.0–134.9 cm	—	—	—	—	—	—	—	—	—	—	—	—
135.0–139.9 cm	—	—	—	—	—	—	—	—	—	—	—	—
140.0–144.9 cm	—	—	—	—	—	—	—	—	—	—	—	—
145.0–149.9 cm	1	2	*	*	*	*	*	*	*	*	*	*
150.0–154.9 cm	10	30	45.72	8.582	3.550	35.7	39.2	42.6	44.7	46.0	48.7	76.1
155.0–159.9 cm	34	99	52.81	10.552	1.695	40.3	43.1	46.7	49.2	56.7	69.6	76.3
160.0–164.9 cm	71	206	53.01	8.417	0.986	42.7	44.1	46.9	51.5	56.3	65.3	68.8
165.0–169.9 cm	132	404	57.72	8.503	0.819	48.0	48.8	53.1	56.4	61.3	67.1	73.3
170.0–174.9 cm	176	574	62.88	8.464	0.633	51.6	53.4	56.7	61.9	67.2	72.9	78.1
175.0–179.9 cm	118	374	65.80	9.457	1.045	53.1	55.6	59.7	64.3	69.5	80.2	89.2
180.0–184.9 cm	51	144	72.00	11.928	1.724	54.6	60.3	64.4	70.2	78.4	84.4	96.6
185.0–189.9 cm	14	48	74.21	15.035	5.200	58.3	58.5	62.9	70.7	84.6	92.4	110.8
190.0–194.9 cm	6	15	83.39	16.431	10.332	66.4	66.7	69.6	73.8	103.0	105.7	106.2
195.0 cm and over	—	—	—	—	—	—	—	—	—	—	—	—
FEMALE												
Under 130 cm	—	—	—	—	—	—	—	—	—	—	—	—
130.0–134.9 cm	—	—	—	—	—	—	—	—	—	—	—	—
135.0–139.9 cm	—	—	—	—	—	—	—	—	—	—	—	—
140.0–144.9 cm	2	5	*	*	*	*	*	*	*	*	*	*
145.0–149.9 cm	15	51	47.91	7.875	3.623	36.0	39.4	42.1	45.4	52.7	55.7	66.3
150.0–154.9 cm	69	242	49.69	8.895	1.190	39.1	40.6	44.3	48.1	52.8	60.5	68.3
155.0–159.9 cm	111	400	51.52	8.473	0.934	41.4	43.5	46.3	50.8	55.1	59.8	65.2
160.0–164.9 cm	137	509	57.03	10.828	0.875	45.1	47.3	50.2	55.0	60.2	71.7	77.7
165.0–169.9 cm	109	398	60.71	10.357	1.053	47.5	49.3	55.1	58.4	65.7	74.1	81.0
170.0–174.9 cm	49	188	65.27	10.730	1.880	49.7	53.6	57.2	61.2	71.6	85.3	86.4
175.0–179.9 cm	7	23	63.30	8.872	4.807	49.7	49.9	53.8	62.4	71.1	71.9	79.2
180.0–184.9 cm	3	26	*	*	*	*	*	*	*	*	*	*
185.0–189.9 cm	1	3	*	*	*	*	*	*	*	*	*	*
190.0–194.9 cm	—	—	—	—	—	—	—	—	—	—	—	—
195.0 cm and over	—	—	—	—	—	—	—	—	—	—	—	—

From National Center for Health Statistics: Height and Weight of Youths 12–17 Years, United States. In Vital and Health Statistics, Series 11, no. 124. Health Services and Mental Health Administration. Washington, DC, US Government Printing Office, 1973.

Note: n = sample size; N = estimated number of youths in population in thousands; $\bar{X}$ = mean; s = standard deviation; $s_{\bar{x}}$ = standard error of the mean.

APPENDIX 8 Percentiles for Weight for Height of Youths Aged 12 to 17 Years *Continued* (Weight in kg of Youths Aged 16 Years at Last Birthday)

Sex and Height	n	N	X̄	s	s_x̄	Percentile 5th	10th	25th	50th	75th	90th	95th
MALE												
Under 130 cm	—	—	—	—	—	—	—	—	—	—	—	—
130.0–134.9 cm	—	—	—	—	—	—	—	—	—	—	—	—
135.0–139.9 cm	—	—	—	—	—	—	—	—	—	—	—	—
140.0–144.9 cm	—	—	—	—	—	—	—	—	—	—	—	—
145.0–149.9 cm	1	1	*	*	*	*	*	*	*	*	*	*
150.0–154.9 cm	4	12	*	*	*	*	*	*	*	*	*	*
155.0–159.9 cm	11	33	49.89	7.323	3.572	42.0	42.2	44.7	46.8	54.4	59.8	67.2
160.0–164.9 cm	32	108	53.09	6.459	1.273	44.2	44.9	48.2	51.4	58.0	60.9	66.1
165.0–169.9 cm	87	275	59.39	9.178	0.981	48.5	49.8	52.7	58.0	63.9	69.3	75.9
170.0–174.9 cm	166	552	62.66	7.556	0.629	51.6	53.8	57.5	61.6	67.1	73.1	78.0
175.0–179.9 cm	149	511	67.33	9.018	0.856	56.3	58.2	61.0	65.4	72.5	80.1	83.8
180.0–184.9 cm	72	227	72.38	12.485	1.993	50.3	59.3	61.1	68.9	76.5	90.2	96.9
185.0–189.9 cm	29	95	81.06	14.268	3.265	63.7	66.6	69.7	78.4	90.3	97.0	111.4
190.0–194.9 cm	3	10	*	*	*	*	*	*	*	*	*	*
195.0 cm and over	2	7	*	*	*	*	*	*	*	*	*	*
FEMALE												
Under 130 cm	—	—	—	—	—	—	—	—	—	—	—	—
130.0–134.9 cm	—	—	—	—	—	—	—	—	—	—	—	—
135.0–139.9 cm	—	—	—	—	—	—	—	—	—	—	—	—
140.0–144.9 cm	2	5	*	*	*	*	*	*	*	*	*	*
145.0–149.9 cm	10	33	52.58	8.198	3.191	43.9	44.1	44.9	51.0	54.5	72.0	72.1
150.0–154.9 cm	57	178	51.79	10.457	1.053	41.4	42.0	45.8	48.9	54.1	61.5	83.3
155.0–159.9 cm	117	354	53.20	7.766	0.734	44.0	45.6	48.4	51.6	56.4	61.9	69.0
160.0–164.9 cm	160	547	57.71	11.129	1.246	46.1	47.3	51.5	55.5	61.2	69.5	75.1
165.0–169.9 cm	122	450	61.72	11.998	0.802	47.1	48.8	53.3	59.1	67.3	78.7	86.7
170.0–174.9 cm	53	170	63.61	8.734	1.126	52.9	53.8	58.1	62.1	66.8	73.8	84.2
175.0–179.9 cm	14	45	72.55	15.012	5.224	58.6	58.8	61.7	65.9	80.6	99.1	105.5
180.0–184.9 cm	1	2	*	*	*	*	*	*	*	*	*	*
185.0–189.9 cm	—	—	—	—	—	—	—	—	—	—	—	—
190.0–194.9 cm	—	—	—	—	—	—	—	—	—	—	—	—
195.0 cm and over	—	—	—	—	—	—	—	—	—	—	—	—

From National Center for Health Statistics: Height and Weight of Youths 12–17 Years, United States. In Vital and Health Statistics, Series 11, no. 124. Health Services and Mental Health Administration. Washington, DC, US Government Printing Office, 1973.

Note: n = sample size; N = estimated number of youths in population in thousands; $\bar{X}$ = mean; s = standard deviation; $s_{\bar{x}}$ = standard error of the mean.

Table continued on following page

APPENDIX 8 Percentiles for Weight for Height of Youths Aged 12 to 17 Years *Continued* (Weight in kg of Youths Aged 17 Years at Last Birthday)

Sex and Height	n	N	$\bar{X}$	s	$s_{\bar{x}}$	Percentile						
						5th	10th	25th	50th	75th	90th	95th
MALE												
Under 130 cm	—	—	—	—	—	—	—	—	—	—	—	—
130.0–134.9 cm	—	—	—	—	—	—	—	—	—	—	—	—
135.0–139.9 cm	—	—	—	—	—	—	—	—	—	—	—	—
140.0–144.9 cm	—	—	—	—	—	—	—	—	—	—	—	—
145.0–149.9 cm	—	—	—	—	—	—	—	—	—	—	—	—
150.0–154.9 cm	1	3	*	*	*	*	*	*	*	*	*	*
155.0–159.9 cm	11	39	54.63	9.397	3.414	43.8	46.4	48.2	49.7	57.8	69.9	73.2
160.0–164.9 cm	25	81	57.75	6.503	1.355	49.7	51.1	52.5	56.9	61.6	70.1	70.8
165.0–169.9 cm	63	248	62.57	8.344	1.224	50.2	53.2	56.4	61.5	66.9	72.7	77.3
170.0–174.9 cm	115	396	67.06	11.163	0.704	53.3	55.5	59.5	64.6	71.9	80.9	91.6
175.0–179.9 cm	151	537	68.37	9.907	0.831	56.9	58.9	61.5	66.5	73.6	79.4	88.4
180.0–184.9 cm	80	297	73.31	12.454	1.335	59.6	61.0	65.1	71.2	78.4	91.8	102.7
185.0–189.9 cm	36	133	76.03	9.171	1.301	62.4	66.3	70.5	75.3	80.8	90.3	92.9
190.0–194.9 cm	7	25	81.40	10.985	7.588	62.9	62.9	67.8	87.3	90.3	90.6	90.6
195.0 cm and over	—	—	—	—	—	—	—	—	—	—	—	—
FEMALE												
Under 130 cm	—	—	—	—	—	—	—	—	—	—	—	—
130.0–134.9 cm	—	—	—	—	—	—	—	—	—	—	—	—
135.0–139.9 cm	—	—	—	—	—	—	—	—	—	—	—	—
140.0–144.9 cm	2	5	*	*	*	*	*	*	*	*	*	*
145.0–149.9 cm	8	26	43.49	3.939	1.604	38.6	38.8	40.1	45.1	45.7	51.1	51.2
150.0–154.9 cm	43	151	49.96	6.508	0.827	41.6	42.3	44.6	48.9	53.5	59.2	64.1
155.0–159.9 cm	103	385	54.71	9.903	0.775	44.4	45.5	48.7	53.2	57.7	61.6	76.2
160.0–164.9 cm	133	506	57.79	10.620	1.028	46.8	48.0	50.2	55.4	61.5	72.3	82.3
165.0–169.9 cm	116	433	60.63	10.117	1.182	47.9	50.3	55.1	59.3	65.1	69.4	71.6
170.0–174.9 cm	51	186	62.18	9.132	1.407	50.6	52.9	55.5	60.2	65.7	76.1	82.7
175.0–179.9 cm	12	47	65.76	8.405	2.229	54.9	56.7	60.1	61.7	75.2	75.9	83.0
180.0–184.9 cm	1	2	*	*	*	*	*	*	*	*	*	*
185.0–189.9 cm	—	—	—	—	—	—	—	—	—	—	—	—
190.0–194.9 cm	—	—	—	—	—	—	—	—	—	—	—	—
195.0 cm and over	—	—	—	—	—	—	—	—	—	—	—	—

From National Center for Health Statistics: Height and Weight of Youths 12–17 Years, United States. In Vital and Health Statistics, Series 11, no. 124. Health Services and Mental Health Administration. Washington, DC, US Government Printing Office, 1973.

Note: n = sample size; N = estimated number of youths in population in thousands; $\bar{X}$ = mean; s = standard deviation; $s_{\bar{x}}$ = standard error of the mean.

Level II Screen

Complete the following screen by interviewing the patient directly and/or by referring to the patient chart. If you do not routinely perform all of the described tests or ask all of the listed questions, please consider including them but do not be concerned if the entire screen is not completed. Please try to conduct a minimal screen on as many older patients as possible, and please try to collect serial measurements, which are extremely valuable in monitoring nutritional status. Please refer to the manual for additional information.

Anthropometrics

Measure height to the nearest inch and weight to the nearest pound. Record the values below and mark them on the Body Mass Index (BMI) scale to the right. Then use a straight edge (paper, ruler) to connect the two points and circle the spot where this straight line crosses the center line (body mass index). Record the number below; healthy older adults should have a BMI between 22 and 27; check the appropriate box to flag an abnormally high or low value.

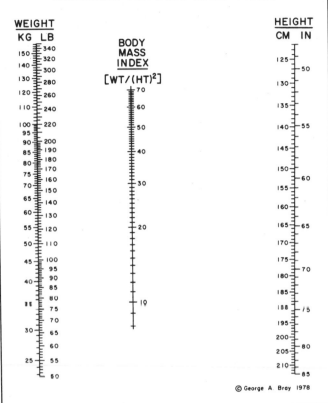

NOMOGRAM FOR BODY MASS INDEX

BODY MASS INDEX $[WT/(HT)^2]$

© George A. Bray 1978

Height (in):_____
Weight (lbs):_____
Body Mass Index
(weight/height^2):_____

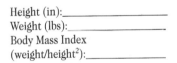

Please place a check by any statement regarding BMI and recent weight loss that is true for the patient.

☐ Body mass index <22

☐ Body mass index >27

☐ Has lost or gained 10 pounds (or more) of body weight in the past 6 months

Record the measurement of mid-arm circumference to the nearest 0.1 centimeter and of triceps skinfold to the nearest 2 millimeters.

Mid-Arm Circumference (cm):_____
Triceps Skinfold (mm):_____
Mid-Arm Muscle Circumference (cm):_____

Refer to the table and check any abnormal values:

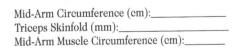

☐ Mid-arm muscle circumference <10th percentile

☐ Triceps skinfold <10th percentile

☐ Triceps skinfold >95th percentile

Note: mid-arm circumference (cm) - {0.314 x triceps skinfold (mm)}= mid-arm *muscle* circumference (cm)

For the remaining sections, please place a check by any statements that are true for the patient.

Laboratory Data

☐ Serum albumin below 3.5 g/dl

☐ Serum cholesterol below 160 mg/dl

☐ Serum cholesterol above 240 mg/dl

Drug Use

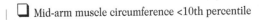

☐ Three or more prescription drugs, OTC medications, and/or vitamin/mineral supplements daily

Appendix continued on following page

Clinical Features

Presence of (check each that apply):

- ❑ Problems with mouth, teeth, or gums
- ❑ Difficulty chewing
- ❑ Difficulty swallowing
- ❑ Angular stomatitis
- ❑ Glossitis
- ❑ History of bone pain
- ❑ History of bone fractures
- ❑ Skin changes (dry, loose, nonspecific lesions, edema)

Percentile	*Men* 55-65 y	65-75 y	*Women* 55-65 y	65-75 y
Arm circumference (cm)				
10th	27.3	26.3	25.7	25.2
50th	31.7	30.7	30.3	29.9
95th	36.9	35.5	38.5	37.3
Arm muscle circumference (cm)				
10th	24.5	23.5	19.6	19.5
50th	27.8	26.8	22.5	22.5
95th	32.0	30.6	28.0	27.9
Triceps skinfold (mm)				
10th	6	6	16	14
50th	11	11	25	24
95th	22	22	38	36

From: Frisancho AR. New norms of upper limb fat and muscle areas for assessment of nutritional status. Am J Clin Nutr 1981; 34:2540-2545. © 1981 American Society for Clinical Nutrition.

Eating Habits

- ❑ Does not have enough food to eat each day
- ❑ Usually eats alone
- ❑ Does not eat anything on one or more days each month
- ❑ Has poor appetite
- ❑ Is on a special diet
- ❑ Eats vegetables two or fewer times daily
- ❑ Eats milk or milk products once or not at all daily
- ❑ Eats fruit or drinks fruit juice once or not at all daily
- ❑ Eats breads, cereals, pasta, rice, or other grains five or fewer times daily
- ❑ Has more than one alcoholic drink per day (if woman); more than two drinks per day (if man)

Living Environment

- ❑ Lives on an income of less than $6000 per year (per individual in the household)
- ❑ Lives alone
- ❑ Is housebound
- ❑ Is concerned about home security
- ❑ Lives in a home with inadequate heating or cooling
- ❑ Does not have a stove and/or refrigerator
- ❑ Is unable or prefers not to spend money on food (<$25-30 per person spent on food each week)

Functional Status

Usually or always needs assistance with (check each that apply):

- ❑ Bathing
- ❑ Dressing
- ❑ Grooming
- ❑ Toileting
- ❑ Eating
- ❑ Walking or moving about
- ❑ Traveling (outside the home)
- ❑ Preparing food
- ❑ Shopping for food or other necessities

Mental/Cognitive Status

- ❑ Clinical evidence of impairment, e.g. Folstein<26
- ❑ Clinical evidence of depressive illness, e.g. Beck Depression Inventory>15, Geriatric Depression Scale>5

Patients in whom you have identified one or more major indicator (see pg 2) of poor nutritional status require immediate medical attention; if minor indicators are found, ensure that they are known to a health professional or to the patient's own physician. Patients who display risk factors (see pg 2) of poor nutritional status should be referred to the appropriate health care or social service professional (dietitian, nurse, dentist, case manager, etc.).

From Nutrition Screening Initiative, American Academy of Family Physicians, American Dietetic Association, National Council on Aging, Ross Products Division, Abbott Laboratories.

APPENDIX 10 Equations for Estimating Stature from Knee Height for Various Groups

Age*	Equation†	Error‡
BLACK FEMALES		
>60	$S = 58.72 + (1.96\ KH)$	8.26 cm
19–60	$S = 68.10 + (1.86\ KH) - (0.06\ A)$	7.60 cm
6–18	$S = 46.59 + (2.02\ KH)$	8.78 cm
WHITE FEMALES		
>60	$S = 75.00 + (1.91\ KH) - (0.17\ A)$	8.82 cm
19–60	$S = 70.25 + (1.87\ KH) - (0.06\ A)$	7.20 cm
6–18	$S = 43.21 + (2.14\ KH)$	7.80 cm
BLACK MALES		
> 60	$S = 95.79 + (1.37\ KH)$	8.44 cm
19–60	$S = 73.42 + (1.79\ KH)$	7.20 cm
6–18	$S = 39.60 + (2.18\ KH)$	9.16 cm
WHITE MALES		
>60	$S = 59.01 + (2.08\ KH)$	7.84 cm
19–60	$S = 71.85 + (1.88\ KH)$	7.94 cm
6–18	$S = 40.54 + (2.22\ KH)$	8.42 cm

Adapted from Chumlea WC, Guo SS, Steinbaugh ML. 1994. Predication of stature from knee height for black and white adults and children with application to mobility-impaired or handicapped persons. J Am Diet Assoc 1994;94: 1385. Copyright The American Dietetic Association. Reprinted by permission from Journal of The American Dietetic Association.

* Age in years rounded to the nearest year.

† S = stature; KH = knee height; A = age in years.

‡ Estimated stature will be within this value for 95% of persons within each age, sex, race group.

INDEX

Note: Page numbers in *italics* indicate figures; those followed by t indicate tables.